Probiotics

Probiotics: A Comprehensive Guide to Enhance Health and Mitigate Disease is an indispensable resource for a deeper understanding of the intricate world of probiotics and their profound impact on human health. This book unravels the complex science behind probiotics, providing a comprehensive exploration of their roles in maintaining a healthy microbiome, fortifying the immune system, and mitigating various diseases. It presents insights into how probiotics influence not only digestive health but also extend their benefits to systemic well-being.

The book provides practical guidance, offering evidence-based recommendations for selecting and incorporating probiotics into daily life. From decoding probiotic strains and understanding their mechanisms of action to exploring the symbiotic relationship between gut health and overall wellness, this resource is for both beginners and seasoned enthusiasts in the field. With a focus on demystifying the often-confusing landscape of probiotics, the book empowers the reader to make informed choices to optimize their health.

Probiotics: A Comprehensive Guide to Enhance Health and Mitigate Disease is an essential reference for healthcare professionals, researchers, and individuals keen on harnessing the potential of probiotics for their well-being. Whether you are a healthcare practitioner looking to enhance patient care or a health-conscious reader eager to navigate the world of probiotics, this guide is a valuable asset that bridges the gap between cutting-edge science and practical application.

Probiotics

A Comprehensive Guide to Enhance Health and Mitigate Disease

Edited by
Gowhar Rashid, Luxita Sharma, and Nihad Ashraf Khan

CRC Press
Taylor & Francis Group
Boca Raton London New York

CRC Press is an imprint of the
Taylor & Francis Group, an **informa** business

First edition published 2024
by CRC Press
2385 NW Executive Center Drive, Suite 320, Boca Raton FL 33431

and by CRC Press
4 Park Square, Milton Park, Abingdon, Oxon, OX14 4RN

CRC Press is an imprint of Taylor & Francis Group, LLC

ISBN: 978-1-032-58694-6 (hbk)
ISBN: 978-1-032-58947-3 (pbk)
ISBN: 978-1-003-45224-9 (ebk)

DOI: 10.1201/9781003452249

Typeset in Times
by Apex CoVantage, LLC

Contents

Introduction

In an era characterized by constant advancements in science and technology, the quest for optimal health and the prevention of disease has become a central pillar of our modern lives. In *Probiotics: A Comprehensive Guide to Enhance Health and Mitigate Disease* we embark on a journey into the intricate web of human well-being, exploring the latest scientific insights, time-tested wisdom, and practical strategies to empower you to take control of your health.

This book is a roadmap for those seeking not only to live longer but also to live better. We'll delve into the fascinating interplay of genetics, lifestyle, nutrition, and environmental factors that shape our health outcomes. As we navigate the complex terrain of human biology, we will uncover the tools and techniques that can transform our lives, allowing us to flourish in a world fraught with health challenges.

From the fundamentals of nutrition to the significance of physical fitness, from the psychology of wellness to the importance of preventive care, *Probiotics: A Comprehensive Guide to Enhance Health and Mitigate Disease* offers a holistic approach to health that is both comprehensive and actionable. We'll explore the latest breakthroughs in medical science and demystify the buzzwords, so you can make informed choices about your health and well-being.

Join us on this expedition into the realms of health enhancement and disease mitigation. Together, we'll uncover the knowledge and strategies that can help you lead a vibrant, healthy life while mitigating the risks that often come with it. Whether you are a seasoned health enthusiast or just beginning your journey to wellness, this book promises to be your trusted companion on the path to a healthier, happier, and more fulfilling life.

Editor Biographies

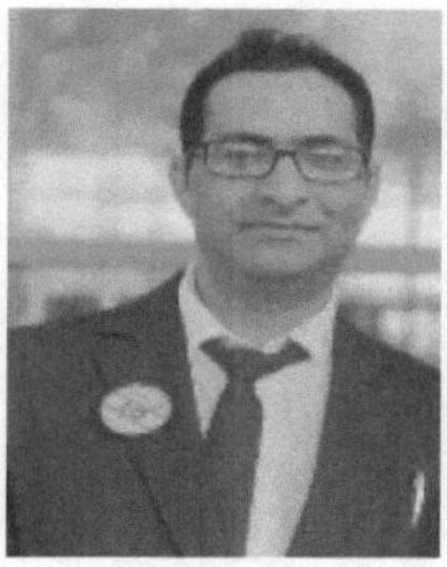

Dr. Gowhar Rashid is Assistant Professor at the Amity Medical School at Amity University Haryana, India. Born and raised in the beautiful region of Srinagar, Kashmir, Dr. Rashid has developed a passion for advancing the field of medical science. His educational journey led him to complete his BSc, MSc, and PhD in Biochemistry from the prestigious Sher I Kashmir Institute of Medical Sciences in Kashmir, India.

With a specialization in diagnostics and cancer research, Dr. Gowhar Rashid has become a recognized expert in his field. His in-depth knowledge and dedication to his work have earned him recognition and respect from both his peers and students. His research focuses on finding innovative solutions and breakthroughs in cancer diagnostics, aiming to improve patient outcomes and contribute to the field's advancements.

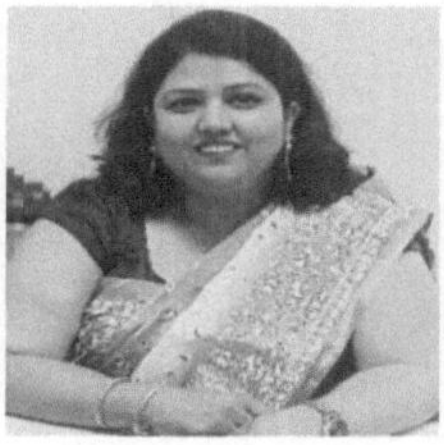

Dr. Luxita Sharma is Associate Professor and Head of the Department of Dietetics and Applied Nutrition at Amity University, Haryana, India. She has 18+ years of experience as a researcher and an academician. She is UGC-NET qualified and has earned a PhD in Food and Nutrition. She is a Fellow Member of Eudoxia Research University, USA, and Executive Director (Hon.) at the Hindustan Agricultural Research Welfare Society. She is a life member of the Indian Dietetics Association and IAPEN India Association.

She has received an International Award in the category of Contribution to Education Community and Outstanding Accomplishments by Asian Education Awards and IAPEN—Indian Association of Enteral and Parenteral Nutrition—and many more awards from reputed organizations like ICAR, IIMR, and MGA, and from the actor Rushad Rana. She has published ten patents with patents and copyrights granted. She has published 90 research papers in national and international journals. She has published 13 books and several book chapters with national and international publishers. She has been a speaker at many national and international conferences and seminars.

Nihad Ashraf Khan is an alumna of Jamia Millia Islamia, New Delhi, India, from where she completed her master's in Biosciences. She completed her bachelor's from India's most reputed university, Delhi University, Ramjas College, in 2020. She has been part of several projects during her bachelor's and master's and has gained expertise in bio-informatics, a booming platform for scientific research. Her research interests include Microbiology, Cell and Molecular Biology, and Bioinformatics. She has worked on a research project during her master's on "Mechanistic Insight into Anti-candidal Effects of Methyl Eugenol" and even done a computational study on Alzheimer's Disease, an approach toward phytochemicals for drug designing. She is interested in contributing to scientific research through her novel ideas.

Contributors

Adarsh Jha
Faculty of Pharmacy, Parul Institute of Pharmacy and Research
Parul University
Waghodia, Vadodara, India

Akanksha Bhattacharya
Department of Biotechnology
Institute for Excellence in Higher Education
Bhopal, Madhya Pradesh, India

Akanksha Yadav
Department of Nutrition and Dietetics, SGT University
Gurgaon, Haryana, India

Anuvab Dey
Department of Biosciences and Bioengineering, IIT Guwahati
North Guwahati, Assam, India

Atharva A. Mahajan
Advanced Centre for Treatment, Research and Education in Cancer
Mumbai, India

Barkha Bhatnagar
Department of Nutrition & Dietetics, SGT University
Gurugram, Haryana, India

Debasrita Banerjee
Department of Dietetics and Nutrition, Nimas College, MAKAUT
West Bengal, India

Deepak Sharma
Institute of Pharmacy, Assam Don Bosco University
Tapesia, Kamarkuchi, Guwahati
Assam, India

Deepika Pal
Amity Medical School, Dietetics and Applied Nutrition, Amity University
Gurgaon, Haryana, India

Dhananjay Sharma
Amity Medical School, Dietetics and Applied Nutrition, Amity University
Gurgaon, Haryana, India

Diksha Bisht
Amity Medical School, Dietetics and Applied Nutrition, Amity University
Gurgaon, Haryana, India

Dorsa Hosseinzadeh
Department of Food Science and Technology, Faculty of Agriculture
University of Tabriz
Tabriz, Iran

Farheen Khan
Department of Biotechnology Era University
Lucknow, India

Gowhar Rashid
Amity Medical School, Amity University
Gurgaon, Haryana, India

Himanshu Chaurasia
Quantum School of Health Sciences
Quantum University
Roorkee, Uttarakhand, India

Himanshu Kumar
Department of Pharmacology, School of Chemical Sciences and Pharmacy
Central University of Rajasthan
Ajmer, Rajasthan, India

Janki Patel
Faculty of Pharmacy, Parul Institute of Pharmacy and Research
Parul University
Waghodia, Vadodara, India

Jyoti Goyat
Department of Nutrition & Dietetics SGT University
Gurugram, Haryana, India

Luciana Gama de Mendonça
Federal University of Ceará, Food Engineering Department, Fortaleza
Ceará, Brazil

Luxita Sharma
Amity Medical School, Dietetics and Applied Nutrition, Amity University, Gurgaon
Haryana, India

Madan Mohan Gupta
School of Pharmacy, Faculty of Medical Sciences University of the West Indies St. Augustine
Trinidad and Tobago, West Indies

Madhurima Majumdar
Department of Biotechnology, Heritage Institute of Technology
Kolkata, India

Mulye Kalpita
Tata Memorial Hospital, Parel
Mumbai, India

Naseem Fatima
Department of Biochemistry
Era's Lucknow Medical College & Hospital
Lucknow, India

Nishma Singh
Swami Vivekanand Subharti University
Meerut, India

Pawar Jayashree
Department of Biotechnology and Microbiology, VPM's B. N. Bandodkar College of Science (Autonomous)
Thane, Maharashtra, India

Pinkal H. Patel
Faculty of Pharmacy, Parul Institute of Pharmacy and Research, Parul University
Waghodia, Vadodara, India

Priscila Ximenes Moreira
Federal Institute of Ceará, Baturité, Ceará, Brazil

Rafael Audino Zambelli
Federal University of Ceará
Food Engineering Department
Fortaleza, Ceará, Brazil

Renesa Dasgupta
Department of Biotechnology, Heritage Institute of Technology
Kolkata, India

Renu Shrestha
Amity Medical School, Dietetics and Applied Nutrition, Amity University, Gurgaon
Haryana, India

Reza Karimi
Department of Food Science and Technology, Faculty of Agricultural Sciences, University of Guilan
Rasht, Iran

Rizwan Ahamad
Department of Pharmacology, School of Pharmaceutical Education and Research, Jamia Hamdard
New Delhi, India

Sadma Parveen
Department of Pharmacology, School of Pharmaceutical Education and Research, Jamia Hamdard
New Delhi, India

Saliha Rizvi
Department of Biotechnology, Era University
Lucknow, India

Shatakshi
Quantum School of Health Sciences
Quantum University
Roorkee, Uttarakhand, India

Shrimanti Das
Department of Biotechnology, Heritage Institute of Technology
Kolkata, India

Shubha Dhyani
Quantum School of Health Sciences
Quantum University
Roorkee, Uttarakhand, India

Subhrojyoti Ghosh
Department of Biotechnology
IIT Madras, India

Sunita Roy Chowdhury
Nutritionist, Nutrition Educator and Director
S. S. Guiding Stars Pvt. Ltd, India

Suryakshi Bhunia
Department of Chemistry
IIT Madras, India

Swati Sharma
Swami Vivekanand Subharti University
Meerut, India

Syed Tasleem Raza
Department of Biochemistry
Era's Lucknow Medical College & Hospital
Lucknow, India

Talker Judith
Department of Biochemistry
All India Institute of Medical Sciences
Bhopal, Madhya Pradesh, India

Abbreviations

AAD	Antibiotic-associated diarrhea
ABT	*Acidophilus, Bifidobacterium, Thermophilus*
ACE	Angiotensin-converting enzyme
ACE2	Angiotensin-converting enzyme 2
AD	Alzheimer's disease
AD	Atopic dermatitis
ADR-1	Adrenergic receptor-1
AFS	Aflatoxin synthesis
AIDS	Acquired immuno deficiency syndrome
ALS	Amyotrophic lateral sclerosis
AMP	Adenosine monophosphate
AMPk	Adenosine monophosphate kinase
ANGPTL4	Angiopoietin-like 4
ANS	Autonomic nervous system
AP	Acute pancreatitis
AS	Atherosclerosis
ASD	Autism spectrum disorder
ASF	Altered Schaedler flora
ATCC53103	American type culture collection strain 53103
ATP	Adenosine triphosphate
B. fragilis	*Bifidobacterium fragilis*
B. longum	*Bifidobacterium longum*
B.	*Bifidobacterium*
BB	*Bifidobacterium bifidum*
BCAAs	Branched-chain amino acids
BCG	Bacillus Calmette-Guerin
BGs	Bacterial ghosts
BMI	Body mass index
BMVs	Bacterial membrane vesicles
BSH	Bile salt hydrolase
C. difficile	*Clostridium difficile*
CAD	Coronary artery disease
CAT	Catalase
CD	Crohn's disease
CD4	Cluster of differentiation 4
CD-95	Cluster of differentiation 95
CDI	*Clostridium difficile* infections
CFU	Colony-forming unit
CIP10448	Collection Institut Pasteur strain 104448
CLRs	C-type lectin receptors
CMVs	Cytoplasmic membrane vesicles
CNS	Central nervous system
CoA	Coenzyme A
COVID-19	Coronavirus disease 2019
COX-2	Cyclooxygenase 2
CRC	Colorectal cancer
CRISPRi	CRISPR interference

CRP	C-reactive protein
CSF	Cerebrospinal fluid
CVD	Cardiovascular disease
DART	DNA-editing all-in-one RNA-guided CRISPR–Cas transposase
DCA	Deoxycholic acid
DCs	Dendritic cells
DHCP	6-Hydroxylmethyl-7,8-dihydropterin pyrophosphate
DM	Diabetes mellitus
DNA	Deoxyribonucleic acid
DP	Degree of polymerization
DSBs	Double-strand DNA breaks
DSHEA	Dietary Product Health and Education Act
DSM	*Diagnostic and Statistical Manual of Mental Disorders*
E. coli	*Escherichia coli*
EcN	*Escherichia coli* Nissle
EFSA	European Food Safety Authority
ELS	Early life stress
ENS	Enteric nervous system
EOMVs	Explosive outer-membrane vesicles
EPS	Exopolysaccharides
ER	Endoplasmic reticulum
ERK1/2	Extracellular signal-regulated kinase 1 and 2
ESBL	Extended spectrum beta lactamase
ET-Seq	Environmental transformation sequencing
EUs	European Unions
F/B ratio	Firmicutes to Bacteroides ratio
FAD	Flavin adenine dinucleotide
FAO	Food and Agriculture Organization
FBS	Fasting blood sugar
FDA	Food and drug administration
FFAR	Free fatty acid receptor
FFAR3	Free fatty acid receptor 3
FMN	Flavin mononucleotide
FMT	Fecal microbiota transplantation
FNB	Food and Nutrition Board
FOS	Fructo-oligosaccharides
G-	Gram-negative bacteria
g/kg	Gram per kilogram
G+-	Gram-positive bacteria
GABA	Gamma-aminobutyric acid
GALT	Gut-associated lymphoid tissue
GBA	Gut–brain axis
GCK	Glucokinase
GDCA	Glycodeoxycholic acid
GIT	Gastrointestinal tract
GLP	Glucagon-like peptide
GLP-1	Glucagon-like peptide 1
GLUT2	Glucose transporter 2 (GLUT2)
GM	Genetically modified
GPCR	G protein-coupled receptors

GPX	Glutathione peroxidase
GQD	Gegen Qinlian decoction
GRAS	Generally recognized as safe
GTP	Guanosine-50-triphosphate
GUDCA	Glucourodeoxycholic acid
H. pylori	*Helicobacter pylori*
HbA1c	Hemoglobin A1c
HCC	Hepatocellular carcinoma
Hcl	Hydrochloric acid
HFD	High-fat diet
HITS	High-throughput insertion tracking by deep sequencing
HIV	Human immunodeficiency virus
HLA	Human leukocyte antigen
HMP	Human Microbiome Project
HMs	Heavy metals
HNF1A	Hepatocyte nuclear factor 1 homeobox A
HOMO-IR	Homeostatic Model Assessment of Insulin Resistance
HPA	Hypothalamic–pituitary–adrenal
HT-29	Human colorectal adenocarcinoma cell line-29
IBD	Inflammatory bowel disease
IBS	Irritable bowel syndrome
ICCs	Interstitial cells of Cajal
ICEs	Integrative and conjugative elements
ICU	Intensive care unit
IDFGD	International Diabetes Federation Global Diabetes
IEC	Intestinal epithelial cells
IFN	Interferon
iHMP	Integrative Human Microbiome Project
IL-6	Interleukin-6
ILSI	International Life Sciences Institute
INF	Interferon
INSeq	Insertion sequencing
IRS-1	Insulin receptor substrate 1
IS	Insertion sequence
ISAPP	International Scientific Association for Probiotics and Prebiotics
IT	Information technology
JNK	Jun N-terminal kinase
KOLs	Key Opinion Leaders
LA	*Lactobacillus acidophilus*
LAB	Lactic acid bacteria
LBPs	Live biotherapeutic products
LG2055	*Lactobacillus gasseri* SBT2055
LGG	*Lactobacillus rhamnosus*
LMW	Low molecular weight
LPS	Lipopolysaccharide
LPXTG	Leu–Pro-X–Thr–Gly
MAM	Microbial anti-inflammatory molecule
MAMPs	Microbe-associated molecular patterns
MAPK	Mitogen-activated protein kinase
MDR	Multi-drug resistant

MeT	Metabolic syndrome
MetaHit	Metagenomics of the human intestinal tract
MGBA	Microbiota–gut–brain axis
MODY	Maturity onset diabetes of the young
MPM	Malignant pleural mesothelioma
mTORC1	Mechanistic target of rapamycin complex 1
MUC	Mucin
MUC2	Mucin 2
MVs	Membrane vesicles
NAD	Nicotinamide adenine dinucleotide
NAFLD	Non-alcoholic fatty liver disease
NAPEs	*N*-acyl phosphatidylethanolamines
NASH	Non-alcoholic steatohepatitis
NE	Necrotizing enterocolitis
NEC	Necrotizing enterocolitis
NF-Kb	Nuclear factor kappa-light-chain-enhancer of activated B cells
NF-kB	Nuclear factor kappa B
NGP	Next-generation probiotics
NiaR	Niacin responsive repressor
NICE	NIsin controlled gene expression
NICU	Neonatal intensive care unit
NIR	Near infrared
NKT	Natural killer T cells
NLRs	Nucleotide binding oligomerization domain (NOD)-like receptors
NOD	Nucleotide binding oligomerization domain
NODLRs	NOD-like intracellular receptors
NSCs	Neural stem cells
OIMVs	Outer inner membrane vesicles
OMVs	Outer-membrane vesicles
OTA	Ochratoxin A
P. copri	*Prevotella copri*
PABA	Para aminobenzoic acid
PAH	Phenylalanine hydroxylase
PAM	Protospacer-adjacent motif
PAMPs	Pathogen-associated molecular patterns
PBMC	Peripheral blood mononuclear cells
PCOS	Polycystic ovary syndrome
PDX1	Pancreatic and duodenal homeobox 1
PET	Positron emission tomography
PFO	Perfringolysin O
PFT	Probiotic fermentation technology
PI	Phosphoinositide 3-kinase
PKB	Protein kinase B
PKC	Protein kinase C
PKU	Phenyketonuria
PL	Pyridoxal
PLP	Pyridoxal phosphate
PM	Pyridoxamine
PMNs	Polymorphonuclear neutrophils
PMP	Pyridoxamine phosphate

PN	Pyridoxine
PNP	Pyridoxine phosphate
PRRs	Pattern-recognition receptors
PsA	Psoriatic arthritis
PUFA	Polyunsaturated fatty acids
PYY	Peptide YY
RA	Rheumatoid arthritis
RAAS	Renin–angiotensin–aldosterone system
RAS	Raman activated microbial cell sorting
RBS	Ribosome binding sites
RCT	Randomized controlled trial
RM	Restriction modification
RNA	Ribonucleic acid
RNS	Reactive nitrogen species
ROS	Reactive oxygen species
S. typhimurium	*Salmonella typhimurium*
SAM	*S*-adenosyl methionine
SARS-CoV-2	Severe acute respiratory syndrome coronavirus 2
SCFA	Short-chain fatty acids
SGOC	serine–glycine–one-carbon
sgRNA	Single-guide RNA
SGZ	Subgranular zone
SIDS	Sudden infant death syndrome
SiRNA	Small interfering ribonucleic acid
SLE	Lupus/systemic lupus erythematosus
SPF	Specific pathogen free
Spp.	Species
STAT	Signal transducer and activator of transcription
STDs	Sexually transmitted diseases
SVZ	Subventricular zone
T1D	Type 1 diabetes
T2DM	Type 2 diabetes mellitus
TCA	Tricarboxylic acid
TCBS	Thiosulfate–citrate–bile–salt sucrose agar
TGF	Transforming growth factor
THTR1	Thaimine transporters 1
THTR2	Thaimine transporters 2
TIMP3	Tissue inhibitor of metalloproteinase 3
TIS	Transposon-insertion sequencing
TLR	Toll-like receptor
TMA	Trimethylamine
TMAO	Trimethylamine-*N*-oxide
TNF-α	Tumor necrosis factor-alpha
TPP	Thiamine pyrophosphate
TraDIS	Transposon-directed insertion site sequencing
TUDCA	Tauroursodeoxycholic acid
UC	Ulcerative colitis
UV	Ultraviolet
UVC	Ultraviolet C
VAP	Ventricular associated pneumonia

VSC	Volatile sulfur compounds
WCFS1	Wageningen Centre for Food Sciences strain 1
WHO	World Health Organization
XOS	Xylo-oligosaccharides
ZO-1	Zonula occludens-1

1 Introduction to Probiotics, Prebiotics, and Synbiotics
A Holistic Approach

Diksha Bisht, Deepika Pal, and Renu Shrestha

1.1 INTRODUCTION

The GI tract in humans boasts the most extensive surface area among all organs, spanning a range of 250–400 m^2, and, additionally, it represents the most significant intersection point between host and environmental influences. Throughout the life span, the human gut processes a large number of foods along with loads of microorganisms coming from the environment (Bengmark, 1998). Some of the microorganisms coming through the food are pathogenic and can produce toxins in the human body and cause infection and inflammation, while a few are found to have beneficial effects on the human body. The bacteria that establish themselves in the GI tract are commonly referred to as gut microbiota. These microbiotas share a complex and mutually advantageous relationship with their host. The number of these inhabiting microorganisms is estimated to outnumber the human body cells. The researchers have well established the beneficial role of this microbiota in the host body. The precise definition is difficult to find, and there is a lot of confusion regarding these terminologies, such as "microbiota" and "microbiome," which are generally used synonymously. The term "microbiota" is used for microbial taxa related to humans, while the term "microbiome" is used as a catalog of these microbial taxa and their genes (Gill et al., 2006). Microbiome was first described by Nobel Laureate Dr. Joshua Lederberg in 2001 as an ecological system of symbiotics and even pathogenic microorganisms inhabiting in human body. However, the study of the microbiome is far more ancient than these scientific discoveries. The research started as early as 1680 with Antonie Van Leuwenhoek, who started a comparison between microbiota residing in different parts of the human body such as oral and fecal microbiota. He also started observing these microbiotas in different health conditions and found that there was remarkable variation in every condition. Various research confirmed the large number of interpersonal variations in microbiomes in healthy individuals. The microbes that are beneficially associated with the host are undoubtedly obtained from the outside environment, but surprisingly the microbial composition of the mammalian gut is significantly different from the environmental microbial species. This chapter includes all the areas defining microbiome and its significance in human health. It also incorporates the introduction of probiotics, prebiotics, and synbiotics and their role in the attainment of health and well-being by different mechanisms.

1.1.1 Understanding Gut Microbiota

The evolution of humans was not solitary. They evolved with a number of microorganisms that reside in the human body and are capable of creating an intricate ecosystem within the human gut, which can change with changing host physiology. Any change in this intricate ecosystem results in dysbiosis in the microbiome. Dysbiosis of the microbial ecosystem can be defined as the disruption in the balanced ecology of inhabiting microorganisms and is associated with multiple disorders such as diabetes mellitus, allergies, IBD, and cancer. Even among healthy individuals, there is a huge variation in the microbiome ecosystem. A few years back, laborious culture-based methods

DOI: 10.1201/9781003452249-1

were used to understand the human gut microbiota. But recently culture-independent methods like low-cost sequencing methods and high-throughput approaches have replaced these labor-intensive methods. Various research has confirmed that gut microbiota shows a high degree of functional superfluity. In a study done by Li et al. (2014), it was suggested that the composition of gut microbiota is affected by multiple environmental factors like diet and genetics of the host. This information could be utilized for the formation of therapeutic strategies in which, according to the disease condition of the host, the microbial community can be modified accordingly.

1.1.2 Microbiota and Microbiome

The most common definition of microbial communities is the group of microorganisms living together. These microbial communities are the assembly of multiple species in which there is continuous interaction of these organisms to create a coterminous environment. The very first scientific definition of the term "microbiome" was established by the scientific team of Whipps and his colleagues in 1988. They characterized the microbiome as a "distinct microbial community inhabiting a reasonably well-defined habitat with specific physio-chemical attributes, often referred to as the theatre of activity." The definition given by Whipps et al. (1988) was a considerable upliftment of previous definitions as it not only defines the microbial community with definite properties and functions but also clearly defines its interaction with the environment (Berg et al., 2020).

The terms "microbiota" and "microbiome" are used synonymously but, as a matter of fact, have a huge difference. The microbiota contains the living members, which form the microbiome. The term "microbiome" has been taken from the ancient Greek word: "micro" means small, and "biome" word is taken from the word "bios," which means life. Microbiota refers to the living microorganisms of a specific ecosystem and is described as the collection of living microorganisms existing within a particular habitat (Marchesi & Ravel, 2015). The movable genetic elements like viroids, free DNA, phages, viruses, plasmids, and prions do not come under the category of microbiota, as they are not considered living microorganisms by the scientific communities (Dupré & O'Malley, 2009). Microbiome involves the whole range of the molecules produced by the microorganisms such as molecules, metabolites, and structural elements produced by simultaneously associated hosts.

1.1.3 Development of Gut Microbiota

Various types of research have proved the initiation of microbiota development just after the birthing process, but very few studies still believe that this development process started from the fetal stage and proved the detection of microbes in womb tissues such as the placenta. The colonization process is rapid after the delivery because of various factors like illness, vaccines, and antibiotic treatments (Rodriguez et al., 2015). Not only the aforementioned factors but also the mode of delivery defines the microbial composition of the infants. In babies delivered through vaginal birth, a thriving number of lactobacilli have been found for the first few days. Contrary to vaginal birth, microbiota in newborns delivered through the cesarean method is significantly lower and colonized by *Clostridium* species instead of *Lactobacillus* (Aagaard et al., 2012). At the beginning of life, microbial diversity is absent or predominated by Proteobacteria and Actinobacteria. During the first few years of life, there is a remarkable increase in microbial diversity, and by the age of two and a half years, the composition, diversity, and functional abilities of the microbiome are similar to adults. Though the gut microbiota composition is otherwise constant during the adult stage of life, there could be an inevitable impact of various life events. The difference in both stages of life can also be sensed by changes in the microbial community. Over the age of 65, there is an excess of two phyla: Bacteroidetes and Clostridium cluster IV. The functional capacity of microbiota in the elderly in amylolysis and the production of SCFAs is reduced, while there is a significant increase in proteolytic activities. The decrease in SCFA production may lead to an inflammation process in the intestines of the elderly population (Biagi et al., 2013).

1.1.4 Importance of a Healthy Gut Microbiota

The correlation between human well-being and the gut has been recognized for centuries, as Hippocrates eloquently put it, "Death sits in the bowls" around 400 B.C. The human intestines harbor a multitude of microorganisms that constitute a complex microbial community. The gut, with its collection of microorganisms, known as the gut microbiota, functions as a vital organ and establishes a multidirectional connection with other bodily organs. This axis involving the gut microflora has a significant role in interactions between the microorganisms and the host. It achieves this by communicating through various pathways including the immunological, endocrine, humoral, neural, and metabolic routes. The microbes, which establish themselves in the human gut, which are primarily non-harmful, maintain a mutually beneficial relationship with the host, contributing to a positive impact on the immune system of the host and its ability to defend against invasive pathogens. Any disruption in the balance of the gut microbiota, referred to as dysbiosis, has been associated with a range of human ailments (Figure 1.1). These include ailments such as depression, high blood pressure, cardiac problems, high blood sugar levels, IBD, obesity, and cancer. Significant worldwide research efforts have concentrated on understanding the considerable influence of the microbial residents within the gut on health and disease development phenomena (AboNahas et al., 2022). The interplay between the host and these microorganisms plays a central role in determining health and susceptibility to disease. The diversity of the gut microbiota is notably shaped by numerous factors related to the host, which include lifestyle, age of the host, dietary pattern, and other environmental components. Among these, diet is presently acknowledged as a leading factor in molding the configuration of the gut microflora (Simões et al., 2022). The human microbiota has the potential to influence appetite, enhance nutrient extraction, and derive energy from numerous constituents of the diet.

Furthermore, microorganisms play an indispensable role in the metabolism of foreign compounds (xenobiotics). In this context, specific gut microorganisms make alterations to the chemical

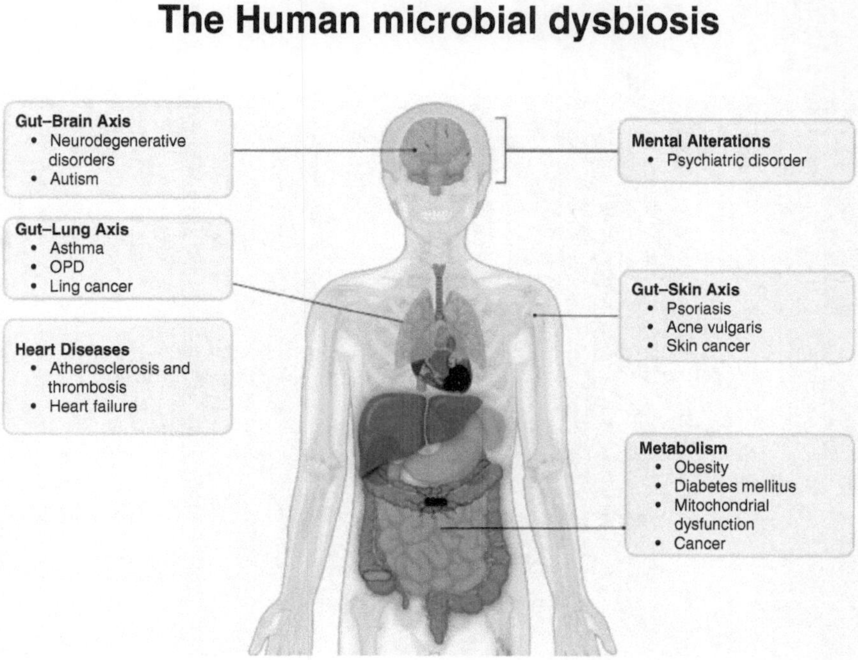

FIGURE 1.1 Diagrammatic representation of human microbial dysbiosis in human diseases.

structures of dietary components, medications, pesticides, and pollutants (Nakov & Velikova, 2020). Extensive clinical investigations have been conducted to explore the equilibrium of microbiota, referred to as eubiosis, and its relevance to various pathological conditions. Maintaining conditions of eubiosis is effective in managing diseases stemming from microorganisms. A balanced and healthful diet, along with the promotion of eubiosis, is beneficial for human health. The overuse of antibiotics disrupts the equilibrium of gut microbiota, predisposing the body to systemic illnesses (Santacroce et al., 2021). Numerous studies based on the population, have highlighted the advantageous role of the human gut microbiota in maintaining health among individuals, underscoring the significance of understanding its structure and the determinants of its composition. These determinants include dietary choices, age, geographical location, and medication use (Wang et al., 2017; Rowland et al., 2018).

1.2 PROBIOTICS: THE BENEFICIAL BACTERIA

The term "probiotic" originating from the modern era carries the meaning of "for life." It is employed to describe the association of bacteria with advantageous impacts on the well-being of humans and animals. A panel of experts appointed by the FAO and the WHO provided a definition for probiotics as "live microorganisms" that, when administered in sufficient quantities, provide a health advantage to the host. The prevalent bacterial genera utilized in probiotic formulations encompass *Bifidobacterium*, *Lactobacillus*, *Escherichia*, *Streptococcus*, *Bacillus*, and *Enterococcus*. In addition, certain strains of fungi belonging to *Saccharomyces* have also been employed for this purpose. The microorganisms listed as probiotics are various strains of *Lactobacillus*, *Streptococcus*, *Saccharomyces*, and *Bifidobacterium* species. Besides these species, *Bacillus cereus*, *Propionibacterium*, *E. coli*, *Enterococcus*, and *Freudenreichii* have also come under the category of probiotics (Jin et al., 2000; Gibson, 1995; Alvarez-Olmos & Oberhelman, 2001).

All the beneficial microorganisms cannot be termed as probiotics, as an ideal probiotic requires some specific properties (Figure 1.2). Microorganisms utilized in probiotic formulations must come under the category of GRAS. These microbes should demonstrate resilience against HCl, bile, and

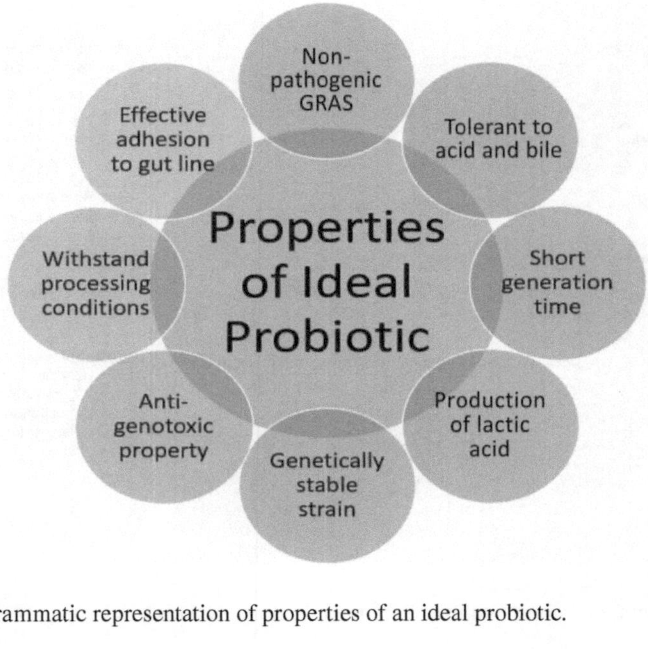

FIGURE 1.2 Diagrammatic representation of properties of an ideal probiotic.

pancreatic juice; exhibit anticarcinogenic properties; and enhance the activity of the immune system. Moreover, they should contribute to reduced intestinal permeability and lactic acid production along with the capability to endure the acidic environment of the stomach and the alkaline condition of the duodenum. Foods intended for human consumption that predominantly incorporate lactic acid bacteria consist of fermented dairy products, wine, sausages, and fruit juices. Probiotic preparations encompass both single and mixed cultures of life microorganisms.

1.2.1 History

The notion of probiotics likely traces its origins to 1908, when Eli Metchnikoff, a Nobel Prize laureate, proposed that the extended lifespan of Bulgarian villagers could be attributed to their consumption of fermented dairy products. In the early 1990s, Metchnikoff introduced the concept of probiotics in a scientific manner, referring to the amendment in microbial diversity within the human body to replace harmful microorganisms with beneficial ones. Nonetheless, a significant breakthrough emerged from the research of Henry Tissier, who noted that a specific type of bacteria was noticeably diminished in the stool samples of children suffering from diarrhea compared to their healthy counterparts. Tissier initiated oral administration of beneficial live organisms such as bifidobacteria to children with diarrhea (infantile diarrhea) to reinstate a healthy gut microbial environment—a pioneering approach. The contemporary interpretation of probiotics was formalized by Havenaar and Huistin Veld. They defined probiotics as viable cultures of bacteria either single or mixed, which, when introduced to animals or humans, confer beneficial effects by enhancing the characteristics of the existing flora within the host. In 1965 Lilly and Stillwell introduced the term "probiotic" to describe the substances, which are released by one organism to encourage the growth of another. In 2002, Marteau et al. defined probiotics as microbial preparations or elements of microbial cells that exert positive effects on health and overall well-being. *Lactobacillus rhamnosus GG* (LGG) stands as the initial probiotic strain to garner significant clinical attention up until the present time. The traditional *Lactobacillus* strain utilized in daily fermentation could not establish itself in the gut. Consequently, the *L. rhamnosus GG* (LGG) was identified in 1985 by establishing a set of desired characteristics for probiotics. This particular strain of *L. rhamnosus GG* has demonstrated advantageous effects on intestinal immunity. It enhances the population of cells that secrete immunoglobulins including IGA, within the intestinal mucosa. Furthermore, it triggers the localized release of interferons and aids in transporting antigens to the underlying lymphoid cells. This mechanism serves to augment the uptake of antigens within Peyer's patches (Aziz et al., 2013).

1.2.2 Global Categorization of Probiotics

There are different categorizations of probiotics in various countries. They are grouped into specific categories such as live biotherapeutic agents; biological agents in the USA; natural health products in Canada; dietary supplements, medical food, and drugs in other European countries. In nations like Japan, China, Malaysia, and India, they are classified as functional food, whereas in Finland, Sweden, and Denmark they are considered food supplements. Furthermore, countries like Germany and Belgium considered them as biotherapeutics or pharmaceuticals. These diverse categorizations for probiotics are individually outlined by various countries, and a comprehensive overview can be found in Table 1.1.

1.2.3 Clinical Significance of Probiotics

The exploration of probiotics for potential clinical health advantages remains a captivating realm of investigation in the current era. The distinctive attributes of probiotics encompassing their ability to combat pathogens, address diabetes and obesity, mitigate inflammation, counteract cancer, alleviate allergies, promote angiogenesis, and influence the brain and central nervous system are discussed in the brief.

TABLE 1.1
International Categories of Probiotics with Definitions

S. No.	Category	Definition
1	Probiotics	Microorganisms that, when consumed in adequate amounts, exert a beneficial influence on the host's overall health.
2	Functional foods	Foods that possess psychological functions extending beyond their nutritional role, encompassing biorhythmic regulation, support for the nervous system, enhancement of the immune system, and fortification of the body's defenses.
3	Dietary supplements	These products are designed to complement one's diet, comprising one or more dietary components (such as vitamins, minerals, and herbs) or their constituents. They are formulated to be ingested orally in the form of a capsule, pill, and tablet/liquid and are identified on the front label as dietary supplements.
4	Drugs	An item intended for the alleviation, management, therapy, diagnosis, or prevention of a medical condition.
5	Biological product	A product that includes a virus, serum, or toxin designed for use in preventing, treating, or curing a disease.
6	Medical food	Items designed for extraneous application in the nutritional management of a disease/condition that has specific dietary needs determined through medical evaluation, and these products are formulated for use under the supervision of a medical professional.
7	Live biotherapeutic agent	A product that encompasses living organisms like bacteria and is utilized in the treatment, prevention, or remedy of human diseases or conditions excluding vaccines.
8	Natural health products	It is described as a substance or a mixture of substances, which can be a homeopathic or traditional medicine, with the intention of exerting a pharmacological effect or another direct influence by: • Treating, diagnosing, preventing, or alleviating a disease; abnormal physiological circumstances; or associated symptoms in humans. • Restoring or rectifying bodily functions in humans. • Altering bodily functions in humans including modifying them in a way that sustains or enhances overall health.

1.2.3.1 Antimicrobial Properties of Probiotics

Extensive research has been dedicated to uncovering the non-pathogenic attributes of probiotics and probiotic combinations. In a study conducted by Islam in 2016, it was proposed that various probiotics produce an array of anti-pathogenic substances, including bacteriocins, hydrogen peroxide, organic acids, diacetyl, ethanol, acetaldehyde, and peptides. Notably, bacteriocins and peptides play a pivotal role in enhancing the permeability of target cell membranes, initiating the disruption of membrane potential, and ultimately leading to cell death.

Additionally, a study by Tejero-Sarinena et al. in 2013 revealed that probiotics exert their inhibitory effects on pathogens through the synthesis of SCFAs such as acetic, butyric, propionic, and lactic acids. These SCFAs play a crucial role in maintaining the appropriate pH levels within the colon, supporting enzymatic activity, and participating in the metabolism of foreign compounds and carcinogens in the intestinal tract. Furthermore, probiotics exhibit antimicrobial activity through competition for binding and receptor sites, as well as for available nutrients essential for growth.

1.2.3.2 Anti-diabetic Activity of Probiotics

The gut microenvironment is notably shaped mainly by two bacterial phyla, gram-negative bacteriodetes, and gram-positive fermicutes (Kobyliak et al., 2016; Hu et al., 2015). Recent investigations have highlighted a connection between obesity and an escalating prevalence of bacteriodetes over time, coupled with a decline in fermicutes. To delve further individuals afflicted with type 2 diabetes exhibit a marked reduction in the abundance of fermicutes species, leading to an elevated ratio of bacteriodetes to fermicutes (Barrett et al., 2012). This elevated ratio corresponds positively with plasma sugar levels. A likewise trend has been implicated in the emergence of conditions like type 1 diabetes, which are autoimmune disorders. Furthermore, modification in the microbiome fosters an increased infiltration of opportunistic pathogens that display resistance to oxidative stress.

1.2.3.3 Anti-allergic Properties of Probiotics

The majority of investigations into probiotic utilization in allergies have centered on patients dealing with atopic eczema. Additionally, research efforts have been directed toward examining the effect of beneficial microbiota on allergies like asthma. Experimental studies propose that particular probiotic strains might exert influence on the intestinal mucosa, thereby potentially modulating allergic responses (Isolauri et al., 2001)

1.2.3.4 Anti-cancerous Properties of Probiotics

Lactobacilli contribute to the prevention or postponement of intestinal tumor development by binding to mutagenic substances present in the intestine. Additionally, they inhibit the growth of bacteria responsible for transforming carcinogenic substances into carcinogens (Orrhage et al., 1994). The capacity of lactobacilli to mitigate the risk of having cancer is further suggested due to their capacity to modify the gut microflora and reduce levels of beta-glucuronidase and other carcinogens. Investigations also indicate that the recurrence of urinary bladder cancers might decrease through the internal administration of probiotics like *Lactobacillus casei* Shirota, although this observation requires validation (Aso et al., 1995).

1.2.3.5 Effect of Probiotics on Urogenital Health

An imbalance in vaginal microbiota predisposes females to experiencing symptomatic vaginal or bladder infections. Two bacterial strains namely *L. rhamnosus GR-1* and *Lactobacillus GG*, demonstrate effectiveness in colonizing and safeguarding the urogenital tract (Saxelin et al., 1995). These strains produce various metabolic byproducts that exhibit antagonistic effects against urinary and vaginal pathogens. These generated substances encompass biosurfactants, which hinder the adhesion of hydrogen peroxide, acids, and bacteriocins, which inhibit growth, and coaggregation molecules that hinder the spread of pathogens (Reid et al., 2001).

Besides these, several studies confirmed the significant effect of probiotics on obesity and their role in the prevention of the transmission of AIDS and STDs, *Helicobacter pylori*, and rotavirus diarrhea. A few strains of *Lactobacillus* are also found to be reducing the mortality rate in infants suffering from necrotizing enterocolitis.

1.2.4 Natural Strains versus Commercial Strains of Probiotics

Natural Strains: Natural strains of microorganisms are those that are found in the environment without any human intervention. These strains have developed naturally through evolution and adaptation to their specific habitats. They may have diverse characteristics and genetic variations due to their exposure to various ecological factors. Natural strains can be isolated from environments (soil, water, plants, and animals). In some cases, they might be unique to certain geographic locations or ecological niches. Yogurt, curd, cheeses, kombucha (fermented tea), miso (a fermented soybean-based paste), kimchi (a Korean dish produced from fermented cabbage), sauerkraut (fermented cabbage), raw unfiltered apple cider vinegar extracted from fermented apple sugars, and pickles are a few examples (Green et al., 2018).

Commercial Strains: Commercial strains, on the other hand, are microorganisms (*Lactobacillus*, *Bifidobacterium*, *Enterococcus*, *Streptococcus*, *Saccharomyces*, *Bacillus*, and *Escherichia*) that have been selected, isolated, and cultivated for specific industrial or commercial purposes. These strains are often chosen on the basis of desirable traits such as high productivity, specific flavor profiles, disease resistance, or other properties that are beneficial for various applications (Sharma et al., 2013). Commercial strains are typically optimized through selective breeding, genetic modification, or other techniques to enhance their performance in industrial processes. The differences between natural and commercial strains of probiotics are listed in Table 1.2.

In both natural and commercial, the aim is to promote a healthy balance of gut microbiota, which has been related to various health benefits. However, the choice between natural and commercial strains often depends on factors such as the desired health effects, convenience of consumption, and regulatory considerations. Some commercial probiotic strains, which are available in India and worldwide, are listed in Table 1.3.

Probiotic Mechanism: As the positive effects of probiotics have been identified, their usage in daily medication for the treatment of gastrointestinal problems is growing nowadays. It is necessary to assess the probiotic mechanism (Figure 1.3) to ameliorate gut health (Latif et al., 2023).

Probiotic strains produce some beneficial compounds like hydrogen peroxide, SCFAs, and various components like bacteriocins that support gut health and immune function in our body. Probiotics help strengthen the intestinal barrier, preventing the leakage of harmful substances from the gut into the bloodstream. Various species of the genus *Lactobacillus* have been identified as producing a number of bacteriocins. These bacteriocins have different levels of inhibitory activity; some are prominent against a considerably larger variety of gram-positive and gram-negative bacteria as well as yeasts and molds (Ahire et al., 2021). Probiotics can also outcompete pathogenic bacteria for nutrients and attachment sites in the gut, reducing the colonization of harmful microbes (Plaza-Diaz et al., 2019). The mechanism of probiotics can influence the immune system, promoting a balanced immune response and reducing inflammation. Additionally, probiotics control the adaptive and innate immune system by modifying macrophages, dendritic cells, and B- and T lymphocytes. Probiotics interact with intestinal epithelial cells, draw macrophages, and mononuclear cells

TABLE 1.2
Differences between Natural and Commercial Strains of Probiotics

Key Differences	Natural Strain	Commercial Strain
Origin	Natural probiotic strains come from the existing microbiota in the environment and humans.	Commercial probiotic strains are isolated, cultured, and often modified for specific applications.
Purpose	Natural probiotic strains contribute to the overall gut microbiota and have evolved alongside their host for various mutual benefits.	Commercial probiotic strains are formulated and marketed with the specific goal of providing health benefits to consumers.
Consistency and Control	Natural strains may vary in their effects due to individual variations, environmental factors, and interactions with other microorganisms.	Commercial strains are carefully selected and manufactured to ensure consistent potency and viability.
Availability	Natural probiotic strains are present in various traditional fermented foods.	Commercial strains are available in the form of cultured dairy products, supplements, and other functional foods.
Regulations	Not required.	Regulatory authorities may require evidence of efficacy and safety before approving the consumption of commercial strains of probiotics in products.

TABLE 1.3
Some Commercial Probiotic Strains Available Globally and in India

S. No.	Commercial Name	Probiotic Culture Used
	Some Commercial Strains in the World	
1.	Valio Gefilus	*Lactobacillus rhamnosus GG*
2.	Welo (probiotic cold pressed drink)	*Bacillus coagulans*
3.	Tropicana Essentials Probiotics	*Bacillus lactis*
4.	GoodBelly	*Lactobacillus plantarum*
5.	Macrolife Macrogreens Superfood Bars	*Lactobacillus acidophilus, Bifidobacterium breve, Lactobacillus bulgaricus, L. rhamnosus*
6.	Welo Probiotic Bar	*B. coagulans*
7.	Biola	*L. rhamnosus*
	Some Commercial Strains in India	
8.	Eubioz	*L. acidophilus, Streptococcus thermophilus, L. rhamnosus,* Bifidobacterium bifidum, Saccharomyces boulardii, Bifidobacterium longum
9.	Bifilac	*Lactobacillus sporogenes, Streptococcus faecalis, Bacillus mesentricus, Clostridium butyricum*
10.	Econova	*Lactobacillus reuteri, L. rhamnosus*
11.	Goodlac	*L. rhamnosus, S. boulardii,* B. longum, L. acidophilus
12.	Actigut	*B. longum, B. bifidum, S. thermophilus, L. rhamnosus, S. boulardii, and L. acidophilus*
13.	Becelac	*L. acidophilus*

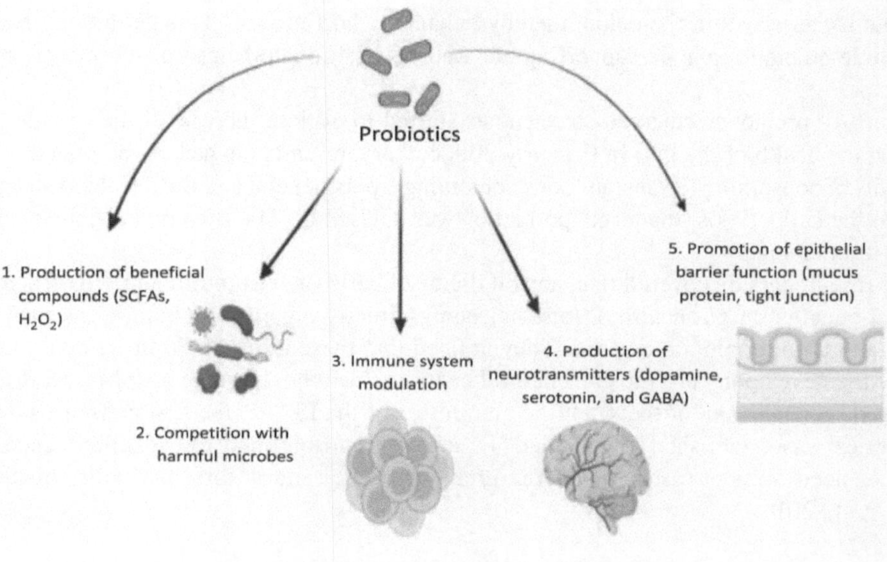

FIGURE 1.3 Diagrammatic representation of the mechanism of action of probiotics.

and boost the production of anti-inflammatory cytokines (Petruzziello et al., 2023). The gut–brain axis allows bacteria to create neurotransmitters in the gut. Certain probiotic strains can alter the levels of serotonin, GABA, and dopamine, which has an impact on gut motility, stress-related pathways, behavior, and mood (Gangaraju et al., 2022; Srivastav et al., 2019; Sajedi & Shabani, 2021). Moreover, Probiotics support epithelial hurdle function by aggregating the production of mucus and tight junction protein expression, which inhibits the transfer of pathogens from the intestine into the blood (Chang et al., 2021). Various systems, including mucus production, water, chloride secretion, and the connection of epithelial cells at their apical junctions by tight junction proteins, work together to maintain the function of the intestinal barrier. In addition to IBD, both active and inactive, enteric infections and autoimmune disorders such as type 1 diabetes mellitus, celiac disease, and interruption of epithelial barrier function are observed in a number of situations (Hemaiswarya et al., 2013).

1.3 PREBIOTICS: FUELING THE GUT MICROBIOTA

> Prebiotics, often defined as non-digestible dietary fibers, play a pivotal role in fostering the proliferation and vitality of beneficial bacteria within the gut ecosystem. These beneficial microorganisms, primarily probiotics, consist of live bacteria and yeasts known for their advantageous effects on our overall health.
>
> **(Gibson et al., 2004)**

Unlike probiotics, which are the beneficial bacteria themselves, prebiotics serve as the nourishment that sustains these microorganisms. Typically, prebiotics take the form of carbohydrates that remain indigestible by the body, such as resistant starches and soluble fibers. Instead, they undergo fermentation by gut bacteria once they reach the colon, largely unaltered in structure.

The term "prebiotic" was coined in 1995 by Marcel Roberfroid, a Belgian professor of biochemistry, during a meeting of the ISAPP. Roberfroid et al., 2010 characterized prebiotics as "non-digestible food ingredients that positively influence the host by promoting the growth and/or activity of specific bacteria within the colon, thereby enhancing host health." This definition underscores the vital role prebiotics play in supporting our well-being through their targeted impact on the gut microbiome.

The idea of prebiotics emerged as scientists started to explore the role of dietary fiber and its impact on the health of the gut. In the early 20th century, researchers had already begun studying the benefits of consuming fermented foods containing live beneficial bacteria (probiotics) on human health. In the early 1900s, the term "probiotic" was devised by Elie Metchnikoff, a Nobel Prize–winning immunologist.

Many researchers discovered that several dietary fibers, such as inulin and oligofructose, had beneficial benefits on gut health despite not being directly digested by humans as their knowledge of the gut microbiota increased. They noticed that these indigestible fibers could favorably influence the development of the gut's helpful bacteria. In 1999, the same year Marcel Roberfroid was named the chairman of the scientific committee of the ISAPP, the first consensus definition of prebiotics was established. It clarified the concept and outlined the specific standards that substances need to meet to be considered prebiotics. The criteria for a prebiotic substance are (Gibson et al., 2010):

1. Fermentation by intestinal microbiota.
2. Resistance to gastrointestinal absorption, gastric acidity, and hydrolysis.
3. Selective stimulation of beneficial bacteria in the colon especially bifidobacteria and lactobacilli.
4. Beneficial effects on the host's body.

1.3.1 Types of Prebiotics

There are various types of prebiotics. Mostly prebiotics belong to carbohydrate groups, and the majority are from oligosaccharides.

Fructans: Fructans are composed of insulin and FOSs or oligofructoses combined with β (2→1) linkage with the glucose. Insulin is present in the form of chain length with a DP of more than 60, while oligofructose has less than 10 DP. FOSs can be synthesized enzymatically from insulin (Gibson et al., 2010). They are mainly found in many vegetables like Jerusalem artichoke, chicory root, and agave, but they are also present in cereals like wheat but in smaller quantities. In Western countries, due to the high intake of cereals products, fructans consumption also increased (Whelan, 2013).

Galacto-oligosaccharides: By enzymatic transglycosylation of lactose, GOS is produced, which gives tri- to pentasaccharides with galactose in β (1→3), β (1→4), and β (1→6) linkage. These trans-galacto-oligosaccharides are also known as TOS (Macfarlane et al., 2008; Gibson et al., 2010). Natural galacto-oligosaccharides (GOS) with the extension of sucrose are found in pulses. Human milk is rich in GOS with extra galactose residue at C_3, C_4, or C_6.

Because it contains two DP and is a synthetic disaccharide made by isomerizing lactose, lactulose is not regarded as dietary fiber but rather as a prebiotic instead. GOS has a significant positive impact on bifidobacteria and lactobacilli. It also stimulates other bacteria like *Bacteroidetes*, *Enterobacteria*, and *Firmicutes* but to a lesser extent (Marín-Manzano et al., 2013).

Starch and Glucose-Derived Oligosaccharides: Due to its physicochemical properties, resistant starch is a category of starch that is difficult to digest in the upper region of the stomach. The extent of RS varies with distinctive foods (such as cereals, potatoes, and legumes) and different treatment techniques. It produces a high level of butyrate; that's why it is considered a prebiotic (Fuentes-Zaragoza et al., 2011). Glucose-derived oligosaccharide is polydextrose. It is composed of glucan with many branches and glycosidic bonds (Costabile et al., 2012).

Non-carbohydrates and other oligosaccharides: Although some carbohydrates do not have to meet the criteria for non-digestibility and selective fermentability to be prebiotics, they seem to be the most likely to do so. Due to their stimulatory effects on lactic acid bacteria both in vitro and in vivo, flavanols from cocoa have also been considered prebiotics (Tzounis et al., 2011).

Other oligosaccharides: Some oligosaccharides are formed from pectin, a polysaccharide; these types of oligosaccharides are called pectic oligosaccharides (POS). They are based on the elongation of rhamnose (rhamnogalacturonan I) or galacturonic acid. The structure of POS can be acetylated at C2 or C3 and the carboxyl groups and converted to methyl ester. The side chains are joined to several sugars, including arabinose, galactose, and xylose. Depending on where POSs came from, their topologies vary greatly.

Mechanism of Action of Prebiotics: There have been notable advancements in the field of prebiotics, but the active mechanism of these prebiotics has not yet been fully explored. Prebiotics play a potent role in our overall health through the mechanisms (Figure 1.4).

- **Selective Promotion of Beneficial Bacteria:** Prebiotics are non-digestible dietary fibers that permit the GI tract intact and reach the colon. They provide a source of nourishment specifically for good microorganisms such as bifidobacteria and lactobacilli. These bacteria have the necessary enzymes to break down and ferment the prebiotic fibers (You et al., 2022).
- **Fermentation:** Beneficial bacteria ferment prebiotic fibers through a process called fermentation. During fermentation, bacteria metabolize prebiotics to produce SCFAs like propionate, butyrate, and acetate (Ríos-Covián et al., 2016). SCFAs act as an energy source for colonic cells and have various benefits for overall health.
- **The pH Regulation:** The process of fermentation of prebiotics by beneficial bacteria leads to the production of SCFAs, which lowers the pH in the colon. This mild acidification

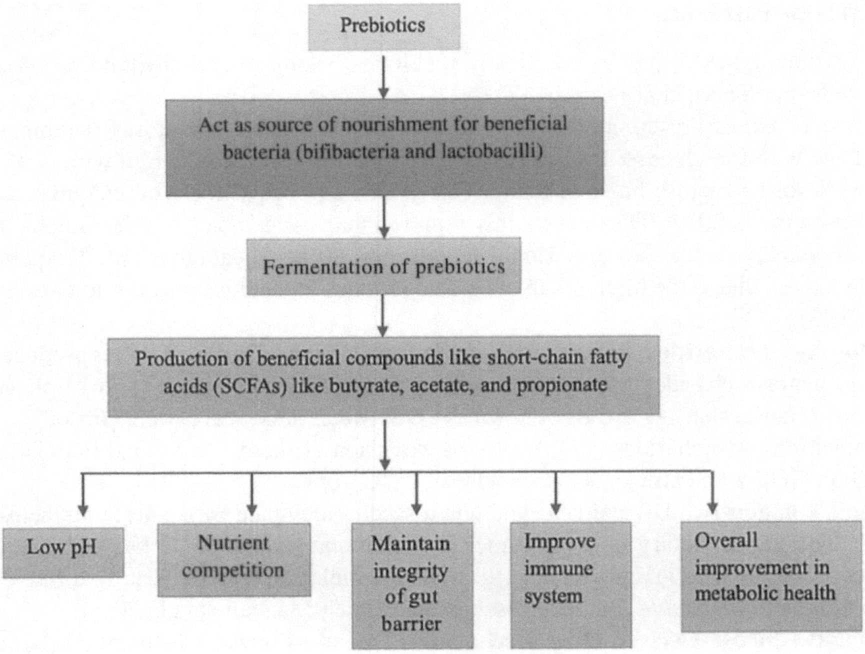

FIGURE 1.4 Flow chart of the mechanism of action of prebiotics.

creates an environment less favorable for the growth of harmful bacteria, thereby promoting a balanced and healthy gut microbiota (De Keersmaecker et al., 2006).

- **Nutrient Competition:** The presence of prebiotics encourages the growth of beneficial bacteria, creating competition for energy sources and sites of attachment in the colon. This competition prevents the spread of dangerous bacteria and preserves a variety of microorganisms (Louis et al., 2016).
- **Modulation of Gut Barrier Function:** SCFAs produced during prebiotic fermentation can stimulate the production of mucin, a substance that lines the intestinal walls and acts as a shielding barrier. Additionally, SCFAs influence tight junctions between intestinal cells, to maintain the reliability of the gut barrier (Whelan, 2013).
- **Immune System Modulation:** A balanced microbiota of the gut plays a potent role in the improvement and functions of the immune system. Prebiotics can influence immune responses by interacting with immune cells and promoting the formation of anti-inflammatory cells.
- **Metabolic Benefits:** Some prebiotics have been associated with metabolic benefits, including improved insulin sensitivity and reduced inflammation. SCFAs produced from prebiotic fermentation can also influence metabolic processes (Figure 1.5) and potentially contribute to overall metabolic health (Marteau et al., 2002).

1.4 SYNBIOTICS: THE POWER OF COMBINING PROBIOTICS AND PREBIOTICS

The microbiome is succinctly described as "the collective genetic material of microorganisms inhabiting a particular environment." Within the context of the human body, the human microbiome encompasses communities of bacteria, fungi, and viruses that coexist and interact with the host, playing pivotal roles in a wide spectrum of functions and interactions, influencing both states of health and disease. According to the Human Microbiome Project Consortium (2012), the human

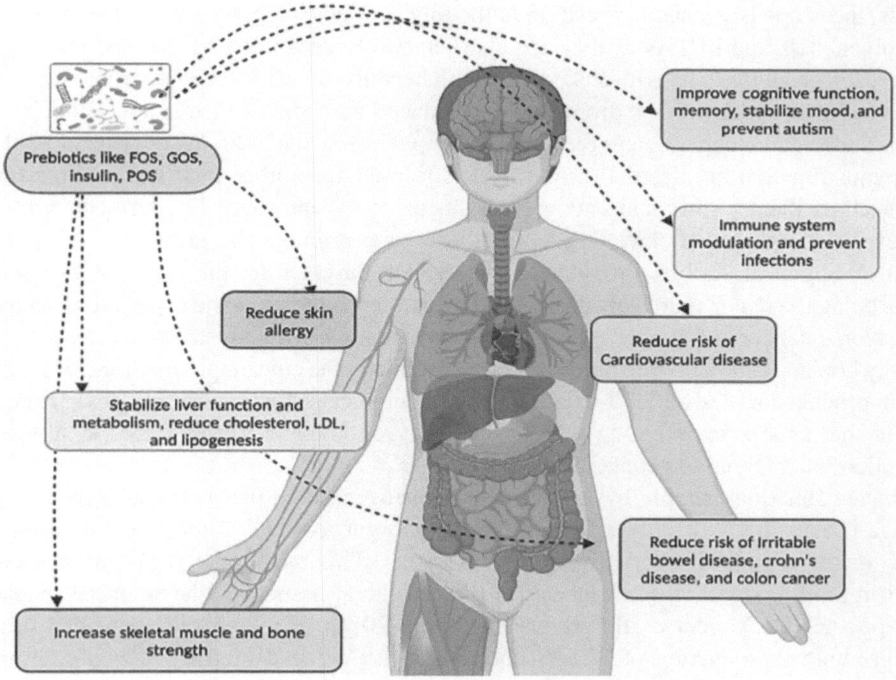

FIGURE 1.5 Diagrammatic representation of metabolic benefits of prebiotic.

microbiome has about one hundred trillion microbes, most of which live in the gut and this various microbe's community is as distinctive to an individual as a fingerprint.

Over the years the impact of the gastrointestinal microbiome on health and disease has been explicated; many influences such as physiological conditions of the host, food intake, the standard of living, and the surrounding environment affect the composition and type of gut microbiome. In one study, the role of food and its potential to modulate the microbiota, as well as being a vital source of nutrients for gut bacteria, sparked attention to using food as a useful tool for changing body composition (Singh et al., 2015; Conlon & Bird, 2015).

The beneficial impact of microbiota is mediated by metabolites produced by microorganisms during fermentation SCFAs, primarily propionate, acetate, butyrate, hydrogen sulfide (HS), ammonia (NH_3), hydrogen, methane (CH_4), CO, and CO_2 gases (Oleskin & Shenderov, 2016). SCFAs are made anaerobically inside the intestine by dietary fibers fermentation (Flint et al., 2008) and have several beneficial effects on an individual besides being a passive source of energy, such as maintaining various vital parameters in the blood to attain homeostasis, controlling inflammatory and immune-based responses, regulating several hormones that have a role in neoplasm suppression, controlling appetency, and handling central and peripheral nervous systems.

Through regulation and interaction with gut microorganisms, probiotics and prebiotics have recently attracted much interest and evidence has accumulated supporting their beneficial effects in various diseases by prebiotics and probiotics. *Bifidobacterium* and *Lactobacillus* strains of probiotics have been extensively studied in animal and human studies for improving lactose intolerance, facilitating immune regulations, preventing cancer and GIT disturbances such as constipation and diarrhea, and maintaining a balance of gut microbiota and tissue barrier integrity (Kumar et al., 2013).

All currently known non-digestible oligosaccharides, polysaccharides, and prebiotics, which are also major carbohydrate compounds, are being researched with great interest because of their health-favorable functions for the host. However, with the latest agreement on the definition of prebiotics, the scope is widened in relation to the aspect of how carbohydrates contain certain beneficial polyphenols and PUFAs as they are also selectively consumed by the host microbiota and could be responsible for the possible claimed health benefits to the host. Gut microbiome makeup in patients with impaired bowel syndrome showed reduced numbers of Firmicutes, Bifidobacterium, and Bacteroidetes in comparison to the control group (Gibson et al., 2017; Boccia et al., 2017).

The major function of intestinal or gut flora is to offer the ability to ferment indigestible substances such as dietary fiber and endogenous mucus of the intestine. The fermentation of these substrates yields compounds like SCFAs and gases that promote the growth of specialized gut microbes (Wong et al., 2006). Propionate, acetate, and butyrate are the major SCFAs produced. Butyrate, being the major source of energy for the gut microbiome, has the potential to induce apoptosis in colonic cancer and trigger intestinal gluconeogenesis, with constructive effects on glucose and energy homeostasis. Butyrate plays an important role in the consumption of significant amounts of oxygen produced as a result of ß-oxidation by epithelial cells and creates a hypoxic environment in the gut that aids in maintaining the optimum oxygen balance required for the sustenance of healthy microbiota (Byndloss et al., 2017).

Propionate functions mainly by regulating gluconeogenesis in the liver and helps in signaling satiety via interacting with fatty acid receptors in the gut. Acetate is the most important SCFA required for the growth of alternative microorganisms. This metabolite is primarily used in the metabolism of cholesterol and lipogenesis in the peripheral tissues and helps in the regulation of central appetite (De Vedder et al., 2014; Frost et al., 2014). "Randomized controlled trials have shown that higher production of SCFAs correlates with reduced intake of dietary fat and with reduced insulin resistance." The microbial enzymes in the gut are also involved in the metabolism of bile acid and lead to the production of several metabolites such as secondary and unconjugated bile acids, which have an important role in the regulation of several pathways in the host by signaling molecules and metabolic regulators (Lin et al., 2012; Long et al., 2017).

1.4.1 Synbiotic

The term "synbiotic" is used to describe a product that exerts a beneficial effect on the host by promoting the presence and colonization of live bacterial nutritional supplements in the GI. It achieves this by explicitly enhancing the overall growth and stimulating the metabolic activities of beneficial bacteria in the gut. The term "synbiotics" derives its significance from the concept of synergism, and it should be reserved for food products in which prebiotic compounds are specifically tailored to support the growth of probiotic organisms (Cencic & Chingwaru, 2010).

The scientific documentation of probiotic use may be recent, but it has been well known through the ages that good microbes can be consumed through food. The tradition of preparation of fermented foods with beneficial microbes runs very deep in the Indian culture. "Takre" or fermented milk/yogurt states the first line of a cure for a disease related to the stomach known as "Jatharagni" (fire in the stomach) in the treatise of Ayurvedic medicine "Charaka" Samhita in 1000 BC. The tradition of using a synbiotic product called "Panchamrit" (fermented milk + honey+ sugar + clarified butter) has been in practice since Vedic times in Hindu culture due to its health benefits.

The concept of prebiotics was introduced by Gibson and Roberfroid (1995). They believed that synbiotics are nothing but a simple combination of probiotics and prebiotics. ISAPP specified some other criteria for describing synbiotics and mainly emphasized the synergistic or complementary effects of synbiotics. The panel-agreed definition of a symbiotic is "a mixture of viable microorganisms and substrates that are selectively utilized by host microorganisms and confer a health benefit on the host" (ISAPP, 2023). The committee carefully considered the microorganisms that should be the symbiotic target of the substrate and concluded by mainly presenting two types of synergistic and complementary specific host microbes, which are the microbes that were previously present in the host (autochthonous microbes) and the one which are co-administered (allochthonous microbes).

In a "synergistic symbiotic" the substrate must be used specifically by the microorganism being administered at the same time and there is no need to be a separate probiotic or prebiotic if the synbiotic is working effectively in the host. A complementary synbiotic is one having a combination of a proven probiotic with a proven prebiotic that targets native microorganisms, such that both two components of the "complementary symbiotic" must fulfill the minimum criteria for probiotics and prebiotics (ISAPP).

1.4.2 Synbiotic Selection Criteria

The choice of a suitable prebiotic and probiotic, yielding a considerable advantageous effect on human health when utilized separately, is the first characteristic to be considered in the design of a symbiotic composition. The most appropriate way would be to determine the particular properties that a prebiotic must have to achieve a favorable outcome compared to a probiotic. The prebiotic must be able to significantly accelerate the growth of specially selected microorganisms and at the same time exert a beneficial effect on the host's health; the prebiotic must promote the gut microbial growth with health-favorable effects, without promoting the growth of other microorganisms. Here, Table 1.4 shows the combination of probiotics and prebiotics used as synbiotics.

1.4.3 Mechanism of Action of Synbiotics

The synergistic effect can be observed with the combination of probiotics and prebiotics; it is known that probiotic specifically affects the intestinal zone, and prebiotics are particularly functioning in the large intestine. The selected prebiotic serves as a nutrient medium for the probiotic strain; the growth and multiplication of the probiotic microbe, its fermentation, and course in the gut depend on the selected prebiotic that helps in the cultivation of the probiotic organisms (Hamasalim,

TABLE 1.4
List of Synbiotics

Synbiotics		
Probiotics	**Prebiotics**	**References**
Peptostreptococcaceae, bifidobacteria, Klebsiellae, *Bacteroides fragilis*	Fructooligosacchrides (FOS)	Dixit et al. (2016)
Bifidobacterium animalis, *Lactobacillus acidophilus*, *Lacticaseibacillus paracasei*	Inulin	Patel and Goyal (2012)
Bafidobacteria, *Bacteriodes fragilis* group	Isomaltooligosacchrides	Oliveira et al. (2011)
Bifidobacterium lactis, *L. acidophilus*, *Lactobacillus bulgaricus*, and *Lactobacillus rhamnosus*	Lactulose	Han et al. (2009)
Zymomonas mobilis	Lactosurcose	Aachary and Prapulla (2011)
Bifidobacterium adolescentis, *Lactiplantibacillus plantarum*	Xygooligosacchrides (XOS)	Macfarlane et al. (2008)
Bifidobacterium longum, *Bifidobacterium catenulatum*	Galactooligosacchrides (GOS)	Bartosch et al. (2005)
Bifidobacterium bifidum, *Bifidobacterium lactis*	Fructooligosacchrides (FOS)	Le Barz et al. (2015)
Bifidobacterium sp.	Arabinoxylan and arabinoxylan oligosaccharides	Bird et al. (2000)
Bacteriodes, *Eubacterium rectale*	Resistant starch 1, 2, 3, 4	Hamasalim (2016)

2016). Several scientific reports denoted that probiotic microbial strain develops advanced tolerance toward unfavorable environmental situations such as high temperature, pH, and O_2 levels in the gut of a particular individual in the presence of prebiotics (Sekhon & Jairath, 2010). Figure 1.6 shows the formation of SCFAs and certain organic acids, which lower the pH of light, improve mineral absorption, and inhibit the growth of pathogens through the selective use of prebiotics from part of the commensal microflora.

By cross-feeding mechanism, the growth of butyrate-forming bacteria increases by the utilization of metabolites from probiotics. Phagocytic activity, modulation of the production of immunoglobulins that promotes immune response enhancement, also promotes the organism's modulation by competing for nutrients and adhesion sites against pathogens and improvement in the barrier functions with the help of probiotics (Ballan et al., 2020).

The cell wall of gram-negative bacteria produces LPS-endotoxins which are released into the systemic circulation and responsible for metabolic endotoxemia. As a result of the increased inflammatory response, $NF\text{-}_{K}B$ is activated and cytokines (TNF-α) are produced ultimately, leading to a rise in insulin resistance due to serine phosphorylation of IRS-1 (Ballan et al., 2020).

The SCFA can signal through GPCRs on the cell surface; pathways related to insulin sensitivity enhancement are GPR41 and GPR43, which are displayed in Figure 1.6, through secretion of hormones such as peptide YY (PYY) and GLP-1, regulation of energy intake happens, and satiety by enhancing the levels of leptin. For metabolic and intestinal diseases, improving the levels of organic acids in the intestinal lumen appears to be an advantageous strategy (Ballan et al., 2020).

The mechanisms of action of the synbiotics that allow a high tolerance, toward factors, are not sufficiently studied. The two mechanisms of action that are used by the synbiotics are as follows (Manigandan et al., 2012):

1. Through increased viability of probiotic organisms
2. By defining distinct beneficial health

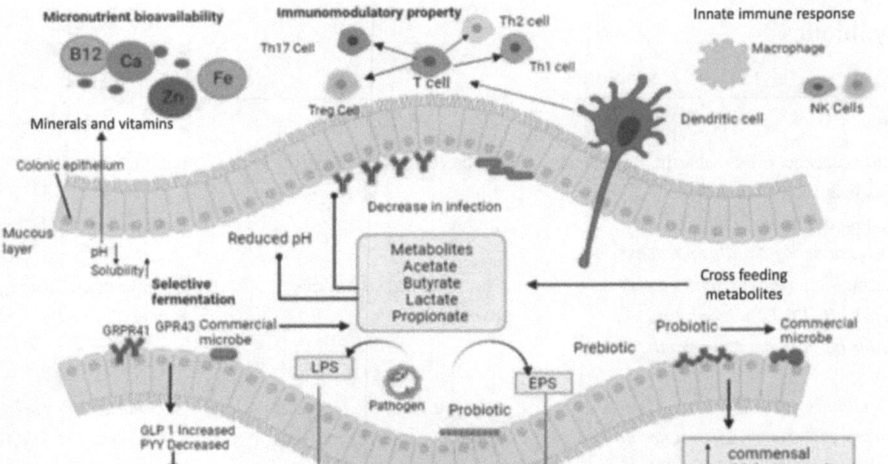

FIGURE 1.6 Mechanisms of action of prebiotics and probiotics.

1.4.4 Synbiotic Products for Humans

1.4.4.1 Synbiotic Yogurt

In this study, they produced synbiotic yogurt (Figure 1.7) with different concentrations of inulin such as 1, 2, 5, and 5 % (w/v). Tarkhineh (Iranian cereal-dairy fermented food) derived from *L. brevis* was used for the preparation of symbiotic yogurt. Results show that there is an increase in the production of antimicrobial compounds with antimicrobial effects on *Salmonella typhimurium.* The physiochemical properties were unchanged, but a significant reduction in the amount of fat in synbiotic yogurt was observed. A novel synbiotic yogurt can be used as an excellent delivery carrier for obtaining the beneficial health effects of probiotic strain *L. brevis*, which can exert the required properties in the yogurt and exert its beneficial health effects (Falah et al., 2021).

1.4.4.2 Synbiotic Yogurt from Camel Milk

In this study, various quality parameters of symbiotic yogurt (Figure 1.8) were analyzed such as organoleptic properties, physicochemical properties, and rheological properties. The yogurt was prepared from camel milk with banana fiber and banana peel fiber as a source of probiotic bacteria (*Lactobacillus gasseri* and *L. casei*) and prebiotics. The major analytical findings of the yogurt were improvement in viscosity, increased rate of survival of beneficial microbial strains, and improved consistency of the product. On the other hand, parameters such as rate of syneresis, pH, and surface tension were decreased. The organoleptic properties such as texture, flavor, color, and overall acceptability were greatly acceptable. The results obtained for banana peel fiber were significantly better than those of banana fiber in all the samples. It can finally be concluded that both forms of fiber have beneficial effects on the human body in their own distinguished ways (Safdari et al., 2021).

1.4.4.3 Synbiotic Ice Cream

In this study, different twenty-seven volatile compounds were reported in the formulations of ice cream (Figure 1.9). It has been observed that the synbiotic ice cream prepared using inulin @ 2%

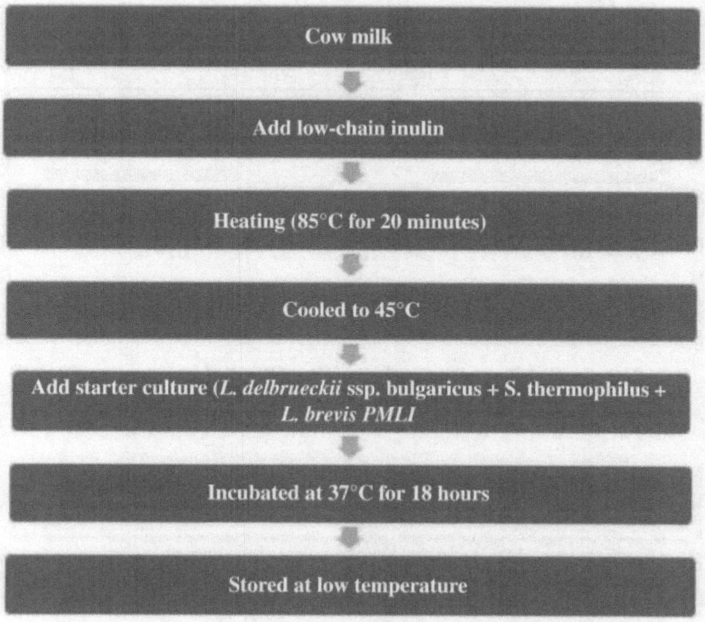

FIGURE 1.7 Synbiotic yogurt with different concentrations of inulin.

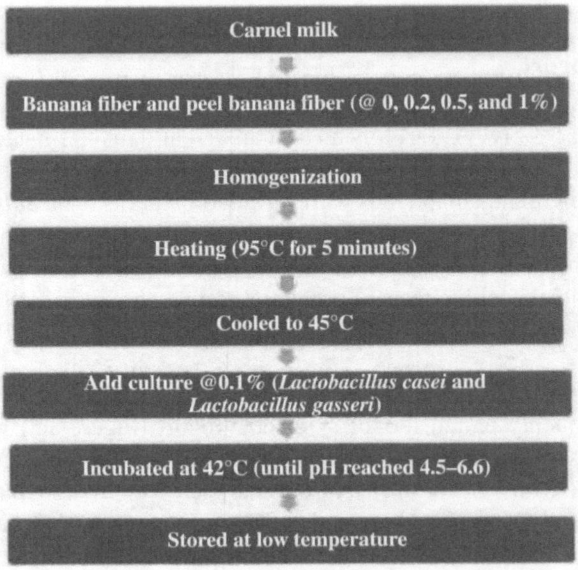

FIGURE 1.8 Preparation of synbiotic yogurt using camel milk with banana fiber and banana peel fiber.

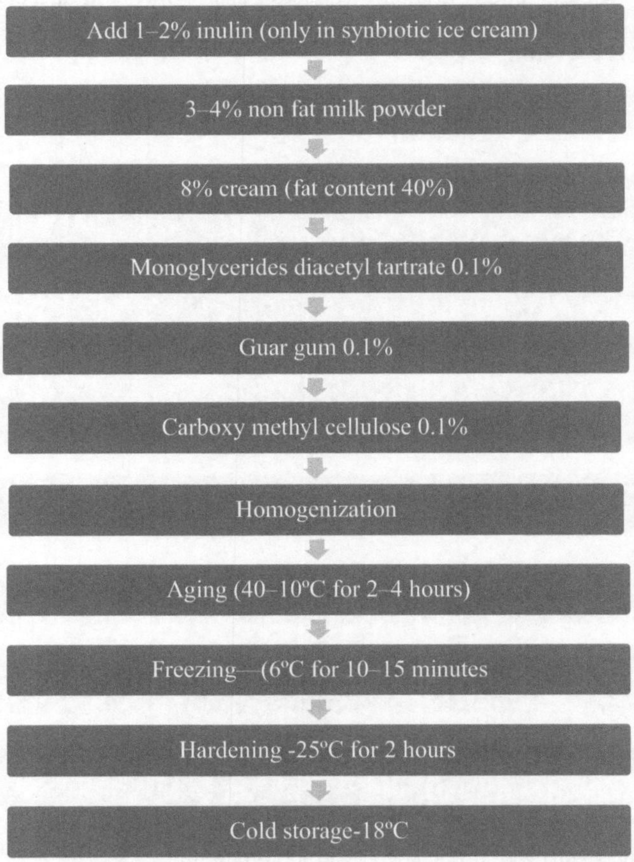

FIGURE 1.9 Synbiotic ice cream.

included higher concentrations (3,983 μg/L) than ice cream prepared only with probiotic strain *S. boulardii* at the rate of 0.5% (1,479 μg/L) and control ice cream (616.1 μg/L). The synbiotic ice cream formulated has the potential to be included in the category of novel functional product with probiotic yeast *S. boulardii* and prebiotic inulin (Sarwar et al., 2021). Table 1.5 shows the list of synbiotic products with probiotics and prebiotics used.

TABLE 1.5
The List of Synbiotic Products with Probiotics and Prebiotics Used

Products	Probiotics	Prebiotics	Result	Reference
Synbiotic semihard cheese	*Lactobacillus paracasei*	Fructo-oligosaccharides (FOS)	*L. paracesei* viability was not affected by FOS in the cheese even after 28 days of ripening. During the testing of this synbiotic cheese in the colonic model higher viability of *L. paracasei* strain was attained in the presence of FOS. The addition of FOS in the cheese has an advantageous impact by enhancing the viability of probiotic strain in the host.	Langa et al. (2019)
Synbiotic yogurt	*Lactobacillus rhamnosus* and *Lactobacillus reuteri*	Inulin, lactulose, and oligofructose	Lowest acidity: control and inulin-contained samples. Highest acidity: Lactulose-containing samples. Lowest syneresis: Inulin and lactulose-containing samples. Highest viscosity: Inulin-containing samples. In inulin-containing samples, *L. rhamosus and L. reuteri* showed the best viability. Best taste: Oligofructose-containing samples. Best texture: Oligofructose and inulin-containing samples.	Shaghaghi et al. (2013)
Synbiotic yogurt	*L. rhamnosus*	Fiber (0.5% oat flour)	The viability of the probiotic strain was good in the yogurt made with prebiotic fiber source (0.5% oat flour) and probiotic strain *L. rhamnosus* up to 3 weeks of storage. Compared to all other yogurts, acidity; protein, fat, and crude fiber content; and the pH of the synbiotic yogurt were high. It works as a functional food and a good transporter for probiotics to the gut and increases gut health to decrease the chances of illnesses.	Ranjitham and Poornakala (2020)
Synbiotic mousse	*L. acidophilus*	Inulin and FOS	Significant decrease in immunoglobulin, total cholesterol, as well as interleukin-1ß in both treatment and control groups.	Xavier-Santos et al. (2018)

1.5 ROLE OF PROBIOTICS, PREBIOTICS, AND SYNBIOTICS IN HUMAN HEALTH

Studies conducted as part of the European Union–funded SYNCAN project have confirmed the anticarcinogenic properties of synbiotics. The patient's health with the risk of colorectal cancer was analyzed with the intervention of two probiotic strains (*L. rhamnosus* and *B. animalis* subsp. *lactic*) blended with FOS as a prebiotic. As an outcome, they observe a change in biomarkers (interferon γ, labeled cells/crypt, necrosis, transepithelial resistance, IL-2, labeling index, genotoxicity), showing disease growth in patients with cancer (Rafter et al., 2007). It was concluded that the studied synbiotic formulation (*L. rhamnosus* GG + *B. animalis* subsp. *lactis* Bb12 4. FOS) helps reduce the risk of colorectal cancer (Van Loo et al., 2005).

The commercial interest in synbiotic food products has also increased with increased awareness of GI health wellness, disorder prevention, and treatment of the disease. Currently, research is focused on screening potential microbes capable of inhabiting the human gut, along with their capability to utilize new prebiotics for the formulations of novel functional foods (Kerry et al., 2018).

Probiotic strains commonly used in synbiotic compositions are *Saccharomyces boulardii*, *Bifidobacterium* sp., *Lactobacillus* spp., and *Bacillus coagulant*, and commonly used prebiotics in synbiotic compositions are XOS, oligosaccharides, FOS, GM, and inulin (Pandey et al., 2015).

1.5.1 Inflammatory Bowel Disease

The two main chronic forms of inflammatory disorders of the GI tract include UC and Crohn's disease (CD) (Haller et al., 2010). The etiology of inflammatory bowel disease has been extensively studied, but the pathogenesis of the disease is not completely understood (Goyel et al., 2014). The attributes of inflammation are different in CD and UC. The inflammation of UC is usually limited to the lining of the colon, while CD occurs throughout the digestive tract and usually leads to inflammation of the distal small intestine and colon (Ardizzone & Porro, 2005; Molodecky et al., 2012).

In one clinical study, the impact of synbiotics having GOS and *Bifidobacterium breve* on patients with gentle to medium UC was evaluated (Ishikawa et al., 2011). Forty-one patients were provided with a synbiotic or a placebo treatment for 12 weeks. During the study, both endoscopic groups were subjected to underdo endoscopic analysis, and the findings revealed that the myeloperoxidase levels in the washout statements were significantly reduced.

Fecal microbiome analysis was also done by plate count method before and after treatment for subjects in the symbiotic group. Of all the microbes evaluated, only the Bacteriodaceae were significantly reduced after synbiotic therapy. *Bifidobacterium* levels were reported to be the same, and *B. breve* was observed in culture only after treatment (5.75 ± 1.65 $\log_{10}$ CFU/g stool). We can therefore say that *B. breve* survived through the GI (Akiyama et al., 2015).

1.5.2 Diarrhea

Generally, infectious agents are responsible for diarrheal diseases, which cause watery stools with high volume. Globally, diarrhea is the leading cause of hospitalizations, which if overlooked for a long time may result in mortality as well (Dinleyici et al., 2013). In one identical investigation, treatment with *Lactobacillus*, *Streptococcus*, and *Bifidobacterium* species (1×10^9 total CFU) and FOS (0.99 g) was done on children with acute rotavirus diarrhea (Dewi et al., 2015). Thirty-five kids were registered for the symbiotic treatment, which resembled a control treatment. The period of acute rotavirus diarrhea was extremely shorter in the symbiotic treatment, and healing of the intestinal mucosa was noted 50 hours after symbiotic administration. Analysis of gut microbiota was not performed. No additional description was provided as to why the synbiotic treatment group reacted to treatment.

The *L. paracasei* (2.5×10^9 CFU) was used to develop a synbiotic that also contained a mixture of arabinogalactan (0.5 g) and XOS (0.7 g). The study contained fifty-five kids with acute diarrhea who had been given therapy with an oral rehydration solution. After the first 72 hours, a higher resolution rate was reported in the symbiotic group in comparison to the placebo group (Terrin et al., 2012). This analysis also permitted other therapies administered after the first 72 hours by the parents, which may affect the complete period of diarrhea.

To control diarrhea and vomiting and various diseases in children, the capability of a mixture of probiotic strains *Streptococcus thernophilus*, *B. animalis* subsp. *lactis*, *Lactobacillus bulgaricus*, and prebiotic inulin (1 g) was estimated (Ringel-Kulka et al., 2015). After the treatment of 16 weeks, children treated with synbiotics had extremely fewer days of fever but extremely more time with liquid stools.

1.5.3 Irritable Bowel Syndrome

Irritable bowel syndrome (IBS) is a disease related to the intestine described by pain in the abdomen, constipation, diarrhea, bloating, or alternating times of these signs. There can be various factors that can contribute to elevating the symptoms of IBS like hyperactivity, anxiety, genetics, gut microbiome, inflammation, and surroundings, but the major cause of IBS has not been proven (Ford et al., 2014). Dietary modifications, medications, physiological interventions, yoga, exercise, and changes in the gut microbiota are aspects of the most popular therapies suggested for IBS (Gibson et al., 2015).

In a study by Matijašić et al. (2016), the effect of the mixture of prebiotic, which includes 90% inulin and 10% oligofructose and multiple probiotic strains of *Lactobacillus acidophillus*, *Bifidobacterium animalis* subspecies *lectis*, and *Streptococcus thermophilus* in fermented milk, was evaluated on the gut microbiome of thirty grown-up patients with IBS.

There was no considerable dissimilarity observed in the number of bacteria tested within the experimental group; in the control group, the number of strains was detected. In another study, extremely decreased laxative use after 4 weeks in adults with constipation was observed due to synbiotic treatment containing psyllium fiber and inulin as prebiotics and *L. acidophilus*, *Bifidobacterium bifidum*, *Lactobacillus plantarum*, *Lactobacillus bulgaricus*, and *L. rhamnosus* as a probiotic (Cudmore et al., 2017).

1.5.4 Ulcerative Colitis

UC is an idiopathic intestinal inflammatory disease characterized mainly by diarrhea with blood and mucous, abdominal discomfort, and rectal bleeding (Judge & Lichtenstein, 2003). Inflammation in UC is usually limited to the mucosal layer. The infection begins in the rectum but soon spreads throughout the proximities of the intestine. No ideal cure for UC has been discovered yet, and the medicinal therapies that are available are limited to maintaining remission (Su et al., 2003).

In this study, for 12 months, 21 patients having mild to average UC were given the probiotic—Yakult, which is a fermented milk of bifidobacterial strain and GOS (10^9 CFU/g bacteria + 53 g GOS/day). Scientists discovered a significant reduction of myeloperoxidase and increased production of desirable SCFA with the synbiotic treatment also observed a reduction in the count of Barteroidaceae and fecal pH and progress in the UC situation.

One randomized crossover analysis was performed on eight patients with UC; oral treatment was done with specific strains of probiotics, *B. animalis* subsp. *lactis*, *L. delbrueckii* subsp. *bulgaricus*, *S. thermophilus*, and *L. acidophilus*, and at the concentration of 4×10^9 organisms per capsule with 15 g of oligofructose powder per day in synbiotic formulation for the period of 1 month.

Therapy did not induce modifications in fecal microbial composition. The scientists concluded that the results were due to restrictions of the analysis, like a smaller number of volunteers for the treatments, the shorter duration of symbiotic treatment, and the shortage of a washout duration in the testing of protocol (Ahmed et al., 2013).

1.6 FUTURE DIRECTIONS AND CONCLUSION

Ongoing progress in modeling and analyzing gut microbiota will enrich our understanding of their impact on health and morbid conditions and equip us to adapt forthcoming and recent therapeutic and preventive strategies. Grasping the precise functions fulfilled by the gut microbiota in growth and development and its intricate involvement in health and morbidity holds the capacity to enhance various aspects of our daily lives. This spans from defining infant formulas to introducing innovative approaches to tackling health challenges like obesity, cancer, diabetes, and other degenerative diseases. Given the complexity of the gut microbiota, future research should adopt a multidisciplinary approach incorporating recent breakthroughs from diverse scientific fields.

1.6.1 Current Research and Emerging Trends

The pivotal role of probiotics, prebiotics, and symbiotics in the realms of health, morbidity, and nutrition has amplified their significance both scientifically and in marketing endeavors worldwide. The emphasis has transitioned from prospective studies toward clinical trials, aimed at yielding a deeper comprehension of how the microbiota intricately interacts with human health and illness.

Emerging technologies like bioinformatics and in silico methodologies can contribute significantly to enhancing our comprehensive understanding of beneficial microorganisms, enabling precise utilization and safety evaluation. Affordability of whole genome sequencing can help in introducing novel probiotic strains. Genetic manipulations such as the use of isogenic mutant strains can prove to be an important tool for studying probiotic mechanisms of action and creating potentially improved strains (Smits, 2019).

Recent advancements in in vitro and ex vivo techniques, leveraging human cells and tissues, transcend the conventional use of in vitro cell lines and animal models. Reproducible human organoids have demonstrated their utility in replicating the manifestations of IBS and elucidating the therapeutic impacts of *L. rhamnosus GG* (Han et al., 2019). Furthermore, cutting-edge organs-on-chips technology amalgamates progress in human cell culture with microelectronics and microfluidics, presenting a platform for exploring the anticancer effects of probiotics and synbiotic formulations.

1.6.2 Conclusion and Key Takeaways

This chapter comprehensively delves into the impact of probiotics, prebiotics, and synbiotics on the host's health. These elements collectively exert systemic effects on the host's health, metabolism, and immune system. When considering symbiotic selection, it is essential to ensure the utilization of prebiotics by probiotics, establishing a prerequisite for maintaining optimal synergy between them to maximize their advantageous outcomes.

By unraveling the underlying mechanism of probiosis and prebiosis, researchers gain the ability to craft improved functional foods aimed at enhancing host health. Manipulating the microbiota's composition through dietary prebiotic substances and probiotic microorganisms presents an intriguing avenue for controlling and treating significant diseases. Recent strides in technology, enabling the in-depth analysis and sequencing of the unexpected microbial diversity within the GI, hold the potential to prevent diseases and promote overall well-being. While numerous reports on probiotic uses in humans are already present, information on prebiotics and synbiotics remains relatively sparse. Furthermore, health claims require substantiation and robust confirmation through appropriately designed clinical trials on a large scale. The ability to target specific organisms within the colon for precise health-promoting purposes holds substantial promise. It is important to note significant variations in bacterial carbohydrate utilization patterns among diverse strains and species, a crucial consideration in the development of novel synbiotics.

BIBLIOGRAPHY

Aachary, A. A., & Prapulla, S. G. (2011). Xylooligosaccharides (XOS) as an emerging prebiotic: Microbial synthesis, utilization, structural characterization, bioactive properties, and applications. *Comprehensive Reviews in Food Science and Food Safety, 10*(1), 2–16.

Aagaard, K., Riehle, K., Ma, J., Segata, N., Mistretta, T. A., Coarfa, C., Raza, S., Rosenbaum, S., Van den Veyver, I., Milosavljevic, A., Gevers, D., Huttenhower, C., Petrosino, J., & Versalovic, J. (2012). A metagenomic approach to characterization of the vaginal microbiome signature in pregnancy. *PLoS One*, *7*(6), e36466. https://doi.org/10.1371/journal.pone.0036466

AboNahas, H. H., Darwish, A. M., Abd El-kareem, H. F., AboNahas, Y. H., Mansour, S. A., Korra, Y. H., Sayyed, R. Z., Abdel-Azeem, A. M., & Saiyed, E. M. (2022). Trust your gut: The human gut microbiome in health and disease. *Microbiome-Gut-Brain Axis: Implications on Health*, 53–96. https://doi.org/10.1007/978-981-16-1626-6_3

Ahire, J. J., Jakkamsetty, C., Kashikar, M. S., Lakshmi, S. G., & Madempudi, R. S. (2021). In vitro evaluation of probiotic properties of lactobacillus plantarum UBLP40 isolated from traditional indigenous fermented food. *Probiotics and Antimicrobial Proteins, 13*(5), 1413–1424. https://doi.org/10.1007/S12602-021-09775-7/METRICS

Ahmed, J., Reddy, B. S., Mølbak, L., Leser, T. D., & MacFie, J. (2013). Impact of probiotics on colonic microflora in patients with colitis: A prospective double blind randomised crossover study. *International Journal of Surgery, 11*(10), 1131–1136.

Akiyama, T., Kimura, K., & Hatano, H. (2015). Diverse galactooligosaccharides consumption by bifidobacteria: Implications of β-galactosidase—LacS operon. *Bioscience, Biotechnology, and Biochemistry, 79*(4), 664–672.

Alvarez-Olmos, M. I., & Oberhelman, R. A. (2001). Probiotic agents and infectious diseases: A modern perspective on a traditional therapy. *Clinical Infectious Diseases*, 32, 1567–1576.

Ardizzone, S., & Porro, G. B. (2005). Biologic therapy for inflammatory bowel disease. *Drugs, 65,* 2253–2286.

Aso, Y., Akaza, H., Kotake, T., Tsukamoto, T., Imai, K., & Naito, S. (1995). Preventive effect of a *Lactobacillus casei* preparation on the recurrence of superficial bladder cancer in a double–blind trial. The BLP study group. *European Urology*, *27*, 104–109.

Azcarate-Peril, M. A., Ritter, A. J., Savaiano, D., Monteagudo-Mera, A., Anderson, C., Magness, S. T., & Klaenhammer, T. R. (2017). Impact of short-chain galactooligosaccharides on the gut microbiome of lactose-intolerant individuals. *Proceedings of the National Academy of Sciences, 114*(3), E367–E375.

Aziz, Q., Dore, J., Emmanuel, A., Guarners, F., & Quigley, E. M. M. (2013). Gut microbiota and gastrointestinal health: Current concepts and future directions. *Neurogastroenterology & Motility, 25,* 4–15.

Ballan, R., Battistini, C., Xavier-Santos, D., & Saad, S. M. I. (2020). Interactions of probiotics and prebiotics with the gut microbiota. *Progress in Molecular Biology and Translational Science, 171,* 265–300.

Barrett, H. L., Callaway, L. K., & Nitert, M. D. (2012). Probiotics: A potential role in the prevention of gestational diabetes? *Acta Diabetologica*, *49*, 1–13.

Bartosch, S., Woodmansey, E. J., Paterson, J. C., McMurdo, M. E., & Macfarlane, G. T. (2005). Microbiological effects of consuming a synbiotic containing Bifidobacterium bifidum, Bifidobacterium lactis, and oligofructose in elderly persons, determined by real-time polymerase chain reaction and counting of viable bacteria. *Clinical Infectious Diseases*, *40*(1), 28–37.

Bengmark, S. (1998). Ecological control of the gastrointestinal tract. The role of probiotic flora. *Gut*, *42*(1), 2–7. https://doi.org/10.1136/gut.42.1.2

Berg, G., Rybakova, D., Fischer, D., Cernava, T., Vergès, M. C. C., Charles, T., Chen, X., Cocolin, L., Eversole, K., Corral, G. H., & Kazou, M. (2020). Microbiome definition re-visited: Old concepts and new challenges. *Microbiome,* 8, 103. https://doi.org/10.1186/s40168-020-00875-0

Biagi, E., Candela, M., Turroni, S., Garagnani, P., Franceschi, C., & Brigidi, P. (2013). Ageing and gut microbes: Perspectives for health maintenance and longevity. *Pharmacological Research*, *69,* 11–20. https://doi.org/10.1016/j.phrs.2012.10.005

Bird, A. R., Brown, I. L., & Topping, D. L. (2000). Starches, resistant starches, the gut microflora and human health. *Current Issues in Intestinal Microbiology, 1*(1), 25–37.

Boccia, S., Torre, I., Santarpia, L., Iervolino, C., Del Piano, C., Puggina, A., & Pasanisi, F. (2017). Intestinal microbiota in adult patients with short bowel syndrome: Preliminary results from a pilot study. *Clinical Nutrition, 36*(6), 1707–1709.

Byndloss, M. X., Olsan, E. E., Rivera-Chavez, F., Tiffany, C. R., Cevallos, S. A., Lokken, K. L., Torres, T. P., Byndloss, A. J., Faber, F., Gao, Y., & Litvak, Y. (2017). Microbiota-activated PPAR-γ signaling inhibits dysbiotic Enterobacteriaceae expansion. *Science*, *357*(6351), 570–575.

Cencic, A., & Chingwaru, W. (2010). The role of functional foods, nutraceuticals, and food supplements in intestinal health. *Nutrients, 2*(6), 611–625.

Chang, Y., Jeong, C., & Cheng, W., Y. C.-J. (2021). *Quality characteristics of yogurts fermented with short-chain fatty acid-producing probiotics and their effects on mucin production and probiotic adhesion onto*. Elsevier. Retrieved August 24, 2023, from https://www.sciencedirect.com/science/article/pii/S0022030221004835

Conlon, M. A., & Bird, A. R. (2015). The impact al' diet and lifestyle on gut microbiota and human health. *Nutrients*, *7*(1), 17–44.

Costabile, A., Fava, F., Röytiö, H., Forssten, S. D., Olli, K., Klievink, J., Rowland, I. R., Ouwehand, A. C., Rastall, R. A., Gibson, G. R., & Walton, G. E. (2012). Impact of polydextrose on the faecal microbiota: A double-blind, crossover, placebo-controlled feeding study in healthy human subjects. *British Journal of Nutrition, 108*(3), 471–481. https://doi.org/10.1017/S0007114511005782

Cudmore, S., Doolan, A., Lacey, S., & Shanahan, F. (2017). A randomised, double-blind, placebo-controlled clinical study: The effects of a synbiotic, Lepicol, in adults with chronic, functional constipation. *International Journal of Food Sciences and Nutrition, 68*(3), 366–377.

Davis, L. M. G., Martinez, I., Walter, J., & Hutkins, R. (2010). A dose dependent impact of prebiotic galactooligosaccharides on the intestinal microbiota of healthy adults. *International Journal of Food Microbiology, 144*(2), 285–292.

De Keersmaecker, S. C. J., Verhoeven, T. L. A., Desair, J., Marchal, K., Vanderleyden, J., & Nagy, I. (2006). Strong antimicrobial activity of Lactobacillus rhamnosus GG against Salmonella typhimurium is due to accumulation of lactic acid. *FEMS Microbiology Letters, 259*(1), 89–96. https://doi.org/10.1111/J.1574-6968.2006.00250.X

De Vedder, F., Kovatcheva-Datchary, P., Goncalves, D., Vinera, J., Zitoun, C., Duchampt, A., Bäckhed, F., & Mithieux, G. (2014). Microbiota—generated metabolites promote metabolic benefits via gut-brain neural circuits. *Cell, 156*(1–2), 84–96.

Dewi, M. R., Soenarto, Y., & Karyana, I. P. G. (2015). Efficacy of synbiotic treatment in children with acute rotavirus diarrhea. *Paediatrica Indonesiana, 55*(2), 74–78.

Dinleyici, E. C., Dalgic, N., Guven, S., Ozen, M., Kara, A., Arica, V., & Vandenplas, Y. (2013). The effect of a multispecies synbiotic mixture on the duration of diarrhea and length of hospital stay in children with acute diarrhea in Turkey: Single blinded randomized study. *European Journal of Pediatrics, 172,* 459–464.

Dixit, Y., Wagle, A., & Vakil, B. (2016). Patents in the field of probiotics, prebiotics, synbiotics: A review. *Journal of Food: Microbiology, Safety & Hygiene, 1*(2), 1–13.

Dupré, J. O., & O'Malley, M. A. (2009). Varieties of living things: Life at the intersection of lineage and metabolism. In S. Normandin & C. Wolf (Eds.), *Vitalism and the scientific image in post-enlightenment life science; history, philosophy and theory of the life sciences* (pp. 1800–2010). Springer.

Falah, F., Vasiee, A., Yazdi, F. T., & Behbahani, B. A. (2021). Preparation and functional properties of synbiotic yogurt fermented with Lactobacillus brevis PML1 derived from a fermented cereal-dairy product. *BioMed Research International, 2021.*

Flint, H. J., Bayer, E. A., Rincon, M. T., Lamed, R., & White, B. A. (2008). Polysaccharide utilization by gut bacteria: Potential for new insights from genomic analysis. *Nature Reviews Microbiology*, *6*(2), 121–31.

Ford, A. C., Quigley, E. M., Lacy, B. E., Lembo, A. J., Saito, Y. A., Schiller, L. R., Soffer, E. E., Spiegel, B. M., & Moayyedi, P. (2014). Efficacy of prebiotics, probiotics, and synbiotics in irritable bowel syndrome and chronic idiopathic constipation: Systematic review and meta-analysis. *Official Journal of the American College of Gastroenterology | ACG, 109*(10), 1547–1561.

Frost, G., Sleeth, M. L., Sahuri-Arisoylu, M., Lizarbe, B., Cerdan, S., Brody, I., Anastasovska, J., Ghourab, S., Hankir, M., Zhang, S., & Carling, D. (2014). The short-chain fatty acid acetate reduces appetite via a central homeostatic mechanism. *Nature Communications*, *5*(1), 1–11.

Fuentes-Zaragoza, E., Sánchez-Zapata, E., Sendra, E., Sayas, E., Navarro, C., Fernández-Lõpez, J., & Pérez-Alvarez, J. A. (2011). Resistant starch as prebiotic: A review. *Starch—Stärke, 63*(7), 406–415. https://doi.org/10.1002/STAR.201000099

Gangaraju, D., Raghu, A. V., Siddalingaiya Gurudutt, P., & Anjanapura Raghu, C. V. (2022). Green synthesis of γ-aminobutyric acid using permeabilized probiotic Enterococcus faecium for biocatalytic application. *Wiley Online LibraryD Gangaraju, AV Raghu, P Siddalingaiya GuruduttNano Select, 2022•Wiley Online Library, 3*(10), 1436–1447. https://doi.org/10.1002/nano.202200059

Gibson, G. R., Probert, H. M., Van Loo, J., Rastall, R. A., & Roberfroid, M. B. (2004). Dietary modulation of the human colonic microbiota: Updating the concept of prebiotics. *Nutrition Research Reviews, 17*(2), 259–275. https://doi.org/10.1079/nrr200479

Gibson, G. R., & Roberfroid, M. B. (1995). Dietary modulation of the human colonic microbiota: Introducing the concept of prebiotics. *The Journal of Nutrition*, *125*, 1401–1412.

Gibson, G. R., Scott, K. P., Rastall, R. A., Tuohy, K. M., Hotchkiss, A., Dubert-Ferrandon, A., . . . & Buddington, R. (2010). Dietary prebiotics: current status and new definition. *Food Sci. Technol. Bull. Funct. Foods, 7*(1), 1–19.

Gibson, P. R., Varney, J., Malakar, S., & Muir, J. G. (2015). Food components and irritable bowel syndrome. *Gastroenterology, 148*(6), 1158–1174.

Gibson, W. I., Hutkins, R., Sanders, M. E., Prescott, S. L., Reimer, R. A., Salminen, S. J., Scott, K., Stanton, C., Swanson, K. S., Cani, P. D., & Verbeke, K. (2017). Expert consensus document: The international scientific association for probiotics and prebiotics (SAPP) consensus statement on the definition and scope of prebiotics. *Nature Reviews Gastroenterology & Hepatology, 14*(8), 491–502.

Gill, S. R., Pop, M., DeBoy, R. T., Eckburg, P. B., Turnbaugh, P. J., Samuel, B. S., Gordon, J. I., Relman, D. A., Fraser-Liggett, C. M., & Nelson, K. E. (2006). Metagenomic analysis of the human distal gut microbiome. *Science, 312,* 1355–1359. https://doi.org/10.1126/science.1124234

Goyal, N., Rana, A., Ahlawat, A., Bijjem, K. R. V., & Kumar, P. (2014). Animal models of inflammatory bowel disease: A review. *Inflammopharmacology, 22*(4), 219–233.

Green, C., Corner, G. I. A. P. P., & Pediatric, G. I. (2018). Probiotics: A review for clinical use. Modified on MAY 26, 2021, Retrieved from https://www.gastroendonews.com/Review-Articles/Article/05-21/Probiotics-for-Clinical-Use/63435

Haller, D., Antoine, J. M., Bengmark, S., Enck, P., Rijkers, G. T., & Lenoir-Wijnkoop, I. (2010). Guidance for substantiating the evidence for beneficial effects of probiotics: Probiotics in chronic inflammatory bowel disease and the functional disorder irritable bowel syndrome. *The Journal of Nutrition, 140*(3), 690S–697S.

Hamasalim, H. J. (2016). Synbiotic as feed additives relating to animal health and performance. *Advances in Microbiology, 6*(4), 288–302.

Han, W. C., Byun, S. H., Kim, M. H., Sohn, E. H., Lim, J. D., Um, B. H., & Jang, K. H. (2009). Production of lactosucrose from sucrose and lactose by a levansucrase from Zymomonas mobilis. *Journal of Microbiology and Biotechnology, 19*(10), 1153–1160.

Han, X., Lee, A., Huang, S., Gao, J., Spence, J. R., & Owyang, C. (2019). Lactobacillus rhamnosus GG prevents epithelial barrier dysfunction induced by interferon-gamma and fecal supernatants from irritable bowel syndrome patients in human intestinal enteroids and colonoids. *Gut Microbes, 10,* 59–76. https://doi.org/10.1080/19490976.2018.1479625

Hemaiswarya, S., Raja, R., Ravikumar, R., & Carvalho, I. S. (2013). Mechanism of action of probiotics. *Brazilian Archives of Biology and Technology, 56,* 113–119.

HMP. *Human microbiome project* [online]. Retrieved February 2023, from https://hmpdacc.org

Hoseinifar, S. H., Ahmadi, A., Raeisi, M., Hoseini, S. M., Khalili, M., & Behnampour, N. (2017). Comparative study on immunomodulatory and growth enhancing effects of three prebiotics (galactooligosaccharide, fructooligosaccharide and inulin) in common carp (Cyprinus carpio). *Aquaculture Research, 48*(7), 3298–3307.

Hu, C., Wong, F. S., & Wen, L. (2015). Type 1 diabetes and gut microbiota: Friend or foe? *Pharmacological Research, 98,* 9–15.

ISAPP. *International scientific association for probiotics and prebiotics* [online]. Retrieved February 2023, from isappscience.org

Ishikawa, H., Matsumoto, S., & Ohashi, Y. (2011). Digestion: Beneficial effects of probiotic Bifidobacterium and galacto-oligosaccharide in patients with ulcerative colitis: A randomized controlled study. *Alternative Medicine Review, 16*(2), 201–202.

Islam, S. U. (2016). Clinical uses of probiotics. *Medicine (Baltimore), 95,* 1–5.

Isolauri, E., Sutas, Y., Kankaanpaa, P., Arvilommi, H., & Salminen, S. (2001). Probiotics: Effect on immunity. *The American Journal of Clinical Nutrition, 73,* 444S–450S.

Jin, L. Z., Marquardt, R. R., & Zhao, X. (2000). A strain of Enterococcus faecium (18C23) inhibits adhesion of enterotoxigenic Escherichia coli K88 to porcine small intestine mucus. *Applied and Environmental Microbiology, 66,* 4200–4204.

Judge, T. A., & Lichtenstein, G. R. (2004). Treatment of fistulizing Crohn's disease. *Gastroenterology Clinics, 33*(2), 421–454.

Kerry, R. G., Patra, J. K., Gouda, S., Park, Y., Shin, H. S., & Das, G. (2018). Benefaction of probiotics for human health: A review. *Journal of Food and Drug Analysis, 26*(3), 927–939.

Kobyliak, N., Conte, C., Cammarota, G., Haley, A. P., Styriak, I., Gaspar, L., Fusek, J., Rodrigo, L., & Kruzliak, P. (2016). Probiotics in prevention and treatment of obesity: A critical view. *Nutrition & Metabolism, 13,* 1–13.

Kolida, S., & Gibson, G. R. (2011). Synbiotics in health and disease. *Annual Review of Food Science and Technology, 2,* 373–393.

Kumar, S., Bansal, A., Chakrabarti, A., & Singhi, S. (2013). Evaluation of efficacy of probiotics prevention of Candida colonization in a PICU—a randomized controlled trial. *Critical Care Medicine, 41*(2), 565–572.

Langa, S., Van Den Bulck, E., Peirotén, A., Gaya, P., Schols, H. A., & Arqués, J. L. (2019). Application of lactobacilli and prebiotic oligosaccharides for the development of a synbiotic semi-hard cheese. *LWT, 114,* 108361.

Latif, A., Shehzad, A., Niazi, S., Zahid, A., Ashraf, W., Iqbal, M. W., & Korma, S. A. (2023). Probiotics: Mechanism of action, health benefits and their application in food industries. *Frontiers in Microbiology, 14,* 1216674.

Le Barz, M., Anhê, F. F., Varin, T. V., Desjardins, Y., Levy, E., Roy, D., & Marette, A. (2015). Probiotics as complementary treatment for metabolic disorders. *Diabetes & Metabolism Journal, 39*(4), 291–303.

Li, J., Jia, H., Cai, X., Zhong, H., Feng, Q., Sunagawa, S., Arumugam, M., Kultima, J. R., Prifti, E., Nielsen, T., & Juncker, A. S. (2014). An integrated catalog of reference genes in the human gut microbiome. *Nature Biotechnology, 32,* 834–841. https://doi.org/10.1038/nbt.2942

Lin, H. V., Frassetto, A., Kowalik Jr, E. J., Nawrocki, A. R., Lu, M. M., Kosinski, J. R., & Marsh, D. J. (2012). Butyrate and propionate protect against diet-induced obesity and regulate gut hormones via free fatty acid receptor 3-independent mechanisms. *PLoS One, 7*(4), e35240.

Long, S. L., Gahan, C. G., & Joyce, S. A. (2017). Interactions between gut bacteria and bile in health and disease. *Molecular Aspects of Medicine, 56,* 54–65.

Louis, P., Flint, H. J., & Michel, C. (2016). How to manipulate the microbiota: Prebiotics. *Advances in Experimental Medicine and Biology, 902,* 119–142. https://doi.org/10.1007/978-3-319-31248-4_9/COVER

Macfarlane, G. T., Steed, H., & Macfarlane, S. (2008). Bacterial metabolism and health-related effects of galacto-oligosaccharides and other prebiotics. *Journal of Applied Microbiology, 104*(2), 305–344.

Manigandan, T., Mangaiyarkarasi, S. P., Hemalatha, R., Hemalatha, V. T., & Murali, N. P. (2012). Probiotics, prebiotics and synbiotics-a review. *Biomedical & Pharmacology Journal, 5*(2), 295.

Marchesi, J. R., & Ravel, J. (2015). The vocabulary of microbiome research: A proposal. *Microbiome, 3,* 31.

Marín-Manzano, M. C., Abecia, L., Hernández-Hernández, O., Sanz, M. L., Montilla, A., Olano, A., Rubio, L. A., Moreno, F. J., & Clemente, A. (2013). Galacto-oligosaccharides derived from lactulose exert a selective stimulation on the growth of Bifidobacterium animalis in the large intestine of growing rats. *Journal of Agricultural and Food Chemistry, 61,* 7560–7567.

Marteau, P., Cuillerier, E., Meance, S., Gerhardt, M. F., Myara, A., Bouvier, M., Bouley, C., Tondu, F., Bommelaer, G., & Grimaud, J. C. (2002). Bifidobacterium animalis strain DN-173 010 shortens the colonic transit time in healthy women: A double-blind, randomized, controlled study. *Alimentary Pharmacology & Therapeutics, 16*(3), 587–593. https://doi.org/10.1046/J.1365-2036.2002.01188.X

Matijašić, B. B., Obermajer, T., Lipoglavšek, L., Sernel, T., Locatelli, I., Kos, M., Šmid, A., & Rogelj, I. (2016). Effects of synbiotic fermented milk containing Lactobacillus acidophilus La-5 and Bifidobacterium animalis ssp. lactis BB-12 on the fecal microbiota of adults with irritable bowel syndrome: A randomized double-blind, placebo-controlled trial. *Journal of Dairy Science, 99*(7), 5008–5021.

Molodecky, N. A., Soon, S., Rabi, D. M., Ghali, W. A., Ferris, M., Chernoff, G., Benchimol, E. I., Panaccione, R., Ghosh, S., Barkema, H. W., & Kaplan, G. G. (2012). Increasing incidence and prevalence of the inflammatory bowel diseases with time, based on systematic review. *Gastroenterology, 142*(1), 46–54.

Nakov, R., & Velikova, T. (2020). Chemical metabolism of xenobiotics by Gut Microbiota. *Current Drug Metabolism*, *21*(4), 260–269. https://doi.org/10.2174/1389200221666200303113830. PMID: 32124693.

Oleskin, A. V., & Shenderov, B. A. (2016). Neuromodulator effects and targets of the SCFAs and gasotransmitters produced by the human symbiotic microbiota. *Microbial Ecology in Health and Disease*, *27*(1), 30971.

Oliveira, R. P. D. S., Florence, A. C. R., Perego, P., De Oliveira, M. N., & Converti, A. (2011). Use of lactulose as prebiotic and its influence on the growth, acidification profile and viable counts of different probiotics in fermented skim milk. *International Journal of Food Microbiology, 145*(1), 22–27.

Orrhage, K., Sillerstrom, E., Gustafsson, J. A., Nord, C. E., & Rafter, J. (1994). Binding of mutagenic heterocyclic amines by intestinal and lactic acid bacteria. *Mutation Research*, *311*, 239–248.

Pandey, K. R., Naik, S. R., & Vakil, B. V. (2015). Probiotics, prebiotics and synbiotics-a review. *Journal of Food Science and Technology, 52,* 7577–7587.

Patel, S., & Goyal, A. (2012). The current trends and future perspectives of prebiotics research: A review. *3 Biotech, 2,* 115–125.

Petruzziello, C., Saviano, A., & Ojetti, V. (2023). Probiotics, the immune response and acute appendicitis: A review. *Vaccines, 11*(7), 1170. https://doi.org/10.3390/VACCINES11071170

Plaza-Diaz, J., Ruiz-Ojeda, F. J., Gil-Campos, M., & Gil, A. (2019). Mechanisms of action of probiotics. *Advances in Nutrition, 10*(suppl_1), S49–S66. Retrieved August 24, 2023, from https://academic.oup.com/advances/article-abstract/10/suppl_1/S49/5307225

Rafter, J., Bennett, M., Caderni, G., Clune, Y., Hughes, R., Karlsson, P. C., & Collins, J. K. (2007). Dietary Synbiotics reduce cancer risk factors in polypectomized and colon cancer patients. *The American Journal of Clinical Nutrition, 85*(2), 488–496.

Ranjitham, A., & Poornakala, S. J. (2020). Standardization and evaluation of synbiotic yoghurt. *International Journal of Current Microbiology and Applied Sciences, 9*(3), 404–418.

Reid, G., Bruce, A. W., Fraser, N., Heinemann, C., Owen, J., & Henning, B. (2001). Oral probiotics can resolve urogenital infections. *FEMS Immunology and Medical Microbiology, 30*, 49–52.

Ringel-Kulka, T., Kotch, J. B., Jensen, E. T., Savage, E., & Weber, D. J. (2015). Randomized, double-blind, placebo-controlled study of synbiotic yogurt effect on the health of children. *The Journal of Pediatrics, 166*(6), 1475–1481.

Ríos-Covián, D., Ruas-Madiedo, P., Margolles, A., Gueimonde, M., De los Reyes-Gavilán, C. G., & Salazar, N. (2016, February). Intestinal short chain fatty acids and their link with diet and human health. *Frontiers in Microbiology, 7*, 180861. https://doi.org/10.3389/FMICB.2016.00185/BIBTEX

Roberfroid, M., Gibson, G. R., Hoyles, L., McCartney, A. L., Rastall, R., Rowland, I., Wolvers, D., Watzl, B., Szajewska, H., Stahl, B., Guarner, F., Respondek, F., Whelan, K., Coxam, V., Davicco, M. J., Léotoing, L., Wittrant, Y., Delzenne, N. M., Cani, P. D., & Meheust, A. (2010). Prebiotic effects: Metabolic and health benefits. *British Journal of Nutrition, 104*(suppl_2), S1–S63. https://doi.org/10.1017/s0007114510003363

Rodriguez, J. M., Murphy, K., Stanton, C., Ross, R. P., Kober, O. I., Juge, N., Avershina, E., Rudi, K., Narbad, A., Jenmalm, M. C., & Marchesi, J. R. (2015). The composition of the gut microbiota throughout life, with an emphasis on early life. *Microbial Ecology in Health and Disease, 26,* 26050.

Rowland, I., Gibson, G., Heinken, A., Scott, K., Swann, J., Thiele, I., & Tuohy, K. (2018). Gut microbiota functions: Metabolism of nutrients and other food components. *European Journal of Nutrition, 57*, 1–24. https://doi.org/10.1007/s00394-017-1445-8

Safdari, Y., Vazifedoost, M., Didar, Z., & Hajirostamloo, B. (2021). The effect of banana fiber and banana peel fiber on the chemical and rheological properties of symbiotic yogurt made from camel milk. *International Journal of Food Science, 2021.*

Sajedi, D., & Shabani, R. (2021). *Changes in leptin, serotonin, and cortisol after eight weeks of aerobic exercise with probiotic intake in a cuprizone-induced demyelination mouse model of multiple*. Elsevier. Retrieved August 24, 2023, from https://www.sciencedirect.com/science/article/pii/S1043466621001733

Santacroce, L., Man, A., Charitos, I. A., Haxhirexha, K., & Topi, S. (2021). Current knowledge about the connection between health status and gut microbiota from birth to elderly. A narrative review. *Frontiers in Bioscience-Landmark, 26*(6), 135–148.

Sarwar, A., Aziz, T., Al-Dalali, S., Zhang, J., ud Din, J., Chen, C., & Yang, Z. (2021). Characterization of synbiotic ice cream made with probiotic yeast Saccharomyces boulardii CNCM I-745 in combination with inulin. *LWT, 141,* 110910.

Saxelin, M., Pessi, T., & Salminen, S. (1995). Fecal recovery following oral administration of Lactobacillus strain GG (ATCC 53103) in gelatin capsules to healthy volunteers. *International Journal of Food Microbiology, 25*, 199–203.

Sekhon, B. S., & Jairath, S. (2010). Prebiotics, probiotics and synbiotics: An overview. *Journal of Pharmaceutical Education & Research, 1*(2).

Shaghaghi, M., Pourahmad, R., & Adeli, H. M. (2013). Synbiotic yogurt production by using prebiotic compounds and probiotic lactobacilli. *International Research Journal of Applied and Basic Sciences, 5*(7), 839–846.

Sharma, S., Arora, M., & Baldi, S. (2013). Probiotics in India: Current status and future prospects. *Pharm Aspire, 1,* 1–12. https://www.researchgate.net/publication/257537041_Probiotics_in_India_Current_status_and_future_prospects

Simões, C. D., Maganinho, M., & Sousa, A. S. (2022). FODMAPs, inflammatory bowel disease and gut microbiota: Updated overview on the current evidence. *European Journal of Nutrition, 61*, 1187–1198. https://doi.org/10.1007/s00394-021-02755-1

Singh, R. K., Chang, H. W., Yan, D. I., Lee, K. M., Ucmak, D., Wong, K., Abrouk, M., Farahnik, B., Nakamura, M., Zhu, T. H., & Bhutani, T. (2015). Influence of diet on the gut microbiome and implications for human health. *Journal of Translational Medicine, 15*(1), 1–17.

Smits, T. H. M. (2019). The importance of genome sequence quality to microbial comparative genomics. *BMC Genomics, 20,* 662. https://doi.org/10.1186/s12864-019-6014-5

Srivastav, S., Neupane, S., Bhurtel, S., Katila, N., & Hong, J. T. (2019). *Probiotics mixture increases butyrate, and subsequently rescues the nigral dopaminergic neurons from MPTP and rotenone-induced neurotoxicity*. Elsevier. Retrieved August 24, 2023, from https://www.sciencedirect.com/science/article/pii/S0955286318312828

Su, C., Lewis, J. D., Deren, J. J., Judge, T., Hoops, T., Wu, G. D., & Lichtenstein, G. R. (2003). Peroxisome proliferators-activated receptor ligand rosiglitazone for the treatment of active Crohn's disease. *Gastroenterology, 4*(124), A380.

Terrin, G., Passariello, A., & Canani, R. B. (2012). Drugs and tight junctions: Adverse effects and opportunities for new therapeutic approaches. *Journal of Pediatric Gastroenterology and Nutrition, 54*(4), 444–445.

Tzounis, X., Rodriguez-Mateos, A., Vulevic, J., Gibson, G. R., Kwik-Uribe, C., & Spencer, J. P. (2011). Prebiotic evaluation of cocoa-derived flavanols in healthy humans by using a randomized, controlled, double-blind, crossover intervention study. *The American Journal of Clinical Nutrition, 93*(1), 62–72. Retrieved August 15, 2023, from https://academic.oup.com/ajcn/article-abstract/93/1/62/4597700

Van Loo, J., Clune, Y., Bennett, M., & Collins, J. K. (2005). The SYNCAN project: Goals, set-up, first results and settings of the human intervention study. *British Journal of Nutrition, 93*(S1), S91–S98.

Wang, B., Yao, M., Lv, L., Ling, Z., & Li, L. (2017). The human microbiota in health and disease. *Engineering, 3,* 71–82. https://doi.org/10.1016/J.ENG.2017.01.008

Whelan, K. (2013). Mechanisms and effectiveness of prebiotics in modifying the gastrointestinal microbiota for the management of digestive disorders. *Proceedings of the Nutrition Society, 72*(3), 288–298. https://doi.org/10.1017/S0029665113001262

Whipps, J., Lewis, K., & Cooke, R. (1988). Mycoparasitism and plant disease control. In M. Burge (Ed.), *Fungi in biological control systems* (pp. 161–187). Manchester University Press.

Wong, J. M., De Souza, R., Kendall, C. W., Emam, A., & Jenkins, D. J. (2006). Colonic health: Fermentation and short chain fatty acids. *Journal of Clinical Gastroenterology, 40*(3), 235–243.

Xavier-Santos, D., Lima, E. D., Simão, A. N. C., Bedani, R., & Saad, S. M. I. (2018). Effect of the consumption of a synbiotic diet mousse containing Lactobacillus acidophilus La-5 by individuals with metabolic syndrome: A randomized controlled trial. *Journal of Functional Foods, 41,* 55–61.

You, S., Ma, Y., Yan, B., Pei, W., Wu, Q., Ding, C., & Huang, C. (2022). The promotion mechanism of prebiotics for probiotics: A review. *Frontiers in Nutrition, 9,* 1000517. https://doi.org/10.3389/FNUT.2022.1000517/BIBTEX.

2 An Overview of Our Gut Microbiome
Mechanism Involved and Role of Probiotics

Shatakshi, Shubha Dhyani, Himanshu Chaurasia, and Himanshu Kumar

2.1 INTRODUCTION

A number of studies have shown that the human body contains approximately 30 trillion cells, 40 trillion microorganisms, and 20–30 trillion other cells. Due to this, several experts have even stated that just half of the human body will be regarded as human (Diwan & Harke, 2021).

A significant variety of microorganisms (bacteria, viruses, fungi, and archaea) colonize the human body. They outnumber human cells and exist alongside us, in our body tissues or within certain parts of them, mostly in the gut. They are referred to collectively as "microbiota" or "microbiome" (Riccio & Rossano, 2020). If we leave aside fungi, viruses, and archaea and focus only on bacteria, then about a thousand types of bacteria are available in the intestine within the human body. Every aspect of the human body, with the exception of some internal organs and fluids, contains bacteria. If all the bacteria discovered in the human body were combined, only the gut would contain 95% of all the microorganisms (Figure 2.1). That is why the intestine of the human body is called its home (Zhuang et al., 2017). If microbiota is defined in one way, then the definition would be "the group of all types of microbes found in the body is called microbiota" (Deo & Deshmukh, 2019). Today we all know that life is not possible on the earth without a symbiotic relationship, and there is a symbiotic relationship between the human body and bacteria. It means there is a good, positive, and mutually beneficial relationship (Gilbert & Neufeld, 2014). Microbes colonize a wide range of anatomical body areas, including the skin, mucosa, gastrointestinal system, respiratory tract, urogenital tract, and mammary gland. They produce a distinct and sophisticated ecosystem that adjusts to the environmental circumstances of each area (Ogunrinola et al., 2020). After carefully examining all the prior information on microbiomes, it was discovered that, up until 2010, little was known about the significant functions that human bacteria play in various body areas with regard to health. As an illustration, the relevance of the gut microbiota in treating disorders connected to neuroinflammatory diseases has never been acknowledged; i.e., it was regarded as entirely fictitious (Riccio & Rossano, 2020). But things have altered dramatically in just a couple of years. According to https://pubmed.ncbi.nlm.nih.gov/, the number of publications published on gut microbiota has increased exponentially from 2010 to 2020, totaling over 32,000 papers, although with just 466 in 2010 as compared to 7,747 in 2019. This increased interest in the human microbiota is also attributable to significant research programs like the Human Microbiome Project-1 and Human Microbiome Project-2 as well as the equivalent European Microbiome Support project, and these projects helped learn how important microbiome is for the health of various parts of the human body ("A Review of 10 Years of Human Microbiome Research Activities at the US National Institutes of Health, Fiscal Years 2007–2016," 2019). Then the belief that gut microbiota affects only the functions of the intestines has become outdated, but it has been announced that it has a

DOI: 10.1201/9781003452249-2

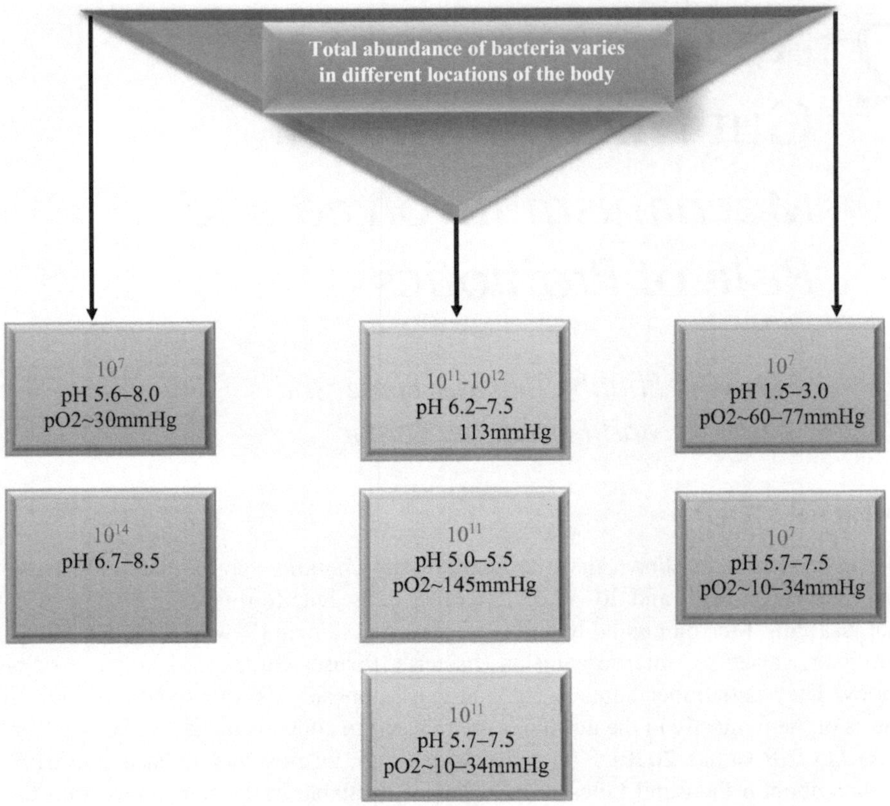

FIGURE 2.1 Total abundance of bacteria varies in different locations of the body. The number of bacteria in all the different organs of the human body depends on the concentration and volume of the bacteria.

much greater impact on the other organs within the human body. Because the human body's gut microbiota is so significant, many earlier researchers have also referred to it as another "Important Organ" of the human body (Marchesi et al., 2016). Rather, it was described in many other terms such as microbial organ and an organ-shaped group of microbes, etc. But the latest term used among these is "meta-organism." That's because meta-organisms reflect the mutual relationship between the gut microbiota of the human body and the human brain (Byndloss & Bäumler, 2018). The gut microbiomes present in the human body vary from person to person according to their different age, diet, stress, and health conditions (Cresci & Bawden, 2015). They start forming in children as soon as they are born, and the gut microbiome of children gradually changes according to their age and physical health. Although some limited studies have rejected that the gut microbiome starts forming in children after birth, they believe that it starts in the mother's womb itself. The composition of the microbiota depends on many other things such as suffering from any disease, the way of eating and drinking, what type of nutrition is taken, the manner in which the delivery was conducted, whether any antibiotic was used, etc. (Nuriel-Ohayon et al., 2016; Martin et al., 2016).

Gradually, by continuing research and digging out more information about it, it was concluded that the gut microflora acts as an extraordinary health weapon in the body, which acts as a shield to protect the human body from many chronic diseases. Once the gut microbiota begins to develop a fault or go wrong, significant and noticeable effects and changes begin to be seen in both the structure and the function of the intestinal flora and these adverse changes also gradually lead to chronic diseases in the body (Figure 2.2).

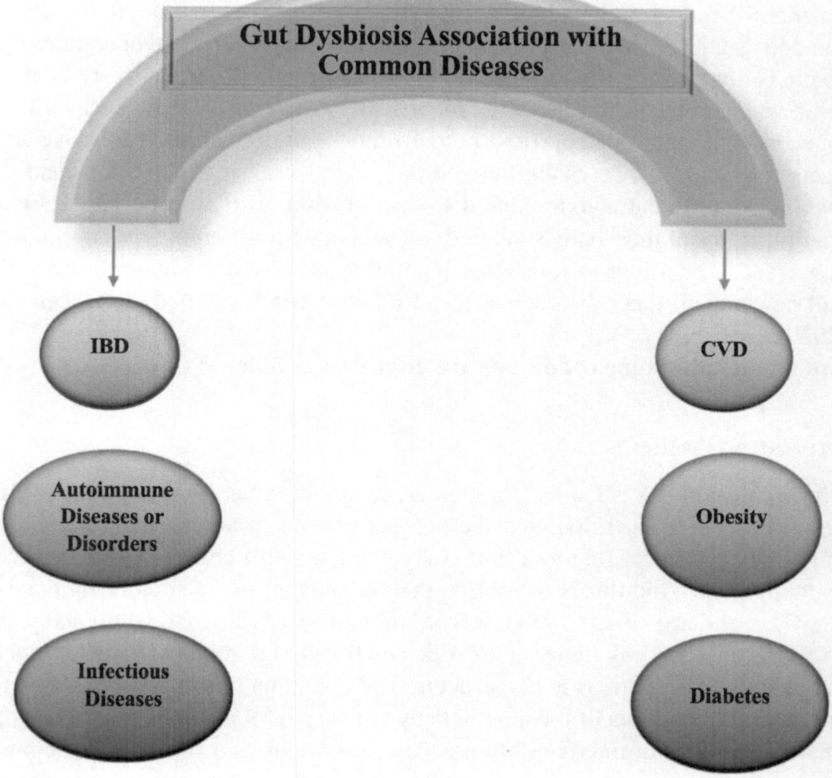

FIGURE 2.2 The process of dysbiosis (imbalance state in good and bad bacteria in the human gut) is interlinked with all these diseases: neurodisorders, heart disease, metabolic disorders, RA, T1D, atopic eczema, atopic asthma, IBS, IBD, etc. This creates a favorable environment for bad bacteria to grow in the human intestinal area, which has a deep impact on the immunity of the body and starts attracting all these diseases such as autoimmune diseases, CVD, diabetes, IBS, IBD, metabolic diseases, and infectious diseases.

In the past few years, there has been a rapid increase in the research on gut microbiota and, through these researches, it has been proved that gut microbiota not only plays an important role in balancing the internal structure of the intestines of the human body. Rather, it is effective in keeping the body away from many chronic diseases like neurodisorders, heart disease, metabolic disorders, RA, T1D, atopic eczema, atopic asthma, IBS, and IBD (Thaiss et al., 2016; Ding et al., 2019; Fan & Pedersen, 2021).

The links between the makeup of the gut microbiome and a number of chronic illnesses are briefly discussed in this chapter such that it is possible to comprehend the function and significance of the gut microbiota (Figure 2.3).

2.2 RELATION BETWEEN GUT MICROBIOME AND AUTOIMMUNE DISORDERS

If seen in today's era, autoimmune disease is becoming a common disease occurring in the human body. Autoimmune diseases are such diseases in which the human body's own immune system gives it a signal that foreign cells have entered the body and the body needs to protect itself from it, so it attacks those foreign cells. But, in reality, they are not foreign cells but healthy cells of our own body that the body's immune system considers as foreign cells and eats them. This happens because the body's immune system becomes unable to tell which cells of the body are healthy and which are harmful cells. The environment and the internal health of the human body have a role in the development of the autoimmune disease, in addition to genetics. Instead, it also strongly relies on the human body's gut microbiome. An imbalance in the composition and operations of the intestinal microbiota is a major contributor to autoimmune disorders. Whenever there is an imbalance between these two internal characteristics, a process of dysbiosis will occur, which will confuse the body's immune system. And this confused body's immune system appears to cause autoimmune diseases. According to all the research done on this topic so far, it has become clear that different people who have different autoimmune disorders or diseases have different types of internal structures and functions of their body's gut microbiota and even different types of imbalances also have been observed. According to research, about 80 types of autoimmune disorders have been accounted till now and all these disorders affect different parts of the body (Shaheen et al., 2022; Jiao et al., 2020).

Some common autoimmune conditions are discussed as follows:

2.2.1 Rheumatoid Arthritis

Nowadays the problem of RA is increasing a lot, especially in India. More than 180 million people in India are suffering from arthritis, and the number of women among them is more than men (Tantuway et al., 2023). According to a new study, there are full chances of India becoming the arthritis capital by 2025. And this is the reason that the number of research being done about RA is increasing (Garg & Garg, 2023). In fact, according to a lot of research, additionally, it has been shown that there is a strong link between arthritis and the gut microbiota. Arthritis can develop if there are any unsuitable alterations to the structure and operation of the gut microbiota (Guerreiro et al., 2018). The gut microbiota of the human body is made up of millions of trillions of bacteria, and because these trillions of microbes are crucial to the health and function of the human body, they also have a significant influence on the inflammation that takes place there. The imbalance occurring in the gut microbiota of the human body is known as the term dysbiosis, and this action of dysbiosis is able to trigger a reaction that leads a damage and inflammation in human joints and this is where arthritis starts. And the beginning of the RA can also be called the predisposition of arthritis. Arthritis is an autoimmune disease, so it cannot be cured permanently, but it can definitely be prevented. Therefore, it is very important that more research be done about the relationship between the gut microbiome and RA and whatever therapeutic nutrition is required for its prevention so that it can be treated through a therapeutic diet. The pace of prevention can be increased to manage RA (Wells et al., 2020; Scher et al., 2013).

2.2.2 Psoriasis

Psoriasis is an autoimmune disorder that directly results in skin disorder or skin disease. This is also directly related to the gut microbiota because it is an autoimmune disease, and that is why a lot of research about it has been going an extended period of time. And this is taking place to collect additional data for its therapy. This is a chronic skin condition that affects a lot of individuals worldwide. That's why the process of its prevention takes a long time. In this condition, different types of red scaly spots appear on the skin of different parts of the body, mostly on the elbows, knees, etc. These scaly red spots on the body's skin are also called plaques. If we throw light on the research done so far on this subject, it comes to light that psoriasis is a complex condition occurring in the skin of the human body that is caused by a combination of not only genetic but also immune and environmental factors (Sikora et al., 2020). Many interesting recent research also reveal that it is directly related to stomach health. The gut microbiome is a group of microorganisms living in the gastrointestinal tract, and, up to this point, we have learned that this group is very important for the structure and inherent functions of our body's internal organs. For that reason, it is very important to maintain the balance in the microbiome of the body because if its balance gets disturbed then the

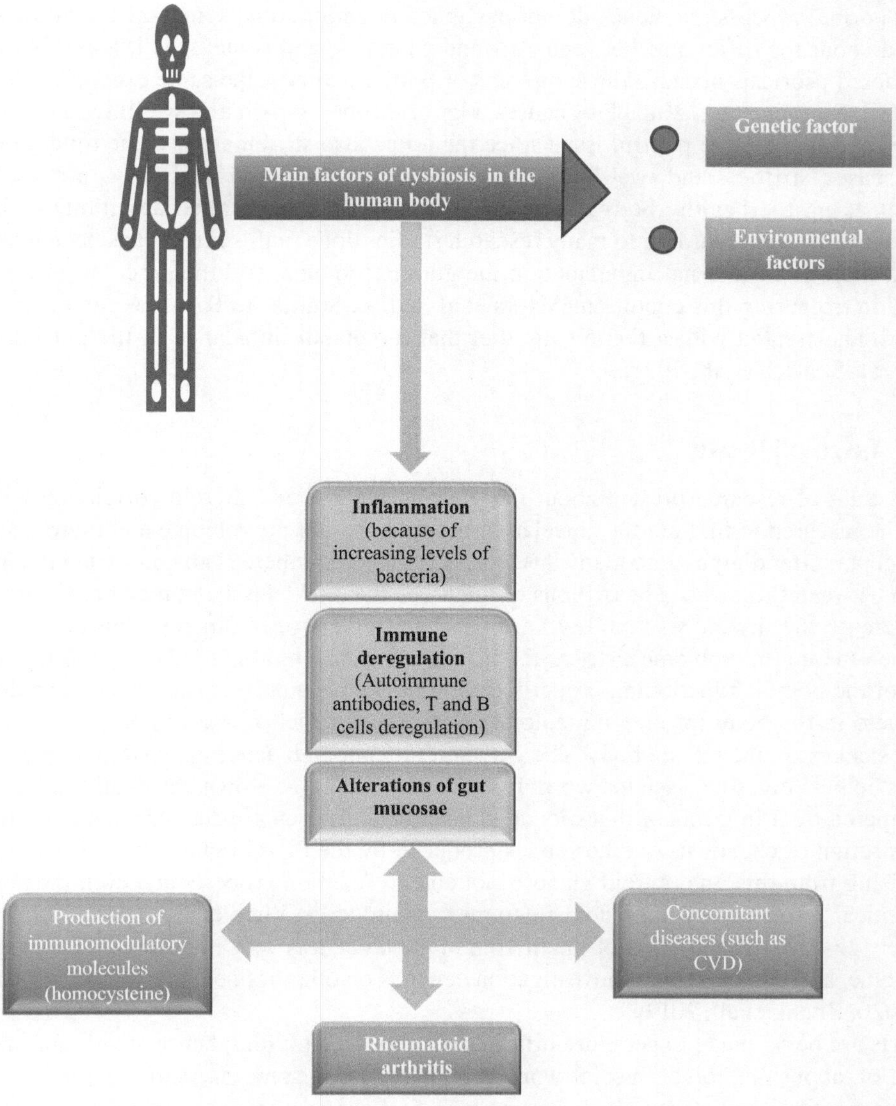

FIGURE 2.3 (i) Genetic factors and (ii) environmental factors. These are the two main causes of dysbiosis. Dysbiosis in the body increases the bacteria that promote gut inflammation. After increasing these bacteria, it creates immune deregulation that causes inflammation and alteration in gut mucosae, and this whole phenomenon is associated with rheumatoid arthritis and other chronic diseases.

process of dysbiosis will occur, which causes turmoil in various internal organs of the body and one of the results of this is an autoimmune disease like psoriasis. This is the reason to indulge in some more research, and more authentic scientific work should be done to collect information about its treatment or prevention to better understand which additional therapeutic dietary changes can be successful in treating this condition (Polak et al., 2021; Thye et al., 2022).

2.2.3 Psoriatic Arthritis

PsA is also an autoimmune disease like RA. The interesting thing is that this disease keeps growing in the human body and most people are not aware of its symptoms. People think that this is a normal process and hence do not pay much attention to its symptoms. Most people get confused about the difference between PsA and psoriasis, and sometimes it happens that PsA is considered psoriasis because the symptoms of both are almost the same except for joint pain (Olejniczak-Staruch et al., 2021) PsA causes a lot of throbbing pain and swelling in the joints of the body, and it is a more painful issue since the joints also stiffen at the same time. In each of these diseases, stiffness and swelling in the joints are common and the body's immune system keeps attacking the healthy body cells, which is why these are called autoimmune diseases (Myers et al., 2019). According to many research studies done in this area, it has been found that, like RA, there is an internal imbalance in the gut microbiome, and the process of dysbiosis is involved in triggering this condition (Myers et al., 2019). Similar to RA, PsA can be prevented, managed, and treated with a therapeutic diet that targets an imbalance in the gut microbiota (Olejniczak-Staruch et al., 2021).

2.2.4 Thyroid Diseases

There is a lot of research present about the gut microbiome and thyroid correlation with each other. The research to find out the correlation between the gut microbiome and thyroid started a little late, but, after digging into many layers, it was found that there is an honest and intense relationship between these two. The trillions of microbes that make up the human body's gut microbiota increase the thyroid's suitability and its capacity for proper function, but this is possible only when the gut microbiome's structure and functions are in proper balance, and the immune system of the body is functioning properly. And that state is a perfect state to create a favorable atmosphere in the body for creating autoimmune diseases such as Hashimoto's thyroiditis and Graves' sickness in the human body. The gut's microbiome imbalance also has an impact on how well our bodies' digestive systems work. Even the thyroid gland's own chemicals and hormones are hampered by it in terms of digestion and absorption. It even creates hindrances in digestion and absorption of chemicals and hormones produced by the thyroid gland and, due to the problems arising from this, the thyroid gland is not able to function properly and even the hormones and chemicals produced by it are not able to respond properly (Virili et al., 2021). That is why, to accurately observe the condition of the thyroid in the body, it is very important to investigate the microbiome, and the direction of investigation depends on other influencing components also (Su et al., 2020; Zhang et al., 2019).

Efforts are being made to get more information about the thyroid; hence, continuous research is going on about this topic. Special work is being done on some particular components present in the stomach, and efforts are being made to find out how these components present in the stomach affect the ability and capability of the thyroid to function (Virili et al., 2021; Knezevic et al., 2020).

Research in this space is progressing, and keeping in mind that particular components are as yet being clarified, a few expected jobs of the stomach microbiome in thyroid capability have been recognized.

2.2.4.1 Thyroid Hormone Metabolism

We all know that the thyroid gland works to streamline metabolic processes in the human body by secreting beneficial hormones. When there are any kind of changes and alterations in the functioning of the thyroid gland, which is not good for our body, the problem arising from it is called thyroid disorder. These thyroid disorders can range from a small problem to a big disease, such as ranging from a small goiter to a fatal disease like cancer. According to studies conducted to date, the thyroid gland is impacted by the makeup of the gut microbiota because healthy activities inside the gut are impacted when dysbiosis develops in the gut microbiota. Because of this, immunological illnesses and metabolic problems begin to coexist. It may be summed up simply as dysbiosis in the gut microbiota that impairs thyroid hormone metabolism (Ejtahed et al., 2020).

2.2.4.2 Inflammation and Autoimmunity

Dysbiosis in the stomach microbiome can advance aggravation, which is frequently connected with immune system conditions. Ongoing irritation can compound immune system thyroid sicknesses by impacting the insusceptible reaction against the thyroid organ (Gong et al., 2021).

2.2.4.3 Hormonal Regulation

The human body has the hypothalamus–pituitary gland, which functions to control thyroid hormone by aiding in its synthesis and release. The functioning of the hypothalamus–pituitary gland is most significantly impacted when the process of gut microbiome dysbiosis takes place in the human body, and, when such a condition emerges, it is possible to generate a situation of thyroid hormone imbalance. So, it has been proven by many previous researches that thyroid hormonal regulation occurs due to an imbalance in the structure and functions of the gut microbiome (Wang et al., 2023).

2.2.4.4 Thyroid Autoimmunity

Previous research has revealed a connection between the gut microbiota and autoimmune illnesses including Hashimoto's thyroiditis and Graves' disease. These illnesses have the same connection to the gut microbiota as all the others we've spoken about so far. Dysbiosis of the gut microbiome triggers autoimmune diseases that start attacking the thyroid gland itself, due to which the thyroid gland is unable to perform its function properly and autoimmune diseases start occurring. Symptoms of these diseases are seen differently in each person according to genetic and environmental factors (Bogusławska et al., 2022)

Thyroid disease can be prevented through a therapeutic diet, but this is possible only if the complex relationship between gut flora and thyroid function is better understood. Dietary modifications, probiotics and prebiotics intervention, and fecal microbiota transplants (FMTs) are also factors by which gut microbiome altering can be prevented and thyroid problems can be treated in the future. More future research is needed to check the efficiency of the therapies used now for thyroid health and to understand its mechanism more closely, and, among these, the most needed is clinical trials (Trofimiuk-Müldner & Bała, 2023).

2.2.5 Type 1 Diabetes

Diabetes is a very common metabolic disease, and, in this disease, the amount of sugar in the blood increases significantly. There are three types of sugar: T1D mellitus, type 2 diabetes mellitus, and gestational diabetes mellitus. The reasons for the occurrence of these three are different, but in all three the amount of sugar in the blood increases. Much of such evidence has been found, which proves that the gut microbiome has proved to be a factor in the origin of diabetes. T1D will be defined in such a way that it is diabetes in which the human body is insulin-dependent (Pan et al., 2018). Many things about it are still unclear. Even how it originates has not yet been scientifically proven with certainty. But it has been proved that it is caused by both genetic and environmental factors, but, if diabetes is genetically prevalent in a family, it is not necessary that every member of the family in every generation has to face the problem of diabetes. It depends on the body's gut microbiome since several scientific research have revealed that there is a significant difference between the gut microbiomes of persons with T1D and those who are physically healthy (Zheng et al., 2018; Zhou et al., 2020).

Insulin plays an important role in T1D. Insulin is produced by the beta cells of a small organ of our body called the pancreas and in T1D; these beta cells of the pancreas are destroyed. Diabetes is an autoimmune disease. When our body's immune system mistakenly starts destroying parts of our body called the pancreas, due to which the beta cells are not able to produce insulin as per the requirement of the body, insulin deficiency starts. This entire process is the cause of T1D (Yang et al., 2010). In T1D, the T-lymphocytes of the body are also destroyed (Boldison & Wong, 2016).

1. **Autoimmune Activation:** When there are significant changes in the composition and diversity of the gut microflora, it results in T1D, an autoimmune disease in which the amount of sugar in the body's blood increases excessively (Itariu & Stulnig, 2014)
2. **Immune Modulation:** Before the onset of T1D, changes in the gut microbiota of the body begin, resulting in the manipulation of the immune system and this is how T1D begins (Wu et al., 2019).
3. **Metabolic Influence:** We have already discussed earlier that the microbiome and metabolic processes are related and this relationship is directly related to the breakdown and utilization of the dietary components consumed by the body. The reaction of digestion, breakdown, and utilization of dietary components in the body after eating has a direct impact on insulin sensitivity and glucose regulation (Han et al, 2018).
4. **Early Life Influences:** According to the previous research done, it has been mentioned that the composition or shape of the gut microbiome depends on the method of delivery of the child (vaginal birth vs. cesarean section), the food and nutrition that had been taken by the mother at that time, the physical health of the mother, and also the mental health, as well as on the child's mental health also depends on environmental factors. And all these factors can provoke T1D in the future (Stewart et al., 2018; Vatanen et al., 2018).

All the factors that are involved in the cause of an imbalanced gut microbiome are capable of producing T1D; they need to be identified and controlled by therapeutic methods and other preventive methods. The imbalanced gut microbiome can be controlled by changing dietary patterns, adding some prebiotics and probiotics, etc. in the diet even FMT is also very beneficial so that the risk of T1D in the future can be reduced or prevented (Table 2.1) (Gülden et al., 2015; Knip & Siljander, 2016; Bibbò et al., 2017).

2.2.6 Lupus/Systemic Lupus Erythematosus

Lupus is a chronic autoimmune disease, and this disease lasts for a long time. Lupus is called a multisystem disease because it does not damage just one organ of the body but multiple organs of the body. That is why the other medical name for lupus is SLE. It is a life-threatening disease and is very common and mostly found in women whose age ranges from 15 to 45 years. If we look at the statistics, this disease is found more in women than in men by 9% to 10%. It is not necessary that this cannot happen before 15 years of age. This disease is also found in girls below 15 years of age, which is called childhood lupus, and this childhood lupus is much more serious than normal lupus. Sometimes it is also seen in women above 45 years of age, but this number is very low. Lupus is rarely seen in males, but, if lupus is found in males, then it is more dangerous than in female patients. It is also called "the Great Imitator" in medical language because mixed symptoms of almost all diseases are found in the patient suffering from it. The common symptoms of lupus are light fever, red patches on the skin, headache, itching, chest pain, weakness, lack of hunger, and weight loss. These are very commonly found symptoms that can easily be found in another common disease. Microbiome, digestive health, and lupus share a relationship. We all know that the gut microbiome trains our body's immune system. Although not much research has been done regarding the relationship between the gut microbiome and lupus, some of the research that has been done has made it clear that an imbalanced gut microbiota may trigger the development of lupus (Zhang, L., et al., 2021).

TABLE 2.1
Human studies Conducted in the Past 10 Years on the Effect of Gut Microbiota on Type 1 Diabetes (T1D)

Authors and Year	Sample Population	Final Study Results
Demirci et al. (2020)	53 T1D vs.53 health-wise sound participants	1. Firmicutes: Bacteroidetes ratio dropped in the T1D group when compared with the healthy group. TLR4 and TLR2 levels were associated with this.
Huang et al. (2018)	12 T1D vs. 10 healthy group	1. The group of T1D was identified with lower Firmicutes: Bacteroidetes ratios 2. Fecal bacterium levels and HbA1c had a negative correlation. 3. Anti-islet cell autoantibodies had a strong correlation with *Bacteroides* concentrations.
Gürsoy et al. (2018)	42 starting T1D vs. 42 nondiabetic healthy group	1. When T1D patients receive their diagnosis, they have higher amounts of intestinal *Candida albicans* species, which indicates that the normal gut microbiota is compromised.
Leiva-Gea et al. (2018)	15 T1D and 15 maturity-onset diabetes of the young 2 vs. 13 nondiabetic healthy group	1. In contrast to other groups, the T1D group demonstrated higher permeability of the intestinal tract and decreased microbial diversity. 2. When contrasted against the control group and patients having MODY2 (other non-autoimmune diabetes), the T1D group had more strains of the genera *Bacteroides*, *Veillonella*, *Ruminococcus*, *Blautia*, and *Streptococcus* and lower concentrations of *Bifidobacterium*, *Roseburia*, *Lachnospira*, and *Faecalibacterium*.
Higuchi et al. (2018)	20 T1D vs. 28 nondiabetic healthy group	1. Gram-negative *Bacteroides* (*vulgatus*, *xylanisolvens*, and *rodentium*) and *Prevotella copri* were more prevalent in T1D patients along with elevated IL-6 and poor glycemic control.
Pellegrini et al. (2017)	19 T1D vs. 16 nondiabetic healthy group	1. Firmicutes: the proportion of Bacteroidetes rose while proportions of the Proteobacteria phyla went down in the T1D group. 2. A significant tie between the microbiome and seven inflammatory genes expressed in T1D patients has been found to be valid.
Pinto et al. (2017)	3 T1D vs. 3 nondiabetic healthy children group	1. In children with T1D, *Bacteroides* and *Clostridium* clusters XVa and IV were prevalent. 2. The healthier category had a significant amount of *Bifidobacterium* spp. 3. Discovered 21 additional significant proteins in children without T1D and 26 additional abundant proteins in T1D patients. These genes' precise protein-dependent functions have been established.
De Goffau et al. (2014)	28 children (1–5 years old) with new-onset T1D vs. 27 nondiabetic healthy group	1. Demonstrated 26 unexpected prominent proteins in T1D patients and 21 novel vital proteins in children without T1D. The exact protein-dependent activities of these genes have been identified. 2. When compared to children who were in good health, T1D children under the age of 2.9 years demonstrated higher levels of the *Bacilli* class (*Streptococci*) and Bacteroidetes phylum, while children who were in good health had higher amounts of butyrate-producing species (*Clostridium* clusters IV and XIVa).
Soyucen et al. (2014)	35 starting T1D vs. 35 nondiabetic healthy group	1. Children with T1D under 2.9 years of age showed greater numbers of the Bacilli class (*Streptococci*) and Bacteroidetes phylum than children in good health, but those who were healthy had higher levels of butyrate-producing species (*Clostridium* clusters IV and XIVa).
Murri et al. (2013)	16 children with T1D vs. 16 nondiabetic healthy group	1. The overall proportion of Firmicutes: Bacteroidetes was much lower in T1Ds, and there were also lower concentrations of the group *Blautia coccoides–Eubacterium rectal* (engaged in butyrate generation and gut integrity maintenance). 2. Children with T1D also showed increased *Clostridium*, *Bacteroides*, and *Veillonella* families and decreased *Lactobacillus*, *Prevotella*, and *Bifidobacterium* genera.

1. **Immune Dysregulation:** The gut microbiome is a main instructor of the body's immune system in other language; we can say that the gut microbiome helps regulate the immune system. Again, dysbiosis is the reason to aggregate the lupus problem in the body (Li et al., 2021).
2. **Inflammation:** It is also clear from some previous research that some gut microbes promote inflammatory environments in the body by releasing inflammatory compounds in the gut area (Ma et al., 2019).
3. **Leaky Gut:** Dysbiosis promotes the problem of a leaky gut, and it also helps to enhance the permeable capacity of the intestine. For this reason, microbial compounds can easily infiltrate the human bloodstream, and this proves to be a major factor in the failure of the immune response system. The whole game is about the failure of the immune response system. As soon as the body's immune system does not respond properly to any problem, it starts attacking the body itself and this triggers lupus (Christovich & Luo, 2022).
4. **Metabolite Production:** The immune system is particularly susceptible to being influenced by the metabolites generated by gut bacteria. The fatty acids that are consumed through food are first broken down into tiny bits by these metabolites generated by gut microorganisms. It does this by converting long-chain fatty acids into SCFAs, and the body uses the latter to control immunity (Russo et al., 2019). Another way to put it is that SCFAs have immunomodulatory effects, and these immunomodulatory effects regulate the body's immunity. That instance, the information discovered indicates that SCFAs can affect the autoimmune response in conditions like lupus (Yao et al., 2022; Islam et al., 2020).
5. **Genetic Interactions:** It is clear from many previous researches that no single specific cause of lupus disease is yet clear. According to the research till now, its causes have been divided into two parts. At number one are genetic causes, and at number two are environmental causes. It is believed that a combination of these two factors triggers or causes lupus disease (Doaty et al., 2016). For example, in a study, it has been explained in this way that if there are two identical twins and one of them has lupus, then the probability of the other's suffering from this disease is up to 24%. Due to the relationship between genetic variables and the makeup of the gut microbiota, the gut microbiome plays a significant role in this illness. Genetic factors greatly influence how the gut microbiota is structured; hence they also influence how the gut microbiota is structured. And how well the human body will be able to fight infections and maintain immunity relies on how healthy and balanced its structure is (Zhang et al., 2021; Tincati et al., 2016).

2.2.7 Atopic Eczema

Atopic eczema is a very common disorder, especially found in children, which is also known as atopic dermatitis. This is as common a disorder as its symptoms are, such as dry skin, red rashes on the skin, or cracks in the middle of the skin. It is an autoimmune disorder that starts during childhood and lasts until adolescence. If we look at the reasons for this, then one of the biggest reasons for its occurrence is genetic factor. This is mostly found in those people who have a lot of allergic conditions in their family history. It means there are some members in the house who have allergic conditions like asthma, fever, and sneezing.

Atopic eczema is a condition in which there is inflammation in the skin. If we look at the statistics, it is found in up to 20% of children and the chances of its occurrence in adults are only 2% to 5%, which is much less than that of children. Recently, there has been a lot of research going on on the relationship between gut microbiota and atopic eczema (Petersen et al., 2019). Heterogeneity of gut microbiota increases significantly in children's first 5 years of life. It has been clearly stated in the available research that the composition of the gut microbiota is unique and individual in every human being. In one study, which was conducted on humans, it was clearly stated that adolescence is the only period in which the gastrointestinal tract of the body harbors a considerable number of microbial cells.

The number of these microwave cells is in trillions. In fact, in some previous research done on humans, the number of these microbial genes has also been given, which is approximately 9.9 million. According to the study, these 9.9 million microbial genes are found only in the intestine during adolescence. That is why it is proven that there is the presence of microorganisms in our entire body and the intestine is the organ that has the maximum number of microorganisms, about 95%. In this disorder too, there is a lot of diversity and imbalance in the composition of the gut microbiome and this is one of the reasons that in this condition the body cells start eating their own healthy cells. That's why atopic eczema is also called an autoimmune disorder (Abrahamsson et al., 2012; Petersen et al., 2019).

2.3 GUT INFLAMMATION AND BOWEL DISORDERS

The problem of gut inflammation or bowl disorders is gradually increasing day by day. Microbes are found in every part of the human body except a few parts. Most of the microbes are found in the intestine, but, apart from the intestine, a good number of microbes are also present in the rest parts of the body. The microbes present in the entire digestive tract are known as gut microbiomes. The microbiome present in the digestive tract is very valuable and useful for the health of the whole human body, especially for gut health. The gut microbiome is very valuable for the health of the human body. Therefore, it is very important to have a balance of gut microbiome in the body. If the problem of imbalance starts arising, i.e., dysbiosis starts in the body, it spoils the health of our gut the most. Dysbiosis is the only reason that gut inflammation starts, and this inflammation causes different types of bowel illnesses in the body. That's why it is very important and necessary to understand why this process of dysbiosis is occurring in the body or what other reasons it may have so that this process can be understood well and its treatment can be done. For its treatment, medicines can be prepared or precautions can be taken through diet (Matsuoka & Kanai, 2015; Salim et al., 2014).

Some inflammatory bowel disorders will be discussed in the next subsections.

2.3.1 Irritable Bowel Syndrome

Nowadays IBS patients are seen mostly. Although this is a common disorder, it is also a serious problem. One cannot be too careless in this problem. Because once this problem increases, it becomes a little difficult to control it. This is a painful disorder, and its symptoms are as follows: frequent abdominal pain, discomfort, bloating, and most importantly the visible change in motion habits. According to experimental research, it has been proved that it causes so much pain that it affects the quality of life in a very serious manner. As we have discussed earlier, there is a close relationship between gut microbiomes and gut health, and the gut microbiome is directly related to bowel disease. That is why the problem of IBS is also directly caused by an imbalance of the gut microbiome. The problem of dysbiosis not only causes the origin of IBS but also helps in increasing it rapidly (Shukla et al., 2018).

Even it has been proven according to previous research that there is a huge difference in the composition of the gut microbiome between a person who has IBS and a person who does not. That is why changes in diet are very important for its treatment (Chey et al., 2015).

2.3.2 Inflammatory Bowel Disease

IBD, like IBS, is a gastrointestinal inflammatory disease that has the potential to cause many physical problems. People who are suffering from IBD also have some common symptoms like IBS. During IBD, there is so much inflammation in the body that long-lasting swelling occurs in the digestive system itself. However, people suffering from IBD mostly suffer from fatigue, stress, diarrhea, cramps, etc. This is also a disease caused by other digestive system problems like microbial imbalance. Therefore, in its treatment, what you are eating or your diet is very important and the patient suffering from IBD will have to change their eating habits and diet according to IBD so that they can get some relief from the inflammation caused by it (Lee & Chang, 2021; DeVoss & Diehl, 2014). Whenever the problem of dysbiosis arises in the body, it has a direct impact on the bacteria and immunity of the body. In fact, in the problem of dysbiosis, the number of harmful bacteria in the body increases and the number of good bacteria decreases, due to which there is a disturbance in the balance of body cells. And, due to the imbalance of these body cells, the gut faces the biggest problem. That means the gut starts getting inflamed and becoming sick. Because of this, the gut is not able to take care of physical harmony. It does not have enough ability to increase the immunity of our body or protect it. Also, due to the problem of dysbiosis, the gut is not able to fulfill its other responsibilities properly such as the gut microbiome helps in the production of different microorganisms and SCFAs in the body. But when the gut is inflamed, it cannot perform this function properly, due to which intestinal health and immune response are deeply affected because microorganisms and SCFAs have an impact on both of these functions (Santana et al., 2022; Lo Sasso et al., 2021). Researchers are continuously doing new research from their side regarding what kind of dietary modifications should be used to manage this disorder and to heal the whole human gut. Among these, most research is being done on the role of probiotics and prebiotics. At the same time, the role of FMT is also being paid more attention. In the process of FMT, part of the healthy stool is taken from a healthy person and transferred to a patient who is suffering from IBD. This is done so that the microbiome of healthy stool can enter the gut of the patient suffering from IBD and generate a healthy, diverse, and balanced microbiome. The gist of all of it is that the gut microbiome is an important part of our body that plays a special role in our health, especially as it plays a central role in the pathogenesis and progression of IBD (McIlroy et al., 2018; Fehily et al., 2021; Qazi et al., 2017).

2.4 RELATION BETWEEN GUT MICROBIOME COMPOSITION AND CARDIOMETABOLIC DISEASES

The relationship between gut microbiome composition and cardiometabolic diseases, in conjunction with such conditions as cardiovascular disease, obesity, type 2 diabetes, and metabolic syndrome, has acquired symbolic attention in modern years. Ascending evidence advocates that the gut microbiome performs a critical role in changing the tone of various physiological processes related to cardiometabolic health.

2.4.1 Metabolism and Obesity

Many previous researchers have proved that there is a special relationship between obesity and metabolism. Metabolism depends on the daily routine and diet of the person. If a person has an irregular unhealthy routine with an unhealthy diet, then his metabolism automatically starts slowing down, due to which symptoms of obesity start appearing directly in the body.

Actually, metabolism is a chemical process of the body that is very helpful in keeping the body healthy (Hulver et al., 2003). It also provides energy to the body so that it can perform its daily routine well. If understood in simple words, researchers have defined it in such a way that metabolism is the process in which the food entered into the body is converted into energy. And this energy is also used in the body to create new cells and repair old cells. The entire internal structure and parts of the body are interconnected. That is why gut microbiome and metabolism are also related to each other. The gut microbiome also plays a role in influencing metabolism. The gut microbiome also works to regulate fat storage, and, with its help, some bacteria increase the energy storage in the body manifold, due to which obesity keeps increasing in the body. That is why the body's imbalanced gut microbiome, obesity, and metabolic disturbance are interlinked with each other (Lee et al., 2020).

2.4.2 Inflammation and Cardiovascular Disease

Whenever the process of dysbiosis starts in the gut microbiome, due to this imbalance, the number of bad bacteria in the body increases and they first increase the penetration of the gut and try to get into the bloodstream directly. This creates a situation of systemic inflammation, and, at the same time, the situation becomes such that the progressions of atherosclerosis and other cardiovascular conditions increase manifold (Witkowski et al., 2020).

2.4.3 Diet and Gut Microbiome

One's body health can be determined by looking at what you eat and how you eat it because food is directly related to the body. Body means not only the external body but how healthy the internal organs are also depending on the diet. And this is the reason that the composition of the gut microbiome largely depends on food. The increase in harmful bacteria in the body and the reduction in microbial diversity are largely caused by excessive consumption of a diet that is high in fat, rich in highly processed food and packed food, and rich in spices. Therefore, to protect the body from harmful bacteria, it is very important to construct such a diet in which the consumption of whole grains, vegetables, and fruits is high, which means that a fiber-rich diet should be consumed as much as possible. Such a diet helps good bacteria to flourish in the body and prevents many diseases (Horn et al., 2022).

2.4.4 Short-Chain Fatty Acids

SCFAs have many health benefits in the human body such as maintaining gut barrier integrity, reducing internal inflammation, and influencing metabolic processes. Actually, one of the functions of gut bacteria is to ferment and break down the dietary fiber reaching the body and convert it into SCFAs, such as acetate, propionate, and butyrate. All these components help in reducing inflammation in the body (Portincasa et al., 2022).

2.4.5 Insulin Resistance and Type 2 Diabetes

The gut microbiome can also influence pancreatic secretion, which has a profound impact on insulin sensitivity and glucose metabolism, which is the main reason for type 2 diabetes. As we have already discussed earlier in this chapter, these out-of-balance microbiomes are a major cause of insulin resistance through different mechanisms that include inflammation and modulation of gut hormone secretions, and, when our body does not utilize its own insulin properly, diabetes begins. So overall, imbalanced microbiomes are a major cause of diabetes (Yang et al., 2021).

So far in this chapter, we have discussed the gut microbiome and its mechanisms. Along with this, it is also known how much the microbiome is useful in the human body and the different types of diseases, occurring in the body, and microbiome, both are somehow related to each other.

2.5 ROLE AND FUNCTION OF PROBIOTICS

Probiotics are a tiny but essential unit that is a precious boon for the human body. It has a lot of health benefits. Many researchers have stated that it is a valuable treasure of the body that gives its benefits only when the time comes; that is why probiotics are also called "good bacteria," which we discussed earlier in this chapter. Basically, these good bacteria keep their shadow on gut health, which means that most of the time they are eager to keep the gut healthy (Li et al., 2016). According to the research done, it has been demonstrated that probiotics are essential for the health of the digestive system (Shin et al., 2019). So, if you want to keep your digestive system healthy, you will have to be friends with these living microorganisms, that is, probiotics (Rahmah et al., 2021). As we already learned from the earlier discussion, there are millions of microbes in our body and these microbes affect our body physically, nutritionally, and metabolically and even affect our immune system. Most of these affect the gastrointestinal tract, which means its main role is to improve the health-related functions of the digestive system (Koga, 2022). So, if you want to understand what probiotics are and what their functions and roles are, then it is important that you have to understand the entire digestive system. Understanding probiotics and their role without understanding the digestive system is absurd.

The digestive system starts with the human mouth and ends in the intestine. The entire process of digesting the food that enters the body starts and ends from the mouth to the intestine. If seen stepwise, the digestion of food first starts from the mouth. As soon as food enters, the process of chewing it is done through the mouth only. After that, the food is chewed properly and mixed with saliva in the mouth and reaches the stomach area, which contains a lot of acids. The reason for the presence of a high amount of acid in the stomach is that the food entered into the stomach is broken down into smaller molecules by the acid present in the stomach. After that, the food divided into molecules passes from the stomach to the intestine. The food reaching the intestine is absorbed by the body (Sensoy, 2021; Mackie et al., 2020). In simple words, by the time the food reaches the intestine, it has become highly nutritious because it has undergone a lot of breakdowns. It gets filtered in the intestine. And this is also a reason for the presence of bacteria in the intestines and the pH of the intestine of the human body is very low. This is the reason that the human intestine has a good atmosphere for the growth of most bacteria. The bacteria present in the intestines are very beneficial for the human body and human health. Some particular bacteria are selected from the gut bacteria and tested to see how important they are for the body. After this, by separating those tested and selected bacteria, a commercial bacterial suspension is made, and the solution of these beneficial selected bacteria is called a probiotic. In short, probiotics are nothing but microbiome, which means these are some selected good bacteria found in the human gut. *Lactobacillus*, *Lactococcus*, *Bifidobacterium*, *Streptococcus thermophilus*, and yeast are the most important and healthy gut bacteria present in probiotics that are beneficial for gut health (Cosme et al., 2022).

We all know that microbiomes and probiotics are associated with each other, which means both of them are interconnected. Probiotics have such toughening abilities to reform the composition and functions of the microbiome, which is why it has been considered beneficially valuable for the health of the human body, notably for the health of the digestive system. Despite having so many health benefits of probiotics, they are consumed in proper amounts, and this amount depends on the physical capacity of the human being, which is decided by the doctor or dietitian as to how much amount, at what time, and what type of the probiotic is to be taken (Miller et al., 2016). Probiotics have many health benefits, and their special feature is that it is available in many natural foods and humans can easily consume them through these natural foods; hence depending on any supplement is not necessary. Probiotics improve digestive health, strengthen the immune system, help in nutrient absorption, and even help in overall well-being. Tables 2.2 and 2.3 list the functions of probiotics that are described in some points.

2.5.1 Microbial Balance

It has been proven in recent research that probiotic is an essential component of gut health. The gastrointestinal tract of the human body is littered with innumerable bacteria from all sides. Among these bacteria, there are both types of bacteria: good bacteria and bad bacteria. But to have a healthy body, it is important to maintain a balance between these two bacteria. If there is an imbalance in these bacteria, the intestines suffer the most damage (El-Saadony et al., 2021). Probiotics are beneficial bacteria that are effective in maintaining the balance of both types of bacteria in the human body. It produces antibacterial substances in the human intestines that help regulate the pH of the gut so that harmful bacteria do not get a favorable environment to grow because whenever the pH level of any body's part increases, harmful bacteria start growing there. An increase in pH creates a favorable environment for harmful bacteria. One among all the functions of probiotics is that it helps strengthen the gut barrier so that no pollution can easily enter the gut and cause damage to the digestive tract. This function of probiotics not only makes the digestive system healthy but also

TABLE 2.2
Role of Different Types of Probiotics in Different Types of Diseases and Disorders

Important Strains of Probiotics	Associated Diseases and Disorders	Impacts on Human Body	References
Oxalobacter formigenes, *Lactobacillus*, and *Bifidobacterium* species (*Lactobacillus plantarum* PBS067, *Lactobacillus acidophilus* LA-14, *Bifidobacterium breve* PBS077, *Bifidobacterium longum* PBS078)	Stones of kidney and gallbladder	1. Prevent kidney and urinary stone formation. 2. Having oxalate degradation properties.	Wigner et al. (2022); Lieske (2017)
Lactobacillus GG, *Lactobacillus rhamnosus* Lactis, *Lactobacillus fermentum*, *Bifidobacterium bifidum*, *Bifidobacterium lactis*, *L. acidophilus*, *Lactobacillus casei*, *L. salivarius*, and *Lactobacillus lactis*	Hypersensitive diseases	1. After the intervention of probiotics, it was observed that it helps to reduce the symptoms of all atopic diseases like atopic eczema and other skin problems. 2. The study also proved that probiotics eliminate the symptoms of atopic dermatitis in children.	Meneghin et al. (2012); Jiang et al. (2020)
L. casei, *L. rhamnosus*, *Streptococcus thermophilus*, *B. breve*, *L. acidophilus*, *B. infantis*, *L. delbrueckii* subsp. *Bulgaricus*, and *Lactobacillus reuteri* DSM 17938	Cramps	It helps a lot in fighting cramps-related diseases in children who are breastfed and also provides the body with the ability to avoid diseases.	Shirazinia et al. (2021); Zermiani et al. (2021)
Lactobacillus, *Bifidobacterium*, and *L. johnsonii*	Bacterial infection	It prevents the growth of bad bacteria in the body and maintains alkaline pH, which helps in preventing the side effects caused by *Helicobacter pylori* infection.	Kamiya et al. (2019)
L. rhamnosus, *L. rhamnosus GG*, *B. animalis* subsp. Lactis alone or in combination with *Streptococcus thermophiles*, *L. reuteri*, *L. rhamnosus* (not GG), and *L. acidophilus*, *Saccharomyces boulardii*, and *L. casei*	Infections linked to antibiotics	It works to prevent the growth of pathogens, thereby supporting the immune response, which helps the good bacteria to heal the body. It promotes substances that help inactivate viruses.	Kopacz and Phadtare (2022)
L. rhamnosus, *L. reuteri*, and *Propionibacterium freudenreichii*	Fungal infection	It acts as a medicine for fungal infections. Therefore, it is very beneficial to the treatment of *Candida* infection.	Demin et al. (2021)

(Continued)

TABLE 2.2 (*Continued*)
Role of Different Types of Probiotics in Different Types of Diseases and Disorders

Important Strains of Probiotics	Associated Diseases and Disorders	Impacts on Human Body	References
Bifidobacterium species, *B. lactis*, *B. longum*, *B. breve*, *B. infantis*, *L. casei*, *L. rhamnosus*, *S. thermophilus*, *L. acidophilus*, and *Lactobacillus bulgaricus*	Costiveness, dyschezia	It works to regulate fecal gut microbiota by managing gut transition time, thereby promoting intestinal organic acids and getting rid of constipation.	Zhang et al. (2021)
L. acidophilus, *L. plantarum*, *L. casei*, *B. lactis*, and *S. cerevisiae*	IBS	Probiotics work on epithelial cells and enhance skin mobility. It also enhances stool frequency and works on stool consistency, which leads to improvement in IBS symptoms.	Kumar et al. (2022)
Lactobacillus GG, *L. casei Shirota*, *L. acidophilus*, *B. bifidum*, *L. rhamnosus*, *L. plantarum*, and *L. paracase*, *Streptococcus salivarius*, and *B. animalis* subsp. *lactis*	Respiration problems or infections	Probiotics help to a great extent in eliminating acute viral upper respiratory infections. It enhances the cytokine plasma level present in the body by protecting the epithelial cells from pathogens, due to which reduction is seen in these respiratory infections and viral infections.	Lehtoranta et al. (2020)
B. animalis subsp. *lactis*, *L. lactis* subsp. *lactis*	Alterations to the gut–brain axis	It helps to build up an improvement in brain activities and neurohealth, and it even plays a vital role in enhancing and developing cognitive behavior in children by directly affecting the central nervous system.	Rajanala et al. (2021)
Lactic acid bacteria	Cancer of the colon	According to the research done so far, it has been proved that probiotics are beneficial in curing cancer. It helps inhibit the progression of cancer by creating a pure and balanced environment between the bacteria living in the intestine.	Śliżewska et al. (2021)
L. acidophilus NCFM, *Lactobacillus gasseri* SBT2055, and *L. rhamnosus* CGMCC1.3724	Diabetes and obesity	It plays a pivotal role in controlling and decreasing the risk of both types of diabetes and enhancing insulin sensitivity. It helps to reduce metabolic diseases by both creating a balanced state in bacteria and reducing the risk of obesity.	Cerdó et al. (2019); Mallappa et al. (2022)

TABLE 2.3
The Names of All Good Bacterial Species That Are Utilized as a Probiotic

Name of All Good Bacterial Species Used As Probiotics	References
Lactobacillus acidophilus, Lactobacillus bulgaricus, Lactobacillus casei, Lactobacillus fermentum, Lactobacillus lactis, Lactobacillus paracasei, Lactobacillus rhamnosus, Lactobacillus delbrueckii subsp. *bulgaricus, Lactobacillus brevis, Lactobacillus johnsonii, Lactobacillus plantarum, Lactobacillus salivarius, Lactobacillus fermentum, Lactobacillus kefiri*	Juturu and Wu (2016)
Enterococcus faecalis, Enterococcus faecium, Escherichia coli, Streptococcus thermophilus, Propionibacterium	Pérez-Díaz et al. (2019); Lagat (2022)
Bifidobacterium adolescentis, Bifidobacterium bifidum, Bifidobacterium breve, Bifidobacterium lactis, Bifidobacterium longum, Bifidobacterium infantis, Bifidobacterium animalis subsp. *animalis, B. nimalis* subsp. *lactis*	Dogra et al. (2021); Alessandri et al. (2021)
Saccharomyces boulardii	Last (2021); Ray (2021)
Coccobacillus, Lactobacillus, Streptococcus, Leuconostoc, L. lactis subsp. *lactis, Pediococcus, Propionibacterium, Enterococcus, Enterococcus durans, Bifidobacterium, Bacillus, Bacillus coagulans, Bacillus subtilis, Saccharomyces cerevisiae, Candida pintolopesii, Aspergillus niger, Aspergillus oryzae, Bacillus lichenformis, Bacillus cereus* var. *toyoi, Bacillus clausii, Bacillus laterosporus, Bacillus pumilus, Bacillus racemilacticus, S. thermophilus*	El Houari et al. (2023)

promotes the process of digestion, increases metabolism, increases the speed of nutrient absorption, and improves overall gastrointestinal support (Peng et al., 2020).

2.5.2 Optimizing Digestive Functions: Strategies for a Healthier Gut

According to the study, probiotics work to strengthen the digestive system and further enhance its functions. Probiotics balance the microbial imbalance in the body and prevent the process of dysbiosis, which allows good bacteria to flourish in the body and does not allow the right environment to be created for bad bacteria.

This mechanism of probiotics promotes the health of the gastrointestinal tract and improves the digestive process. Consuming probiotics increases the quality of smoothness in the stool, due to which the bowel movement becomes normal and the symptoms of some diseases like diarrhea and constipation are relieved. In short, probiotics help to improve gut mobility (Ibrahim et al., 2020).

Probiotics also help in improving the functioning of the digestive system, and there are many examples of this such as probiotics helping in the breakdown of carbohydrates, fiber, proteins, and different nutrients that reach the intestines for digestion. Some specific probiotics produce their own digestive enzymes to maintain the breakdown process and helps to promote easy and quick absorption of these dietary components in the human body. All these actions by probiotics prove that they promote nutrient absorption in the body (Judkins et al., 2020).

2.5.3 Enhancing Gut Barrier Function

To understand how probiotics improve the functions of the gut barrier or what the relationship between the two is, it is important to first understand what the gut barrier is. In a way, the gut barrier can also be seen as a controlled and protective gate that separates the gastrointestinal tract from the rest of the body. Its other name is an intestinal barrier. It acts as a defensive shield barrier by controlling and managing the overall passage of nutrients, water, and electrolytes into the bloodstream and preventing harmful and hazardous substances from entering the body. In short, as per the conclusion of many studies, this is simply clear that the proper functioning of the gut barrier and its strengthening are also essential for the human body (Ma et al., 2022).

As it is clear from the headline, probiotics help in strengthening and functioning of the gut barrier and provide a positive effect. In simple words, it has become clear from many studies that probiotics have this relation with the intestinal barrier, and probiotics are good bacteria present in the intestine and these good bacteria greatly improve the integrity or virtue of the tight junction between the cells of the intestinal lining. Actually, tight junctions are a type of protein complexes that are most specific. They are closely interconnected to their neighboring epithelial cells and generate a tight and strong seal between them. This tight junction anticipates and stops the leakage of molecules and bacteria into the gut lining and bloodstream by a tight and strong seal (Martel et al., 2022). Therefore, tight junction is very important for gut health and the strength of tight junction and its regulation function depends on probiotics. In addition, probiotics prepare a kind of mucus barrier and it does this by stimulating mucus production. Overall, probiotics play an important and essential role in human digestive health by strengthening the gut barrier (Serek & Oleksy-Wawrzyniak, 2021).

2.5.4 Balancing the Immune Response

The immune response of the human body depends on the health of the gut, which means the condition of the gut microbiome in the intestine completely regulates the immune response and probiotics are used only to manage the condition of the gut microbiome. If seen clearly, it means that probiotics can leave a deep impact on physical immunity, which has been demonstrated in all the research conducted till now. According to a study, probiotics have a great continuous interaction with lymphocyte tissues and immune cells in the gut and this whole process plays a huge role by which probiotics are able to regulate the immune response, especially in the gut because the gut is the only significant and valuable place where a convincing and powerful portion of the immune system is positioned (Rousseaux et al., 2023; Begum et al., 2021).

According to the fact of a study, it has been proven that cytokines are the fundamental molecules that are responsible for signaling the immune system, and probiotics are such important friendly bacteria that have a deep impact on the production of cytokines. In another study, it was described in this way that one of the roles of probiotics in gut health is that they work to control or regulate the production of cytokines (Maldonado Galdeano et al., 2019; Kany et al., 2019).

As per a study, gut-associated lymphoid tissue (GALT) plays a vital role in the immune system because it is a valuable part of the human body's immune system with great immune cells and lymphoid structures, positioned in the gut, and the probiotics collaborate with GALT to have a beneficial and positive effect on immunity in the gastrointestinal tract (Barati et al., 2022; Mörbe et al., 2021).

2.5.5 Boosting Metabolism and Nutrient Absorption for Optimal Health

From the research so far, we have learned that probiotics have a major role in keeping the entire intestines healthy. That means it mainly works to keep the gut healthy. Due to the good bacterial properties of probiotics, they eliminate the process of dysbiosis in the gut and maintain a balance, and, by creating that balance, the pH value of the gut remains normal. Due to normal pH value, bad bacteria do not get such an environment where they can flourish or cause any harm to the gut. Due to this harmony of good and bad bacteria in the intestines, the immune system also remains healthy and responds positively. Normally the pH value of the gut is 7–8.5, and this pH value depends on the bacteria present in the intestines (Chen et al., 2022). When compared with the stomach, the human gut is alkaline in nature. The alkaline nature of the intestine is a symbol of a healthy gut, which completely depends on the harmony of bacteria, and the entire credit for this goes to probiotics. If bad bacteria start replacing good bacteria in the gut, then the gut starts becoming acidic, and the gut becoming acidic means it suffers from diseases (Gomaa, 2020). Studies have suggested that when dietary components like fats, carbs, and proteins enter the intestines, probiotics play a major role in their absorption. Probiotics begin the fermentation process of dietary fiber and complex carbohydrates to produce SCFAs, and the production of the SCFA is an essential step for overall gut health and also aids in energy metabolism (Ashaolu et al., 2021). Probiotics also have an effective effect on cholesterol levels by metabolizing bile acids. Apart from impacting cholesterol in the human body, probiotics change polyphenols into bioactive compounds by converting them, and, by doing so, they also help in the synthesis of some vitamins that are essential for the human body. Probiotic also makes an important contribution in absorbing and digesting the nutrients reaching the intestines by utilizing dietary sugar, degrading polysaccharides, and metabolizing essential amino acids (You et al., 2022).

2.6 CONCLUSION

As per the available research data it has been proven that the gut microbiome is identified as a pivotal organ in improving human overall health; it has demonstrated that its benefits are not limited to gut health only. That is the reason it is defined as a fundamental component of human biology and physiology. First of all, gut microbiomes work to improve digestion and metabolism in the human body. It divides the components of food reaching the intestine into smaller pieces and also increases the speed of its digestion absorption because the human body is not capable of digesting many complex components on its own. Its most important function in digestion is that it produces SCFAs through the fermentation process, and this is the only reason that these act as a fuel for good gut health. These SCFAs help in balancing the internal environment of the intestines in the human body. In addition, they help in providing proper energy to the human body.

In many researches, it has been declared as a driver of the human body's immune system. Actually, in simple language, it helps in increasing the proportion of good bacteria in the gut, due to which bad bacteria do not get huge space to grow, and maintaining the balance between good and bad bacteria in the human gut is essential. The body's immunity totally depends on the gut because the major part of the immune system is positioned in the gut. In short, the state of the balance in the gut microbiome is necessary to enhance immunity, regulate the gut barrier function profoundly, and improve digestion and metabolism, and achieving all these easily depends on the combination of probiotics.

The areas that may have future exploration are discovering new probiotic strains and providing particular probiotics according to individual microbiome composition.

BIBLIOGRAPHY

Abrahamsson, T. R., Jakobsson, H. E., Andersson, A. F., Björkstén, B., Engstrand, L., & Jenmalm, M. C. (2012). Low diversity of the gut microbiota in infants with atopic eczema. *Journal of Allergy and Clinical Immunology, 129*(2), 434–440. https://doi.org/10.1016/j.jaci.2011.10.025

Adorini, L., Gregori, S., & Harrison, L. C. (2002). Understanding autoimmune diabetes: insights from mouse models. *Trends in Molecular Medicine*, *8*(1), 31–38.

Alessandri, G., van Sinderen, D., & Ventura, M. (2021). The genus Bifidobacterium: From genomics to functionality of an important component of the mammalian gut microbiota running title: Bifidobacterial adaptation to and interaction with the host. *Computational and Structural Biotechnology Journal, 19,* 1472–1487. https://doi.org/10.1016/j.csbj.2021.03.006

Ashaolu, T. J., Ashaolu, J. O., & Adeyeye, S. A. O. (2021). Fermentation of prebiotics by human colonic microbiota in vitro and short-chain fatty acids production: A critical review. *Journal of Applied Microbiology, 130*(3), 677–687. https://doi.org/10.1111/jam.14843

Barati, M., Jabbari, M., Abdi Ghavidel, A., Nikmehr, P., Arzhang, P., Aynehchi, A., Babashahi, M., Mosharkesh, E., Roshanravan, N., Shabani, M., & Davoodi, S. H. (2022). The engineered probiotics for the treatment of chronic diseases: A systematic review. *Journal of Food Biochemistry, 46*(10), e14343. https://doi.org/10.1111/jfbc.14343

Begum, J., Buyamayum, B., Lingaraju, M. C., Dev, K., & Biswas, A. (2021). Probiotics: Role in immunomodulation and consequent effects: Probiotics and immunity. *Letters in Animal Biology, 1*(1), 1–6.

Bibbò, S., Dore, M. P., Pes, G. M., Delitala, G., & Delitala, A. P. (2017). Is there a role for gut microbiota in type 1 diabetes pathogenesis? *Annals of Medicine, 49*(1), 11–22. https://doi.org/10.1080/07853890.2016.1222449

Bogusławska, J., Godlewska, M., Gajda, E., & Piekiełko-Witkowska, A. (2022). Cellular and molecular basis of thyroid autoimmunity. *European Thyroid Journal, 11*(1). https://doi.org/10.1530/ETJ-21-0024

Boldison, J., & Wong, F. S. (2016). Immune and pancreatic β cell interactions in type 1 diabetes. *Trends in Endocrinology and Metabolism, 27*(12), 856–867. https://doi.org/10.1016/j.tem.2016.08.007

Byndloss, M. X., & Bäumler, A. J. (2018). The germ-organ theory of non-communicable diseases. *Nature Reviews. Microbiology, 16*(2), 103–110. https://doi.org/10.1038/nrmicro.2017.158

Cerdó, T., García-Santos, J. A., G Bermúdez, M., & Campoy, C. (2019). The role of probiotics and prebiotics in the prevention and treatment of obesity. *Nutrients, 11*(3), 635. https://doi.org/10.3390/nu11030635

Charitos, I. A., Topi, S., Gagliano-Candela, R., De Nitto, E., Polimeno, L., Montagnani, M., & Santacroce, L. (2022). The toxic effects of endocrine disrupting chemicals (EDCs) on gut microbiota: Bisphenol A (BPA) A review. *Endocrine, Metabolic & Immune Disorders-Drug Targets (Formerly Current Drug Targets-Immune, Endocrine & Metabolic Disorders), 22*(7), 716–727.

Chen, S., Zhu, F. D., Li, B. L., Yang, J. M., Yang, T., Liu, X. Q., Zhang, J., & Zhao, Y. (2022). Alkaline media-sensitive nanocarrier based on carboxylated cyclodextrin for targeted delivery of anti-colon drug. *Journal of Applied Polymer Science, 139*(46), e53163. https://doi.org/10.1002/app.53163

Chey, W. D., Kurlander, J., & Eswaran, S. (2015). Irritable bowel syndrome: A clinical review. *JAMA, 313*(9), 949–958. https://doi.org/10.1001/jama.2015.0954

Christovich, A., & Luo, X. M. (2022). Gut microbiota, leaky gut, and autoimmune diseases. *Frontiers in Immunology, 13*, 946248.

Cosme, F., Inês, A., & Vilela, A. (2022). Consumer's acceptability and health consciousness of probiotic and prebiotic of non-dairy products. *Food Research International, 151,* 110842. https://doi.org/10.1016/j.foodres.2021.110842

Cresci, G. A., & Bawden, E. (2015). Gut microbiome: What we do and don't know. *Nutrition in Clinical Practice, 30*(6), 734–746. https://doi.org/10.1177/0884533615609899

De Goffau, M. C., Fuentes, S., van den Bogert, B., Honkanen, H., de Vos, W. M., Welling, G. W., Hyöty, H., & Harmsen, H. J. (2014). Aberrant gut microbiota composition at the onset of type 1 diabetes in young children. *Diabetologia, 57*(8), 1569–1577. https://doi.org/10.1007/s00125-014-3274-0

De Vos, W. M., Tilg, H., Van Hul, M., & Cani, P. D. (2022). Gut microbiome and health: mechanistic insights. *Gut, 71*(5), 1020–1032.

Dedrick, S., Sundaresh, B., Huang, Q., Brady, C., Yoo, T., Cronin, C., Rudnicki, C., Flood, M., Momeni, B., Ludvigsson, J., & Altindis, E. (2020). The role of gut microbiota and environmental factors in type 1 diabetes pathogenesis. *Frontiers in Endocrinology, 11,* 78. https://doi.org/10.3389/fendo.2020.00078

Demin, K. A., Refeld, A. G., Bogdanova, A. A., Prazdnova, E. V., Popov, I. V., Kutsevalova, O. Y., Ermakov, A. M., Bren, A. B., Rudoy, D. V., Chistyakov, V. A., Weeks, R., & Chikindas, M. L. (2021). Mechanisms of Candida resistance to antimycotics and promising ways to overcome it: The role of probiotics. *Probiotics and Antimicrobial Proteins, 13*(4), 926–948. https://doi.org/10.1007/s12602-021-09776-6

Demirci, M., Bahar Tokman, H., Taner, Z., Keskin, F. E., Çağatay, P., Ozturk Bakar, Y., Özyazar, M., Kiraz, N., & Kocazeybek, B. S. (2020). Bacteroidetes and Firmicutes levels in gut microbiota and effects of hosts TLR2/TLR4 gene expression levels in adult type 1 diabetes patients in Istanbul, Turkey. *Journal of Diabetes and Its Complications, 34*(2), 107449. https://doi.org/10.1016/j.jdiacomp.2019.107449

Deo, P. N., & Deshmukh, R. (2019). Oral microbiome: Unveiling the fundamentals. *Journal of Oral and Maxillofacial Pathology: JOMFP, 23*(1), 122–128. https://doi.org/10.4103/jomfp.JOMFP_304_18

DeVoss, J., & Diehl, L. (2014). Murine models of inflammatory bowel disease (IBD) challenges of modeling human disease. *Toxicologic Pathology, 42*(1), 99–110. https://doi.org/10.1177/0192623313509729

Ding, R. X., Goh, W. R., Wu, R. N., Yue, X. Q., Luo, X., Khine, W. W. T., Wu, J. R., & Lee, Y. K. (2019). Revisit gut microbiota and its impact on human health and disease. *Journal of Food and Drug Analysis*, *27*(3), 623–631. https://doi.org/10.1016/j.jfda.2018.12.012

Diwan, A. D., & Harke, S. N. (2021). Bank on microbiome to keep the Body Healthy. *Journal of Nutrition and Food Sciences, 2*(2), 1–5.

Doaty, S., Agrawal, H., Bauer, E., & Furst, D. E. (2016). Infection and lupus: Which causes which? *Current Rheumatology Reports, 18*(3), 13. https://doi.org/10.1007/s11926-016-0561-4

Dogra, S. K., Martin, F. P., Donnicola, D., Julita, M., Berger, B., & Sprenger, N. (2021). Human milk oligosaccharide-stimulated Bifidobacterium species contribute to prevent later respiratory tract infections. *Microorganisms, 9*(9). https://doi.org/10.3390/microorganisms9091939

Ejtahed, H. S., Angoorani, P., Soroush, A. R., Siadat, S. D., Shirzad, N., Hasani-Ranjbar, S., & Larijani, B. (2020). Our little friends with big roles: Alterations of the gut microbiota in thyroid disorders. *Endocrine, Metabolic and Immune Disorders—Drug Targets (Formerly Current Drug Targets-Immune, Endocrine & Metabolic Disorders), 20*(3), 344–350. https://doi.org/10.2174/1871530319666190930110605

El Houari, A., Carpenter, M., Chaplin, D., Golyshin, P., & McDonald, J. E. (2023). Lutisporasaccharofermentans sp. nov., a mesophilic, non-spore-forming bacterium isolated from a lab-scale methanogenic landfill bioreactor digesting anaerobic sludge, and emendation of the genus Lutispora to include species which are non-spore-forming and mesophilic. *International Journal of Systematic and Evolutionary Microbiology, 73*(1). https://doi.org/10.1099/ijsem.0.005683

El-Saadony, M. T., Alagawany, M., Patra, A. K., Kar, I., Tiwari, R., Dawood, M. A. O., Dhama, K., & Abdel-Latif, H. M. R. (2021). The functionality of probiotics in aquaculture: An overview. *Fish and Shellfish Immunology, 117,* 36–52. https://doi.org/10.1016/j.fsi.2021.07.007

Fan, Y., & Pedersen, O. (2021). Gut microbiota in human metabolic health and disease. *Nature Reviews. Microbiology*, *19*(1), 55–71. https://doi.org/10.1038/s41579-020-0433-9

Fehily, S. R., Basnayake, C., Wright, E. K., & Kamm, M. A. (2021). Fecal microbiota transplantation therapy in Crohn's disease: Systematic review. *Journal of Gastroenterology and Hepatology, 36*(10), 2672–2686. https://doi.org/10.1111/jgh.15598

Fenneman, A. C., Bruinstroop, E., Nieuwdorp, M., van der Spek, A. H., & Boelen, A. (2023). A comprehensive review of thyroid hormone metabolism in the gut and its clinical implications. *Thyroid, 33*(1), 32–44.

Garg, R., & Garg, A. (2023). The research trends and scientometric assessment of rheumatoid arthritis in India during 2016–2021. *Current Rheumatology Reviews, 19*(1), 26–35. https://doi.org/10.2174/1573397118666220804162313

Gilbert, J. A., & Neufeld, J. D. (2014). Life in a world without microbes. *PLoS Biology, 12*(12), e1002020. https://doi.org/10.1371/journal.pbio.1002020

Gomaa, E. Z. (2020). Human gut microbiota/microbiome in health and diseases: A review. *Antonie van Leeuwenhoek, 113*(12), 2019–2040. https://doi.org/10.1007/s10482-020-01474-7

Gong, B., Wang, C., Meng, F., Wang, H., Song, B., Yang, Y., & Shan, Z. (2021). Association between gut microbiota and autoimmune thyroid disease: A systematic review and meta-analysis. *Frontiers in Endocrinology, 12,* 774362. https://doi.org/10.3389/fendo.2021.774362

Guerreiro, C. S., Calado, Â., Sousa, J., & Fonseca, J. E. (2018). Diet, microbiota, and gut permeability—the unknown triad in rheumatoid arthritis. *Frontiers in Medicine, 5,* 349. https://doi.org/10.3389/fmed.2018.00349

Gülden, E., Wong, F. S., & Wen, L. (2015). The gut microbiota and type 1 diabetes. *Clinical Immunology, 159*(2), 143–153. https://doi.org/10.1016/j.clim.2015.05.013

Gürsoy, S., Koçkar, T., Atik, S. U., Önal, Z., Önal, H., & Adal, E. (2018). Autoimmunity and intestinal colonization by Candida albicans in patients with type 1 diabetes at the time of the diagnosis. *Korean Journal of Pediatrics, 61*(7), 217–220. https://doi.org/10.3345/kjp.2018.61.7.217

Han, H., Li, Y., Fang, J., Liu, G., Yin, J., Li, T., & Yin, Y. (2018). Gut microbiota and type 1 diabetes. *International Journal of Molecular Sciences*, *19*(4), 995.

Higuchi, B. S., Rodrigues, N., Gonzaga, M. I., Paiolo, J. C. C., Stefanutto, N., Omori, W. P., Pinheiro, D. G., Brisotti, J. L., Matheucci, E., Mariano, V. S., & De Oliveira, G. L. V. (2018). Intestinal dysbiosis in autoimmune diabetes is correlated with poor glycemic control and increased interleukin-6: A pilot study. *Frontiers in Immunology, 9,* 1689. https://doi.org/10.3389/fimmu.2018.01689

Horn, J., Mayer, D. E., Chen, S., & Mayer, E. A. (2022). Role of diet and its effects on the gut microbiome in the pathophysiology of mental disorders. *Translational Psychiatry, 12*(1), 164. https://doi.org/10.1038/s41398-022-01922-0

Huang, Y., Li, S. C., Hu, J., Ruan, H. B., Guo, H. M., Zhang, H. H., Wang, X., Pei, Y. F., Pan, Y., & Fang, C. (2018). Gut microbiota profiling in Han Chinese with type 1 diabetes. *Diabetes Research and Clinical Practice, 141,* 256–263. https://doi.org/10.1016/j.diabres.2018.04.032

Hulver, M. W., Berggren, J. R., Cortright, R. N., Dudek, R. W., Thompson, R. P., Pories, W. J., . . . Houmard, J. A. (2003). Skeletal muscle lipid metabolism with obesity. *American Journal of Physiology-Endocrinology and Metabolism, 284*(4), E741–E747.

Ibrahim, A., Ali, R. A. R., Manaf, M. R. A., Ahmad, N., Tajurruddin, F. W., Qin, W. Z., Desa, S. H. M., & Ibrahim, N. M. (2020). Multi-strain probiotics (Hexbio) containing MCP BCMC strains improved constipation and gut motility in Parkinson's disease: A randomised controlled trial. *PLoS One, 15*(12), e0244680. https://doi.org/10.1371/journal.pone.0244680

Islam, M. A., Khandker, S. S., Kotyla, P. J., & Hassan, R. (2020). Immunomodulatory effects of diet and nutrients in systemic lupus erythematosus (SLE): A systematic review. *Frontiers in Immunology, 11,* 1477. https://doi.org/10.3389/fimmu.2020.01477

Itariu, B. K., & Stulnig, T. M. (2014). Autoimmune aspects of type 2 diabetes mellitus-a mini-review. *Gerontology, 60*(3), 189–196. https://doi.org/10.1159/000356747

Jiang, W., Ni, B., Liu, Z., Liu, X., Xie, W., Wu, I. X. Y., & Li, X. (2020). The role of probiotics in the prevention and treatment of atopic dermatitis in children: An updated systematic review and meta-analysis of randomized controlled trials. *Paediatric Drugs, 22*(5), 535–549. https://doi.org/10.1007/s40272-020-00410-6

Jiao, Y., Wu, L., Huntington, N. D., & Zhang, X. (2020). Crosstalk between gut microbiota and innate immunity and its implication in autoimmune diseases. *Frontiers in Immunology, 11,* 282. https://doi.org/10.3389/fimmu.2020.00282

Judkins, T. C., Archer, D. L., Kramer, D. C., & Solch, R. J. (2020). Probiotics, nutrition, and the small intestine. *Current Gastroenterology Reports, 22*(1), 2. https://doi.org/10.1007/s11894-019-0740-3

Juturu, V., & Wu, J. C. (2016). Microbial production of lactic acid: The latest development. *Critical Reviews in Biotechnology, 36*(6), 967–977. https://doi.org/10.3109/07388551.2015.1066305

Kamiya, S., Yonezawa, H., & Osaki, T. (2019). Role of probiotics in eradication therapy for Helicobacter pylori infection. *Helicobacter Pylori in Human Diseases: Advances in Microbiology, Infectious Diseases and Public Health Volume, 11,* 243–255.

Kany, S., Vollrath, J. T., & Relja, B. (2019). Cytokines in inflammatory disease. *International Journal of Molecular Sciences, 20*(23), 6008. https://doi.org/10.3390/ijms20236008

Knezevic, J., Starchl, C., Tmava Berisha, A., & Amrein, K. (2020). Thyroid-gut-axis: How does the microbiota influence thyroid function? *Nutrients, 12*(6), 1769. https://doi.org/10.3390/nu12061769

Knip, M., & Siljander, H. (2016). The role of the intestinal microbiota in type 1 diabetes mellitus. *Nature Reviews. Endocrinology, 12*(3), 154–167. https://doi.org/10.1038/nrendo.2015.218

Koga, Y. (2022). Microbiota in the stomach and application of probiotics to gastroduodenal diseases. *World Journal of Gastroenterology, 28*(47), 6702–6715. https://doi.org/10.3748/wjg.v28.i47.6702

Köhling, H. L., Plummer, S. F., Marchesi, J. R., Davidge, K. S., & Ludgate, M. (2017). The microbiota and autoimmunity: Their role in thyroid autoimmune diseases. *Clinical Immunology, 183,* 63–74.

Kopacz, K., & Phadtare, S. (2022, August). Probiotics for the prevention of antibiotic-associated diarrhea. In *Healthcare* (Vol. 10, No. 8, p. 1450). MDPI.

Kumar, L. S., Pugalenthi, L. S., Ahmad, M., Reddy, S., Barkhane, Z., & Elmadi, J. (2022). Probiotics in irritable bowel syndrome: A review of their therapeutic role. *Cureus, 14*(4).

Lagat, M. K. (2022). *Biological and chemical extraction of chitin and chitosan from the black soldier fly (Hermetiaillucens) exoskeleton and antimicrobial activity against selected human pathogenic microbes* [Doctoral dissertation, JKUAT-COPAS].

Last, A. (2021). *Interactions of Candida albicans with nonpathogenic gut bacteria* [Doctoral dissertation, Friedrich-Schiller-Universität Jena].

Lee, C. J., Sears, C. L., & Maruthur, N. (2020). Gut microbiome and its role in obesity and insulin resistance. *Annals of the New York Academy of Sciences, 1461*(1), 37–52. https://doi.org/10.1111/nyas.14107

Lee, M., & Chang, E. B. (2021). Inflammatory bowel diseases (IBD) and the microbiome—searching the crime scene for clues. *Gastroenterology, 160*(2), 524–537.

Lehtoranta, L., Latvala, S., & Lehtinen, M. J. (2020). Role of probiotics in stimulating the immune system in viral respiratory tract infections: A narrative review. *Nutrients, 12*(10), 3163. https://doi.org/10.3390/nu12103163

Leiva-Gea, I., Sánchez-Alcoholado, L., Martín-Tejedor, B., Castellano-Castillo, D., Moreno-Indias, I., Urda-Cardona, A., Tinahones, F. J., Fernández-García, J. C., & Queipo-Ortuño, M. I. (2018). Gut microbiota differs in composition and functionality between children with type 1 diabetes and MODY2 and healthy control subjects: A case-control study. *Diabetes Care, 41*(11), 2385–2395.

Li, D., Wang, P., Wang, P., Hu, X., & Chen, F. (2016). The gut microbiota: A treasure for human health. *Biotechnology Advances, 34*(7), 1210–1224. https://doi.org/10.1016/j.biotechadv.2016.08.003

Li, M., & Wang, F. (2021). Role of intestinal microbiota on gut homeostasis and rheumatoid arthritis. *Journal of Immunology Research, 2021*.

Li, R., Meng, X., Chen, B., Zhao, L., & Zhang, X. (2021). Gut microbiota in lupus: A butterfly effect? *Current Rheumatology Reports, 23*(4), 27. https://doi.org/10.1007/s11926-021-00986-z

Lieske, J. C. (2017). Probiotics for prevention of urinary stones. *Annals of Translational Medicine, 5*(2), 29. https://doi.org/10.21037/atm.2016.11.86

Lo Sasso, G., Khachatryan, L., Kondylis, A., Battey, J. N. D., Sierro, N., Danilova, N. A., Grigoryeva, T. V., Markelova, M. I., Khusnutdinova, D. R., Laikov, A. V., Salafutdinov, I. I., Romanova, Y. D., Siniagina, M. N., Vasiliev, I. Y., Boulygina, E. A., Solovyeva, V. V., Garanina, E. E., Kitaeva, K. V., Ivanov, K. Y., . . . Abdulkhakov, S. R. (2021). Inflammatory bowel disease–associated changes in the gut: Focus on Kazan patients. *Inflammatory Bowel Diseases, 27*(3), 418–433. https://doi.org/10.1093/ibd/izaa188

Ma, X. Y., Son, Y. H., Yoo, J. W., Joo, M. K., & Kim, D. H. (2022). Citation: Tight junction protein expression-inducing probiotics alleviate TNBS-induced cognitive impairment with colitis in mice. *Nutrients, 14*(14), 2975. https://doi.org/10.3390/nu14142975

Ma, Y., Xu, X., Li, M., Cai, J., Wei, Q., & Niu, H. (2019). Gut microbiota promote the inflammatory response in the pathogenesis of systemic lupus erythematosus. *Molecular Medicine, 25*(1), 35. https://doi.org/10.1186/s10020-019-0102-5

Mackie, A., Mulet-Cabero, A. I., & Torcello-Gómez, A. (2020). Simulating human digestion: Developing our knowledge to create healthier and more sustainable foods. *Food and Function, 11*(11), 9397–9431. https://doi.org/10.1039/d0fo01981j

Maldonado Galdeano, C., Cazorla, S. I., Lemme Dumit, J. M., Vélez, E., & Perdigón, G. (2019). Beneficial effects of probiotic consumption on the immune system. *Annals of Nutrition and Metabolism, 74*(2), 115–124. https://doi.org/10.1159/000496426

Mallappa, R. H., Balasubramaniam, C., Amarlapudi, M. R., Kelkar, S., Adewumi, G. A., Kadyan, S., Pradhan, D., & Grover, S. (2022). Role of probiotics in the prevention and management of diabetes and obesity. In *Probiotics in the prevention and management of human diseases* (pp. 321–336). Academic Press.

Marchesi, J. R., Adams, D. H., Fava, F., Hermes, G. D., Hirschfield, G. M., Hold, G., Quraishi, M. N., Kinross, J., Smidt, H., Tuohy, K. M., Thomas, L. V., Zoetendal, E. G., & Hart, A. (2016). The gut microbiota and host health: A new clinical frontier. *Gut, 65*(2), 330–339. https://doi.org/10.1136/gutjnl-2015-309990

Martel, J., Chang, S. H., Ko, Y. F., Hwang, T. L., Young, J. D., & Ojcius, D. M. (2022). Gut barrier disruption and chronic disease. *Trends in Endocrinology and Metabolism, 33*(4), 247–265. https://doi.org/10.1016/j.tem.2022.01.002

Martin, R., Makino, H., Cetinyurek Yavuz, A., Ben-Amor, K., Roelofs, M., Ishikawa, E., Kubota, H., Swinkels, S., Sakai, T., Oishi, K., Kushiro, A., & Knol, J. (2016). Early-life events, including mode of delivery and type of feeding, siblings and gender, shape the developing gut microbiota. *PLoS One, 11*(6), e0158498. https://doi.org/10.1371/journal.pone.0158498

Matsuoka, K., & Kanai, T. (2015, January). The gut microbiota and inflammatory bowel disease. In *Seminars in immunopathology* (Vol. 37, pp. 47–55). Springer.

McIlroy, J., Ianiro, G., Mukhopadhya, I., Hansen, R., & Hold, G. L. (2018). The gut microbiome in inflammatory bowel disease—avenues for microbial management. *Alimentary Pharmacology and Therapeutics, 47*(1), 26–42. https://doi.org/10.1111/apt.14384

Meneghin, F., Fabiano, V., Mameli, C., & Zuccotti, G. V. (2012). Probiotics and atopic dermatitis in children. *Pharmaceuticals, 5*(7), 727–744. https://doi.org/10.3390/ph5070727

Miller, L. E., Zimmermann, A. K., & Ouwehand, A. C. (2016). Contemporary meta-analysis of short-term probiotic consumption on gastrointestinal transit. *World Journal of Gastroenterology, 22*(21), 5122–5131. https://doi.org/10.3748/wjg.v22.i21.5122

Mörbe, U. M., Jørgensen, P. B., Fenton, T. M., von Burg, N., Riis, L. B., Spencer, J., & Agace, W. W. (2021). Human gut-associated lymphoid tissues (GALT); diversity, structure, and function. *Mucosal Immunology, 14*(4), 793–802. https://doi.org/10.1038/s41385-021-00389-4

Murri, M., Leiva, I., Gomez-Zumaquero, J. M., Tinahones, F. J., Cardona, F., Soriguer, F., & Queipo-Ortuño, M. I. (2013). Gut microbiota in children with type 1 diabetes differs from that in healthy children: A case-control study. *BMC Medicine, 11*, 46. https://doi.org/10.1186/1741-7015-11-46

Myers, B., Brownstone, N., Reddy, V., Chan, S., Thibodeaux, Q., Truong, A., Bhutani, T., Chang, H. W., & Liao, W. (2019). The gut microbiome in psoriasis and psoriatic arthritis. *Best Practice and Research. Clinical Rheumatology, 33*(6), 101494. https://doi.org/10.1016/j.berh.2020.101494

NIH Human Microbiome Portfolio Analysis Team. (2019). A review of 10 years of human microbiome research activities at the US National Institutes of Health, fiscal years 2007–2016. *Microbiome*, *7*(1), 31. https://doi.org/10.1186/s40168-019-0620-y

Nuriel-Ohayon, M., Neuman, H., & Koren, O. (2016). Microbial changes during pregnancy, birth, and infancy. *Frontiers in Microbiology*, *7*, 1031. https://doi.org/10.3389/fmicb.2016.01031

Ogunrinola, G. A., Oyewale, J. O., Oshamika, O. O., & Olasehinde, G. I. (2020). The human microbiome and its impacts on health. *International Journal of Microbiology, 2020*, 8045646. https://doi.org/10.1155/2020/8045646

Olejniczak-Staruch, I., Ciążyńska, M., Sobolewska-Sztychny, D., Narbutt, J., Skibińska, M., & Lesiak, A. (2021). Alterations of the skin and gut microbiome in psoriasis and psoriatic arthritis. *International Journal of Molecular Sciences, 22*(8), 3998. https://doi.org/10.3390/ijms22083998

Pan, W., Zhang, Y., Zeng, C., Xu, F., Yan, J., & Weng, J. (2018). miR192 is upregulated in T1DM, regulates pancreatic β-cell development and inhibits insulin secretion through suppressing -GLP-1 expression. *Experimental and Therapeutic Medicine, 16*(3), 2717–2724. https://doi.org/10.3892/etm.2018.6453

Pellegrini, S., Sordi, V., Bolla, A. M., Saita, D., Ferrarese, R., Canducci, F., Clementi, M., Invernizzi, F., Mariani, A., Bonfanti, R., Barera, G., Testoni, P. A., Doglioni, C., Bosi, E., & Piemonti, L. (2017). Duodenal mucosa of patients with type 1 diabetes shows distinctive inflammatory profile and microbiota. *Journal of Clinical Endocrinology and Metabolism, 102*(5), 1468–1477. https://doi.org/10.1210/jc.2016-3222

Peng, M., Tabashsum, Z., Anderson, M., Truong, A., Houser, A. K., Padilla, J., Akmel, A., Bhatti, J., Rahaman, S. O., & Biswas, D. (2020). Effectiveness of probiotics, prebiotics, and prebiotic-like components in common functional foods. *Comprehensive Reviews in Food Science and Food Safety, 19*(4), 1908–1933. https://doi.org/10.1111/1541-4337.12565

Pérez-Díaz, I. M., Hayes, J. S., Medina, E., Webber, A. M., Butz, N., Dickey, A. N., Lu, Z., & Azcarate-Peril, M. A. (2019). Assessment of the non-lactic acid bacteria microbiota in fresh cucumbers and commercially fermented cucumber pickles brined with 6% NaCl. *Food Microbiology, 77,* 10–20. https://doi.org/10.1016/j.fm.2018.08.003

Petersen, E. B. M., Skov, L., Thyssen, J. P., & Jensen, P. (2019). Role of the gut microbiota in atopic dermatitis: A systematic review. *Acta Dermato-Venereologica, 99*(1), 5–11. https://doi.org/10.2340/00015555-3008

Pinto, E., Anselmo, M., Calha, M., Bottrill, A., Duarte, I., Andrew, P. W., & Faleiro, M. L. (2017). The intestinal proteome of diabetic and control children is enriched with different microbial and host proteins. *Microbiology*, *163*(2), 161–174.

Polak, K., Bergler-Czop, B., Szczepanek, M., Wojciechowska, K., Frątczak, A., & Kiss, N. (2021). Psoriasis and gut microbiome—current state of art. *International Journal of Molecular Sciences, 22*(9), 4529. https://doi.org/10.3390/ijms22094529

Portincasa, P., Bonfrate, L., Vacca, M., De Angelis, M., Farella, I., Lanza, E., Khalil, M., Wang, D. Q., Sperandio, M., & Di Ciaula, A. (2022). Gut microbiota and short chain fatty acids: Implications in glucose homeostasis. *International Journal of Molecular Sciences, 23*(3), 1105. https://doi.org/10.3390/ijms23031105

Pot, B., Salvetti, E., Mattarelli, P., & Felis, G. E. (2019). The potential impact of the Lactobacillus name change: The results of an expert meeting organised by the lactic acid bacteria industrial platform (LABIP). *Trends in Food Science and Technology, 94,* 105–113. https://doi.org/10.1016/j.tifs.2019.07.006

Qazi, T., Amaratunga, T., Barnes, E. L., Fischer, M., Kassam, Z., & Allegretti, J. R. (2017). The risk of inflammatory bowel disease flares after fecal microbiota transplantation: Systematic review and meta-analysis. *Gut Microbes, 8*(6), 574–588. https://doi.org/10.1080/19490976.2017.1353848

Rahmah, P. A., Khairani, A. F., Atik, N., Arisanti, N., & Fatimah, S. N. (2021). Correlation of knowledge, attitude, and practice toward probiotics for the digestive system among health science students. *Journal of Multidisciplinary Healthcare, 14*, 1135–1144. https://doi.org/10.2147/JMDH.S305670

Rajanala, K., Kumar, N., & Chamallamudi, M. R. (2021). Modulation of gut-brain axis by probiotics: A promising anti-depressant approach. *Current Neuropharmacology, 19*(7), 990–1006. https://doi.org/10.2174/1570159X19666201215142520

Ray, K. (2021). Yeast probiotics for the treatment of IBD. *Nature Reviews. Gastroenterology and Hepatology, 18*(9), 594–594. https://doi.org/10.1038/s41575-021-00497-3

Riccio, P., & Rossano, R. (2020). The human gut microbiota is neither an organ nor a commensal. *FEBS Letters, 594*(20), 3262–3271. https://doi.org/10.1002/1873-3468.13946

Rousseaux, A., Brosseau, C., & Bodinier, M. (2023). Immunomodulation of B lymphocytes by prebiotics, probiotics and synbiotics: Application in pathologies. *Nutrients, 15*(2), 269. https://doi.org/10.3390/nu15020269

Russo, E., Giudici, F., Fiorindi, C., Ficari, F., Scaringi, S., & Amedei, A. (2019). Immunomodulating activity and therapeutic effects of short chain fatty acids and tryptophan post-biotics in inflammatory bowel disease. *Frontiers in Immunology, 10,* 2754. https://doi.org/10.3389/fimmu.2019.02754

Salim, S. Y., Kaplan, G. G., & Madsen, K. L. (2014). Air pollution effects on the gut microbiota: A link between exposure and inflammatory disease. *Gut Microbes, 5*(2), 215–219. https://doi.org/10.4161/gmic.27251

Santana, P. T., Rosas, S. L. B., Ribeiro, B. E., Marinho, Y., & de Souza, H. S. P. (2022). Dysbiosis in inflammatory bowel disease: Pathogenic role and potential therapeutic targets. *International Journal of Molecular Sciences, 23*(7), 3464. https://doi.org/10.3390/ijms23073464

Scher, J. U., Sczesnak, A., Longman, R. S., Segata, N., Ubeda, C., Bielski, C., Rostron, T., Cerundolo, V., Pamer, E. G., Abramson, S. B., Huttenhower, C., & Littman, D. R. (2013). Expansion of intestinal Prevotella copri correlates with enhanced susceptibility to arthritis. *eLife, 2,* e01202. https://doi.org/10.7554/eLife.01202

Sensoy, I. (2021). A review on the food digestion in the digestive tract and the used in vitro models. *Current Research in Food Science, 4,* 308–319. https://doi.org/10.1016/j.crfs.2021.04.004

Serek, P., & Oleksy-Wawrzyniak, M. (2021). The effect of bacterial infections, probiotics and zonulin on intestinal barrier integrity. *International Journal of Molecular Sciences, 22*(21), 11359. https://doi.org/10.3390/ijms222111359

Shaheen, W. A., Quraishi, M. N., & Iqbal, T. H. (2022). Gut microbiome and autoimmune disorders. *Clinical and Experimental Immunology, 209*(2), 161–174. https://doi.org/10.1093/cei/uxac057

Shin, D., Chang, S. Y., Bogere, P., Won, K., Choi, J. Y., Choi, Y. J., Lee, H. K., Hur, J., Park, B. Y., Kim, Y., & Heo, J. (2019). Beneficial roles of probiotics on the modulation of gut microbiota and immune response in pigs. *PLoS One, 14*(8), e0220843. https://doi.org/10.1371/journal.pone.0220843

Shirazinia, R., Golabchifar, A. A., & Fazeli, M. R. (2021). Efficacy of probiotics for managing infantile colic due to their anti-inflammatory properties: A meta-analysis and systematic review. *Clinical and Experimental Pediatrics, 64*(12), 642–651. https://doi.org/10.3345/cep.2020.01676

Shukla, R., Ghoshal, U., Ranjan, P., & Ghoshal, U. C. (2018). Expression of toll-like receptors, pro-, and anti-inflammatory cytokines in relation to gut microbiota in irritable bowel syndrome: The evidence for its micro-organic basis. *Journal of Neurogastroenterology and Motility, 24*(4), 628–642. https://doi.org/10.5056/jnm18130

Sikora, M., Stec, A., Chrabaszcz, M., Knot, A., Waskiel-Burnat, A., Rakowska, A., Olszewska, M., & Rudnicka, L. (2020). Gut microbiome in psoriasis: An updated review. *Pathogens, 9*(6), 463. https://doi.org/10.3390/pathogens9060463

Śliżewska, K., Markowiak-Kopeć, P., & Śliżewska, W. (2021). The role of probiotics in cancer prevention. *Cancers, 13*(1), 20. https://doi.org/10.3390/cancers13010020

Soyucen, E., Gulcan, A., Aktuglu-Zeybek, A. C., Onal, H., Kiykim, E., & Aydin, A. (2014). Differences in the gut microbiota of healthy children and those with type 1 diabetes. *Pediatrics International, 56*(3), 336–343. https://doi.org/10.1111/ped.12243

Stewart, C. J., Ajami, N. J., O'Brien, J. L., Hutchinson, D. S., Smith, D. P., Wong, M. C., Ross, M. C., Lloyd, R. E., Doddapaneni, H., Metcalf, G. A., Muzny, D., Gibbs, R. A., Vatanen, T., Huttenhower, C., Xavier, R. J., Rewers, M., Hagopian, W., Toppari, J., Ziegler, A. G., . . . Petrosino, J. F. (2018). Temporal development of the gut microbiome in early childhood from the TEDDY study. *Nature, 562*(7728), 583–588. https://doi.org/10.1038/s41586-018-0617-x

Su, X., Zhao, Y., Li, Y., Ma, S., & Wang, Z. (2020). Gut dysbiosis is associated with primary hypothyroidism with interaction on gut-thyroid axis. *Clinical Science, 134*(12), 1521–1535. https://doi.org/10.1042/CS20200475

Tantuway, V., Thomas, W., Parikh, M. B., Sharma, R., Jeyaraman, N., & Jeyaraman, M. (2023). Clinical outcome of minimally manipulated, mechanically isolated autologous adipose tissue-derived stromal vascular fraction (Sahaj Therapy®) in knee osteoarthritis—randomized controlled trial. *Indian Journal of Orthopaedics*, *57*(10), 1646–1658. https://doi.org/10.1007/s43465-023-00981-9

Thaiss, C. A., Itav, S., Rothschild, D., Meijer, M. T., Levy, M., Moresi, C., Dohnalová, L., Braverman, S., Rozin, S., Malitsky, S., Dori-Bachash, M., Kuperman, Y., Biton, I., Gertler, A., Harmelin, A., Shapiro, H., Halpern, Z., Aharoni, A., Segal, E., & Elinav, E. (2016). Persistent microbiome alterations modulate the rate of post-dieting weight regain. *Nature, 540*(7634), 544–551. https://doi.org/10.1038/nature20796

Thye, A. Y. K., Bah, Y. R., Law, J. W. F., Tan, L. T. H., He, Y. W., Wong, S. H., Thurairajasingam, S., Chan, K. G., Lee, L. H., & Letchumanan, V. (2022). Gut–skin axis: Unravelling the connection between the gut microbiome and psoriasis. *Biomedicines, 10*(5), 1037. https://doi.org/10.3390/biomedicines10051037

Tincati, C., Douek, D. C., & Marchetti, G. (2016). Gut barrier structure, mucosal immunity and intestinal microbiota in the pathogenesis and treatment of HIV infection. *AIDS Research and Therapy, 13*(1), 19. https://doi.org/10.1186/s12981-016-0103-1

Topi, S., Bottalico, L., Charitos, I. A., Colella, M., Di Domenico, M., Palmirotta, R., & Santacroce, L. (2022). Biomolecular mechanisms of autoimmune diseases and their relationship with the resident microbiota: Friend or foe? *Pathophysiology, 29*(3), 507–536.

Trofimiuk-Müldner, M., & Bała, M. M. (2023). Are probiotics, prebiotics, and synbiotics beneficial in primary thyroid diseases? A systematic review with meta-analysis. *Annals of Agricultural and Environmental Medicine, 30*(2), 217–223. https://doi.org/10.26444/aaem/162732

Vatanen, T., Franzosa, E. A., Schwager, R., Tripathi, S., Arthur, T. D., Vehik, K., Lernmark, Å., Hagopian, W. A., Rewers, M. J., She, J. X., Toppari, J., Ziegler, A. G., Akolkar, B., Krischer, J. P., Stewart, C. J., Ajami, N. J., Petrosino, J. F., Gevers, D., Lähdesmäki, H., . . . Xavier, R. J. (2018). The human gut microbiome in early-onset type 1 diabetes from the TEDDY study. *Nature, 562*(7728), 589–594. https://doi.org/10.1038/s41586-018-0620-2

Virili, C., Stramazzo, I., & Centanni, M. (2021). Gut microbiome and thyroid autoimmunity. *Best Practice and Research. Clinical Endocrinology and Metabolism, 35*(3), 101506. https://doi.org/10.1016/j.beem.2021.101506

Wang, J., Liu, S., Xie, Y., & Xu, C. (2023). Association analysis of gut microbiota-metabolites-neuroendocrine changes in male rats acute exposure to simulated altitude of 5500 m. *Scientific Reports, 13*(1), 9225. https://doi.org/10.1038/s41598-023-35573-y

Wells, P. M., Adebayo, A. S., Bowyer, R. C. E., Freidin, M. B., Finckh, A., Strowig, T., Lesker, T. R., Alpizar-Rodriguez, D., Gilbert, B., Kirkham, B., Cope, A. P., Steves, C. J., & Williams, F. M. K. (2020). Associations between gut microbiota and genetic risk for rheumatoid arthritis in the absence of disease: A cross-sectional study. *Lancet. Rheumatology, 2*(7), e418–e427. https://doi.org/10.1016/S2665-9913(20)30064-3

Wigner, P., Bijak, M., & Saluk-Bijak, J. (2022). Probiotics in the prevention of the calcium oxalate urolithiasis. *Cells, 11*(2), 284. https://doi.org/10.3390/cells11020284

Witkowski, M., Weeks, T. L., & Hazen, S. L. (2020). Gut microbiota and cardiovascular disease. *Circulation Research, 127*(4), 553–570. https://doi.org/10.1161/CIRCRESAHA.120.316242

Wu, C., Pan, L. L., Niu, W., Fang, X., Liang, W., Li, J., Li, H., Pan, X., Chen, W., Zhang, H., Lakey, J. R. T., Agerberth, B., de Vos, P., & Sun, J. (2019). Modulation of gut microbiota by low methoxyl pectin attenuates type 1 diabetes in non-obese diabetic mice. *Frontiers in Immunology, 10,* 1733. https://doi.org/10.3389/fimmu.2019.01733

Yang, L., Luo, S., Huang, G., Peng, J., Li, X., Yan, X., Lin, J., Wenzlau, J. M., Davidson, H. W., Hutton, J. C., & Zhou, Z. (2010). The diagnostic value of zinc transporter 8 autoantibody (ZnT8A) for type 1 diabetes in Chinese. *Diabetes/Metabolism Research and Reviews, 26*(7), 579–584. https://doi.org/10.1002/dmrr.1128

Yang, R., Jia, Q., Mehmood, S., Ma, S., & Liu, X. (2021). Genistein ameliorates inflammation and insulin resistance through mediation of gut microbiota composition in type 2 diabetic mice. *European Journal of Nutrition, 60*(4), 2155–2168. https://doi.org/10.1007/s00394-020-02403-0

Yao, H., Yang, H., Wang, Y., Xing, Q., Yan, L., & Chai, Y. (2022). Gut microbiome and fecal metabolic alteration in systemic lupus erythematosus patients with depression. *Frontiers in Cellular and Infection Microbiology, 12,* 1040211. https://doi.org/10.3389/fcimb.2022.1040211

Yoo, J. Y., Groer, M., Dutra, S. V. O., Sarkar, A., & McSkimming, D. I. (2020). Gut microbiota and immune system interactions. *Microorganisms, 8*(10), 1587.

You, S., Ma, Y., Yan, B., Pei, W., Wu, Q., Ding, C., & Huang, C. (2022). The promotion mechanism of prebiotics for probiotics: A review. *Frontiers in Nutrition, 9,* 1000517. https://doi.org/10.3389/fnut.2022.1000517

Zermiani, A. P. D. R. B., de Paula, A. L. P. P., Miguel, E. R. A., Lopes, L. D. G., Santana, N. D. C. S., da Silva Santos, T., Demarchi, I. G., & Teixeira, J. J. (2021). Evidence of Lactobacillus reuteri to reduce colic in breastfed babies: Systematic review and meta-analysis. *Complementary Therapies in Medicine, 63,* 102781. https://doi.org/10.1016/j.ctim.2021.102781

Zhang, J., Zhang, F., Zhao, C., Xu, Q., Liang, C., Yang, Y., Wang, H., Shang, Y., Wang, Y., Mu, X., Zhu, D., Zhang, C., Yang, J., Yao, M., & Zhang, L. (2019). Dysbiosis of the gut microbiome is associated with thyroid cancer and thyroid nodules and correlated with clinical index of thyroid function. *Endocrine, 64*(3), 564–574. https://doi.org/10.1007/s12020-018-1831-x

Zhang, L., Qing, P., Yang, H., Wu, Y., Liu, Y., & Luo, Y. (2021). Gut microbiome and metabolites in systemic lupus erythematosus: Link, mechanisms and intervention. *Frontiers in Immunology, 12*, 686501.

Zhang, S., Wang, R., Li, D., Zhao, L., & Zhu, L. (2021). Role of gut microbiota in functional constipation. *Gastroenterology Report, 9*(5), 392–401. https://doi.org/10.1093/gastro/goab035

Zheng, P., Li, Z., & Zhou, Z. (2018). Gut microbiome in type 1 diabetes: A comprehensive review. *Diabetes/Metabolism Research and Reviews, 34*(7), e3043. https://doi.org/10.1002/dmrr.3043

Zhou, H., Zhao, X., Sun, L., Liu, Y., Lv, Y., Gang, X., & Wang, G. (2020). Gut microbiota profile in patients with type 1 diabetes based on 16S rRNA gene sequencing: A systematic review. *Disease Markers, 2020*, 3936247. https://doi.org/10.1155/2020/3936247

Zhuang, X., Xiong, L., Li, L., Li, M., & Chen, M. (2017). Alterations of gut microbiota in patients with irritable bowel syndrome: A systematic review and meta-analysis. *Journal of Gastroenterology and Hepatology, 32*(1), 28–38. https://doi.org/10.1111/jgh.13471

3 Gut Microbiota and Nutrient Enrichment

Mechanism and Production of Vitamins

Rizwan Ahamad and Sadma Parveen

3.1 INTRODUCTION

The gastrointestinal system has significant importance as a fundamental component of the human body. It serves as a means of transportation and assimilation for the nutrients ingested (Thursby & Juge, 2017). The environment in question is a habitat for several categories of microorganisms, including archaea, bacteria, and eukarya. These bacteria are well recognized as the "gut microbiota". The major phyla in this composition are Firmicutes and Bacteroidetes, whereas Actinobacteria, Proteobacteria, and Verrucomicrobia are present as minority members (Marchesi, 2010; Arumugam et al., 2011). The organisms establish a mutually beneficial association with the host and defend against detrimental infections (Bäumler & Sperandio, 2016). Intestinal fermentation is known to promote energy usage (den Besten et al., 2013) and alter host immunological activity and signaling molecules (Gensollen et al., 2016). The human gut microbiota has distinct characteristics and exhibits a notable level of stability, rendering it very resistant to alterations (Dogra et al., 2020). However, it is important to note that these entities are not static; rather, they exhibit a dynamic nature and undergo changes in their composition across various phases of our lives (O'Toole & Claesson, 2010). Numerous variables, including the mode of childbirth (Neu & Rushing, 2011), the age of the individual (Odamaki et al., 2016), lifestyle choices, medication use, and notably, dietary patterns (Heiman & Greenway, 2016), have a substantial impact on the makeup of the gut microbiota.

However, it is important to note that the human gut also contains bacteria that are capable of synthesizing certain B vitamins, such as biotin, cobalamin, folate, niacin, pantothenate, PN, riboflavin, and thiamine. It should be noted, however, that the production of these vitamins by gut bacteria is restricted (Uebanso et al., 2020). Certain gut bacteria have a dependency on certain vitamins to facilitate their development. Concurrently, the presence of auxotrophic bacteria engenders a competitive environment among these bacterial species. The insufficiency of these vitamins hinders the regular functioning of cellular ingestion and initiates the progression of various chronic illnesses in the human body. Hence, B vitamins are important for both the host organism and the resident gut bacteria. The provision of these vitamins in one's food is crucial to fulfill the daily needs of the host, as stated by Hossain et al. (2022). B vitamins are known to have significant impacts on the composition and abundance of the gut flora. There is a substantial body of information indicating that the maintenance of a healthy gut is closely associated with a balanced and thriving microbial ecosystem. Hence, it is essential to delineate the connection between the gut microbiota and its impact on gut health.

The presence of around 10^{14}–10^{15}microbial cells inside the human body has been estimated (Sender et al., 2016). It is believed that these microbial cells exceed the permissive cells in the adult body by an amount of minimum ratio of 10:1. This claim was subsequently challenged since a more recent estimate suggests that the ratio is far closer to a 1:1 proportion (Sender et al., 2016). Significantly, the diversity of the human gut flora surpasses that of human cells, hence contributing to the intricacy involved in comprehending the impact of microorganisms and their inhalation on haleness and the modulation of ailment development (McFall-Ngai et al., 2013).

DOI: 10.1201/9781003452249-3

3.2 THE IMPACT OF NUTRITIOUS MICRONUTRIENTS ON GUT FLORA MODULATION

3.2.1 Polyphenols

Polyphenols, including stilbenes, phenolic acids, flavonoids, and lignans, derived from many sources such as tea, fruits, vegetables, coffee, cereals, and wine, have garnered significant attention in study owing to their prospective antioxidant, anti-inflammatory, along with anticarcinogenic properties (Williamson, 2017; Puupponen-Pimiä et al., 2002; Han et al., 2007). According to *in-vitro* research, polyphenols could influence the composition of the human gut flora. They may do this by suppressing the development of potentially harmful organisms like *H. pylori* and *Staphylococcus* species while promoting the proliferation of good bacteria such as lactobacillus and Bifidobacteria (Selma et al., 2009).

Previous research conducted in laboratory settings, known as *in-vitro* studies, has demonstrated that certain compounds found in plants called flavonoids, including phenolic acids (such as *p*-coumaric acid, epicatechins, and *o*-coumaric acid), anthocyanins, and other polyphenols like rutin, quercetin, caffeic acid, and chlorogenic acid, have the potential to enhance the presence of beneficial microorganisms in the gut, specifically *Bifidobacterium* and *Lactobacillus*. Additionally, these compounds have been found to reduce the colonization of potentially harmful bacteria in the human gut (Selma et al., 2009; Tabasco et al., 2011). Previous studies have shown that catechins could promote the proliferation of *Escherichia coli*, *Clostridium coccoides*, *Eubacterium rectale* group, and *Bifidobacterium* sp., while concurrently inhibiting the development of a possible pathogenic organism, namely the *Clostridium hystolyticum* group (Tzounis et al., 2008). The process of fermenting polyphenols has been shown to have a fringe benefit on the population of valuable microbiota, like Bifidobacteria. This fermentation process also leads to a decrease in the F/B ratio by facilitating the development of certain individuals belonging to the phylum Bacteroidetes (Parkar et al., 2013). The authors put out the suggestion that the metabolic transformation of polyphenols facilitated the synthesis of SCFAs, which are acknowledged for their significant contribution to gastrointestinal and metabolic well-being (Topping & Clifton, 2001). Through the use of agar plate tests, it was shown that naringenin, a flavone compound found in citrus products, influenced the proliferation and inborn control of gut-associated bacteria (Firrman et al., 2018).

3.2.2 Vitamins

Vitamins are organic chemicals that play a crucial role in maintaining proper physiological function, requiring minimal quantities for optimal support. Co-factors for enzymes play a crucial role in the body, serving a diverse range of functions. Food serves as the main provider of vitamins since our bodies are unable to produce them in sufficient quantities to fulfill our daily requirements. However, it is worth noting that some vitamins, such as phylloquinone and B vitamins, are created by the microbiota present in our GIT (Rowland et al., 2018). The presence of vitamin deficiencies may lead to the development or worsening of chronic health issues. It is often seen that individuals with inadequate intake or immersion of vitamins in the superior GIT might dominate the composition and variety of the gut flora. Multiple vitamin supplements have the capacity to provide significantly elevated levels of individual vitamins. Consequently, the limited assimilation of vitamins in superior GIT might supreme the composition and variety of the gut flora. Figure 3.1 provides a schematic overview of the bacteria capable of synthesizing B vitamins, as well as the consequences of B vitamin deficiencies on gut health.

3.2.2.1 Thiamine (Vitamin B1)

Thiamine is a vital component that is necessary for the proper functioning of several enzymes, including those involved in the TCA cycle, and glycolysis with the pentose phosphate route

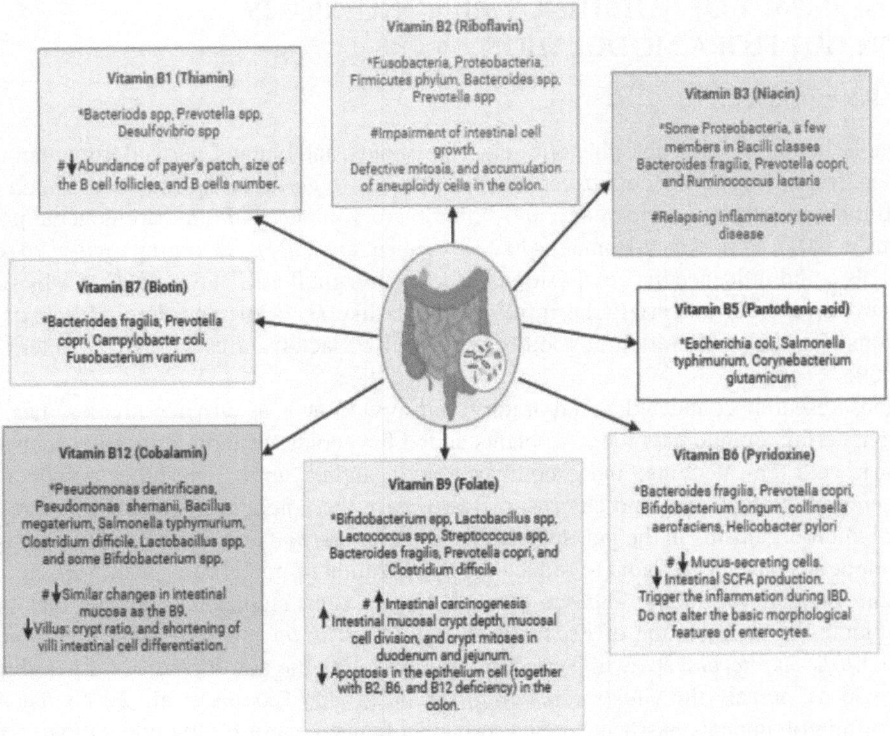

FIGURE 3.1 A schematic representation listing the bacteria that can synthesize B vitamins and the effects of B vitamin deficiencies on gut health.

Note: *Microbes that involved in the biosynthesis of vitamins.

#The impacts of deficiencies.

(Manzetti et al., 2014). Multiple bacterial species can produce unbound thiamine or its biologically vital form, TPP (Said, 2013). Nevertheless, it has been shown that bacteria classified under enterotype 2 have a greater potential for thiamine biosynthesis. The bacterial taxa *Prevotella* and *Desulfovibrio* are seen to have increased expression of four enzymes, namely phosphomethylpyridine kinase, hydroxymethylpyridine kinase, thiaminephosphate pyrophosphorylase, and thiamine-monophosphate kinase. These enzymes play a critical role in manufacturing thiamine (Arumugam et al., 2011). Furthermore, it has been shown that over 90% of other *Bacteroides* sp. that are linked with the stomach have the capacity for thiamine production and contain the genes responsible for thiamine transportation (Costliow & Degnan, 2017). The absorption of dietary thiamine occurs via carrier-mediated delivery mechanisms, namely high-binding THTR-1 and THTR-2, which are found in the membrane and sheath of the small intestine (Manzetti et al., 2014). In the case of dietary thiamine being present in a bound form, such as TPP, it must undergo a conversion process into free thiamine before absorption. Similarly, the aforementioned transporters, namely THTR-1 and THTR-2, play a crucial role in facilitating the uptake of thiamine that is generated by bacteria in the colon (Nabokina et al., 2014). Nevertheless, it has been shown that the TPP generated by the gut flora is taken up directly by the TPP mediator, namely TPPT-1 (Nabokina et al., 2014). This finding suggests a distinction between the absorption of TPP derived from food and that created by bacteria. The precise mechanisms through which thiamine influences intestinal integrity remain unclear. However, an extended body of attestation suggests that thiamine may have a role in regulating immunological activities connected to the gut, maybe via its involvement in energy metabolism.

3.2.2.2 Riboflavin (Vitamin B2)

Riboflavin, a vitamin, has an aspect in the metabolic processes of fats, carbohydrates, and proteins, namely in energy production (Sriram et al., 2012). The conversion of riboflavin to its nimble forms, namely, FAD and FMN, is facilitated by the enzymes riboflavin and FAD integrate, respectively. The production of riboflavin by the human gut bacteria is largely seen in the large intestine (Said, 2013). The ingestion of dietary riboflavin in the form of FAD or FMN necessitates its conversion into free riboflavin before absorption (Home Page, n.d.). The absorption of riboflavin in humans mostly happens in the proximal lower intestine via active carrier-mediated transportation (Steinert et al., 2016). The presence of a fully intact riboflavin operator gene is seen in Fusobacteria and Baceteroidetes, additionally in 92% of Proteobacteria. This suggests that these bacterial groups are the main contributors to riboflavin production inside the GIT. Moreover, it has been estimated that around 50% of the Firmicutes phylum can synthesize riboflavin (Magnúsdóttir et al., 2015). Lactic acid bacteria derived from dairy products have been shown to exhibit the ability to synthesize riboflavin (Thakur et al., 2015). The production of riboflavin in bacteria involves the use of GTP, a molecule via the purine biotransformation route, and ribulose-5-phosphate, an intermediary generated via the pentose phosphate track (García-Angulo, 2017).

3.2.2.3 Niacin (Vitamin B3)

Vitamin B3, sometimes referred to as niacin, nicotinic acid, or nicotinamide, undergoes a conversion process to produce its biologically active form, known as NAD. NAD plays a crucial role as a redox cofactor in several vital metabolic activities (Qi et al., 2019). Intestinal bacteria, like other complex organisms, primarily produce vitamin B3 by metabolizing the amino acid tryptophan via a distinct mechanism (Gazzaniga et al., 2009). Based on the genetic evaluation, it has been shown that the *Bacilli* class has a total of four possible niacin-producing bacteria, while the *Clostridia* class consists of 44 such bacteria. Additionally, the Proteobacteria class has been found to have 29 major niacin-synthesizing germs. *P. copri*, *Bacteroides fragilis*, and *Ruminococcus lactaris* can synthesize vitamin B3 inside the GIT due to the presence of a vitamin B3 biosynthesis pathway (Magnúsdóttir et al., 2015).

Additionally, it should be noted that the NiaR has been identified in a wide range of *Clostridium* and *Bacillus* microbes, indicating their ability to undertake the process of de novo synthesis of NAD (Rodionov et al., 2008). Both human and animal colonic cuticle cells have a very effective, selective, and controlled channel for the absorption of vitamin B3. Niacin, which is generated by bacteria, has a role in providing sustenance to colonocytes in the surrounding environment and preserving the structure of intestinal stem cells (Kumar et al., 2013). The focus cohort conducted research that established a correlation between vitamin B3 and the makeup of gut microbes. A significant correlation was seen between a shortage in vitamin B3 and reduced microbial diversity, as well as decreased levels of Bacteroidetes, among those who are obese. The prevalence of this bacterium was notably greater with a gastrointestinal-focused detained-release administration of nicotinic acid, barring nicotinamide, in individuals with obesity (Hossain et al., 2022). Vitamin B3 is essential in the mitigation of inflammation and is implicated in the expansion of recurrent demagogic bowel illnesses, like ulcerative colitis, in cases of deficiency. The mechanism by which it exerts its anti-inflammatory effects involves the inhibition in intestinal tissues via the activation of the PGD2/DP1 signal in cuticle cells (Li et al., 2017).

3.2.2.4 Pantothenic Acid (Vitamin B5)

Vitamin B5, also known as pantothenic acid, serves as a necessary precursor for the production of CoA and functions as an acyl transporter (Ragaller et al., 2011). The compound has a role in several metabolic pathways, including the cycle of citric acid, cellular development, production of neurotransmitters, and oxidation of fatty acids (Hayflick, 2014). Several bacterial species, such as *S. typhimurium*, *E. coli*, and *Corynebacterium glutamicum*, can biosynthesize pantothenic acid. Aspartate and interposed metabolites derived from valine biogenesis are used in the production of vitamin B5 (Leonardi & Jackowski, 2007). As an example, *S. typhimurium* synthesizes pantothenate by utilizing acetohydroxy acid synthetase, isozyme I, and dihydroxy acid dehydratase catalyst, which convert ketoisovalerate into pantothenate (Epelbaum et al., 1998). In addition, additional bacteria, namely *Lactobacillus helveticus*, rely on vitamin B5 for their Vitamin Hand fatty acid metabolic processes (Yao et al., 2018). The addition of vitamin B5 to the diet has an impact on the structure of gut flora. The intake of pantothenic acid was shown to have a positive effect on the comparative abundance of *Actinobacteria* and *Prevotella*, while simultaneously reducing the quantity of *Bacteroides* in breastfeeding mothers (Carrothers et al., 2015).

3.2.2.5 Pyridoxine (Vitamin B6)

Vitamin B6 is composed of six vitamers, namely PL, PN, PM, and their organic compound counterparts, especially PLP, PMP, and PNP (Parra et al., 2018). PLP is considered the major biologically vigorous form of PN, exhibiting high enzymatic activity. Vitamin B6 functions as a cofactor in several metabolic activities, particularly working in the production and catabolism of amino acids. In addition to these functions, it has a significant function in the biosynthesis of fatty acids and neurotransmitters and exhibits antioxidant properties (Mooney et al., 2009). Within the GIT of mammals, microorganisms can produce vitamin B6 via either de novo biosynthesis or salvage routes. Microorganisms, including *P. copri* and *B. fragilis* from the Bacteroidetes phylum, *B. longum* and *Collinsella aerofaciens* from the Actinobacteria phylum, and *H. pylori* from the Proteobacteria phylum, possess the ability to synthesize vitamin B6 due to their possession of the necessary metabolic pathways (Yoshii et al., 2019).

The majority of nourishing vitamins are taken inside the small intestine. Nevertheless, there is still a certain level of absorption of comestible and bacterially produced PN that happens in the superior intestine. This is due to the presence of PN transporters that are manifest in the human colon. Prokaryotes and single-cell eukaryotes that are unable to synthesize vitamin B6 have a dependency on acquiring this vitamin from their external environment. In contrast, multicellular organisms can transport vitamin B6 to various organs inside their bodies after absorption (Mooney et al., 2009). The endogenous synthesis of vitamin B6 in the GIT is inadequate to meet the daily nutritional needs of the host. The lack of this substance resulted in lower microbial variation and a substantial alteration in intestinal metabolite levels when compared with the normal groups in rats. The presence of a significant number of Lachnospiraceae_NK4A136_group (Mayengbam et al., 2020) and Prevotella was found to be increased in individuals with PN deficiency, whereas the plenty of Bacteroides was seen to be reduced in individuals with high vitamin B6 consumption (Carrothers et al., 2015).

3.2.2.6 Biotin (Vitamin B7)

Biotin acts as a coenzyme in many metabolic activities, including glycolysis (Bistas & Tadi, 2023), as well as in cellular signaling and epigenetic controls (Yao et al., 2018). In addition, it exerts regulatory influence on gene expression, particularly concerning NF-kB, via a histone binding activity. Biotinylation is a process well recognized in the scientific community (Liu et al., 2017), Hence, it is plausible that this particular vitamin has anti-inflammatory properties as well. Biotin is mostly biosynthesized by the use of either malonyl CoA or Pimeloyl-CoA as reported in previous studies (Bi et al., 2016). There is an overrepresentation of enzymes involved in the biotin biosynthesis pathway. Enterotype 1, which is characterized by plenty of Bacteroides (Arumugam et al., 2011), is seen. Bacterial strains capable of synthesizing vitamin B7 including the microorganisms mentioned in the text include *Fusobacterium varium*, *B. fragilis*, *Campylobacter coli*, and *P. copri* (Arumugam et al., 2011).

3.2.2.7 Folate (Vitamin B9)

Folate, or vitamin B9, is a compound resulting from the conjugation of 4-aminobenzoic acid and l-glutamic acid. The primary source of vitamin B9 for the host is derived from dietary intake, with a small contribution from the gut bacteria (Iyer & Tomar, 2009). Folate is a crucial nutrient that serves as a methyl donor, supplying one-carbon units. Additionally, folate works in the production of SAM, which is necessary for cellular biosynthesis and DNA methylation (Alves da Silva et al., 2018). Vitamin deficiency has been proven to have a crucial impact on cell longevity and proliferation due to its crucial role in the replication and restoration of nucleic acids (Stover, 2004). Moreover, folate has a vital role in the regulation of gene activity, the regeneration of the intestinal lining, the production of essential chemicals for optimal brain function, the inhibition of lymphocyte expansion, and the reduction of organic killer cellular cytotoxicity (Gazzali et al., 2016). Therefore, it can be inferred that folate is an essential component for the functioning of all living cells since it is involved in several biochemical and biosynthetic processes. The biological processes under consideration exhibit universality; however, their metabolic pathways exhibit variation across different organisms. Various organisms, including fungi, bacteria, plants, and some archaea, could engage in the process of folate biosynthesis. These organisms use a comparable route with minor adjustments (de Crécy-Lagard et al., 2007).

Several bacterial species have been identified as producers of vitamin B9 in the gut. These comprise *B. fragilis*, *Clostridium difficile*, *Lactobacillus plantarum*, *P. copri*, *L. delbrueckii* sp. *bulgaricus*, *L. reuteri*, *Streptococcus thermophilus*, certain species of *Bifidobacterium*, *Fusobacterium varium*, and *Salmonella enterica* (Magnúsdóttir et al., 2015). Among these bacteria, *Bifidobacterium* spp. have been extensively investigated in academic research. The microorganisms may be classified according to their capacity to create folate. The high vitamin B9 producers include *B. longum* subsp. Infantis and *Bifidobacterium bifidum*, whereas the low folate producers consist of *B. longum* subsp. *Longum B. breve*, and *B. adolescentis*. The process of vitamin B9 synthesis involves the incorporation of a pterin segment derived from DHCP and a PABA. The latter refers to a midway compound that is produced by the process of cleaving pyruvate using the enzyme 4-amino-4-deoxychorismate lyase (*Nutrients | Free Full-Text*, n.d.). The presence of these enzymes is mostly limited to the genes of *Bifidobacterium* sp., namely *B. dentium* Bd1 and *B. adolescentis* (Turroni et al., 2010, p. 210). Consequently, these enzymes are responsible for the synthesis of folate in the presence of DHPP lactobacilli are also among the often-seen bacteria that possess the ability to produce folate. In contrast to *Bifidobacterium*, many species of *Lactobacillus*, like *L. sakei*, *L. plantarum*, *L. reuteri*, *L. delbrueckii*, *L. helveticus*, along with *L. fermentum*, can create DHCP. Consequently, these species are capable of synthesizing folate in the presence of PABA (*Nutrients | Free Full-Text*, n.d.). However, it should be noted that both *Lactococcus* and *Streptococcus* bacteria have a fully functional route for the synthesis of folate from scratch, and as a result, they do not rely on the availability of DHPP or PABA (Makarova & Koonin, 2007).

3.2.2.8 Cobalamin (Vitamin B12)

Cobalamin, or cobalamin, is a vitamin of significant size and complexity (Watanabe, 2007). Other type of this vitamin incorporates methyl-, deoxyadenosyl-, cyano-, and hydroxycobalamin. Cyano form existence is minimal in the food, and it serves as a supplement to the diet (Herrmann & Geisel, 2002). Similar to folate, cobalamin engages in a role in the production of methyl donors, including SAM. The presence of methyl donors is of utmost importance in the processes of nucleic acid synthesis, as well as protein and lipid metabolism (*Present Knowledge in Nutrition 11th Edition*, n.d.). Cobalamin serves as a cofactor in the enzymatic activity of methionine synthase, facilitating the metabolic process of sulfur amino acids. The described enzymatic process is responsible for the conversion of homocysteine to methionine, hence recycling the former compound. This information is supported by references. Cobalamin is essential for the effective operation of the nerve system with the production of red blood corpuscle (Ross et al., 2012).

The human abdomen has a restricted number of bacteria capable of synthesizing vitamin B12, with the majority using precorrin-2 as a precursor (Magnúsdóttir et al., 2015). It has been shown that about 20% of the bacteria residing in the GIT can synthesize vitamin B12, whereas over 80% of the gut bacteria rely on vitamin B12 for their metabolic processes (Kelly et al., 2019). The biosynthesis of vitamin B12 by bacteria encompasses the use of around 30 genes and may occur via either aerobic or opposite metabolic route. The aerobic process was investigated via *Pseudomonas denitrificans*, whereas the anaerobic process was examined in *Bacillus megaterium*, *S. typhimurium*, along with *P. shermanii* (Moore & Warren, 2012). Traditionally, it was believed that *Lactobacillus* spp. lacked the ability to synthesize vitamin B12. Nevertheless, the revelation of the glycerol-to-propanediol conversion in lactic acid bacteria has shown their aptitude for synthesizing vitamin B12 (Kleerebezem & Hugenholtz, 2003).

3.2.3 Minerals and Microelements

Minerals and microelements are crucial micronutrients for human consumption and engage in active interactions with the abdomen microbiota (Skrypnik & Suliburska, 2018; Gîlcă-Blanariu et al., 2018). Both inadequate nutrition and excessive intake of minerals and trace elements have led to the development of many illnesses in the human population.

According to epidemiological statistics, there is an observed correlation between increased calcium consumption and a reduced incidence of obesity. There is a suggestion that increased consumption of calcium is linked to alterations in the abdomen flora, which in turn are connected to a slant phenotype (Zhang et al., 2019; Gomes et al., 2015). In an intervention trial including healthy individuals, the consumption of 1000 mg of calcium per day for a duration of 8 weeks led to an increased presence of *Clostridium* XVIII in the fecal samples of male participants (Trautvetter et al., 2018). Due to its status as an unculturable bacterium, the classification of this bacterial species as either helpful or harmful remains undetermined. However, the presence of calcium and phosphorous in a combined dosage of 1000 mg P and 500 mg Ca has the potential to promote the proliferation of butyrate-producing microorganisms in the fecal matter. Research was done to check out the impact of hypocalcemia on body's weight increase in the offspring throughout several generations (Garg et al., 2018). The presence of excessive nutritious calcium (12 g/kg) in the parental diet was shown to be linked to a reduction in Verrucomicrobia in the gut of the offspring. Conversely, inadequate calcium intake in the parental diet (2.5 g/kg) was related to an elevated ratio of F/B in the descendant (Li et al., 2019).

3.3 THE PERSUASIVENESS OF NUTRITIONAL MACRONUTRIENTS ON MODULATION OF GUT FLORA

The influence of dietary macronutrients on the modulation of intestinal microorganisms has been described in Figure 3.2.

3.3.1 Carbohydrates

Carbohydrates act as the primary source of power for the human body and have a major impact on the modulation and structure of the gut flora. Carbohydrates originating from plants that are not digested in the superior digestive system are categorized as digestible fiber. The structure of these carbohydrates, together with other undigested nutrition, has a role in determining the degree to which they are fermented by the bacteria in the superior intestine. Many previous trials have proven that the Western-style diet, characterized by a comparatively reduced fiber portion, has the capacity to diminish the prevalence of *Bifidobacterium* with the overall variety of the gut microbiota (Schroeder et al., 2018). A persistent deficiency in dietary fiber has the potential to diminish the variety of gut germs (Prajapati et al., 2016). Research has shown that the consumption of a pre-Hispanic Mexican food, which is rich in fiber, may ameliorate gut dysbiosis in rats who are given an HFD supplemented with sucrose. This is proven by a reduction in the ratio of F/B ratio and an increase in the abundance of *Lactobacillus* sp. (Avila-Nava et al., 2017).

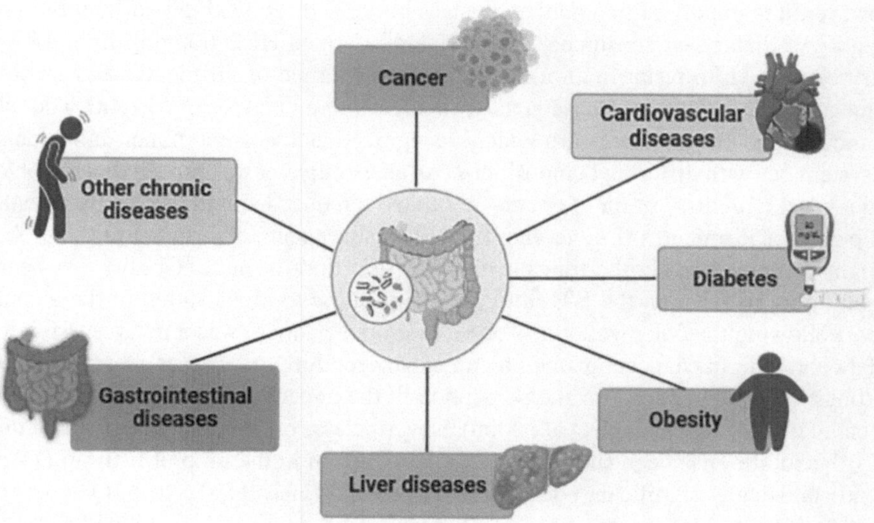

FIGURE 3.2 The role of diet macronutrients in modulating the intestinal microorganisms.

Numerous clinical studies have consistently shown that the implementation of a high-fiber food intervention, including the consumption of inulin, complete grain cereal, along with fructo-oligosaccharide (mixed in a 1:1 ratio), solvable-corn fiber, and forage kernel-rooted bread, leads to an elevation in the presence of various beneficial microbiota in fecal samples. These microbiota include *Bifidobacterium* sp., *Lactobacillus* sp. (García-Peris et al., 2012), *Fecalibacterium* sp., *Akkermansia* sp., *Roseburia* sp., *Bacteroides* sp. (Candela et al., 2016), and *Prevotella* sp. (Kovatcheva-Datchary et al., 2015). Additionally, diets that are loaded with fiber have been indicated to decrease the ratio of F/B ratio (De Filippo et al., 2010) and enhance the variety of gut microbial populations (Candela et al., 2016; De Filippo et al., 2010). The study found that obese individuals had a decreased percentage of Bacteroidetes compared to lean individuals. The percentage of Bacteroidetes exhibited an increase when individuals followed a carbohydrate-sparse low-calorie food for 1 year. This increase was seen in response to weight reduction. In addition, it was shown that obese individuals exhibited an augmentation in the presence of advantageous species such as *Prevotella*, *Parabacteroides distasonis*, and *Fecalibacterium prausnitzii* inside their gut microbiome subsequent to the intake of a high-compound carbohydrate diet (specifically, low-fat with 28% fat content) for 1 year (Haro et al., 2016).

3.3.2 Fat

Research repeatedly demonstrates that a dietary schedule characterized by greater levels of saturated and/or total fat has consistently been associated with negative effects on the gut flora. A total of 15 clinical declaim, consisting of 6 randomized restrained interventional trials and 9 observational reports, have provided evidence indicating that foods that have higher in complete and saturated fat have an adverse impact on the lavishness and multifariousness of gut flora (Wolters et al., 2019). The aforementioned results were substantiated by meticulously conducted feeding experiments on mice. These experiments showed that diets with varying fat content, ranging from 44% to 72%, led to an elevation in the ratio of F/B in gut flora (Ley et al., 2005; Hamilton et al., 2015; Chen et al., 2018; Cowan et al., 2014).

Earlier studies have indicated that alterations in the ratio of F/B within the gut flora are contingent upon both the specific location of the intestine and the length of ingestion (Hamilton et al.,

2015). However, it is important to note that changes in the F/B ratio exhibit variability in response to the quantity of dietary fat consumed. The intake of a mixed HFD (ranging from 44% to 72%) in rats has been shown to result in an increase in the plentitude of Firmicutes and a reduction in the percentage of Bacteroidetes. Consequently, this leads to an elevated F/B ratio. The pathogens phyla Firmicutes and Bacteroidetes are widely recognized as the predominant inhabitants of the digestive system but with differing compositions. As an example, it was proven that the ob/ob mice, which had a genetic predisposition to obesity, exhibited a reduced abundance of Bacteroidetes and increased plenty of Firmicutes (Ley et al., 2005). The study team also found that the obese phenotype might be conveyed via the transplantation of gut flora in mice. Obesity has been shown to contribute to an increase in the F/B ratio, thereby leading to an elevation in the abundance of Firmicutes. Following the colonization of "obese microbiota", there was a notable rise in the overall body fat content in mice, accompanied by an enhanced ability to extract energy from the food. These findings have implications for the perception of the underlying mechanisms involved in the development of obesity (Turnbaugh et al., 2006). Nevertheless, varying the proportion of dietary fat between 20% and 40% has been shown to lead to a reduction in the ratio of F/B ratio (Wan et al., 2019), or no statistically significant alterations in this ratio (Haro et al., 2016; Qiao et al., 2013). Moreover, the gut microbial compositions in rat models caused by a HFD exhibited a higher prevalence of microorganisms belonging to the order Clostridiales, whereas there was a reduction in the prevalence of microbes from the family Lachnospiraceae. This drop in abundance may be linked to its correlation with body fat percentage, as shown by previous research (Collins et al., 2016).

3.3.3 Protein

Animal studies have provided data indicating that the quality of protein has an impact on the makeup of gut bacteria. In a test investigation, it was indicated that the proteins found in cheese whey has the potential to function as growth element for the enumeration of Bifidobacteria and lactobacilli in fecal samples, as compared to casein (Sprong et al., 2010). Additionally, it was proven that the utilization of a diet mostly composed of whey protein resulted in a decrease in the prevalence of *Clostridium* (McAllan et al., 2014) inside the GIT.

The study demonstrated that the protein derived from mung beans successfully reversed the HFD-instigate ratio of F/B in mice. The protein derived from mung beans also showed an increase in the prevalence of the Ruminococcacea family inside HFD mice replicas. Based on the aforementioned result, the scientists formulated a hypothesis suggesting that the metabolism of bile acids by members of the Ruminococcacea family may have had a beneficial effect on mice fed an HFD (Nakatani et al., 2018). In disparity with the findings shown in plant-dependent protein treatments, it was noticed that diets containing casein led to an elevation in fecal Enterobacteriaceae and a reduction in fecal lactobacilli in pigs (Rist et al., 2014). Additionally, it was shown that the abundance of Bacteroidales and Clostridiales was elevated in mice that were given a Western food characterized by a higher content of meat and seafood (Holm et al., 2016). Additionally, research has demonstrated that the consumption of animal-based protein can heighten susceptibility to intestinal inflammation by promoting the growth of potentially harmful gut microbiota, such as *Enterococcus*, *Streptococcus*, *Turicibater*, *Escherichia*, Peptostreptococcaceae, and Ruminococcaceaea genera, in comparison to mice consuming a plant-based protein (Kostovcikova et al., 2019). The findings of a recent clinical investigation have brought attention to the potential risks associated with casein and soy protein diets. It has been seen that these diets may disrupt the regular protein expression in the abdominal mucosa of heavy persons. Therefore, care should be taken when considering the use of these diets. The scientists did not see any alterations in microbial diverseness or shifts in the plenty of certain taxa. However, they were able to identify the presence of both advantageous and deleterious metabolites generated by certain microorganisms. The scientists observed a major increase in metabolites entangled in the degradation of amino acids, accompanied by a notable decrease in the concentration of butyrate. This decrease in butyrate concentration was shown to be strongly associated with certain bacteria belonging to the genera *Oscilospira*, *Clostridia*, *Odoribacter* and *Butyricimonas* (Beaumont et al., 2017).

3.4 THE INFLUENCE OF GUT MICROBIOTA AND DIETARY PATTERNS ON HUMAN DISEASE AND HEALTH

The gut microbiome plays a key role in human health and influences digestion, nutrient absorption, and immune function. Unbalanced gut microbiomes are associated with various diseases which have been shown in Figure 3.3.

The makeup of the human microbiota exhibits variability across people, and this variability is significant enough to distinguish people within a greater population (Franzosa et al., 2015). Research findings have shown major variations in the physiology of the gut microbiome among persons who are in good health. Research findings have shown that around 80% of the gut microbiota in humans remains consistent for a minimum duration of 1 year.

A comparative analysis of 124 individual meta-genomes was conducted to examine the differences between healthy, overweight, and obese persons. The findings of this research indicate that patients diagnosed with IBD exhibit a notable decrease in the number of non-redundant bacterial genes compared to healthy participants (Qin et al., 2010). It is noteworthy that there is a substantial correlation between functional chromosome and gene sum up and a people's clinical condition, suggesting that these factors might potentially serve as interpretation tools for human bowel illnesses. Agrarian communities have a lower prevalence of IBD and added allergens compared to Western civilizations (Lozupone et al., 2012). Significantly, alterations in the bacterial constitution of the human gut flora have been linked to gastrointestinal disorders like IBD, obesity, IBS, and diabetes.

Obesity arises as a result of an extended disparity between the amount of energy consumed and the amount expended, which is influenced by a complex interaction of genetic predisposition, dietary factors, physiological factors, social factors, and environmental variables. There exists a hypothesis suggesting that gut flora might play a crucial role in the evolution and progression of obesity. Individuals classified as obese have reduced alpha diversity in their gut microbiota compared

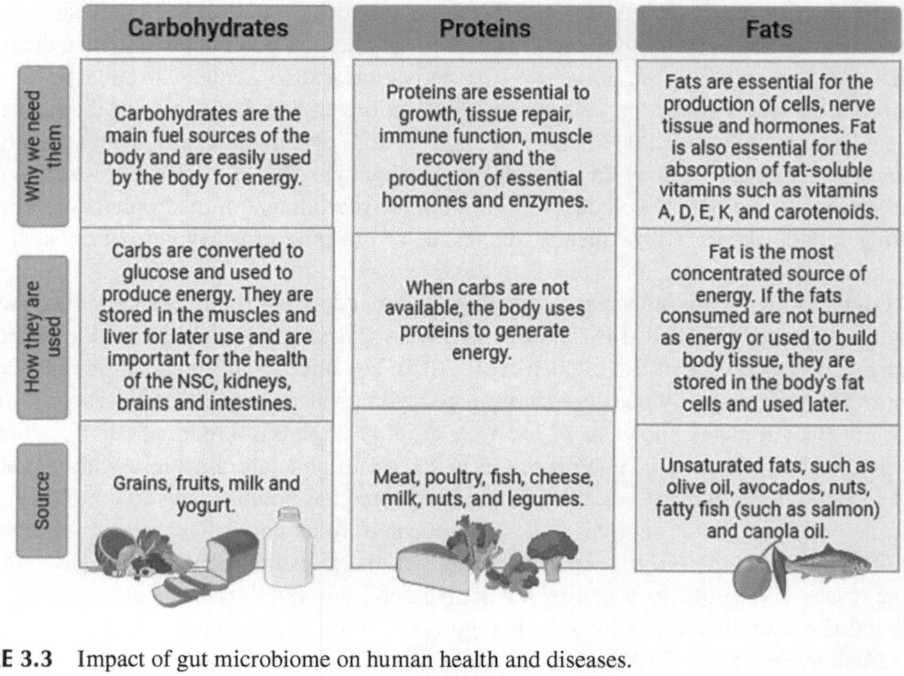

FIGURE 3.3 Impact of gut microbiome on human health and diseases.

to those classified as lean. Furthermore, they display notable disparities in the abundance of certain taxa and functional genes when compared to their lean counterparts (Turnbaugh et al., 2006). There is a notable disparity in the makeup of the intestinal microbiota between individuals who are lean and those who are obese. Specifically, those with obesity have a higher prevalence of gram-negative bacteria and a lower prevalence of gram-positive microbes. The presence of gut flora is likely essential in the evolution of obesity, as shown by the resistance of germ-free mice to obesity caused by an HFD. This suggests that a high-calorie diet alone is insufficient to cause obesity and insulin resistance (Backhed et al., 2007). There has been a proposition suggesting that the microbiota of persons who are fat could possess a higher level of efficiency in extracting power from a particular diet compared to the microbes of those who are lean. To test this idea, a procedure was conducted whereby microbiomes from overweight mice were relocated into germ-free mice. Remarkably, mice that were colonized along with ob/ob microbiomes demonstrated a notably higher rise in human body fat over a span of 2 weeks. nevertheless, it is vital to note that these results did not reach statistical significance in human subjects (Turnbaugh et al., 2006). Obesity and HFD intake are linked with alterations in the composition of gut flora, inflammation, disruption of the gut barrier, and the presence of metabolic endotoxemia, a subclinical inflammatory condition mediated by LPS. The available experimental data indicate that diets rich in fat have the potential to impact the integrity of epithelial cells, resulting in compromised permeability of the gut. This, in turn, may lead to the translocation of TLR ligands, ultimately causing systemic inflammation (Cani et al., 2008). There are two proposed methods for the absorption of LPS from the GIT into the circulatory system. The first mechanism involves the transport assisted by chylomicrons, while the second mechanism involves the extracellular leakage via tight junctions in the epithelial lining. These processes have the potential to operate simultaneously, and both serve as potential connections between the absorption of LPS and the development of metabolic disorders. LPS is taken up by epithelial cells and then transferred to the Golgi partition, where chylomicrons are set aside prior to their production after a high-fat meal. One potential mechanism for the passage of LPS through the gastrointestinal epithelium is by paracellular movement via tight junctions (Caesar et al., 2010). The binding of LPS to the CD14/TLR4 network on the layer of enteroendocrine and gut epithelial tissues induces the release of pro-inflammatory cytokines (Wright et al., 1990). The findings of this study indicate that persons diagnosed with metabolic ailment have notably higher levels of serum LPS compared to those without the disease. It should be noted that these results have not yet been published.

The gut flora after an HFD or in the presence of obesity has the potential to enhance the infiltration of macrophages into adipose tissue via LPS activation and subsequent stimulation of TLR4. Furthermore, it has been shown that elevated concentrations of free fatty acids in the plasma may also induce the activation of TLR4 (Rocha et al., 2016). Adipocyte hypertrophy, a phenomenon seen during obesity, is characterized by an enlargement of adipocyte cells. This process is accompanied by an elevated rate of adipocyte cell death, prompting the recruitment of macrophages to eliminate the resulting cellular debris. Consequently, the rescue of pro-inflammatory cytokines, such as IL6 and TNF-α, occurs as a consequence of this cellular leakage.

TNF-α induces insulin resistance by promoting the breakdown of lipids in adipocytes, therefore activating the JNK and IKKbNF-kB signaling pathways. These pathways then lead to an increase in the serine phosphorylation of IRS1 (Chen et al., 2015). The microbiota composition of individuals recognized with MetS or grisly obesity exhibits a notable prevalence of Prevotellaceae, a particular subdivision of Bacteroidetes known as *P. copri*. Additionally, there is a reduction in the abundance of *Faecalibacterium prausnitzii*. *F. prausnitzii* is known to generate a protein with a molecular weight of 15 kilodaltons, which is referred to as a MAM and has notable anti-inflammation characteristics. The enzymes and/or peptides that are implicated in the anti-inflammation response have the capability to hinder the NF-kB route in the cells of the intestinal epithelium (Quévrain et al., 2016). The levels of *F. prausnitzii* exhibit a negative correlation with inflammatory markers, suggesting that this bacterium has the potential to regulate systemic inflammation and perhaps alleviate diabetes (Medina-Vera et al., 2019).

3.5 INFLUENCING FACTORS ON THE SYNTHESIS OF VITAMIN B BY GUT MICROBIOTA

The production of B vitamins by gut microbiota is influenced by a range of variables, such as free radicals, antibiotics, dietary choices, and an individual's hereditary composition. The effects of antibiotic exposure on B vitamin synthesis exhibit variability depending on the specific kind of antibiotics used. For example, the inclusion of penicillin and aureomycin in the food resulted in an elevation in hepatic vitamin B2 content and an increase in the evacuation of vitamin B2 and vitamin B3 in the urine of male mice (Guggenheim et al., 1953). Nevertheless, the consumption of streptomycin and cycloheximide (Tan et al., 1973) resulted in a decrease in the amounts of vitamin B9 and B12 in the liver. The relationship between antibiotic exposure and the production of vitamins is not well understood, however, it is plausible that the varying reactions seen might be attributed to the selective modifications of the gut microbiota.

On the contrary, free radicals are molecules that are characterized by the presence of an unpaired electron, which has the potential to initiate oxidative stress (Di Meo & Venditti, 2020). An illustrative instance may be seen with nitric oxide, which has the ability to create complexes with metal ions, such as cobalt (Haurani, 1989). Cobalt serves as a crucial structural element in vitamin B12, and as a result, the formation of complexes with nitric oxide renders it inaccessible for microbial vitamin B12 manufacturing. Furthermore, the development of vitamin makers, such as *B. fragilis*, may be suppressed by exposure to free radicals like hydrogen peroxide (Rocha et al., 1996). This suppression ultimately leads to a decrease in the capacity for vitamin biosynthesis.

Furthermore, the gut microbial composition is influenced by factors such as host genetics, dietary choices, and lifestyle. The presence of genetic variations in human genes has been shown to be linked to the structure of the gut and the makeup of the microbiome (Hall et al., 2017). The existence of discrete vitamin B biosynthetic routes within the human microbes of the gut provides evidence for the hypothesis that genetic diversity in humans influences the synthesis of vitamin B (Magnúsdóttir et al., 2015). Bonder et al. (2016) made an intriguing discovery whereby they uncovered a specific genetic variation, known as a single nucleotide variant, that exhibited a correlation with the prevalence of the *Bifidobacterium* genus (Bonder et al., 2016). This species of bacteria is known for its ability to synthesize several B vitamins. Furthermore, the food of a host serves as the feedstock for the bacteria residing in the GIT, and its effects on the composition of gut flora have been widely investigated in previous studies (Flint et al., 2015; Zoetendal & de Vos, 2014). Diets that include prebiotics along with other nutritional elements, such as polyphenols and micronutrients, have been shown to have a substantial impact on the proliferation of beneficial microbes, which include bacteria that create vitamins. Certain vitamins, like riboflavin, function as a redox arbitrator, therefore promoting the proliferation of auxotrophic germs, such as *F. prauznitsii* (Bonder et al., 2016). In contrast, the restriction of these substrates would intensify the competition among the microorganisms as well as between the microorganisms and the host organism in a setting where a symbiotic association is likely to occur (Magnúsdóttir et al., 2015).

3.6 SUMMARY AND FUTURE PERSPECTIVES

There exists a considerable amount of information indicating that polyphenols have a constant and significant impact on enhancing the existence of advantageous microorganisms in the GIT. This phenomenon may potentially contribute to positive health outcomes that extend beyond the confines of the gut. The efficacy of some polyphenols has been proven in animal models to lower the F/B ratio. Furthermore, it has been shown via *in-vitro* studies that some polyphenols possess the capacity to diminish the prevalence of harmful or pathogenic microorganisms. Polyphenols have been shown to exert a favorable modulation on many significant beneficial microorganisms, including *Lactobacillus*, *Bifidobacterium*, *Fecalibacterium* sp., and *Akkermansia*. Certain polyphenols could regulate the presence and activity of various beneficial microorganisms, including *E. dolichum*, *C. coccoides*, *E. rectale* grouping, *Ruminococcus torques*, *Lactococcus lactis*, *Clostridium hathewayi*, *Prevotella* sp., *Bacteroides uniformis*, *Blautia coccoides*, and *Eggerthella lenta*. Vitamins are the secondary prime element that influences the modulation of gut microorganisms that contribute to health benefits. Vitamins have a discernible impact on the modulation of both health-promoting and health-detrimental microorganisms. Specifically, the supplementation of vitamins A, C, D, and E has been shown to exert a favorable effect on health-promoting microorganisms, including *Bifidobacterium*, *Akkermansia*, and *Lactobacillus* spp. The potential therapeutic effects of vitamin A in individuals with ASD and other related conditions are being investigated due to its ability to restore the balance of usual flora in the imbalanced gut. This research aims to study the therapeutic possibility of vitamin A for the treatment of ASD and comparable disorders. Caution should be used while administering vitamin B, since it has the potential to trigger the virulence of pestilential organisms and may also have a beneficial modulating effect on some damaging microorganisms. There is a significant lack of scholarly research that investigates the impact of minerals and microelements on the modulation of gut flora. Nevertheless, the provision of phosphorus, calcium, selenium, magnesium, and zinc has proved potential for promoting favorable gut bacteria such as *Akkermansia*, *Bifidobacterium*, and *Ruminococcus*, although with modest effects. Research studies have shown that the administration of iron supplements to newborns with iron deficiency may effectively regulate harmful and possibly disease-causing microbiota. The addition of iodine to the diet results in a reduction in the prevalence of *F. prausnizii*, whereas the inclusion of selenium in the diet escorts to a drop in the prevalence of *Mucisprillum* and *Dorea*. Further research is required to draw definitive conclusions on these effects.

3.7 CONCLUSIONS

B vitamins serve as co-factors in various cellular metabolic pathways. The primary source of these vitamins is typically the food intake, which is essential for meeting the daily needs of the host and supporting the fitness of the intestinal ecosystem. The gut flora has the capacity to synthesize an unquestionable quantity of B vitamins and their synthesis in the GIT is subject to several circumstances, such as the impact of free radicals and antibiotics, genetic composition, dietary patterns, and lifestyle choices. The vitamins produced by bacteria are insufficient to meet the daily nutritional needs of both the host and gut flora. The interplay between gut microorganisms, the host, and microbe-to-microbe interactions may lead to a potential deficiency of vitamins within the intestinal environment, particularly when food intake is suboptimal. The individual's social standing may have an impact on the makeup of their gut microbiota, the health of their colon, and their overall metabolic processes. The gut microbiota of people exhibits significant diversity, resulting in variations in the production of B vitamins and their respective dietary needs among different individuals. The discovery of the many functions of microbially synthesized metabolites, such as B vitamins, in maintaining intestinal well-being and modulating the host's cellular signaling processes, is an ongoing endeavor. Hence, there are possibilities available for exploring the impression of dietary B vitamins on interactions among the gut and the host.

BIBLIOGRAPHY

Alves da Silva, A. V., de Castro Oliveira, S. B., Di Rienzi, S. C., Brown-Steinke, K., Dehan, L. M., Rood, J. K., Carreira, V. S., Le, H., Maier, E. A., Betz, K. J., Aihara, E., Ley, R. E., Preidis, G. A., Shen, L., & Moore, S. R. (2018). Murine methyl donor deficiency impairs early growth in association with dysmorphic small intestinal crypts and reduced gut microbial community diversity. *Current Developments in Nutrition, 3*(1), nzy070. https://doi.org/10.1093/cdn/nzy070

Arumugam, M., Raes, J., Pelletier, E., Le Paslier, D., Yamada, T., Mende, D. R., Fernandes, G. R., Tap, J., Bruls, T., Batto, J.-M., Bertalan, M., Borruel, N., Casellas, F., Fernandez, L., Gautier, L., Hansen, T., Hattori, M., Hayashi, T., Kleerebezem, M., . . . Bork, P. (2011). Enterotypes of the human gut microbiome. *Nature, 473*(7346), 174–180. https://doi.org/10.1038/nature09944

Avila-Nava, A., Noriega, L. G., Tovar, A. R., Granados, O., Perez-Cruz, C., Pedraza-Chaverri, J., & Torres, N. (2017). Food combination based on a pre-Hispanic Mexican diet decreases metabolic and cognitive abnormalities and gut microbiota dysbiosis caused by a sucrose-enriched high-fat diet in rats. *Molecular Nutrition and Food Research, 61*(1), 1501023. https://doi.org/10.1002/mnfr.201501023

Bäckhed, F., Manchester, J. K., Semenkovich, C. F., & Gordon, J. I. (2007). Mechanisms underlying the resistance to diet-induced obesity in germ-free mice. *PNAS, 104*(3), 979–984. Retrieved October 19, 2023, from https://www.pnas.org/doi/abs/10.1073/pnas.0605374104

Bäumler, A. J., & Sperandio, V. (2016). Interactions between the microbiota and pathogenic bacteria in the gut. *Nature, 535*(7610), 85–93. Retrieved October 18, 2023, from https://www.nature.com/articles/nature18849. https://doi.org/10.1038/nature18849

Bi, H., Zhu, L., Jia, J., & Cronan, J. E. (2016). A biotin biosynthesis gene restricted to Helicobacter. *Scientific Reports, 6*(1), article 1. https://doi.org/10.1038/srep21162

Beaumont M, Portune KJ, Steuer N, Lan A, Cerrudo V, Audebert M, Dumont F, Mancano G, Khodorova N, Andriamihaja M, Airinei G. (2017). Quantity and source of dietary protein influence metabolite production by gut microbiota and rectal mucosa gene expression: a randomized, parallel, double-blind trial in overweight humans. *The American journal of clinical nutrition*, *106*(4), 1005–1019. https://doi.org/10.3945/ajcn.117.158816

Bistas, K. G., & Tadi, P. (2023). Biotin. In *StatPearls*. StatPearls Publishing. http://www.ncbi.nlm.nih.gov/books/NBK554493/

Bonder, M. J., Kurilshikov, A., Tigchelaar, E. F., Mujagic, Z., Imhann, F., Vila, A. V., Deelen, P., Vatanen, T., Schirmer, M., Smeekens, S. P., Zhernakova, D. V., Jankipersadsing, S. A., Jaeger, M., Oosting, M., Cenit, M. C., Masclee, A. A., Swertz, M. A., Li, Y., Kumar, V., . . . Zhernakova, A. (2016). The effect of host genetics on the gut microbiome. *Nature Genetics*, *48*(11), 1407–1412. Retrieved October 19, 2023, from https://www.nature.com/articles/ng.3663; https://doi.org/10.1038/ng.3663

Caesar, R., Fåk, F., & Bäckhed, F. (2010). Effects of gut microbiota on obesity and atherosclerosis via modulation of inflammation and lipid metabolism. *Journal of Internal Medicine—Wiley Online Library, 268*(4), 320–328. Retrieved October 19, 2023, from https://onlinelibrary.wiley.com/doi/full/10.1111/j.1365-2796.2010.02270.x

Candela, M., Biagi, E., Soverini, M., Consolandi, C., Quercia, S., Severgnini, M., Peano, C., Turroni, S., Rampelli, S., Pozzilli, P., Pianesi, M., Fallucca, F., & Brigidi, P. (2016). Modulation of gut microbiota dysbioses in type 2 diabetic patients by macrobiotic Ma-Pi 2 diet. *British Journal of Nutrition, 116*(1), 80–93. https://doi.org/10.1017/S0007114516001045

Cani, P. D., Bibiloni, R., Knauf, C., Waget, A., Neyrinck, A. M., Delzenne, N. M., & Burcelin, R. (2008). Changes in gut microbiota control metabolic endotoxemia-induced inflammation in high-fat diet–induced obesity and diabetes in mice. *Diabetes: American Diabetes Association*, *57*(6), 1470–1481. Retrieved October 19, 2023, from https://diabetesjournals.org/diabetes/article/57/6/1470/40782/Changes-in-Gut-Microbiota-Control-Metabolic. https://doi.org/10.2337/db07-1403

Carrothers, J. M., York, M. A., Brooker, S. L., Lackey, K. A., Williams, J. E., Shafii, B., Price, W. J., Settles, M. L., McGuire, M. A., & McGuire, M. K. (2015). Fecal microbial community structure is stable over time and related to variation in macronutrient and micronutrient intakes in lactating women. *Journal of Nutrition, 145*(10), 2379–2388. https://doi.org/10.3945/jn.115.211110

Chen, G., Xie, M., Wan, P., Chen, D., Dai, Z., Ye, H., Hu, B., Zeng, X., & Liu, Z. (2018). Fuzhuan brick tea polysaccharides attenuate metabolic syndrome in high fat diet induced mice in association with modulation in the gut microbiota. *Journal of Agricultural and Food Chemistry, 66*(11), 2783–2795. https://doi.org/10.1021/acs.jafc.8b00296

Chen, L., Chen, R., Wang, H., & Liang, F. (2015). Mechanisms linking inflammation to insulin resistance. *International Journal of Endocrinology*, *2015*. https://doi.org/10.1155/2015/508409

Collins, B., Hoffman, J., Martinez, K., Grace, M., Lila, M. A., Cockrell, C., Nadimpalli, A., Chang, E., Chuang, C. C., Zhong, W., Mackert, J., Shen, W., Cooney, P., Hopkins, R., & McIntosh, M. (2016). A polyphenol-rich fraction obtained from table grapes decreases adiposity, insulin resistance and markers of inflammation and impacts gut microbiota in high-fat-fed mice. *Journal of Nutritional Biochemistry, 31,* 150–165. https://doi.org/10.1016/j.jnutbio.2015.12.021

Costliow, Z. A., & Degnan, P. H. (2017). Thiamine acquisition strategies impact metabolism and competition in the gut microbe Bacteroides thetaiotaomicron. *mSystems, 2*(5), e00116–e00117. https://doi.org/10.1128/mSystems.00116-17

Cowan, T. E., Palmnäs, M. S. A., Yang, J., Bomhof, M. R., Ardell, K. L., Reimer, R. A., Vogel, H. J., & Shearer, J. (2014). Chronic coffee consumption in the diet-induced obese rat: Impact on gut microbiota and serum metabolomics. *Journal of Nutritional Biochemistry, 25*(4), 489–495. https://doi.org/10.1016/j.jnutbio.2013.12.009

de Crécy-Lagard, V., El Yacoubi, B., de la Garza, R. D., Noiriel, A., & Hanson, A. D. (2007). Comparative genomics of bacterial and plant folate synthesis and salvage: Predictions and validations. *BMC Genomics*, *8*(1), 1–15. https://doi.org/10.1186/1471-2164-8-245

De Filippo, C., Cavalieri, D., Di Paola, M., Ramazzotti, M., Poullet, J. B., Massart, S., Collini, S., Pieraccini, G., & Lionetti, P. (2010). Impact of diet in shaping gut microbiota revealed by a comparative study in children from Europe and rural Africa. *Proceedings of the National Academy of Sciences of the United States of America, 107*(33), 14691–14696. https://doi.org/10.1073/pnas.1005963107

Den Besten, G., van Eunen, K. van Groen, A. K., Venema, K., Reijngoud, D. J., & Bakker, B. M. (2013). The role of short-chain fatty acids in the interplay between diet, gut microbiota, and host energy metabolism. *Journal of Lipid Research, 54*(9), 2325–2340. https://doi.org/10.1194/jlr.R036012

Di Meo, S., & Venditti, P. (2020). Evolution of the knowledge of free radicals and other oxidants. *Oxidative Medicine and Cellular Longevity, 2020*. https://doi.org/10.1155/2020/9829176

Dogra, S. K., Doré, J., & Damak, S. (2020). Gut microbiota resilience: Definition, link to health and strategies for intervention. *Frontiers in Microbiology*, *11*, 572921. Retrieved October 18, 2023, from https://www.frontiersin.org/articles/10.3389/fmicb.2020.572921/full

Epelbaum, S., LaRossa, R. A., VanDyk, T. K., Elkayam, T., Chipman, D. M., & Barak, Z. E. (1998). Branched-chain amino acid biosynthesis in Salmonella typhimurium: A quantitative analysis. *Journal of Bacteriology*, *180*(16), 4056–4067. Retrieved October 19, 2023, from https://pubmed.ncbi.nlm.nih.gov/9696751/

Firrman, J., Liu, L., Argoty, G. A., Zhang, L., Tomasula, P., Wang, M., Pontious, S., Kobori, M., & Xiao, W. (2018). Analysis of temporal changes in growth and gene expression for commensal gut microbes in response to the polyphenol naringenin. *Microbiology Insights, 11*. https://doi.org/10.1177/1178636118775100

Flint, H. J., Duncan, S. H., Scott, K. P., & Louis, P. (2015). Links between diet, gut microbiota composition and gut metabolism. *Proceedings of the Nutrition Society, 74*(1), 13–22. https://doi.org/10.1017/S0029665114001463

Franzosa, E. A., Huang, K., Meadow, J. F., Gevers, D., Lemon, K. P., Bohannan, B. J., & Huttenhower, C. (2015). Identifying personal microbiomes using metagenomic codes. *Proceedings of the National Academy of Sciences*, *112*(22), E2930–E2938. https://doi.org/10.1073/pnas.1423854112

García-Angulo, V. A. (2017). Overlapping riboflavin supply pathways in bacteria. *Critical Reviews in Microbiology, 43*(2), 196–209. https://doi.org/10.1080/1040841X.2016.1192578

García-Peris, P., Velasco, C., Lozano, M. A., Moreno, Y., Paron, L., de la Cuerda, C., Bretón, I., Camblor, M., García-Hernández, J., Guarner, F., & Hernández, M. (2012). Effect of a mixture of inulin and fructo-oligosaccharide on the gut microflora of lactobacillus and bifidobacterium of patients receiving radiotherapy: a randomized, double-blind, placebo-controlled trial. *Hospital Nutrition*, *27*(6), 1908–1915. https://doi.org/10.3305/nh.2012.27.6.5992

Garg, M., Hendy, P., Ding, J. N., Shaw, S., Hold, G., & Hart, A. (2018). The effect of vitamin D on intestinal inflammation and faecal microbiota in patients with ulcerative colitis. *Journal of Crohn's and Colitis, 12*(8), 963–972. https://doi.org/10.1093/ecco-jcc/jjy052

Gazzali, A. M., Lobry, M., Colombeau, L., Acherar, S., Azaïs, H., Mordon, S., Arnoux, P., Baros, F., Vanderesse, R., & Frochot, C. (2016). Stability of folic acid under several parameters. *European Journal of Pharmaceutical Sciences: Official Journal of the European Federation for Pharmaceutical Sciences, 93,* 419–430. https://doi.org/10.1016/j.ejps.2016.08.045

Gazzaniga, F., Stebbins, R., Chang, S. Z., McPeek, M. A., & Brenner, C. (2009). Microbial NAD metabolism: Lessons from comparative genomics. *Microbiology and Molecular Biology Reviews: MMBR, 73*(3), 529–541. https://doi.org/10.1128/MMBR.00042-08

Gensollen, T., Iyer, S. S., Kasper, D. L., & Blumberg, R. S. (2016). How colonization by microbiota in early life shapes the immune system. *Science, 352*(6285), 539–544. Retrieved October 18, 2023, from https://www.science.org/doi/abs/10.1126/science.aad9378. https://doi.org/10.1126/science.aad9378

Gîlcă-Blanariu, G. E., Diaconescu, S., Ciocoiu, M., & Ştefănescu, G. (2018). New insights into the role of trace elements in IBD. *BioMed Research International, 2018,* 1813047. https://doi.org/10.1155/2018/1813047

Gomes, J. M. G., Costa, J. A., & Alfenas, R. C. (2015). Could the beneficial effects of dietary calcium on obesity and diabetes control be mediated by changes in intestinal microbiota and integrity? *British Journal of Nutrition, 114*(11), 1756–1765. https://doi.org/10.1017/S0007114515003608

Guggenheim, K., Halevy, S., Hartmann, I., & Zamir, R. (1953). The effect of antibiotics on the metabolism of certain B vitamins. *Journal of Nutrition, 50*(2), 245–253. https://doi.org/10.1093/jn/50.2.245

Hall, A. B., Tolonen, A. C., & Xavier, R. J. (2017). Human genetic variation and the gut microbiome in disease. *Nature Reviews. Genetics*, *18*(11), 690–699. Retrieved October 19, 2023, from https://www.nature.com/articles/nrg.2017.63 https://doi.org/10.1038/nrg.2017.63

Hamilton, M. K., Boudry, G., Lemay, D. G., & Raybould, H. E. (2015). Changes in intestinal barrier function and gut microbiota in high-fat diet-fed rats are dynamic and region dependent. *American Journal of Physiology, Gastrointestinal and Liver Physiology, 308*(10), G840–G851. https://doi.org/10.1152/ajpgi.00029.2015

Han, X., Shen, T., & Lou, H. (2007). Dietary polyphenols and their biological significance. *International Journal of Molecular Sciences, 8*(9), article 9. https://doi.org/10.3390/i8090950

Haro, C., Montes-Borrego, M., Rangel-Zúñiga, O. A., Alcalá-Díaz, J. F., Gómez-Delgado, F., Pérez-Martínez, P., Delgado-Lista, J., Quintana-Navarro, G. M., Tinahones, F. J., Landa, B. B., López-Miranda, J., Camargo, A., & Pérez-Jiménez, F. (2016). Two healthy diets modulate gut microbial community improving insulin sensitivity in a human obese population. *Journal of Clinical Endocrinology and Metabolism, 101*(1), 233–242. https://doi.org/10.1210/jc.2015-3351

Haurani, F. I. (1989). The effects of free radicals on cobalamin and iron. *Free Radical Research Communications*, *7*(3–6), 241–243. Retrieved October 19, 2023, from https://www.tandfonline.com/doi/abs/10.3109/10715768909087948

Hayflick, S. J. (2014). Defective pantothenate metabolism and neurodegeneration. *Biochemical Society Transactions, 42*(4), 1063–1068. https://doi.org/10.1042/BST20140098

Heiman, M. L., & Greenway, F. L. (2016). A healthy gastrointestinal microbiome is dependent on dietary diversity. *Molecular Metabolism, 5*(5), 317–320. https://doi.org/10.1016/j.molmet.2016.02.005

Herrmann, W., & Geisel, J. (2002). Vegetarian lifestyle and monitoring of vitamin B-12 status. *Clinica Chimica Acta; International Journal of Clinical Chemistry, 326*(1–2), 47–59. https://doi.org/10.1016/S0009-8981(02)00307-8

Holm, J. B., Rønnevik, A., Tastesen, H. S., Fjære, E., Fauske, K. R., Liisberg, U., Madsen, L., Kristiansen, K., & Liaset, B. (2016). Diet-induced obesity, energy metabolism and gut microbiota in C57BL/6J mice fed Western diets based on lean seafood or lean meat mixtures. *Journal of Nutritional Biochemistry, 31,* 127–136. https://doi.org/10.1016/j.jnutbio.2015.12.017

Home Page. (n.d.). *Advances in nutrition*. Retrieved October 19, 2023, from https://advances.nutrition.org/

Hossain, M. K., Hossain, M. M., Mim, Z. T., Khatun, H., Hossain, M. T., & Shahjahan, M. (2022, September). Multi-species probiotics improve growth, intestinal microbiota and morphology of Indian major carp mrigal *Cirrhinus cirrhosus*. *Saudi Journal of Biological Sciences*, *29*(9), 103399. https://doi.org/10.1016/j.sjbs.2022.103399

Iyer, R., & Tomar, S. K. (2009). Folate: A functional food constituent. *Journal of Food Science: Wiley Online Library, 74*(9), R114–R122. Retrieved October 19, 2023, from https://ift.onlinelibrary.wiley.com/doi/full/10.1111/j.1750-3841.2009.01359.x

Kelly, C. J., Alexeev, E. E., Farb, L., Vickery, T. W., Zheng, L., Campbell Eric L., Kitzenberg, D. A., Battista, K. D., Kominsky, D. J., Robertson, C. E., Frank, D. N., Stabler, S. P., & Colgan, S. P. (2019). Oral vitamin B12 supplement is delivered to the distal gut, altering the corrinoid profile and selectively depleting Bacteroides in C57BL/6 mice. *Gut Microbes, 10*(6), 654–662. https://doi.org/10.1080/19490976.2019.1597667

Kleerebezem, M., & Hugenholtz, J. (2003). Metabolic pathway engineering in lactic acid bacteria. *Current Opinion in Biotechnology, 14*(2), 232–237. https://doi.org/10.1016/S0958-1669(03)00033-8

Kostovcikova, K., Coufal, S., Galanova, N., Fajstova, A., Hudcovic, T., Kostovcik, M., Prochazkova, P., Jiraskova Zakostelska, Z., Cermakova, M., Sediva, B., & Kuzma, M. (2019). Diet rich in animal protein promotes pro-inflammatory macrophage response and exacerbates colitis in mice. *Frontiers in Immunology, 10,* 919. Retrieved October 19, 2023, from https://www.frontiersin.org/articles/10.3389/fimmu.2019.00919/full?adb_sid=3703854a-9fca-4240-8d35-9e71054695eb

Kovatcheva-Datchary, P., Nilsson, A., Akrami, R., Lee, Y. S., De Vadder, F., Arora, T., Hallen, A., Martens, E., Björck, I., & Bäckhed, F. (2015). Dietary fiber-induced improvement in glucose metabolism is associated with increased abundance of Prevotella. *Cell Metabolism, 22*(6), 971–982. https://doi.org/10.1016/j.cmet.2015.10.001

Kumar, J. S., Subramanian, V. S., Kapadia, R., Kashyap, M. L., & Said, H. M. (2013). Mammalian colonocytes possess a carrier-mediated mechanism for uptake of vitamin B3 (niacin): Studies utilizing human and mouse colonic preparations. *American Journal of Physiology. Gastrointestinal and Liver Physiology, 305*(3), G207–G213. https://doi.org/10.1152/ajpgi.00148.2013

Leonardi, R., & Jackowski, S. (2007). Biosynthesis of pantothenic acid and coenzyme A. *EcoSal Plus, 2*(2). https://doi.org/10.1128/ecosalplus.3.6.3.4

Ley, R. E., Bäckhed, F., Turnbaugh, P., Lozupone, C. A., Knight, R. D., & Gordon, J. I. (2005). Obesity alters gut microbial ecology. *Proceedings of the National Academy of Sciences of the United States of America, 102*(31), 11070–11075. https://doi.org/10.1073/pnas.0504978102

Li, J., Kong, D., Wang, Q., Wu, W., Tang, Y., Bai, T., Guo, L., Wei, L., Zhang, Q., Yu, Y., Qian, Y., Zuo, S., Liu, G., Liu, Q., Wu, S., Zang, Y., Zhu, Q., Jia, D., Wang, Y., & Yu, Y. (2017). Niacin ameliorates ulcerative colitis via prostaglandin D2-mediated D prostanoid receptor 1 activation. *EMBO Molecular Medicine, 9*(5), 571–588. https://doi.org/10.15252/emmm.201606987

Li, P., Tang, T., Chang, X., Fan, X., Chen, X., Wang, R., Fan, C., & Qi, K. (2019). Abnormality in maternal dietary calcium intake during pregnancy and lactation promotes body weight gain by affecting the gut microbiota in mouse offspring. *Molecular Nutrition and Food Research, 63*(5), e1800399. https://doi.org/10.1002/mnfr.201800399

Liu, T., Zhang, L., Joo, D., & Sun, S. C. (2017). NF-κB signaling in inflammation. *Signal Transduction and Targeted Therapy, 2*(1), article 1. https://doi.org/10.1038/sigtrans.2017.23

Lozupone, C. A., Stombaugh, J. I., Gordon, J. I., Jansson, J. K., & Knight, R. (2012). Diversity, stability and resilience of the human gut microbiota. *Nature, 489*(7415), article 7415. https://doi.org/10.1038/nature11550

Magnúsdóttir, S., Ravcheev, D., de Crécy-Lagard, V., & Thiele, I. (2015). Systematic genome assessment of B-vitamin biosynthesis suggests co-operation among gut microbes. *Frontiers in Genetics, 6*, 148. https://www.frontiersin.org/articles/10.3389/fgene.2015.00148

Makarova, K. S., & Koonin, E. V. (2007). Evolutionary genomics of lactic acid bacteria. *Journal of Bacteriology, 189*(4), 1199–1208. https://doi.org/10.1128/JB.01351-06

Manzetti, S., Zhang, J., & van der Spoel, D. (2014). Thiamin function, metabolism, uptake, and transport. *Biochemistry, 53*(5), 821–835. https://doi.org/10.1021/bi401618y

Marchesi, J. R. (2010). Chapter 2 Prokaryotic and eukaryotic diversity of the human gut. In A. I. Laskin, S. Sariaslani, & G. M. Gadd (Eds.), *Advances in applied microbiology* (Vol. 72, pp. 43–62). Academic Press. https://doi.org/10.1016/S0065-2164(10)72002-5

Mayengbam, S., Chleilat, F., & Reimer, R. A. (2020). Dietary vitamin B6 deficiency impairs gut microbiota and host and microbial metabolites in rats. *Biomedicines, 8*(11), 469. https://doi.org/10.3390/biomedicines8110469

McAllan, L., Skuse, P., Cotter, P. D., Connor, P. O., Cryan, J. F., Ross, R. P., Fitzgerald, G., Roche, H. M., & Nilaweera, K. N. (2014). Protein quality and the protein to carbohydrate ratio within a high fat diet influences energy balance and the gut microbiota in C57BL/6J mice. *PLoS One, 9*(2), e88904. Retrieved October 19, 2023, from https://journals.plos.org/plosone/article?id=10.1371/journal.pone.0088904

McFall-Ngai, M., Hadfield, M. G., Bosch, T. C. G., Carey, H. V., Domazet-Lošo, T., Douglas, A. E., Dubilier, N., Eberl, G., Fukami, T., Gilbert, S. F., Hentschel, U., King, N., Kjelleberg, S., Knoll, A. H., Kremer, N., Mazmanian, S. K., Metcalf, J. L., Nealson, K., Pierce, N. E., & Wernegreen, J. J. (2013). Animals in a bacterial world, a new imperative for the life sciences. *Proceedings of the National Academy of Sciences, 110*(9), 3229–3236. https://doi.org/10.1073/pnas.1218525110

Medina-Vera, I., Sanchez-Tapia, M., Noriega-López, L., Granados-Portillo, O., Guevara-Cruz, M., Flores-López, A., Avila-Nava, A., Fernández, M. L., Tovar, A. R., & Torres, N. (2019). A dietary intervention with functional foods reduces metabolic endotoxaemia and attenuates biochemical abnormalities by modifying faecal microbiota in people with type 2 diabetes. *Diabetes and Metabolism, 45*(2), 122–131. https://doi.org/10.1016/j.diabet.2018.09.004

Mooney, S., Leuendorf, J. E., Hendrickson, C., & Hellmann, H. (2009). Vitamin B6: A long known compound of surprising complexity—PMC. *Molecules, 14*(1), 329–351. Retrieved October 19, 2023, from https://www.ncbi.nlm.nih.gov/pmc/articles/PMC6253932/

Moore, S. J., & Warren, M. J. (2012). The anaerobic biosynthesis of vitamin B12. *Biochemical Society Transactions, 40*(3), 581–586. https://doi.org/10.1042/BST20120066

Nabokina, S. M., Inoue, K., Subramanian, V. S., Valle, J. E., Yuasa, H., & Said, H. M. (2014). Molecular identification and functional characterization of the human colonic thiamine pyrophosphate transporter. *Journal of Biological Chemistry, 289*(7), 4405–4416. https://doi.org/10.1074/jbc.M113.528257

Nakatani, A., Li, X., Miyamoto, J., Igarashi, M., Watanabe, H., Sutou, A., Watanabe, K., Motoyama, T., Tachibana, N., Kohno, M., Inoue, H., & Kimura, I. (2018). Dietary mung bean protein reduces high-fat diet-induced weight gain by modulating host bile acid metabolism in a gut microbiota-dependent manner. *Biochemical and Biophysical Research Communications, 501*(4), 955–961. https://doi.org/10.1016/j.bbrc.2018.05.090

Neu, J., & Rushing, J. (2011). Cesarean versus vaginal delivery: Long-term infant outcomes and the hygiene hypothesis. *Clinics in Perinatology, 38*(2), 321–331. Retrieved October 18, 2023, from https://www.perinatology.theclinics.com/article/S0095-5108(11)00029-7/fulltext https://doi.org/10.1016/j.clp.2011.03.008

Nutrients | Free Full-Text. (n.d.). *Folate production by probiotic bacteria.* Retrieved October 19, 2023, from https://www.mdpi.com/2072-6643/3/1/118

Odamaki, T., Kato, K., Sugahara, H., Hashikura, N., Takahashi, S., Xiao, J. Z., Abe, F., & Osawa, R. (2016). Age-related changes in gut microbiota composition from newborn to centenarian: A cross-sectional study. *BMC Microbiology, 16*(1), 1–12. Retrieved October 18, 2023, from https://bmcmicrobiol.biomedcentral.com/articles/10.1186/s12866-016-0708-5

O'Toole, P. W., & Claesson, M. J. (2010). Gut microbiota: Changes throughout the lifespan from infancy to elderly. *International Dairy Journal, 20*(4), 281–291. https://doi.org/10.1016/j.idairyj.2009.11.010

Parkar, S. G., Trower, T. M., & Stevenson, D. E. (2013). Fecal microbial metabolism of polyphenols and its effects on human gut microbiota. *Anaerobe, 23,* 12–19. https://doi.org/10.1016/j.anaerobe.2013.07.009

Parra, M., Stahl, S., & Hellmann, H. (2018). Vitamin B6 and its role in cell metabolism and physiology—PMC. *Cells, 7*(7), 84. Retrieved October 19, 2023, from https://www.ncbi.nlm.nih.gov/pmc/articles/PMC6071262/

Prajapati, B., Rajput, P., Kumar Jena, P., & Seshadri, S. (2016). Investigation of chitosan for prevention of diabetic progression through gut microbiota alteration in sugar rich diet induced diabetic rats. *Current Pharmaceutical Biotechnology, 17*(2), 173–184. https://doi.org/10.2174/1389201017666151029110505

Present Knowledge in Nutrition—11th Edition. (n.d.). Retrieved October 19, 2023, from https://shop.elsevier.com/books/present-knowledge-in-nutrition/marriott/978-0-323-66162-1

Puupponen-Pimiä, R., Aura, A.-M., Oksman-Caldentey, K.-M., Myllärinen, P., Saarela, M., Mattila-Sandholm, T., & Poutanen, K. (2002). Development of functional ingredients for gut health. *Trends in Food Science and Technology, 13*(1), 3–11. https://doi.org/10.1016/S0924-2244(02)00020-1

Qi, Y., Lohman, J., Bratlie, K. M., Peroutka-Bigus, N., Bellaire, B., Wannemuehler, M., Yoon, K. J., Barrett, T. A., & Wang, Q. (2019). Vitamin C and B3 as new biomaterials to alter intestinal stem cells. *Journal of Biomedical Materials Research. Part A, 107*(9), 1886–1897. https://doi.org/10.1002/jbm.a.36715

Qiao, Y., Sun, J., Ding, Y., Le, G., & Shi, Y. (2013). Alterations of the gut microbiota in high-fat diet mice is strongly linked to oxidative stress. *Applied Microbiology and Biotechnology, 97*(4), 1689–1697. https://doi.org/10.1007/s00253-012-4323-6

Qin, J., Li, R., Raes, J., Arumugam, M., Burgdorf, K. S., Manichanh, C., Nielsen, T., Pons, N., Levenez, F., Yamada, T., Mende, D. R., Li, J., Xu, J., Li, S., Li, D., Cao, J., Wang, B., Liang, H., Zheng, H., & Wang, J. (2010). A human gut microbial gene catalogue established by metagenomic sequencing. *Nature, 464*(7285), article 7285. https://doi.org/10.1038/nature08821

Quévrain, E., Maubert, M. A., Michon, C., Chain, F., Marquant, R., Tailhades, J., Miquel, S., Carlier, L., Bermúdez-Humarán, L. G., Pigneur, B., Lequin, O., Kharrat, P., Thomas, G., Rainteau, D., Aubry, C., Breyner, N., Afonso, C., Lavielle, S., Grill, J.-P., . . . Seksik, P. (2016). Identification of an anti-inflammatory protein from Faecalibacterium prausnitzii, a commensal bacterium deficient in Crohn's disease. *Gut, 65*(3), 415–425. https://doi.org/10.1136/gutjnl-2014-307649

Ragaller, V., Lebzien, P., Südekum, K. H., Hüther, L., & Flachowsky, G. (2011). Pantothenic acid in ruminant nutrition: A review. *Journal of Animal Physiology and Animal Nutrition, 95*(1), 6–16. https://doi.org/10.1111/j.1439-0396.2010.01004.x

Rocha, D. M., Caldas, A. P., Oliveira, L. L., Bressan, J., & Hermsdorff, H. H. (2016). Saturated fatty acids trigger TLR4-mediated inflammatory response. *Atherosclerosis, 244,* 211–215. https://doi.org/10.1016/j.atherosclerosis.2015.11.015

Rist, V. T., Weiss, E., Sauer, N., Mosenthin, R., & Eklund, M. (2014). Effect of dietary protein supply originating from soybean meal or casein on the intestinal microbiota of piglets. *Anaerobe, 25*, 72–79. https://doi.org/10.1016/j.anaerobe.2013.10.003

Rocha, E. R., Selby, T., Coleman, J. P., & Smith, C. J. (1996). Oxidative stress response in an anaerobe, *Bacteroides fragilis*: A role for catalase in protection against hydrogen peroxide. *Journal of Bacteriology, 178*(23), 6895–6903. Retrieved October 19, 2023, from https://journals.asm.org/doi/abs/10.1128/jb.178.23.6895-6903.1996

Rodionov, D. A., Li, X., Rodionova, I. A., Yang, C., Sorci, L., Dervyn, E., Martynowski, D., Zhang, H., Gelfand, M. S., & Osterman, A. L. (2008). Transcriptional regulation of NAD metabolism in bacteria: Genomic reconstruction of NiaR (YrxA) regulon. *Nucleic Acids Research, 36*(6), 2032–2046. https://doi.org/10.1093/nar/gkn046

Ross, A. C., Caballero, B. H., Cousins, R. J., Tucker, K. L., & Ziegler, T. R. (2012). *Modern nutrition in health and disease* (11th ed.). Wolters Kluwer Health Adis (ESP). https://pure.johnshopkins.edu/en/publications/modern-nutrition-in-health-and-disease-eleventh-edition

Rowland, I., Gibson, G., Heinken, A., Scott, K., Swann, J., Thiele, I., & Tuohy, K. (2018). Gut microbiota functions: Metabolism of nutrients and other food components. *European Journal of Nutrition, 57*(1), 1–24. https://doi.org/10.1007/s00394-017-1445-8

Said, H. M. (2013). Recent advances in transport of water-soluble vitamins in organs of the digestive system: A focus on the colon and the pancreas. *American Journal of Physiology. Gastrointestinal and Liver Physiology, 305*(9), G601-G610. https://doi.org/10.1152/ajpgi.00231.2013

Schroeder, B. O., Birchenough, G. M. H., Ståhlman, M., Arike, L., Johansson, M. E. V., Hansson, G. C., & Bäckhed, F. (2018). Bifidobacteria or fiber protects against diet-induced microbiota-mediated colonic mucus deterioration. *Cell Host and Microbe, 23*(1), 27–40.e7. https://doi.org/10.1016/j.chom.2017.11.004

Selma, M. V., Espín, J. C., & Tomás-Barberán, F. A. (2009). Interaction between phenolics and gut microbiota: Role in human health. *Journal of Agricultural and Food Chemistry, 57*(15), 6485–6501. https://doi.org/10.1021/jf902107d

Sender, R., Fuchs, S., & Milo, R. (2016). Are we really vastly outnumbered? Revisiting the ratio of bacterial to host cells in humans. *Cell, 164*(3), 337–340. https://doi.org/10.1016/j.cell.2016.01.013

Skrypnik, K., & Suliburska, J. (2018). Association between the gut microbiota and mineral metabolism. *Journal of the Science of Food and Agriculture, 98*(7), 2449–2460. https://doi.org/10.1002/jsfa.8724

Sprong, R. C., Schonewille, A. J., & van der Meer, R. (2010). Dietary cheese whey protein protects rats against mild dextran sulfate sodium–induced colitis: Role of mucin and microbiota. *Journal of Dairy Science, 93*(4), 1364–1371. https://doi.org/10.3168/jds.2009-2397

Sriram, K., Manzanares, W., & Joseph, K. (2012). Thiamine in nutrition therapy. *Nutrition in Clinical Practice: Official Publication of the American Society for Parenteral and Enteral Nutrition, 27*(1), 41–50. https://doi.org/10.1177/0884533611426149

Steinert, R. E., Sadaghian Sadabad, M., Harmsen, H. J. M., & Weber, P. (2016). The prebiotic concept and human health: A changing landscape with riboflavin as a novel prebiotic candidate? *European Journal of Clinical Nutrition, 70*(12), 1348–1353. https://doi.org/10.1038/ejcn.2016.119

Stover, P. J. (2004). Physiology of folate and vitamin B12 in health and disease. *Nutrition Reviews, 62*(suppl_1), S3–S12. Retrieved October 19, 2023, from https://pubmed.ncbi.nlm.nih.gov/15298442/

Tabasco, R., Sánchez-Patán, F., Monagas, M., Bartolomé, B., Victoria Moreno-Arribas, M., Peláez, C., & Requena, T. (2011). Effect of grape polyphenols on lactic acid bacteria and Bifidobacteria growth: Resistance and metabolism. *Food Microbiology, 28*(7), 1345–1352. https://doi.org/10.1016/j.fm.2011.06.005

Tan, C. H., Blaisdell, S. J., & Hansen, H. J. (1973). Mouse transcobalamin II metabolism: The effects of antibiotics on the clearance of vitamin B12 from the serum transcobalamin II-vitamin B12 complex and the reappearance of the free serum transcobalamin II in the mouse. *Biochimica et Biophysica Acta (BBA)—General Subjects, 320*(2), 469–477. https://doi.org/10.1016/0304-4165(73)90327-9

Thakur, K., Tomar, S. K., & De, S. (2015). Lactic acid bacteria as a cell factory for riboflavin production. *Microbial Biotechnology, 9*(4), 441–451. https://doi.org/10.1111/1751-7915.12335

Thursby, E., & Juge, N. (2017). Introduction to the human gut microbiota. *Biochemical Journal, 474*(11), 1823–1836. https://doi.org/10.1042/BCJ20160510

Topping, D. L., & Clifton, P. M. (2001). Short-chain fatty acids and human colonic function: Roles of resistant starch and nonstarch polysaccharides. *Physiological Reviews, 81*(3), 1031–1064. https://doi.org/10.1152/physrev.2001.81.3.1031

Trautvetter, U., Camarinha-Silva, A., Jahreis, G., Lorkowski, S., & Glei, M. (2018). High phosphorus intake and gut-related parameters—Results of a randomized placebo-controlled human intervention study. *Nutrition Journal, 17*(1), 23. https://doi.org/10.1186/s12937-018-0331-4

Turnbaugh, P. J., Ley, R. E., Mahowald, M. A., Magrini, V., Mardis, E. R., & Gordon, J. I. (2006). An obesity-associated gut microbiome with increased capacity for energy harvest. *Nature, 444*(7122), article 7122. https://doi.org/10.1038/nature05414

Turroni, F., Foroni, E., O'Connell Motherway, M., Bottacini, F., Giubellini, V., Zomer, A., Ferrarini, A., Delledonne, M., Zhang, Z., van Sinderen, D., & Ventura, M. (2010). Characterization of the serpin-encoding gene of Bifidobacterium breve 210B. *Applied and Environmental Microbiology, 76*(10), 3206–3219. https://doi.org/10.1128/AEM.02938-09

Tzounis, X., Vulevic, J., Kuhnle, G. G. C., George, T., Leonczak, J., Gibson, G. R., Kwik-Uribe, C., & Spencer, J. P. E. (2008). Flavanol monomer-induced changes to the human faecal microflora. *British Journal of Nutrition, 99*(4), 782–792. https://doi.org/10.1017/S0007114507853384

Uebanso, T., Shimohata, T., Mawatari, K., & Takahashi, A. (2020). Functional roles of B-vitamins in the gut and gut microbiome. *Molecular Nutrition and Food Research, 64*(18), e2000426. https://doi.org/10.1002/mnfr.202000426

Wan, Y., Wang, F., Yuan, J., Li, J., Jiang, D., Zhang, J., Li, H., Wang, R., Tang, J., Huang, T., Zheng, J., Sinclair, A. J., Mann, J., & Li, D. (2019). Effects of dietary fat on gut microbiota and faecal metabolites, and their relationship with cardiometabolic risk factors: A 6-month randomised controlled-feeding trial. *Gut, 68*(8), 1417–1429. https://doi.org/10.1136/gutjnl-2018-317609

Watanabe, F. (2007). Vitamin B12 sources and bioavailability. *Experimental Biology and Medicine*, *232*(10), 1266–1274. https://doi.org/10.3181/0703-MR-67

Williamson, G. (2017). The role of polyphenols in modern nutrition. *Nutrition Bulletin, 42*(3), 226–235. https://doi.org/10.1111/nbu.12278

Wolters, M., Ahrens, J., Romaní-Pérez, M., Watkins, C., Sanz, Y., Benítez-Páez, A., Stanton, C., & Günther, K. (2019). Dietary fat, the gut microbiota, and metabolic health—A systematic review conducted within the MyNewGut project. *Clinical Nutrition, 38*(6), 2504–2520. https://doi.org/10.1016/j.clnu.2018.12.024

Wright, S. D., Ramos, R. A., Tobias, P. S., Ulevitch, R. J., & Mathison, J. C. (1990). CD14, a receptor for complexes of lipopolysaccharide (LPS) and LPS binding protein *Science*, *249*(4975), 1431–1433. Retrieved October 19, 2023, https://doi.org/10.1126/science.1698311

Yao, C., Chou, J., Wang, T., Zhao, H., & Zhang, B. (2018). Pantothenic acid, vitamin C, and biotin play important roles in the growth of Lactobacillus helveticus. *Frontiers in Microbiology*, *9*, 1194. https://doi.org/10.3389/fmicb.2018.01194

Yoshii, K., Hosomi, K., Sawane, K., & Kunisawa, J. (2019). Metabolism of dietary and microbial vitamin B family in the regulation of host immunity. *Frontiers in Nutrition, 6,* 48. https://doi.org/10.3389/fnut.2019.00048

Zhang, F., Ye, J., Zhu, X., Wang, L., Gao, P., Shu, G., Jiang, Q., & Wang, S. (2019). Anti-obesity effects of dietary calcium: The evidence and possible mechanisms. *International Journal of Molecular Sciences, 20*(12), article 12. https://doi.org/10.3390/ijms20123072

Zoetendal, E. G., & de Vos, W. M. (2014). Effect of diet on the intestinal microbiota and its activity. *Current Opinion in Gastroenterology*, *30*(2), 189–195. Retrieved October 19, 2023, from https://journals.lww.com/co-gastroenterology/abstract/2014/03000/effect_of_diet_on_the_intestinal_microbiota_and.14.aspx https://doi.org/10.1097/MOG.0000000000000048

4 Gut Microbiota and Diseases

Relationship and Impact of Microorganisms in Promoting Various Diseases

Jyoti Goyat and Barkha Bhatnagar

4.1 THE HISTORICAL AND MODERN SIGNIFICANCE OF GUT MICROBIOTA

The strong association between human health and the intestinal microbiota has been long recognized in 400 B.C. Hippocrates says, "Death sits in the bowels." Globally, numerous types of research have emphasized establishing the association between human health and disease due to the significant impact of the intestinal microflora (AboNahas et al., 2022). "Microbiota" term encompasses the total population of microbes residing in specific regions of the gastrointestinal tract in both humans and animals. Notably, the human digestive system hosts a substantially greater diversity of microorganisms and species when compared to other bodily regions (Quigley, 2013). This diverse population consists of thousands of microbes, including a few eukaryotes, bacteria, fungi, and viruses, which establish colonization within the digestive tract shortly after an individual's birth (Sekirov et al., 2010; Passos and Moraes-Filho, 2017).

The human microbiota, often referred to as an "invisible organ," comprises ample genetic information compared to the entire human genome. The words "microbiota" and "microbiome" are generally used interchangeably, but they are distinctive in nature. The term "microbiota" denotes the collection of live microbes present within a given environment, such as the oral and gut microbiota, whereas microbiome encompasses the entirety of the genetic material associated with all the microbes inhabiting that environment. This broader definition not only comprehends to microbial community but also encompasses the structural components, metabolic byproducts, and the environmental factors that influence their existence (Hou et al., 2022).

The human gut microbiota is extremely diverse and consists of trillions of microbes within the digestive tract. The evolution of the gut microbiota and its development begin at birth. The compositional and functional changes depend largely on various factors such as genetics, environmental conditions, nutrition (Gomaa, 2020); type of delivery (Nagpal et al., 2017); antibiotics usage (Hasan & Yang, 2019) age; and dietary habits of the host (Odamaki et al., 2016).

In upholding gut health, the microbiota acts as an important protagonist and plays several key functions, which include reinforcing the integrity of the gut (Natividad & Verdu, 2013), facilitating the extraction of energy (den Besten et al., 2013), safeguarding against opportunistic pathogens (Bäumler & Sperandio, 2016), and overseeing the host's immune response (Gensollen et al., 2016). Nonetheless, disruptions in these mechanisms can transpire due to shifts in microbial composition, commonly referred to as dysbiosis (Chang & Lin, 2016). Even minor alterations in the arrangement of microorganisms can potentially lead to gastrointestinal disturbances and trigger diseases in distant organs (Ahlawat et al., 2021).

The interplay between microorganisms and the host holds a significant sway over both well-being and illness. The microbial diversity of the gut is substantially influenced by a multitude of host-related factors, such as lifestyle, environmental conditions, age, and dietary choices. Among

 DOI: 10.1201/9781003452249-4

these factors, dietary habits are considered the principal modulators swaying the gut microbiota (Simões et al., 2022). Several researchers have a notion that the microbiota plays a pivotal role in influencing aspects of health such as immune function, energy balance, weight regulation, and conditions associated with obesity (Piccioni et al., 2022).

Similarly, the gut microbiota and its metabolic byproducts are linked to numerous diseases affecting multiple organs, including CVDs, alcoholic and non-alcoholic fatty liver diseases, cirrhosis of the liver, IBDs, and chronic kidney diseases (CKDs) (Hsu et al., 2020; Ryma et al., 2021; Jansen et al., 2021; Zhou et al., 2021; Wang et al., 2021; Philips et al., 2022).

4.2 DIVERSITY AND DEVELOPMENT OF HUMAN GUT MICROBIOTA

The composition of human gut microbiota varies from one site to another. Microorganisms of the human gut play an influential role in maintaining good host health (Shreiner et al., 2015). The bacteria living in the gastrointestinal system undertake a range of tasks, which encompass fermentation of food, defense against harmful pathogens, stimulation of the host immune response, and essential vitamin synthesis (Hillman et al., 2017). Typically, gut microbiota consists of six phyla: Firmicutes, Bacteroidetes, Actinobacteria, Proteobacteria, Fusobacteria, and Verrucomicrobia (Laterza et al., 2016). Among these, Bacteroidetes are the most abundant, followed by Firmicutes. Within this particular family, its constituent species constitute roughly 30% of the gut's bacterial population, underscoring the genus's substantial importance within the host organism. The gut microbiota predominantly possesses anaerobic bacteria, consisting of approximately 99% of the total, while the cecum hosts a dense population of aerobic species (Michael, 2016; Gomaa, 2020).

The most extensively studied fungi found in the microbiota include *Candida*, *Saccharomyces*, *Malassezia*, and *Cladosporium* (Auchtung et al., 2018). Beyond fungi and bacteria, the host gut microbiota includes phages, viruses, and archaea, with a notable presence of *Methanobrevibacter smithii* primarily (Lozupone et al., 2012). The gut microbes exhibit differences in the distribution pattern of microorganisms at both the genus level and beyond, which vary over time and space. Variations in both bacterial diversity and abundance become evident when progressing from the esophagus toward the rectum, as illustrated in Figure 4.1. These differences span a wide spectrum, with bacterial counts of 10^1 g^{-1} present in the esophagus and stomach to 10^{12} g^{-1} in the distal gut and colon (Jandhyala et al., 2015).

Although not as widely acknowledged as the gut, microbiota also inhabits different sites of the body like the skin, mouth, respiratory system, and vaginal tract. The microorganisms

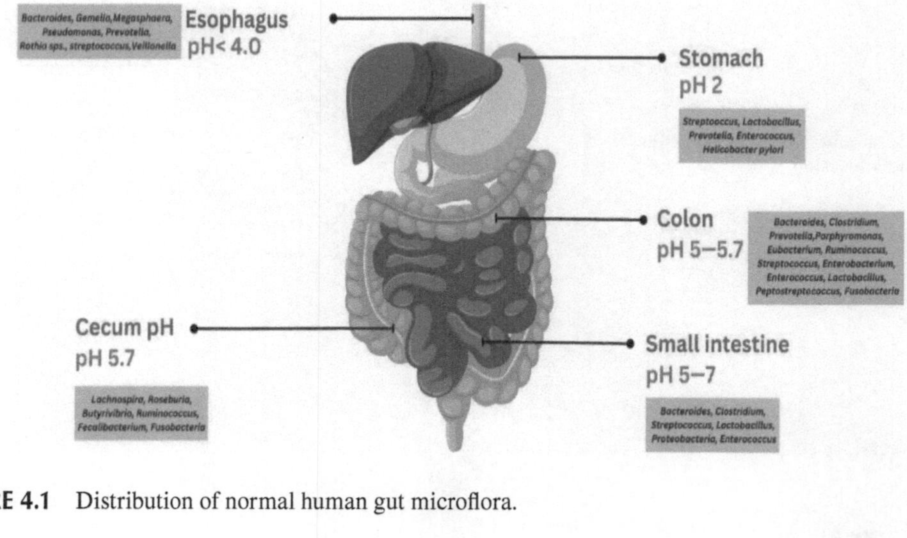

FIGURE 4.1 Distribution of normal human gut microflora.

present in the oral cavity of humans are considered the second-largest microbial biodiversity (Deo & Deshmukh, 2019). Various small habitats present within the oral cavity are saliva, tooth surfaces, tongue, gums, buccal mucosa, palate, and sub- and supra-gingival plaque. These sub-habitats are susceptible to substantial and swift alterations in their composition and functionality, attributed to factors like genetic transformations, pH variations, and bacterial interactions (Segata et al., 2012). The microbial configurations observed in all seven of these locations exhibit a high degree of similarity, with only minor distinctions. Notable bacterial species in the oral cavity encompass Firmicutes, Fusobacteria, Proteobacteria, Actinobacteria, and Bacteroidete.

Studies suggest the presence of microbiota in lung tissues, although healthy human lungs are traditionally considered sterile (Dickson & Huffnagle, 2015). The lung microbiota is primarily composed of Actinobacteria, Firmicutes, Proteobacteria, and Bacteroidetes. The makeup of the lung microbiota is primarily formed by three key factors: the influx of microorganisms, the removal of microorganisms, and the pace at which they reproduce (Dickson et al., 2014). The microbial diversity and its distribution on the human skin vary by geographic region, likely due to the physical and chemical differences in skin regions (Tong et al., 2018).

4.3 THE IMPACT OF GUT MICROBIOTA ON DIGESTIVE HEALTH

The gut microbiota plays a crucial role in maintaining good host health by primarily contributing to its intestinal well-being. Its functions are vital in ensuring optimal digestive processes, energy extraction, reinforcement of mucosal immunity, maintenance of the intestinal mucosal barrier, protection against pathogens, synthesis of essential vitamins, neurotransmitters, and the generation of bioactive compounds especially beneficial molecules like SCFAs (Riccio, 2011; Wahlström et al., 2016; Paone & Cani, 2020; van de Wouw et al., 2018; Tremaroli & Bäckhed, 2012; Lindsay et al., 2020) (see Figure 4.2).

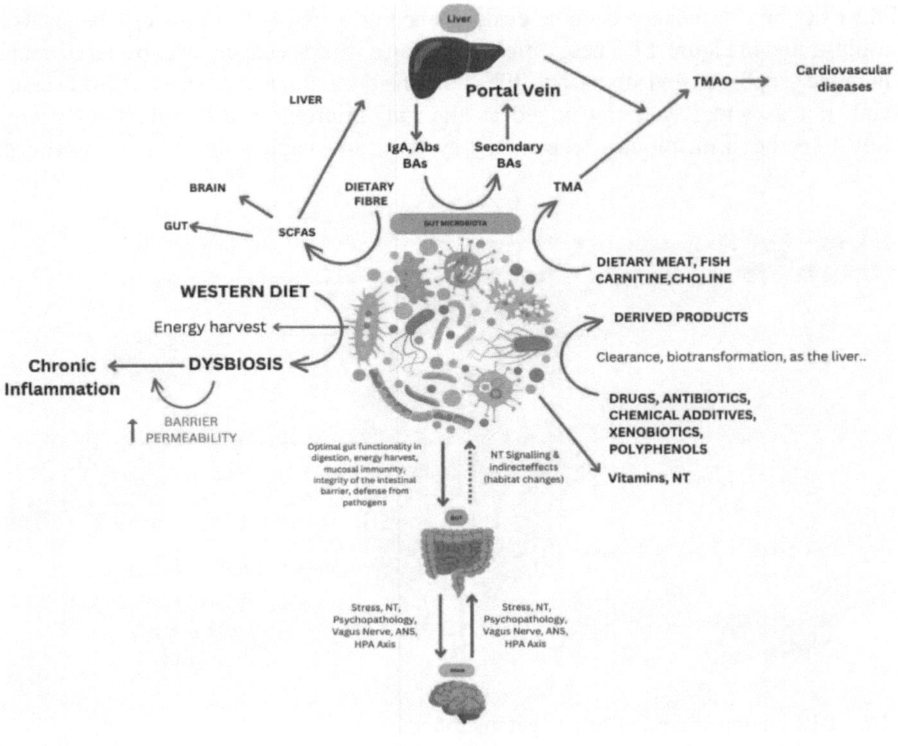

FIGURE 4.2 Interaction of gut microbiota with organs of the host.

Microbiota maintains a symbiotic relationship with the intestine, functioning primarily as a catabolic organism that regulates and protects its habitat against new colonizations. The association between microbiota and intestinal functions is so close that they can be considered interdependent. It is fitting to characterize the gut and its microbiota as constituting a "microbial-assisted digestive system." This system involves the human gut microbes aiding in the breakdown of substances that the intestine is unable to process, particularly fiber, and in extracting extra energy from the ingested food (see Figure 4.2). The host microbiota seems to play a crucial role in buffering the digestive process of food (Riccio & Rossano, 2020).

4.4 BALANCING THE IMMUNE SYSTEM: THE ROLE OF GUT MICROBIOTA

The fundamental role of gut microbiota is well known for the positive maintenance of human health, with a particular emphasis on the immune system, which bestows numerous vital advantages upon the host. Research has illuminated the significance of early development and expansion of the microbial community of the gut in averting autoimmune disorders and ensuring the effectiveness of the host immune system (Lazar et al., 2018; Schluter et al., 2020; Elmassry et al., 2022; Spencer et al., 2019).

The microbiome of the intestine holds a fundamental role in fostering the immune system maturation, encompassing both inherited and adaptive immunity. The inherited immune response relies on epithelial barriers (physical), specialized cells, and circulating molecules capable of promptly recognizing a large spectrum of foreign antigens and responsible for their removal (Thaiss et al., 2016), whereas mucosal immunity operates largely independently of systemic immunity and undergoes substantial alterations followed by bacterial colonization from the intestinal tract. Commensal microbes play a crucial role in nurturing the growth and development of the immune response, aiding it in differentiating between commensal and opportunistic bacteria. Several studies have unveiled the influence of the gastrointestinal microbiome on the behavior and characteristics of neutrophils and its role in the differentiation of T cells into various helper T cell subsets, including regulatory T cells, TH17, Th2, and Th1 (Francino, 2014; Afzaal et al., 2022; Tomkovich & Jobin, 2016; Owaga et al., 2015). Notably, Th17 cells, which is a subset of TCD4+ cells, produce various cytokines that exert an impact on inflammation and the balance of the immune system (Rossi & Bot, 2013). The gut microbiome actively participates in initiating and maturing the immune system's response to pathogens, while also promoting and sustaining tolerance (Pickard et al., 2017). Development and progression of the immunity commences at the time of birth and continues to interact with the microbiota, achieving full maturation in the presence of commensal microflora. This complete progression of the immune system proves crucial in preventing abnormal immune responses that could lead to chronic inflammation and illness (Tibbs et al., 2019).

4.5 DYSBIOSIS AND CONTRIBUTING FACTORS

The "dysbiosis" term refers to the unevenness of gut microbial biodiversity, making the host more susceptible to pro-inflammatory conditions or diseases. Dysbiosis is generally characterized by an imbalance in the microbial population, loss of diversity, or disruption of homeostasis (Hooks and O'Malley, 2017; Brüssow, 2020). A more refined characterization of dysbiosis can be expressed as "an unwavering microbial diversity that actively participates in the development, diagnosis, and disease treatment" (Levy et al., 2017). Since this imbalance is directly linked to detrimental health concerns, it is crucial to understand its causes to prevent pro-inflammatory conditions that may lead to severe diseases. One significant challenge in diagnosing this imbalance is that dysbiosis can be either specific to a single disease or associated with multiple conditions. It is vital to distinguish disease-specific modifications in the microbial community that may lead to the onset of disease from those that result from altered selective pressures created by the disease microenvironment, such as chronic or acute inflammation (Peterson et al., 2015).

4.5.1 Factors Affecting Microbial Biodiversity

Numerous factors play a significant role in swaying or controlling the gut microbial community, which may have an effective impact on the host. These factors are as follows:

1. Age
2. Diet
3. Exercise
4. Host genetics
5. Effect of smoking
6. Antibiotics
7. Geographical influences

4.5.1.1 Age

The age plays an impactful role in molding the gut microbial composition of the host. Colonization of microbiota depends on the mode of childbirth, be it cesarean or vaginal. Initially, intestines are densely occupied by aerobic strains of bacteria like Proteobacteria, but, as the oxygen levels deplete, anaerobic strains such as Actinobacteria, Firmicutes, and Bacteroides establish themselves (Del Chierico et al., 2015). The establishment and progression of the microbial community inside the gut primarily initiate in the first year of an infant's life, with biodiversity increasing gradually over time (Schanche et al., 2015). Gut microbiota starts stabilization between the ages of 2 and 5, marked by an increased presence of Bacteroidetes and Firmicutes (Fouhy et al., 2019). Between ages 7 and 12, the synthesis of folate and vitamin B12 experiences a surge (Hollister et al., 2015). During adolescence (11–18 years), a noteworthy increment has been seen in the genera *Clostridium* and *Bifidobacterium* compared to adults. Nonetheless, Bacteroidetes and Firmicutes continue to dominate the gut microbiota in healthy adults, with smaller proportions of Proteobacteria, Verrucomicrobia, and Actinobacteria (Gomaa, 2020).

In the elderly, gut biodiversity significantly declines, including reductions in *Bacteroides*, *Bifidobacteria*, and along with diminished production of SCFAs and reduction in amylolytic activity. However, the populations of facultative anaerobes like clostridia, fusobacteria, and eubacteria increase (Thompson et al., 2015). The aging process leads to substantial alterations in the configuration and function of the elderly gut microbiota, categorized by reduced microbial diversity, a decline in SCFA-producing species, and a rise in pathogenic bacteria (Biagi et al., 2017). These microbial changes may be influenced by decreased dietary variations and heightened inflammatory factors (Voreades et al., 2014).

4.5.1.2 Diet

The diet also plays a significant role in making a positive or negative impact on the biodiversity of the human gut. It can modulate the microbial content of certain species and regulate the production of metabolites in the gut habitat (Hills et al., 2019). The interaction between hosts and microorganisms begins at birth, and diet plays a critical role in shaping gut microbiota in an infant as it adapts to changing nutrient sources. During infancy, predominantly the gut microbiota possesses genes that are specialized in breaking down the oligosaccharides present in maternal milk. With the introduction of solid foods, the microbiome becomes enriched with genes associated with the digestion of polysaccharides and vitamins (Bäckhed et al., 2015). The choice of food significantly impacts microbial diversity in the infant microbiota, where breastfed infants tend to exhibit overgrowth of Actinobacteria while inhibiting the proliferation of Proteobacteria and Firmicutes. Maternal milk contains oligosaccharides efficiently digested by bacterial species in the microbial pool, increasing SCFA production and immune system activation. In contrast, infants fed formula milk exhibit an increase in clostridia, streptococci, bacteroides, and enterobacteria (Lee et al., 2015; Azad et al.,

2013). Gut microbiota development continues after infancy, with diet becoming a vital factor in shaping its structure and biodiversity. Vegetarians tend to have dominant Bacteroidetes and Firmicutes species in their gut, while dietary fiber consumption is crucial for regulating gut mucosal barrier function (Ray, 2018). High-fiber diets are associated with improved metabolic profiles in individuals with type 2 diabetes by regulating glucose levels (Zhao et al., 2018). Conversely, those consuming high-protein and high-fat diets possess the richness of bile juice–tolerant species in the gut, such as *Alistipes*, *Bilophila*, and *Bacteroides*, and fewer Firmicutes. Such diets can weaken immunity, increase susceptibility to infection, and lead to metabolic syndromes (Jethwani & Grover, 2019).

4.5.1.3 Exercise

Physical activity promotes greater diversity in the gut microbiota and exhibits a positive association with the consumption of protein and levels of creatine kinase in humans (Clarke et al., 2014). Athletes have higher levels of Firmicutes and lower levels of Bacteroidetes compared to non-athletes. Exercise increases the abundance of bacterial genera like *Bifidobacterium*, *Lactobacillus*, and *Akkermansia* in the microbial pool while decreasing Proteobacteria, Turicibacter, and Rikenellaceae (Hughes, 2020). Exercise leads to an elevation in SCFAs, which serve as markers of gut well-being, along with the proliferation of butyrate-producing species like Erysipelotrichaceae, Roseburia, Clostridiales, and Lachnospiraceae. These changes in the gut microbiota are elucidated in the research conducted by Allen et al. (2018). Numerous factors, both within and outside the body, play a role in fostering a robust bacterial community in athletes. Being in natural surroundings and maintaining a wholesome lifestyle can encourage a more diverse microbiota. Furthermore, internal adaptations that occur during endurance training, such as a decrease in blood flow and the availability of less oxygen in tissues, can bring about alterations in the gastrointestinal tract, as highlighted by Gomaa in 2020. Studies suggest that exercise could be used as a therapeutic approach to address dysbiosis-related diseases, including obesity and gastrointestinal diseases (Estaki et al., 2016).

4.5.1.4 Host Genetics

Host genetics significantly affect the richness of microbial species, and the abundances of individual genera, and may modify susceptibility to pathogens. Several correlations have been established between the microbiome and genes associated with the host's innate immunity, which in turn influence the composition of the microbiome and diseases related to it, as demonstrated in the study by Iebba et al. (2016). Numerous studies support the idea that genetic factors or host genetics strongly contribute to shaping the gut microbiota (Kurilshikov et al., 2017; Chen et al., 2018).

4.5.1.5 Antibiotics

Prolonged use of antibiotics has a dual effect, as it eradicates both pathogenic and beneficial microorganisms while also causing an imbalance in the gut microbiota, known as dysbiosis (Klingensmith & Coopersmith, 2016). Antibiotics disrupt the competitive elimination mechanism through which microbes inhibit pathogenic activity. The duration of antibiotics and its type also affect the gut microbiota. For example, prolonged use of clindamycin over two years can lead to alterations in the gut microbiota (Gomaa, 2020). Vancomycin treatment increases the level of Proteobacteria species while decreasing the levels of *Fuminococcus*, Bacteroidetes, and *Faecalibacterium* (Isaac et al., 2016).

4.5.1.6 Effect of Smoking

The composition of gastrointestinal microbes is significantly altered by the habit of smoking. Smoking cessation has been associated with an increase in Actinobacteria and Firmicutes and a decrease in Proteobacteria and Bacteroidetes in the fecal microbiota of healthy individuals. Furthermore, notable distinctions in gut and oral microbiota have been noted when comparing smokers to nonsmokers (Gomaa, 2020).

4.5.1.7 Geographical Impact

Geographic regions exert an influence on the distribution of phyla within the human gut microbiota (Schnorr et al., 2014). Variations in environmental conditions, dietary habits, and lifestyles across different locales contribute to the diversity of gut microbial populations (Martínez et al., 2015). Research findings indicate that, in non-industrialized regions, adults tend to exhibit a higher prevalence of Firmicutes, whereas individuals residing in Westernized societies often show a greater proportion of Bacteroidetes in comparison to Firmicutes (Zhu et al., 2015).

4.6 HOST–MICROBE INTERACTION: THE KEY TO HEALTH AND DISEASE

A complex relationship exists between the human body and its microbial community, and disturbances can have adverse effects on both. When subjected to external fluctuations, the equilibrium of the microbiota community may become disturbed, resulting in the dysregulation of biological functions and the onset of diseases. This alteration of microbial composition, known as dysbiosis, can be critical and is linked to the development and progression of various conditions. As of now, a growing body of evidence indicates that the microbiota is linked to the emergence of cancer, CVDs, respiratory conditions, IBDs, CKDs, neurological disorders, diabetes, and liver ailments (Gomaa, 2020; Hou et al., 2022). A harmonious balance of gut microbiota is essential for maintaining a mutually beneficial relationship between the microbiome and the host.

4.6.1 The Role of Gut Microbiota in Obesity Development

In recent years, the increasing ubiquity of obesity has emerged as a global public health crisis, with a concerning upward trend (Geng et al., 2022). This metabolic disorder is associated with insulin resistance, diabetes, hyperlipidemia, osteoarthritis, cancer, and liver steatosis (Gomaa, 2020). Obesity can result from various factors, including genetic, environmental, and behavioral factors. Researchers found a crucial role of gut microbiota plays in the development of obesity (Villanueva-Millán et al., 2015). The microbiota in overweight individuals displays an increased capacity for fermenting and extracting energy from dietary sources. The presence of an "obesogenic" gut microbiota, characterized by a high Firmicutes to *Bacteroides* ratio, increases the number of microbes involved in polysaccharide breakdown, leading to elevated levels of SCFAs. As a result, this leads to heightened expression of genes that encode enzymes responsible for carbohydrate metabolism and the production of SCFAs (Cao et al., 2019; Andoh et al., 2016). Obese individuals have been found to have a prevalence of *Campylobacter*, *Porphyromonas*, *Bacteroides*, *Parabacteroides*, *Staphylococcus*, *Ruminococcus*, and *Dialister* compared to lean individuals, along with lower proportions of *Faecalibacterium*, *Bifidobacterium*, and *Lactobacillus* (Le Chatelier et al., 2013). The human gut microbiota and its role in obesity and the production of metabolites are also contributed by genetic and epigenetic variations.

Several proposed mechanisms explain the role of the gut microbiota in obesity development. Gut microbes can reduce fatty acid oxidation by inhibiting AMPk, a cellular energy indicator found in muscle fibers and the liver. The suppression of AMPk reduces fatty acid oxidation and leads to increased fat accumulation (López, 2017; Pindjakova et al., 2017). Another mechanism involves the regulation of energy and the microbiome's ability to ferment dietary polysaccharides that humans cannot digest (Khan et al., 2016). Fermentation of fiber releases SCFAs, which initiate lipogenesis and promote triglyceride storage through molecular pathways.

4.6.2 Hypertension

Hypertension is a major health threat and a key risk factor for metabolic syndromes (Shah et al., 2019). It is being reported that by 2025 the global prevalence of hypertension will reach around 1.56 billion. Hypertension has various contributing factors, including genetic and environmental factors such as salt intake, physical inactivity, excessive alcohol consumption, and smoking (Rust & Ekmekcioglu, 2017; Afzaal et al., 2022). Several studies suggest that the progression of hypertension is closely linked to dysbiosis in the gut microbial community (Miremadi et al., 2016; Jose & Raj, 2015). The proportions of Bacteroidetes and Firmicutes in the intestinal microbial habitat have been significantly correlated with hypertension (Yang et al., 2015). In vivo, studies on humans and animals have shown that an abundance of Firmicutes and Bacteroidetes in the gut microbiota is associated with hypertension, as determined by 16S ribosomal RNA sequencing (Moghadamrad et al., 2015).

SCFAs have a crucial role in preserving gut microbiome balance and enhancing the immunity of the host. Recent studies indicate that SCFAs present in the gut microbiota may exert a strong influence on the regulation of hypertension by activating GPCR pathways, which could potentially affect the release of renin (Pluznick et al., 2013; Kang & Cai, 2018). Additionally, studies have shown that *Lactobacillus* can contribute positively to blood pressure maintenance (Gómez-Guzmán et al., 2015). Contemporary investigations, including clinical trials, have unveiled a complex interplay between gut microbiota and hypertension, underscoring the need for further human studies to confirm the pivotal role of gut microbiota in hypertension and to develop viable therapeutic approaches (Afzaal et al., 2022).

4.6.3 Cardiovascular Diseases

Despite the current methodologies employed for athero-thrombosis prevention and management, heart disease remains a significant global cause of death. The incidence of CVDs in low- and middle-income countries continues to rise at an alarming rate, potentially leading to increased mortality (Odutayo et al., 2016). Key factors contributing to the progression of CVD include obesity, hypertension, diabetes, stress, and, notably, diet and physical inactivity (Qian et al., 2022).

The pathophysiology and progression of CVDs are significantly influenced by the intestine, mainly due to reduced intestinal perfusion, leading to dysfunction of the intestinal barrier (Sabatino et al., 2015). The intestinal microbiota of the host constitutes the intestinal epithelial barrier, which plays a pivotal role in regulating immune function, synthesizing vitamins, facilitating nutrient digestion, and safeguarding against the intrusion of pathogenic bacteria, all of which are essential for human well-being (Wu et al., 2020; DeGruttola et al., 2016; Chen et al., 2021; Thomas & Jobin, 2020). Imbalances in the human gut microbiota, arising from unhealthy dietary habits, environmental factors, intestinal infections, and various other influences, can result in intestinal malnutrition, provoke inflammation, and disturb metabolism. These factors contribute to the occurrence and progression of CVDs (Qian et al., 2022). This imbalance of the microbiome is associated with the release of metabolites from intestinal flora, causing disruption of endothelial barriers and their proper functioning (Afzaal et al., 2022).

A strong correlation exists between CAD and the abundance of* Streptococcus *and Enterobacteriaceae in the gut (Jie et al., 2017). Patients with CAD are believed to harbor altered populations of the most predominant bacterial species. Ramírez-Macías et al. (2022) reported a significant decrease in the population of Bacteroidetes and an elevation in Firmicutes. The metabolite known as TMAO plays a pivotal role in atherosclerosis and has the potential to serve as a predictor of cardiovascular risk.

Researchers have put forth various mechanisms to comprehend the substantial influence of gut microbiota in the onset and control of CVDs. There is a strong association between copies of bacterial genes encoding trimethylamine (TMA) lyase and the occurrence of atherosclerotic CVDs (Barrington & Lusis, 2017). TMA lyase plays a role in producing TMAO, which is a metabolite originating from the gut microbiota (Witkowski et al., 2022). TMAO has been demonstrated to play a role in the advancement of atherosclerotic CVD in both in vivo and in vitro research (Tang & Hazen, 2014; Jonsson & Bäckhed, 2017). As a result, there is growing interest in utilizing gut microbiota regulations as an active treatment option for the prompt rise in cardiovascular and other metabolic disorders.

4.6.4 Diabetes Mellitus

Diabetes mellitus exerts a detrimental impact on the global population's health. Risk factors for diabetes include heredity, unhealthy dietary habits, physical inactivity, and obesity. The worldwide surge in diabetes incidence can be attributed in large part to the shift toward Westernized lifestyles, alterations in dietary choices, and the adoption of unhealthy habits. Reports indicate that, in 2019, approximately 463 million people worldwide were afflicted with diabetes, a number projected to surpass 700 million by 2045 (Saeedi et al., 2019). Recent research has confirmed a strong connection between the advancement of diabetes and changes in the makeup of the gut microbiota (Gurung et al., 2020; Sender et al., 2016). Diet emerges as a primary determinant in shaping the intestinal microbiome's composition and plays a significant role in diabetes development (Meijnikman et al., 2018).

The composition and type of diet significantly influence the production of different metabolites in the gut microbiota, and different nutrients contribute to the formation of gut microflora. Afzaal et al. (2022) reported that when transitioning from a diet rich in plant polysaccharides and low in fat to a high-sugar and high-fat diet, there is a rapid alteration in the host's gut microbiota composition. In recent decades, there has been a drastic shift in human eating patterns, with people preferring fats over fibers. These changes in dietary habits have also altered the composition of intestinal microflora. Therefore, it is reasonable to suggest a strong correlation between the incidence of diabetes and systemic alterations in intestinal microflora (Sircana et al., 2018).

Research has proposed that the microbiome can play a role in influencing type 2 diabetes, potentially through mechanisms related to changes in butyrate and incretin secretions (Baothman et al., 2016; Nøhr et al., 2013). Individuals with type 2 diabetes often exhibit a degree of imbalance in their intestinal microbial community, characterized by reduced butyrate levels and an increase in opportunistic pathogens (Baothman et al., 2016). Multiple studies have highlighted the substantial impact of gut microbiota on various aspects of type 2 diabetes, including glucose regulation, inflammation, and insulin signaling (Cani, 2018). Nevertheless, further research is necessary to gain a comprehensive understanding of the underlying mechanisms and the influential role of gut microflora in the onset and progression of diabetes.

4.6.5 The Role of Gut Microbiome in Cancer Development and Prevention

Cancer stands as the second leading cause of death globally (Fitzmaurice et al., 2017). A multitude of risk factors contribute to cancer, encompassing exposure to pathogens, UV radiation, toxic substances, dietary choices, and a sedentary lifestyle. Nevertheless, the magnitude of risk hinges significantly on the dosage, timing, and interplay of these factors, in conjunction with an individual's genetic predisposition (Vivarelli et al., 2019). Recent attention has centered on the composition and functions of the intestinal microbiome, given its intricate relationship with the host (Tao et al., 2020). Research has illuminated that alterations within the gut microbial community play a substantial role in the development of colorectal carcinoma and the genesis of carcinogenic tumors, in both genetic and experimental models (Vivarelli et al., 2019; Arthur et al., 2012). The dual nature of the gut microbiome's impact has been revealed through metabolomics and metagenomics studies, encompassing its influence on cancer risk reduction, tumor progression, and response to anticancer treatments (Bultman, 2014).

In prostate cancer patients, an increased presence of *B. massiliensis* has been detected, whereas species such as *Eubacterium rectale* and *Faecalibacterium prausnitzii* have been observed in diminished quantities, suggesting the potential involvement of these specific microbes in prostate cancer pathogenesis (Chung et al., 2018). Furthermore, there is growing recognition of the roles of *Bacteroides fragilis*, *Fusobacterium nucleatum*, and *Peptostreptococcus* anaerobic species in colorectal cancer development, underscoring the close association between the gut microbiome and colorectal cancer (Hsieh et al., 2018). Similarly, *F. nucleatum* and *Clostridium colicanis*, species inhabiting the gut, are considered indicative markers for gastric cancer carcinogenesis (Mehta et al., 2017). Recent research has unveiled the ability of *F. nucleatum* to suppress the host's immune response and promote cellular proliferation. Conversely, diets rich in whole grains and fiber have been linked to a reduced risk of *F. nucleatum*-driven cancer, suggesting that the gut microbiome plays a pivotal role in mediating interactions between food and colorectal cancer (Hall et al., 2017). The recognition of the significant role of gut microbiota in cancer progression has spurred interest in microbiota-based therapies for cancer management. Nevertheless, further research is imperative to gain a comprehensive understanding of the mechanisms underlying the influence of the gut microbiome on cancer progression and its potential anti-carcinogenic properties (Afzaal et al., 2022).

4.6.6 The Role of Gut Microbiome in Inflammatory Bowel Disease Pathogenesis

IBD constitutes a significant global health concern, with the highest incidence observed in Western countries. Alarmingly, cases of IBD have been on the rise in recently industrialized regions across the Middle East, Asia, Africa, and South America (Kaplan & Ng, 2017). Ascertaining the precise etiology and pathogenesis of IBD is of paramount importance. In recent years, substantial progress has been made in unraveling the complexities of IBD progression. The most pivotal and clinically significant breakthrough in this advancement has been the recognition of the gut microbiome as a critical, multifunctional inflammatory factor. Notably, the role of gut microbiota in the pathogenesis of IBD has come into sharp focus, emphasizing its pivotal role in intestinal inflammation. Multiple studies have affirmed a reduction in microbial diversity among IBD patients (Matsuoka & Kanai, 2015; Afzaal et al., 2022). A substantial decline in the abundance of Proteobacteria and Firmicutes has been observed in the microbiota of IBD patients, possibly contributing to the depletion of the intestinal microbiome. Within the Firmicutes phylum, a decrease in the *Clostridium leptum* group, particularly *F. prausnitzii*, has been noted (Wang et al., 2014). The modulation of the gut microbiome to restore immunological equilibrium is currently under consideration as a potential therapeutic avenue for managing IBD patients (Facciotti, 2022).

Pathogenic bacteria, predominantly belonging to the Proteobacteria phylum, have been prominently identified in IBD cases. An analysis of microbial diversity indicates an expansion in the number of bacterial species within this phylum, suggesting an active role in instigating chronic inflammation among IBD patients (Hold et al., 2014). However, further experimental investigations are requisite to explore and comprehend the mechanisms underpinning the progression of IBD.

4.7 EUBIOSIS AND RELATIONSHIP WITH FOOD

The term "eubiosis" is used in contrast to "dysbiosis," where the eubiotic state refers to the collective genome or microbiota that provides the host with a full range of health benefits and functional properties. Dysbiosis, on the other hand, is an imbalance in microbial biodiversity that leads to small chronic inflammations, as a misbalanced microbiome cannot provide its health properties to the host (Suparan et al., 2022). It is necessary to maintain a healthy microbial ecosystem to access all the health benefits offered by microbes present in the gut microbiota. Maintaining a healthy gut balance is achievable through dietary choices. The impact of diet on the microbiome has been a longstanding subject of human research. Food choices can lead to transient changes in the gut ecosystem, particularly in response to components like meat, fish, and dietary fiber, which can exert lasting effects on the composition of the microbiota (Bajinka et al., 2020). Studies have shown that diets consisting of more than two major nutrients can alter the host's microbiota and metabolic output simultaneously (Qiu et al., 2020). Dietary fiber has been found to have significant progressive benefits on human metabolism by altering the gut microflora and producing beneficial butyrate metabolites (Silva et al., 2020). Alongside the intake of a balanced diet in our daily lives, it is important to include a high-fiber diet to maintain good gut health (Zhang et al., 2013).

A well-balanced composition of the microbiota helps in fermenting undigested carbohydrates that our digestive system cannot process. These undigested complex sugars, known as microbiota-accessible carbohydrates, lead to an increased release of health-effective SCFA metabolites (Seo et al., 2020). Among the undigested carbohydrates in the diet are resistant starch, dietary fiber, and oligosaccharides, which have the potential to enhance gut biodiversity and confer health benefits (Yang et al., 2020). The consumption of unsaturated fats from plant-based sources in the diet often leads to a decrease in detrimental bacteria and may promote the growth of butyrate-producing bacteria and *Bifidobacterium*, which can have positive effects on the individual's well-being (Muralidharan et al., 2019). The positive effect of macronutrients on the gut microbiota is well established. Additionally, studies suggest that micronutrients play a key role in reshaping the gut microflora of the host in a healthy way (Ramos & Martín, 2021). All these significant findings point to a positive association between eubiosis and diet, which has a positive, healthy impact on human physiology and disease progression.

4.8 CONCLUSION

Gut microbiota plays a crucial role in promoting overall health and sustaining a healthy lifestyle. To attain a thriving microbiota, the maintenance of a well-balanced microflora composition, known as eubiosis, becomes paramount. Numerous factors and circumstances can disrupt this equilibrium, leading to an imbalanced microbial composition referred to as dysbiosis. The composition of intestinal flora exhibits substantial variation from person to person and region to region, influenced by factors such as age, dietary patterns, substance use (such as smoking), geographic location, and physical activity, among others. Dysbiosis stands as a significant driver of inflammation and serves as the initiation point for various diseases, given the widespread presence of microbes throughout our body.

Common ailments like obesity, CVD, diabetes, IBD, and neurological disorders often stem from an unhealthy or unbalanced microbial composition in the gut. Fortunately, interventions, particularly dietary ones, can help redress this imbalance. A nourishing, well-balanced diet has the potential to mitigate the impact of dysbiosis. Diets rich in unsaturated fats and dietary fiber can release beneficial metabolites that positively influence the host's physiology by reducing the prevalence of opportunistic microbes.

The intricacies of the microbial ecosystem necessitate comprehensive multidisciplinary research by the scientific community. Such research endeavors promise to yield valuable insights into the intricate relationship between gut microbiota and human health, paving the way for innovative therapeutic approaches and interventions aimed at combating a spectrum of diseases.

In conclusion, the maintenance of healthy gut microbiota through the promotion of eubiosis stands as a cornerstone of overall well-being. Striving for this balance, particularly through dietary choices, can exert a profound impact on both the prevention and management of a wide array of health conditions.

BIBLIOGRAPHY

AboNahas, H. H., Darwish, A. M., El-Kareem, A., H. F., AboNahas, Y. H., Mansour, S. A., Korra, Y. H., Sayyed, R. Z., Abdel-Azeem, A. M., & Saied, E. M. (2022). Trust your gut: The human gut microbiome in health and disease. *Microbiome-Gut-Brain Axis: Implications on Health*, 53–96.

Afzaal, M., Saeed, F., Shah, Y. A., Hussain, M., Rabail, R., Socol, C. T., Hassoun, A., Pateiro, M., Lorenzo, J. M., Rusu, A. V., & Aadil, R. M. (2022). Human gut microbiota in health and disease: Unveiling the relationship. *Frontiers in Microbiology, 13,* 999001. https://doi.org/10.3389/fmicb.2022.999001

Ahlawat, S., Asha, & Sharma, K. K. (2021). Gut–organ axis: A microbial outreach and networking. *Letters in Applied Microbiology, 72*(6), 636–668. https://doi.org/10.1111/lam.13333

Allen, J. M., Mailing, L. J., Niemiro, G. M., Moore, R., Cook, M. D., White, B. A., Holscher, H. D., & Woods, J. A. (2018). Exercise alters gut microbiota composition and function in lean and obese humans. *Medicine and Science in Sports and Exercise, 50*(4), 747–757. https://doi.org/10.1249/MSS.0000000000001495

Andoh, A., Nishida, A., Takahashi, K., Inatomi, O., Imaeda, H., Bamba, S., Kito, K., Sugimoto, M., & Kobayashi, T. (2016). Comparison of the gut microbial community between obese and lean peoples using 16S gene sequencing in a Japanese population. *Journal of Clinical Biochemistry and Nutrition, 59*(1), 65–70. https://doi.org/10.3164/jcbn.15-152

Arthur, J. C., Perez-Chanona, E., Mühlbauer, M., Tomkovich, S., Uronis, J. M., Fan, T. J., Campbell, B. J., Abujamel, T., Dogan, B., Rogers, A. B., Rhodes, J. M., Stintzi, A., Simpson, K. W., Hansen, J. J., Keku, T. O., Fodor, A. A., & Jobin, C. (2012). Intestinal inflammation targets cancer-inducing activity of the microbiota. *Science, 338*(6103), 120–123. https://doi.org/10.1126/science.1224820

Auchtung, T. A., Fofanova, T. Y., Stewart, C. J., Nash, A. K., Wong, M. C., Gesell, J. R., Auchtung, J. M., Ajami, N. J., & Petrosino, J. F. (2018). Investigating colonization of the healthy adult gastrointestinal tract by fungi. *mSphere, 3*(2), 10. https://doi.org/10.1128/mSphere.00092-18

Azad, M. B., Konya, T., Maughan, H., Guttman, D. S., Field, C. J., Chari, R. S., Sears, M. R., Becker, A. B., Scott, J. A., Kozyrskyj, A. L., & CHILD Study Investigators. (2013). Gut microbiota of healthy Canadian infants: Profiles by mode of delivery and infant diet at 4 months. *CMAJ: Canadian Medical Association Journal, 185*(5), 385–394. https://doi.org/10.1503/cmaj.121189

Bäckhed, F., Roswall, J., Peng, Y., Feng, Q., Jia, H., Kovatcheva-Datchary, P., Li, Y., Xia, Y., Xie, H., Zhong, H., Khan, M., Zhang, J., Li, J., Xiao, L., Al-Aama, J., Zhang, D., Lee, Y., Kotowska, D., Colding, C., . . . Wang, J. (2015). Dynamics and stabilization of the human gut microbiome during the first year of life. *Cell Host and Microbe, 17*(5), 690–703. https://doi.org/10.1016/j.chom.2015.04.004

Bajinka, O., Tan, Y., Abdelhalim, K. A., Özdemir, G., & Qiu, X. (2020). Extrinsic factors influencing gut microbes, the immediate consequences and restoring eubiosis. *AMB Express, 10*(1), 130. https://doi.org/10.1186/s13568-020-01066-8

Baothman, O. A., Zamzami, M. A., Taher, I., Abubaker, J., & Abu-Farha, M. (2016). The role of gut microbiota in the development of obesity and diabetes. *Lipids in Health and Disease, 15*(1), 108. https://doi.org/10.1186/s12944-016-0278-4

Barrington, W. T., & Lusis, A. J. (2017). Atherosclerosis: Association between the gut microbiome and atherosclerosis. *Nature Reviews. Cardiology, 14*(12), 699–700. https://doi.org/10.1038/nrcardio.2017.169

Bäumler, A. J., & Sperandio, V. (2016). Interactions between the microbiota and pathogenic bacteria in the gut. *Nature, 535*(7610), 85–93. https://doi.org/10.1038/nature18849

Biagi, E., Rampelli, S., Turroni, S., Quercia, S., Candela, M., & Brigidi, P. (2017). The gut microbiota of centenarians: Signatures of longevity in the gut microbiota profile. *Mechanisms of Ageing and Development, 165*(B), 180–184. https://doi.org/10.1016/j.mad.2016.12.013

Brüssow, H. (2020). Problems with the concept of gut microbiota dysbiosis. *Microbial Biotechnology, 13*(2), 423–434. https://doi.org/10.1111/1751-7915.13479

Bultman, S. J. (2014). Emerging roles of the microbiome in cancer. *Carcinogenesis, 35*(2), 249–255. https://doi.org/10.1093/carcin/bgt392

Cani, P. D. (2018). Human gut microbiome: Hopes, threats, and promises. *Gut, 67*(9), 1716–1725. https://doi.org/10.1136/gutjnl-2018-316723

Cao, S. Y., Zhao, C. N., Xu, X. Y., Tang, G. Y., Corke, H., Gan, R. Y., & Li, H. B. (2019). Dietary plants, gut microbiota, and obesity: Effects and mechanisms. *Trends in Food Science and Technology, 92,* 194–204. https://doi.org/10.1016/j.tifs.2019.08.004

Chang, C., & Lin, H. (2016). Dysbiosis in gastrointestinal disorders. *Best Practice and Research. Clinical Gastroenterology, 30*(1), 3–15. https://doi.org/10.1016/j.bpg.2016.02.001

Chen, C., Huang, X., Fang, S., Yang, H., He, M., Zhao, Y., & Huang, L. (2018). Contribution of host genetics to the variation of microbial composition of cecum lumen and feces in pigs. *Frontiers in Microbiology, 9,* 2626. https://doi.org/10.3389/fmicb.2018.02626

Chen, Z. R., Jin, S. F., Ma, W. B., & Jiang, R. L. (2021). Intestinal microecology: A crucial strategy for targeted therapy of liver diseases. *Hepatobiliary and Pancreatic Diseases International, 20*(5), 499–500. https://doi.org/10.1016/j.hbpd.2021.07.007

Chung, L., Thiele Orberg, E., Geis, A. L., Chan, J. L., Fu, K., DeStefano Shields, C. E., Dejea, C. M., Fathi, P., Chen, J., Finard, B. B., Tam, A. J., McAllister, F., Fan, H., Wu, X., Ganguly, S., Lebid, A., Metz, P., Van Meerbeke, S. W., Huso, D. L., . . . Housseau, F. (2018). *Bacteroides fragilis* toxin coordinates a pro-carcinogenic inflammatory cascade via targeting of colonic epithelial cells. *Cell Host and Microbe, 23*(2), 203–214.e5. https://doi.org/10.1016/j.chom.2018.01.007

Clarke, S. F., Murphy, E. F., O'Sullivan, O., Lucey, A. J., Humphreys, M., Hogan, A., Hayes, P., O'Reilly, M., Jeffery, I. B., Wood-Martin, R., Kerins, D. M., Quigley, E., Ross, R. P., O'Toole, P. W., Molloy, M. G., Falvey, E., Shanahan, F., & Cotter, P. D. (2014). Exercise and associated dietary extremes impact on gut microbial diversity. *Gut, 63*(12), 1913–1920. https://doi.org/10.1136/gutjnl-2013-306541

DeGruttola, A. K., Low, D., Mizoguchi, A., & Mizoguchi, E. (2016). Current understanding of dysbiosis in disease in human and animal models. *Inflammatory Bowel Diseases, 22*(5), 1137–1150. https://doi.org/10.1097/MIB.0000000000000750

Del Chierico, F., Vernocchi, P., Petrucca, A., Paci, P., Fuentes, S., Praticò, G., Capuani, G., Masotti, A., Reddel, S., Russo, A., Vallone, C., Salvatori, G., Buffone, E., Signore, F., Rigon, G., Dotta, A., Miccheli, A., de Vos, W. M., Dallapiccola, B., & Putignani, L. (2015). Phylogenetic and metabolic tracking of gut microbiota during perinatal development. *PLoS One, 10*(9), e0137347. https://doi.org/10.1371/journal.pone.0137347

Den Besten, G., Van Eunen, K., Groen, A. K., Venema, K., Reijngoud, D. J., & Bakker, B. M. (2013). The role of short-chain fatty acids in the interplay between diet, gut microbiota, and host energy metabolism. *Journal of Lipid Research, 54*(9), 2325–2340. https://doi.org/10.1194/jlr.R036012

Deo, P. N., & Deshmukh, R. (2019). Oral microbiome: Unveiling the fundamentals. *Journal of Oral and Maxillofacial Pathology, 23*(1), 122–128. https://doi.org/10.4103/jomfp.JOMFP_304_18

Dickson, R. P., & Huffnagle, G. B. (2015). The lung microbiome: New principles for respiratory bacteriology in health and disease. *PLoS Pathogens, 11*(7), e1004923. https://doi.org/10.1371/journal.ppat.1004923

Dickson, R. P., Martinez, F. J., & Huffnagle, G. B. (2014). The role of the microbiome in exacerbations of chronic lung diseases. *Lancet, 384*(9944), 691–702. https://doi.org/10.1016/S0140-6736(14)61136-3

Elmassry, M. M., Zayed, A., & Farag, M. A. (2022). Gut homeostasis and microbiota under attack: Impact of the different types of food contaminants on gut health. *Critical Reviews in Food Science and Nutrition, 62*(3), 738–763. https://doi.org/10.1080/10408398.2020.1828263

Estaki, M., Pither, J., Baumeister, P., Little, J. P., Gill, S. K., Ghosh, S., Ahmadi-Vand, Z., Marsden, K. R., & Gibson, D. L. (2016). Cardiorespiratory fitness as a predictor of intestinal microbial diversity and distinct metagenomic functions. *Microbiome, 4*(1), 42. https://doi.org/10.1186/s40168-016-0189-7

Facciotti, F. (2022). Modulation of intestinal immune cell responses by eubiotic or dysbiotic microbiota in inflammatory bowel diseases. *Pharma Nutrition, 21,* 100303. https://doi.org/10.1016/j.phanu.2022.100303

Fouhy, F., Watkins, C., Hill, C. J., O'Shea, C. A., Nagle, B., Dempsey, E. M., O'Toole, P. W., Ross, R. P., Ryan, C. A., & Stanton, C. (2019). Perinatal factors affect the gut microbiota up to four years after birth. *Nature Communications, 10*(1), 1517. https://doi.org/10.1038/s41467-019-09252-4

Francino, M. P. (2014). Early development of the gut microbiota and immune health. *Pathogens, 3*(3), 769–790. https://doi.org/10.3390/pathogens3030769

Geng, J., Ni, Q., Sun, W., Li, L., & Feng, X. (2022). The links between gut microbiota and obesity and obesity-related diseases. *Biomedicine and Pharmacotherapy, 147,* 112678. https://doi.org/10.1016/j.biopha.2022.112678

Gensollen, T., Iyer, S. S., Kasper, D. L., & Blumberg, R. S. (2016). How colonization by microbiota in early life shapes the immune system. *Science, 352*(6285), 539–544. https://doi.org/10.1126/science.aad9378

Fitzmaurice, C., Allen, C., Barber, R. M., Barregard, L., Bhutta, Z. A., Brenner, H., Dicker, D. J., Chimed-Orchir, O., Dandona, R., Dandona, L., Fleming, T., Forouzanfar, M. H., Hancock, J., Hay, R. J., Hunter-Merrill, R., Huynh, C., Hosgood, H. D., Johnson, C. O., Jonas, J. B. . . . Naghavi, M. (2017). Global, regional, and national cancer incidence, mortality, years of life lost, years lived with disability, and disability-adjusted life-years for 32 cancer groups, 1990 to 2015: A systematic analysis for the global burden of disease study. *JAMA Oncology, 3*(4), 524–548. https://doi.org/10.1001/jamaoncol.2016.5688

Gomaa, E. Z. (2020). Human gut microbiota/microbiome in health and diseases: A review. *Antonie van Leeuwenhoek, 113*(12), 2019–2040. https://doi.org/10.1007/s10482-020-01474-7

Gómez-Guzmán, M., Toral, M., Romero, M., Jiménez, R., Galindo, P., Sánchez, M., Zarzuelo, M. J., Olivares, M., Gálvez, J., & Duarte, J. (2015). Antihypertensive effects of probiotics Lactobacillus strains in spontaneously hypertensive rats. *Molecular Nutrition and Food Research, 59*(11), 2326–2336. https://doi.org/10.1002/mnfr.201500290

Gurung, M., Li, Z., You, H., Rodrigues, R., Jump, D. B., Morgun, A., & Shulzhenko, N. (2020). Role of gut microbiota in type 2 diabetes pathophysiology. *EBio Medicine, 51*, 102590. https://doi.org/10.1016/j.ebiom.2019.11.051

Hall, A. B., Yassour, M., Sauk, J., Garner, A., Jiang, X., Arthur, T., Lagoudas, G. K., Vatanen, T., Fornelos, N., Wilson, R., Bertha, M., Cohen, M., Garber, J., Khalili, H., Gevers, D., Ananthakrishnan, A. N., Kugathasan, S., Lander, E. S., Blainey, P., . . . Huttenhower, C. (2017). A novel *Ruminococcus gnavus* clade enriched in inflammatory bowel disease patients. *Genome Medicine, 9*(1), 103. https://doi.org/10.1186/s13073-017-0490-5

Hasan, N., & Yang, H. (2019). Factors affecting the composition of the gut microbiota, and its modulation. *PeerJ, 7,* e7502. https://doi.org/10.7717/peerj.7502

Hillman, E. T., Lu, H., Yao, T., & Nakatsu, C. H. (2017). Microbial ecology along the gastrointestinal tract. *Microbes and Environments, 32*(4), 300–313. https://doi.org/10.1264/jsme2.ME17017

Hills, R. D., Pontefract, B. A., Mishcon, H. R., Black, C. A., Sutton, S. C., & Theberge, C. R. (2019). Gut microbiome: Profound implications for diet and disease. *Nutrients, 11*(7), 1613. https://doi.org/10.3390/nu11071613

Hold, G. L., Smith, M., Grange, C., Watt, E. R., El-Omar, E. M., & Mukhopadhya, I. (2014). Role of the gut microbiota in inflammatory bowel disease pathogenesis: What have we learnt in the past 10 years? *World Journal of Gastroenterology, 20*(5), 1192–1210. https://doi.org/10.3748/wjg.v20.i5.1192

Hollister, E. B., Riehle, K., Luna, R. A., Weidler, E. M., Rubio-Gonzales, M., Mistretta, T. A., Raza, S., Doddapaneni, H. V., Metcalf, G. A., Muzny, D. M., Gibbs, R. A., Petrosino, J. F., Shulman, R. J., & Versalovic, J. (2015). Structure and function of the healthy pre-adolescent pediatric gut microbiome. *Microbiome, 3*(1), 36. https://doi.org/10.1186/s40168-015-0101-x

Hooks, K. B., & O'Malley, M. A. (2017). Dysbiosis and its discontents. *mBio, 8*(5), 10–1128. https://doi.org/10.1128/mBio.01492-17

Hou, K., Wu, Z. X., Chen, X. Y., Wang, J. Q., Zhang, D., Xiao, C., Zhu, D., Koya, J. B., Wei, L., Li, J., & Chen, Z. S. (2022). Microbiota in health and diseases. *Signal Transduction and Targeted Therapy, 7*(1), 135. https://doi.org/10.1038/s41392-022-00974-4

Hsieh, Y. Y., Tung, S. Y., Pan, H. Y., Yen, C. W., Xu, H. W., Lin, Y. J., Deng, Y. F., Hsu, W. T., Wu, C. S., & Li, C. (2018). Increased abundance of *Clostridium* and *Fusobacterium* in gastric microbiota of patients with gastric cancer in Taiwan. *Scientific Reports, 8*(1), 158. https://doi.org/10.1038/s41598-017-18596-0

Hsu, C. N., Hou, C. Y., Chang-Chien, G. P., Lin, S., Yang, H. W., & Tain, Y. L. (2020). Perinatal resveratrol therapy prevents hypertension programmed by maternal chronic kidney disease in adult male offspring: Implications of the gut microbiome and their metabolites. *Biomedicines, 8*(12), 567. https://doi.org/10.3390/biomedicines8120567

Hughes, R. L. (2020). A review of the role of the gut microbiome in personalized sports nutrition. *Frontiers in Nutrition, 6*, 191. https://doi.org/10.3389/fnut.2019.00191

Iebba, V., Totino, V., Gagliardi, A., Santangelo, F., Cacciotti, F., Trancassini, M., Mancini, C., Cicerone, C., Corazziari, E., Pantanella, F., & Schippa, S. (2016). Eubiosis and dysbiosis: The two sides of the microbiota. *New Microbiologica, 39*(1), 1–12.

Isaac, S., Scher, J. U., Djukovic, A., Jiménez, N., Littman, D. R., Abramson, S. B., Pamer, E. G., & Ubeda, C. (2016). Short- and long-term effects of oral vancomycin on the human intestinal microbiota. *Journal of Antimicrobial Chemotherapy, 72*(1), 128–136. https://doi.org/10.1093/jac/dkw383

Jandhyala, S. M., Talukdar, R., Subramanyam, C., Vuyyuru, H., Sasikala, M., & Nageshwar Reddy, D. N. (2015). Role of the normal gut microbiota. *World Journal of Gastroenterology, 21*(29), 8787–8803. https://doi.org/10.3748/wjg.v21.i29.8787

Jansen, V. L., Gerdes, V. E., Middeldorp, S., & van Mens, T. E. (2021). Gut microbiota and their metabolites in cardiovascular disease. *Best Practice and Research. Clinical Endocrinology and Metabolism, 35*(3), 101492. https://doi.org/10.1016/j.beem.2021.101492

Jethwani, P., & Grover, K. (2019). Gut microbiota in health and diseases—a review. *International Journal of Current Microbiology and Applied Sciences, 8*(8), 1586–1599. https://doi.org/10.20546/ijcmas.2019.808.187

Jie, Z., Xia, H., Zhong, S. L., Feng, Q., Li, S., Liang, S., Zhong, H., Liu, Z., Gao, Y., Zhao, H., Zhang, D., Su, Z., Fang, Z., Lan, Z., Li, J., Xiao, L., Li, J., Li, R., Li, X.,. . . Kristiansen, K. (2017). The gut microbiome in atherosclerotic cardiovascular disease. *Nature Communications, 8*(1), 845. https://doi.org/10.1038/s41467-017-00900-1

Jonsson, A. L., & Bäckhed, F. (2017). Role of gut microbiota in atherosclerosis. *Nature Reviews. Cardiology, 14*(2), 79–87. https://doi.org/10.1038/nrcardio.2016.183

Jose, P. A., & Raj, D. (2015). Gut microbiota in hypertension. *Current Opinion in Nephrology and Hypertension, 24*(5), 403–409. https://doi.org/10.1097/MNH.0000000000000149

Kang, Y., & Cai, Y. (2018). Gut microbiota and hypertension: From pathogenesis to new therapeutic strategies. *Clinics and Research in Hepatology and Gastroenterology, 42*(2), 110–117. https://doi.org/10.1016/j.clinre.2017.09.006

Kaplan, G. G., & Ng, S. C. (2017). Understanding and preventing the global increase of inflammatory bowel disease. *Gastroenterology, 152*(2), 313–321.e2. https://doi.org/10.1053/j.gastro.2016.10.020

Khan, M. J., Gerasimidis, K., Edwards, C. A., & Shaikh, M. G. (2016). Role of gut microbiota in the etiology of obesity: Proposed mechanisms and review of the literature. *Journal of Obesity, 2016*, 7353642. https://doi.org/10.1155/2016/7353642

Klingensmith, N. J., & Coopersmith, C. M. (2016). The gut is the motor of multiple organ dysfunction in critical illness. *Critical Care Clinics, 32*(2), 203–212. https://doi.org/10.1016/j.ccc.2015.11.004

Kurilshikov, A., Wijmenga, C., Fu, J., & Zhernakova, A. (2017). Host genetics and gut microbiome: Challenges and perspectives. *Trends in Immunology, 38*(9), 633–647. https://doi.org/10.1016/j.it.2017.06.003

Laterza, L., Rizzatti, G., Gaetani, E., Chiusolo, P., & Gasbarrini, A. (2016). The gut microbiota and immune system relationship in human graft-versus-host disease. *Mediterranean Journal of Hematology and Infectious Diseases, 8*(1), e2016025. https://doi.org/10.4084/MJHID.2016.025

Lazar, V., Ditu, L. M., Pircalabioru, G. G., Gheorghe, I., Curutiu, C., Holban, A. M., Picu, A., Petcu, L., & Chifiriuc, M. C. (2018). Aspects of gut microbiota and immune system interactions in infectious diseases, immunopathology, and cancer. *Frontiers in Immunology, 9,* 1830. https://doi.org/10.3389/fimmu.2018.01830

Le Chatelier, E., Nielsen, T., Qin, J., Prifti, E., Hildebrand, F., Falony, G., Almeida, M., Arumugam, M., Batto, J. M., Kennedy, S., Leonard, P., Li, J., Burgdorf, K., Grarup, N., Jørgensen, T., Brandslund, I., Nielsen, H. B., Juncker, A. S., Bertalan, M., . . . Pedersen, O. (2013). Richness of human gut microbiome correlates with metabolic markers. *Nature, 500*(7464), 541–546. https://doi.org/10.1038/nature12506

Lee, S., Lim, J. Y., Kim, B. S., Cho, S. J., Kim, N. Y., Kim, O. B., & Kim, Y. (2015). Comparison of the gut microbiota profile in breast-fed and formula-fed Korean infants using Pyrosequencing. *Nutrition Research and Practice, 9*(3), 242–248. https://doi.org/10.4162/nrp.2015.9.3.242

Levy, M., Kolodziejczyk, A. A., Thaiss, C. A., & Elinav, E. (2017). Dysbiosis and the immune system. *Nature Reviews. Immunology, 17*(4), 219–232. https://doi.org/10.1038/nri.2017.7

Lindsay, E. C., Metcalfe, N. B., & Llewellyn, M. S. (2020). The potential role of the gut microbiota in shaping host energetics and metabolic rate. *Journal of Animal Ecology*, *89*(11), 2415–2426. https://doi.org/10.1111/1365-2656.13327

López, M. (2017). EJE PRIZE 2017: Hypothalamic AMPK: A golden target against obesity? *European Journal of Endocrinology, 176*(5), R235–R246. https://doi.org/10.1530/EJE-16-0927

Lozupone, C. A., Stombaugh, J. I., Gordon, J. I., Jansson, J. K., & Knight, R. (2012). Diversity, stability, and resilience of the human gut microbiota. *Nature, 489*(7415), 220–230. https://doi.org/10.1038/nature11550

Martinez, I., Stegen, J. C., Maldonado-Gómez, M. X., Eren, A. M., Siba, P. M., Greenhill, A. R., & Walter, J. (2015). The gut microbiota of rural Papua New Guineans: Composition, diversity patterns, and ecological processes. *Cell Reports, 11*(4), 527–538. https://doi.org/10.1016/j.celrep.2015.03.049

Matsuoka, K., & Kanai, T. (2015, January). The gut microbiota and inflammatory bowel disease. In *Seminars in immunopathology* (Vol. 37, pp. 47–55). Springer Berlin Heidelberg.

Mehta, R. S., Nishihara, R., Cao, Y., Song, M., Mima, K., Qian, Z. R., Nowak, J. A., Kosumi, K., Hamada, T., Masugi, Y., Bullman, S., Drew, D. A., Kostic, A. D., Fung, T. T., Garrett, W. S., Huttenhower, C., Wu, K., Meyerhardt, J. A., Zhang, X., . . . Ogino, S. (2017). Association of dietary patterns with risk of colorectal cancer subtypes classified by *Fusobacterium nucleatum* in tumor tissue. *JAMA Oncology, 3*(7), 921–927. https://doi.org/10.1001/jamaoncol.2016.6374

Meijnikman, A. S., Gerdes, V. E., Nieuwdorp, M., & Herrema, H. (2018). Evaluating the causality of gut microbiota in obesity and diabetes in humans. *Endocrine Reviews, 39*(2), 133–153. https://doi.org/10.1210/er.2017-00192

Michael, S. (2016). Gut microbiota and host evolution scaling up symbiosis. *Trends in Ecology and Evolution, 31*(7), 539–549.

Miremadi, F., Sherkat, F., & Stojanovska, L. (2016). Hypocholesterolaemic effect and anti-hypertensive properties of probiotics and prebiotics: A review. *Journal of Functional Foods*, *25*, 497–510.

Moghadamrad, S., McCoy, K. D., Geuking, M. B., Sägesser, H., Kirundi, J., Macpherson, A. J., & De Gottardi, A. (2015). Attenuated portal hypertension in germ-free mice: Function of bacterial flora on the development of mesenteric lymphatic and blood vessels. *Hepatology, 61*(5), 1685–1695. https://doi.org/10.1002/hep.27698

Muralidharan, J., Galiè, S., Hernández-Alonso, P., Bulló, M., & Salas-Salvadó, J. (2019). Plant-based fat, dietary patterns rich in vegetable fat and gut microbiota modulation. *Frontiers in Nutrition, 6,* 157. https://doi.org/10.3389/fnut.2019.00157

Nagpal, R., Tsuji, H., Takahashi, T., Nomoto, K., Kawashima, K., Nagata, S., & Yamashiro, Y. (2017). Ontogenesis of the gut microbiota composition in healthy, full-term, vaginally born and breast-fed infants over the first 3 years of life: A quantitative bird's-eye view. *Frontiers in Microbiology, 8,* 1388. https://doi.org/10.3389/fmicb.2017.01388

Natividad, J. M. M., & Verdu, E. F. (2013). Modulation of intestinal barrier by intestinal microbiota: Pathological and therapeutic implications. *Pharmacological Research, 69*(1), 42–51. https://doi.org/10.1016/j.phrs.2012.10.007

Nøhr, M. K., Pedersen, M. H., Gille, A., Egerod, K. L., Engelstoft, M. S., Husted, A. S., Sichlau, R. M., Grunddal, K. V., Poulsen, S. S., Han, S., Jones, R. M., Offermanns, S., & Schwartz, T. W. (2013). GPR41/FFAR3 and GPR43/FFAR2 as cosensors for short-chain fatty acids in enteroendocrine cells vs FFAR3 in enteric neurons and FFAR2 in enteric leukocytes. *Endocrinology, 154*(10), 3552–3564. https://doi.org/10.1210/en.2013-1142

Odamaki, T., Kato, K., Sugahara, H., Hashikura, N., Takahashi, S., Xiao, J. Z., Abe, F., & Osawa, R. (2016). Age-related changes in gut microbiota composition from newborn to centenarian: A cross-sectional study. *BMC Microbiology, 16*(1), 90. https://doi.org/10.1186/s12866-016-0708-5

Odutayo, A., Wong, C. X., Hsiao, A. J., Hopewell, S., Altman, D. G., & Emdin, C. A. (2016). Atrial fibrillation and risks of cardiovascular disease, renal disease, and death: Systematic review and meta-analysis. *BMJ, 354*. https://doi.org/10.1136/bmj.i4482

Owaga, E., Hsieh, R. H., Mugendi, B., Masuku, S., Shih, C. K., & Chang, J. S. (2015). Th17 cells as potential probiotic therapeutic targets in inflammatory bowel diseases. *International Journal of Molecular Sciences, 16*(9), 20841–20858. https://doi.org/10.3390/ijms160920841

Paone, P., & Cani, P. D. (2020). Mucus barrier, mucins, and gut microbiota: The expected slimy partners? *Gut, 69*(12), 2232–2243. https://doi.org/10.1136/gutjnl-2020-322260

Passos, M. D. C. F., & Moraes-Filho, J. P. (2017). Intestinal microbiota in digestive diseases. *Arquivos de Gastroenterologia, 54*(3), 255–262. https://doi.org/10.1590/S0004-2803.201700000-31

Peterson, C. T., Sharma, V., Elmén, L., & Peterson, S. N. (2015). Immune homeostasis, dysbiosis and therapeutic modulation of the gut microbiota. *Clinical and Experimental Immunology, 179*(3), 363–377. https://doi.org/10.1111/cei.12474

Philips, C. A., Augustine, P., Ganesan, K., Ranade, S., Chopra, V., Patil, K., Shende, S., Ahamed, R., Kumbar, S., Rajesh, S., George, T., Mohanan, M., Mohan, N., Phadke, N., Rani, M., Narayanan, A., & Jagan, S. M. (2022). The role of gut microbiota in clinical complications, disease severity, and treatment response in severe alcoholic hepatitis. *Indian Journal of Gastroenterology, 41*(1), 37–51. https://doi.org/10.1007/s12664-021-01157-9

Piccioni, A., Cicchinelli, S., Valletta, F., De Luca, G., Longhitano, Y., Candelli, M., Ojetti, V., Sardeo, F., Navarra, S., Covino, M., & Franceschi, F. (2022). Gut microbiota and autoimmune diseases: A charming real world together with probiotics. *Current Medicinal Chemistry, 29*(18), 3147–3159. https://doi.org/10.2174/0929867328666210922161913

Pickard, J. M., Zeng, M. Y., Caruso, R., & Núñez, G. (2017). Gut microbiota: Role in pathogen colonization, immune responses, and inflammatory disease. *Immunological Reviews, 279*(1), 70–89. https://doi.org/10.1111/imr.12567

Pindjakova, J., Sartini, C., Lo Re, O., Rappa, F., Coupe, B., Lelouvier, B., Pazienza, V., & Vinciguerra, M. (2017). Gut dysbiosis and adaptive immune response in diet-induced obesity vs. systemic inflammation. *Frontiers in Microbiology, 8,* 1157. https://doi.org/10.3389/fmicb.2017.01157

Pluznick, J. L., Protzko, R. J., Gevorgyan, H., Peterlin, Z., Sipos, A., Han, J., Brunet, I., Wan, L. X., Rey, F., Wang, T., Firestein, S. J., Yanagisawa, M., Gordon, J. I., Eichmann, A., Peti-Peterdi, J., & Caplan, M. J. (2013). Olfactory receptor responding to gut microbiota-derived signals plays a role in renin secretion and blood pressure regulation. *Proceedings of the National Academy of Sciences of the United States of America, 110*(11), 4410–4415. https://doi.org/10.1073/pnas.1215927110

Quigley, E. M. (2013). Gut bacteria in health and disease. *Gastroenterology & Hepatology*, *9*(9), 560.

Qian, B., Zhang, K., Li, Y., & Sun, K. (2022). Update on gut microbiota in cardiovascular diseases. *Frontiers in Cellular and Infection Microbiology, 12,* 1059349. https://doi.org/10.3389/fcimb.2022.1059349

Qiu, X., Ye, Q., Sun, M., Wang, L., Tan, Y., & Wu, G. (2020). Saturated hydrogen improves lipid metabolism disorders and dysbacteriosis induced by a high-fat diet. *Experimental Biology and Medicine, 245*(6), 512–521. https://doi.org/10.1177/1535370219898407

Ramírez-Macías, I., Orenes-Piñero, E., Camelo-Castillo, A., Rivera-Caravaca, J. M., López-García, C., & Marín, F. (2022). Novel insights in the relationship of gut microbiota and coronary artery diseases. *Critical Reviews in Food Science and Nutrition, 62*(14), 3738–3750. https://doi.org/10.1080/10408398.2020.1868397

Ramos, S., & Martín, M. Á. (2021). Impact of diet on gut microbiota. *Current Opinion in Food Science, 37,* 83–90. https://doi.org/10.1016/j.cofs.2020.09.006

Ray, K. (2018). Gut microbiota filling up on fibre for a healthy gut. *Nature Reviews Gastroenterology and Hepatology, 15*(2), 67. https://doi.org/10.1038/nrgastro.2018.2

Riccio, P. (2011). The molecular basis of nutritional intervention in multiple sclerosis: A narrative review. *Complementary Therapies in Medicine, 19*(4), 228–237. https://doi.org/10.1016/j.ctim.2011.06.006

Riccio, P., & Rossano, R. (2020). The human gut microbiota is neither an organ nor a commensal. *FEBS Letters, 594*(20), 3262–3271. https://doi.org/10.1002/1873-3468.13946

Rossi, M., & Bot, A. (2013). The Th17 cell population and the immune homeostasis of the gastrointestinal tract. *International Reviews of Immunology, 32*(5–6), 471–474. https://doi.org/10.3109/08830185.2013.843983

Rust, P., & Ekmekcioglu, C. (2017). Impact of salt intake on the pathogenesis and treatment of hypertension. *Hypertension: From Basic Research to Clinical Practice,* 61–84.

Ryma, T., Samer, A., Soufli, I., Rafa, H., & Touil-Boukoffa, C. (2021). Role of probiotics and their metabolites in inflammatory bowel diseases (IBDs). *Gastroenterology Insights, 12*(1), 56–66. https://doi.org/10.3390/gastroent12010006

Sabatino, A., Regolisti, G., Brusasco, I., Cabassi, A., Morabito, S., & Fiaccadori, E. (2015). Alterations of intestinal barrier and microbiota in chronic kidney disease. *Nephrology, Dialysis, Transplantation, 30*(6), 924–933. https://doi.org/10.1093/ndt/gfu287

Saeedi, P., Petersohn, I., Salpea, P., Malanda, B., Karuranga, S., Unwin, N., Colagiuri, S., Guariguata, L., Motala, A. A., Ogurtsova, K., Shaw, J. E., Bright, D., Williams, R., & IDF Diabetes Atlas Committee. (2019). Global and regional diabetes prevalence estimates for 2019 and projections for 2030 and 2045: Results from the international diabetes federation diabetes atlas. *Diabetes Research and Clinical Practice, 157,* 107843. https://doi.org/10.1016/j.diabres.2019.107843

Schanche, M., Avershina, E., Dotterud, C., Øien, T., Storrø, O., Johnsen, R., & Rudi, K. (2015). High-resolution analyses of overlap in the microbiota between mothers and their children. *Current Microbiology, 71*(2), 283–290. https://doi.org/10.1007/s00284-015-0843-5

Schluter, J., Peled, J. U., Taylor, B. P., Markey, K. A., Smith, M., Taur, Y., Niehus, R., Staffas, A., Dai, A., Fontana, E., Amoretti, L. A., Wright, R. J., Morjaria, S., Fenelus, M., Pessin, M. S., Chao, N. J., Lew, M., Bohannon, L., Bush, A., . . . Xavier, J. B. (2020). The gut microbiota is associated with immune cell dynamics in humans. *Nature, 588*(7837), 303–307. https://doi.org/10.1038/s41586-020-2971-8

Schnorr, S. L., Candela, M., Rampelli, S., Centanni, M., Consolandi, C., Basaglia, G., Turroni, S., Biagi, E., Peano, C., Severgnini, M., Fiori, J., Gotti, R., De Bellis, G., Luiselli, D., Brigidi, P., Mabulla, A., Marlowe, F., Henry, A. G., & Crittenden, A. N. (2014). Gut microbiome of the Hadza hunter-gatherers. *Nature Communications, 5,* 3654. https://doi.org/10.1038/ncomms4654

Segata, N., Haake, S. K., Mannon, P., Lemon, K. P., Waldron, L., Gevers, D., Huttenhower, C., & Izard, J. (2012). Composition of the adult digestive tract bacterial microbiome based on seven mouth surfaces, tonsils, throat and stool samples. *Genome Biology, 13*(6), R42. https://doi.org/10.1186/gb-2012-13-6-r42

Sekirov, I., Russell, S. L., Antunes, L. C., & Finlay, B. B. (2010). Gut microbiota in health and disease. *Physiological Reviews, 90*(3), 859–904. https://doi.org/10.1152/physrev.00045.2009

Sender, R., Fuchs, S., & Milo, R. (2016). Revised estimates for the number of human and bacteria cells in the body. *PLoS Biology, 14*(8), e1002533. https://doi.org/10.1371/journal.pbio.1002533

Seo, Y. S., Lee, H. B., Kim, Y., & Park, H. Y. (2020). Dietary carbohydrate constituents related to gut dysbiosis and health. *Microorganisms, 8*(3), 427. https://doi.org/10.3390/microorganisms8030427

Shah, T. G., Sutaria, J. M., & Vyas, M. V. (2019). The association between pulmonary hypertension and stroke: A systematic review and meta-analysis. *International Journal of Cardiology, 295,* 21–24. https://doi.org/10.1016/j.ijcard.2019.07.085

Shreiner, A. B., Kao, J. Y., & Young, V. B. (2015). The gut microbiome in health and in disease. *Current Opinion in Gastroenterology, 31*(1), 69–75. https://doi.org/10.1097/MOG.0000000000000139

Silva, F. M. C. E., Oliveira, E. E. D., Ambrósio, M. G. E., Ayupe, M. C., Souza, V. P. D., Gameiro, J., Reis, D. R. L., Machado, M. A., Macedo, G. C., Mattes, J., & Ferreira, A. P. (2020). High-fat diet-induced obesity worsens TH2 immune response and immunopathologic characteristics in murine model of eosinophilic oesophagitis. *Clinical and Experimental Allergy, 50*(2), 244–255. https://doi.org/10.1111/cea.13533

Simões, C. D., Maganinho, M., & Sousa, A. S. (2022). FODMAPs, inflammatory bowel disease, and gut microbiota: Updated overview on the current evidence. *European Journal of Nutrition, 61*(3), 1187–1198. https://doi.org/10.1007/s00394-021-02755-1

Sircana, A., Framarin, L., Leone, N., Berrutti, M., Castellino, F., Parente, R., De Michieli, F., Paschetta, E., & Musso, G. (2018). Altered gut microbiota in type 2 diabetes: Just a coincidence? *Current Diabetes Reports, 18*(10), 98. https://doi.org/10.1007/s11892-018-1057-6

Spencer, S. P., Fragiadakis, G. K., & Sonnenburg, J. L. (2019). Pursuing human-relevant gut microbiota-immune interactions. *Immunity, 51*(2), 225–239. https://doi.org/10.1016/j.immuni.2019.08.002

Suparan, K., Sriwichaiin, S., Chattipakorn, N., & Chattipakorn, S. C. (2022). Human blood bacteriome: Eubiotic and dysbiotic states in health and diseases. *Cells, 11*(13). https://doi.org/10.3390/cells11132015

Tang, W. H., & Hazen, S. L. (2014). The contributory role of gut microbiota in cardiovascular disease. *Journal of Clinical Investigation, 124*(10), 4204–4211. https://doi.org/10.1172/JCI72331

Tao, J., Li, S., Gan, R. Y., Zhao, C. N., Meng, X., & Li, H. B. (2020). Targeting gut microbiota with dietary components on cancer: Effects and potential mechanisms of action. *Critical Reviews in Food Science and Nutrition, 60*(6), 1025–1037. https://doi.org/10.1080/10408398.2018.1555789

Thaiss, C. A., Zmora, N., Levy, M., & Elinav, E. (2016). The microbiome and innate immunity. *Nature, 535*(7610), 65–74. https://doi.org/10.1038/nature18847

Thomas, R. M., & Jobin, C. (2020). Microbiota in pancreatic health and disease: The next frontier in microbiome research. *Nature Reviews. Gastroenterology and Hepatology, 17*(1), 53–64. https://doi.org/10.1038/s41575-019-0242-7

Thompson, A. L., Monteagudo-Mera, A., Cadenas, M. B., Lampl, M. L., Azcarate-Peril, M. A., McGavin, M. J., & Eckstein, T. (2015). Milk and solid-feeding practices and daycare attendance are associated with differences in bacterial diversity, predominant communities, and metabolic and immune function of the infant gut microbiome. *Frontiers in Cellular and Infection Microbiology, 5,* 3. https://doi.org/10.3389/fcimb.2015.00003

Tibbs, T. N., Lopez, L. R., & Arthur, J. C. (2019). The influence of the microbiota on immune development, chronic inflammation, and cancer in the context of aging. *Microbial Cell, 6*(8), 324–334. https://doi.org/10.15698/mic2019.08.685

Tomkovich, S., & Jobin, C. (2016). Microbiota in pancreatic health and disease: The next frontier in microbiome research. *Nature Reviews. Gastroenterology and Hepatology, 17*(1), 53–64.

Tong, X., Xu, J., Lian, F., Yu, X., Zhao, Y., Xu, L., Zhang, M., Zhao, X., Shen, J., Wu, S., Pang, X., Tian, J., Zhang, C., Zhou, Q., Wang, L., Pang, B., Chen, F., Peng, Z., Wang, J., . . . Zhao, L. (2018). Structural alteration of gut microbiota during the amelioration of human type 2 diabetes with hyperlipidemia by metformin and a traditional Chinese herbal formula: A multicenter, randomized, open label clinical trial. *mBio, 9*(3), e02392–17. https://doi.org/10.1128/mBio.02392-17

Tremaroli, V., & Bäckhed, F. (2012). Functional interactions between the gut microbiota and host metabolism. *Nature, 489*(7415), 242–249. https://doi.org/10.1038/nature11552

van de Wouw, M., Boehme, M., Lyte, J. M., Wiley, N., Strain, C., O'Sullivan, O., Clarke, G., Stanton, C., Dinan, T. G., & Cryan, J. F. (2018). Short-chain fatty acids: Microbial metabolites that alleviate stress-induced brain-gut axis alterations. *Journal of Physiology, 596*(20), 4923–4944. https://doi.org/10.1113/JP276431

Villanueva-Millán, M. J., Pérez-Matute, P., & Oteo, J. A. (2015). Gut microbiota: A key player in health and disease. A review focused on obesity. *Journal of Physiology and Biochemistry, 71*(3), 509–525. https://doi.org/10.1007/s13105-015-0390-3

Vivarelli, S., Salemi, R., Candido, S., Falzone, L., Santagati, M., Stefani, S., Torino, F., Banna, G. L., Tonini, G., & Libra, M. (2019). Gut microbiota and cancer: From pathogenesis to therapy. *Cancers, 11*(1), 38. https://doi.org/10.3390/cancers11010038

Voreades, N., Kozil, A., & Weir, T. L. (2014). Diet and the development of the human intestinal microbiome. *Frontiers in Microbiology, 5,* 494. https://doi.org/10.3389/fmicb.2014.00494

Wahlström, A., Sayin, S. I., Marschall, H. U., & Bäckhed, F. (2016). Intestinal crosstalk between bile acids and microbiota and its impact on host metabolism. *Cell Metabolism, 24*(1), 41–50. https://doi.org/10.1016/j.cmet.2016.05.005

Wang, R., Tang, R., Li, B., Ma, X., Schnabl, B., & Tilg, H. (2021). Gut microbiome, liver immunology, and liver diseases. *Cellular and Molecular Immunology, 18*(1), 4–17. https://doi.org/10.1038/s41423-020-00592-6

Wang, W., Chen, L., Zhou, R., Wang, X., Song, L., Huang, S., Wang, G., & Xia, B. (2014). Increased proportions of Bifidobacterium and the Lactobacillus group and loss of butyrate-producing bacteria in inflammatory bowel disease. *Journal of Clinical Microbiology, 52*(2), 398–406. https://doi.org/10.1128/JCM.01500-13

Witkowski, M., Witkowski, M., Friebel, J., Buffa, J. A., Li, X. S., Wang, Z., Sangwan, N., Li, L., DiDonato, J. A., Tizian, C., Haghikia, A., Kirchhofer, D., Mach, F., Räber, L., Matter, C. M., Tang, W. H. W., Landmesser, U., Lüscher, T. F., Rauch, U., & Hazen, S. L. (2022). Vascular endothelial Tissue Factor contributes to trimethylamine N-oxide-enhanced arterial thrombosis. *Cardiovascular Research, 118*(10), 2367–2384. https://doi.org/10.1093/cvr/cvab263

Wu, J., Guo, Y., Lu, X., Huang, F., Lv, F., Wei, D., Shang, A., Yang, J., Pan, Q., Jiang, B., Yu, J., Cao, H., & Li, L. (2020). Th1/Th2 cells and associated cytokines in acute hepatitis E and related acute liver failure. *Journal of Immunology Research, 2020,* 6027361. https://doi.org/10.1155/2020/6027361

Yang, C., Fei, Y., Qin, Y., Luo, D., Yang, S., Kou, X., Zi, Y., Deng, T., & Jin, M. (2015). Bacterial flora changes in conjunctiva of rats with streptozotocin-induced type I diabetes. *PLoS One, 10*(7), e0133021. https://doi.org/10.1371/journal.pone.0133021

Yang, Q., Liang, Q., Balakrishnan, B., Belobrajdic, D. P., Feng, Q. J., & Zhang, W. (2020). Role of dietary nutrients in the modulation of gut microbiota: A narrative review. *Nutrients, 12*(2), 381. https://doi.org/10.3390/nu12020381

Zhang, C., Li, S., Yang, L., Huang, P., Li, W., Wang, S., Zhao, G., Zhang, M., Pang, X., Yan, Z., Liu, Y., & Zhao, L. (2013). Structural modulation of gut microbiota in life-long calorie-restricted mice. *Nature Communications, 4*(1), 2163. https://doi.org/10.1038/ncomms3163

Zhao, L., Zhang, F., Ding, X., Wu, G., Lam, Y. Y., Wang, X., Fu, H., Xue, X., Lu, C., Ma, J., Yu, L., Xu, C., Ren, Z., Xu, Y., Xu, S., Shen, H., Zhu, X., Shi, Y., Shen, Q., . . . Zhang, C. (2018). Gut bacteria selectively promoted by dietary fibers alleviate type 2 diabetes. *Science, 359*(6380), 1151–1156. https://doi.org/10.1126/science.aao5774

Zhou, J., Tripathi, M., Sinha, R. A., Singh, B. K., & Yen, P. M. (2021). Gut microbiota and their metabolites in the progression of non-alcoholic fatty liver disease. *Hepatoma Research, 7,* 11. https://doi.org/10.20517/2394-5079.2020.134

Zhu, A., Sunagawa, S., Mende, D. R., & Bork, P. (2015). Inter-individual differences in the gene content of human gut bacterial species. *Genome Biology, 16*(1), 82. https://doi.org/10.1186/s13059-015-0646-9

5 Probiotics for Children

Involvement in Ameliorating Children's Health

Swati Sharma and Nishma Singh

5.1 INTRODUCTION

5.1.1 Origins of Probiotics

Probiotics are termed as "living microorganisms in which major portion size comes from bacteria alongside some yeast strains, that is if and when consumed in sufficient amounts possess health advantages on the host body." The thought of a probiotic bacterium is not novel for human beings—the ancient art of fermenting food items and the use of preservatives to preserve foods unintentionally familiarized human beings with these useful microorganisms for consumption long before science could examine and explain their secrets. In the vast landscape of human health, a microscopic world teems with life, influencing our well-being in ways beyond our immediate perception. Among these invisible inhabitants are probiotics, a term that has gained significant recognition in recent years. This comprehensive exploration aims to elucidate the intricate realm of probiotics, delving into their origins, mechanisms, potential benefits, and the evolving research surrounding them.

The probiotics world is unique and full of diversity with a number of microbiome strains subject to different species. There are two specific species such as *Lactobacillus* and *Bifidobacterium* achieved a well-known status among all species. The potential benefits and specific characteristics are the two qualities that each strain possesses. Specifically, the microbiome that aids in lactose digestion is *Lactobacillus acidophilus* and on the other hand intestinal integrity is maintained by *Bifidobacterium bifidum*.

The probiotics microbiome is commonly considered an alive microbiome that has the potential to enrich the health of consumers after consumption of specific and desired quantity. Sometimes they are denoted as "good bacteria" and commonly exist in fermented foods like yogurt, kefir, sauerkraut, and kimchi. Probiotics can shore up the health of GIT, digestion, and the immune system. However, the specific benefits can vary depending on the strains of probiotics used and the individual's health condition.

5.1.2 Characteristics of Probiotics

Probiotics considered as living microbiomes and administered in sufficient measure generated an advantageous effect on the consumer. A probiotic is proven to survive the passage through the gastrointestinal pathway (where it shows the impact on the digestive tract). LAB is a bacterium generally consumed. The utilization of LAB in the food sector is as long as they possess the capability to change sugar including lactose and other carbs into the lactate. The characteristic sour taste found in cultured bovine milk products is because of the existence of LAB; e.g., yogurt and curd, as well as through lowering the pH of a food item, lessen the opportunities for harmful microorganisms to grow inside food medium and thus generating health benefits while minimizing the chances of occurrence of gastrointestinal infections. The delicate balance between human health and the intricate world of microorganisms has captivated the scientific community for centuries. Probiotics,

DOI: 10.1201/9781003452249-5

the "friendly" microorganisms residing in the gut, have emerged as protagonists in this symbiotic relationship. In recent years, extensive research has highlighted the profound role of probiotics in shaping children's health and development. This comprehensive exploration delves into the multifaceted dimensions of a probiotic bacterium, elucidating their mechanisms of action, potential benefits, considerations, and the evolving landscape of pediatric probiotic research.

5.1.3 Species of Probiotics

Species of the classes, *Lactobacillus* and *Bifidobacterium*, are considered as commonly utilized probiotic microbiomes. Probiotic microbiome *Lactobacillus* species include *L. acidophilus, Lactobacillus plantarum, Lactobacillus casei* subspecies *rhamnosus, Lactobacillus brevis* and *Lactobacillus delbreuckii* subspecies *bulgaricus*, and *Bifidobacterium* species includes *Bifidobacterium adolescentis, Bifidobacterium bifidum, Bifidobacterium longum, Bifidobacterium infantis*, and *Bifidobacterium breve.* Other probiotic organisms include *Streptococcus salivarius* sp. *thermophilus, Lactococcus lactis* sp. *lactis, L. lactis* sp. *cremoris, Enterococcus faecium, Leuconostoc mesenteroides* sp. *dextranicum, Saccharomyces boulardii, Propionibacterium freudenreichii*, and *Pediococcus acidilactici.* Probiotic bacteria produce lactic acid, which lowers pH inside the gut and prevents the multiplication of harmful pathogenic bacteria, e.g., *Clostridium, Salmonella, Shigella*, and *Escherichia coli*, through the generation of a large number of antimicrobial substances such as acidophilin and bacteriocin. They assist in the absorption of some new minerals such as calcium by producing increased acidity in the intestine/GIT. They are also responsible for producing vitamins like vitamin B and vitamin K at the time of their proliferation in the GIT. Figure 5.1 shows probiotics functioning inside the gut to maintain immunity.

5.2 DEFINITIONS OF PROBIOTICS

"Probiotics" is obtained from a Greek word that means "pro-life." Researchers reevaluated during the ongoing decade, as well as reexplored scientific evidence as collected in the field of probiotic research, and gained the knowledge that they are not only essential for the well-being of the GIT but are significant as far as the general well-being of humanity concerned.

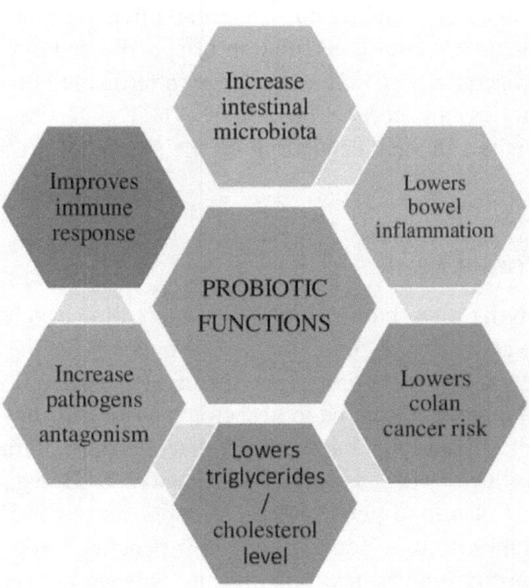

FIGURE 5.1 Probiotics functioning inside the gut to maintain immunity.

Some famous definitions of "probiotics" perceived through decades.

Lilly and Stillwell (1965) explained probiotics as "growth promoting factors produced by microorganisms."

Parker (1974) established collaboration between microbiome and receiver: "Organisms and substances with beneficial effects for animals by influencing the intestinal microflora."

Fuller (1989) explained, "A live microbial feed supplement which beneficially affects the host animal by improving its intestinal microbial balance."

Havenaar and Huis In't Veld (1992) pronounce probiotic bacterium as "a mono- or mixed culture of live microorganisms which, applied to animal or man, affect beneficially the host by improving the properties of the indigenous microflora."

ILSI—International Life Sciences Institute, Europe Working Group (1998) explained, "A feasible microbial food supplement which constructively stimulates the health of the host."

Diplock et al. (1999) elaborated,

> Probiotic food is functional if they have been satisfactorily established to beneficially affect one or more target functions in the body beyond adequate nutritional effects, in a way that is pertinent to either an enhanced state of health and well-being and/or lessening in the risk of diseases.

Naidu et al. (1999) say, "The host physiology was constructively impacted by a microbial dietary ancillary through regulating its mucosal and systematic immunity alongside cultivating nutritional."

Tannock and Brown (2000) found that lasting consumption of probiotics was not related to only major altercations in gastrointestinal microbial composition and thus proposed an alternative definition: "Microbial cells that pass through the intestinal tactile which is performing so, benefit the health condition of the consumer."

Schrezenmeir and de Vrese (2001) defined probiotics as "a preparation of a product containing viable, defined microorganisms in sufficient numbers, which alter the microflora (by implantation or colonization) in a compartment of the host and by that exert beneficial health effects in this host." FAO/WHO (2001) and Reid et al. (2003) concentrated exclusively on its health purpose: "Live microorganisms which when administered in adequate amounts confer a health benefit on the host."

It is clear that these definitions have:

1. Restricted the use of the word probiotic to products that contain live microorganisms.
2. Pointed out the need for providing an adequate dose of probiotic bacteria to exert the desirable effects.

5.2.1 History of Probiotics

The term "probiotic" is a relatively new word meaning "for life," and it is currently used to name bacteria associated with beneficial effects for humans and animals. The original observation of the positive role played by some selected bacteria is attributed to Eli Metchnikoff, the Russian-born Nobel Prize winner working at the Pasteur Institute at the beginning of the past century, who recommended that "the dependence of the intestinal microbes on the food makes it possible to adopt measures to modify the flora in our bodies and to replace the harmful microbes by useful microbes" (Metchnikoff, 1907). The term "probiotic" was first coined in 1965, by Lilly and Stillwell, to describe substances secreted by an organism that stimulate the growth of another.

At this time Henry Tissier, a French pediatrician, observed that children with diarrhea had in their stools a low number of bacteria characterized by a peculiar, Y-shaped morphology. These "bifid" bacteria were, on the contrary, abundant in healthy children (Tissier, 1900). He suggested that these bacteria could be administered to patients with diarrhea to help restore a healthy gut flora. The works of Metchnikoff and Tissier were the initial ones to make scientific recommendations concerning the probiotic use of bacteria, even if the word "probiotic" was not coined until 1960, to name substances produced by microorganisms that promoted the growth of other microorganisms (Lilly & Stillwell, 1965).

A more recent, but probably not the last, definition is "live microorganisms, which when consumed in adequate amounts, confer a health effect on the host" (Guarner & Schaafsma, 1998).

To be categorized under probiotic meaning "for life" a live microbial strain must encounter very stern criteria. According to FAO/WHO, these criteria include being safe for human consumption, being a live and viable organism with strain identification, being of human origin, being restricted to acid or bile, being able to survive the upper intestinal tract environment and reach the distal intestine (ilium and colon) to attach to the intestinal epithelium, and being able to colonize the distal intestine, confer health benefits to the host, and have scientifically proven health benefits (Cresci & Izzo, 2017).

5.2.2 Potential Benefits of Probiotics

The potential benefits of probiotics are listed in Table 5.1.

5.2.3 Anatomy of GI Tract

For the assessment of patients having gastrointestinal disorders, an important step is to be well-versed in the anatomy and physiology of the gastrointestinal system. Scanlon GIT is a tube that started from the mouth to the anus, which is the movement of muscles and release of different enzymes to digest food. Moreover, it has been called the alimentary canal, digestive tract, and GIT. It has three main parts, a lumen, i.e., a hollow tube in the innermost area, in the middle a muscular layer is present and on the outer surface there is a final layer of epithelial cells. The function of these layers is to keep the integrity of mucosa in the GIT (Preston & Wilson, 2013).

TABLE 5.1
Potential Benefits of Probiotics

Benefits	Mode of Action
Lactose intolerance	Conversion of lactose into lactic acid
Lowering blood pressure	Due to ACE (angiotensin-converting enzyme) inhibitor-like peptides produced during fermentation
Improving immune function and preventing infections	Improve immune function by increasing the number of IgA-producing plasma cells, increasing or improving phagocytosis as well as increasing the proportion of T lymphocytes and natural killer cells
Control of diarrhea	Treat various forms of gastroenteritis, by maintaining microbial balance
Reducing inflammation	Modulate inflammatory and hypersensitivity responses, due to the regulation of cytokine function
Irritable bowel syndrome (IBS) and colitis	Prevent the overgrowth of potentially pathogenic organisms such as *Clostridium difficile*
Improving mineral absorption	Correct malabsorption of trace minerals
Antibiotic-associated diarrhea	Microbiota alteration changes carbohydrate metabolism with decreased short-chain fatty acid absorption
Colon cancer	Certain probiotics (*Lactobacillus bulgaricus*) may help prevent colon cancer by preventing the breakdown of enzymes (B-glucuronidase) that contribute to the growth of cancer-causing agents

The parts of GIT include the mouth (for mastication), esophagus, stomach and small intestine, large intestine, rectum, anus, accessory organs liver, gall bladder, and pancreas. The length of an average fully matured digestive tract is about 30 feet long, which is responsible for the passing of food through it and not being in the body (Agans et al., 2011). Significantly the GIT starts with the ingestion of food into the elementary canal while eating food and moving the contents inside the elementary tract. The process of digestion includes the mechanical breakdown of food for example, mastication, i.e., the breakdown of large food particles into smaller particles with the help of enzymes, which are produced and released by glands and other accessory organs of the digestive tract and formerly known as chemical digestion of foods; the second function is absorption process where digested food particles are passing through the walls of few organs of the elementary canal and utilized by the body tissues. And last and final function is the elimination of food, i.e., undigested and not absorbed through the GIT and finally excreted out from the elementary tract in the form of faces through the step known as the defecation process. Here, the large intestine is a home of various complex beneficial microbiomes that are responsible for human health.

Identified areas of the body with normal flora (GIT, urogenital tract, and skin) and the most common types of organisms in these areas and relation to pathogenicity of these organisms owing to the increased prevalence of diseases and disorders associated with gut flora imbalances and the fact that traditional treatments such as antibiotic administration appear to have the potential for long-term disruption, microbial manipulation of the host microbiome to treat chronic diseases has been recently renewed interest (Zhang Y. J., 2015). Manipulation may be elicited through probiotics and prebiotics.

5.2.4 Normal Flora of GI Tract

The gut mucosa of humans includes the epithelial cells, lamina propria, and the muscularis mucosae, which is colonized by 1,014 microbes, which not only include bacteria but also other microorganisms such as mold, archaea, viruses, and protozoans. The main bacteria in the human gut are Firmicutes, Bacteroidetes, Actinobacteria, Proteobacteria, Verrucomicrobia, and Fusobacteria. Firmicutes are gram-positive bacteria with a low G+, including the large class of clostridia and the LAB, i.e., *Lactobacillus*, while Actinobacteria are gram-positive bacteria with a high G+, including *Colinsella* and *Bifidobacterium* species.

The two significantly beneficial kinds of gut microbiome are LAB and *Bifidobacterium*, achieved through digested food and settled in the gut area of the GIT. The prominent LAB found in the human GIT are *Lactobacillus* and *Leuconostoc* species. The keynote bacteria principally exist in the GIT of infants and are also found in low levels in adults or *Bifidobacterium* species.

5.2.5 List of Microorganisms

Table 5.2 displays a comprehensive list of microorganisms utilized as probiotics.

5.2.6 Structure of Different Microorganisms

Figure 5.2 illustrates the diverse structures of various microorganisms.

5.3 PROPERTIES OF PROBIOTICS

An ideal probiotic preparation should have the following properties (Table 5.3). For an adequate amount of health benefits, a dose of 5 billion colony-forming units a day (5×10^9 CFU/day) has been recommended, for at least five days. The microorganisms used in probiotic preparations should be GRAS; they should be resistant to bile, hydrochloric acid, and pancreatic juice; have anticarcinogenic activity and stimulate the immune system; have reduced intestinal permeability; produce

TABLE 5.2
List of Microorganisms Used as Probiotics

***Lactobacillus* Species**	***Bifidobacterium* Species**	***Streptococcus* Species**	***Saccharomyces* Species**	***Others***
L. acidophilus	*B. bifidum*	*S. thermophilus*	*S. boulardii*	*Bacillus cereus*
L. casai (rhamnosus)	*B. breve*	*S. salivarius sub species thermophilus*		*Escherichia coli*
L. fermentum	*B. lactis*			*Enterococcus*
L. gasseri	*B. longum*			*Propionibacterium freudenreichii*
L. johnsonii	*B. infantis*			
L. lactis	*B. adolescentis*			
L. paracasai				
L. plantarum				
L. reuteri				
L. salivarius				
L. bulgaricus				

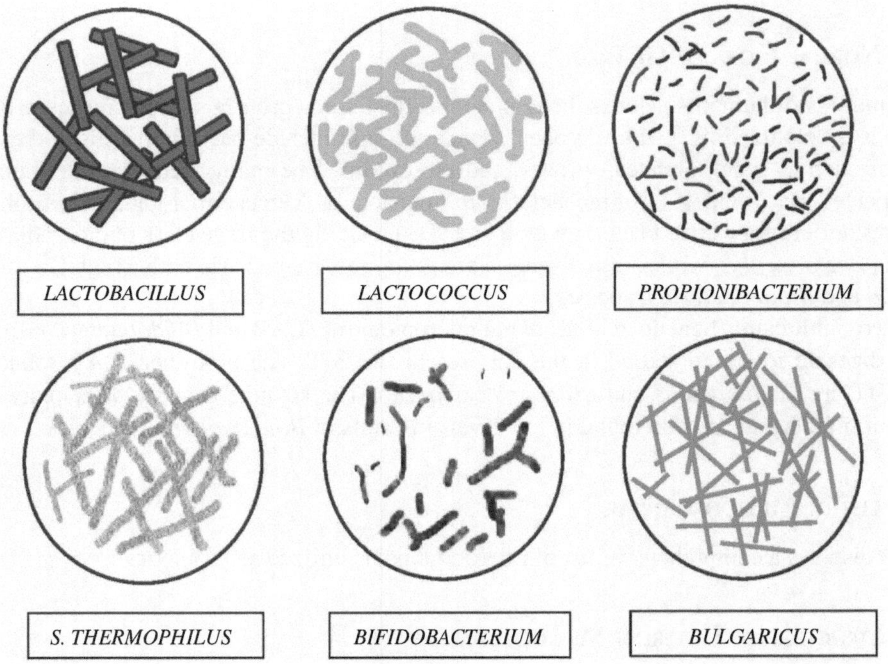

FIGURE 5.2 Structure of different microorganisms.

lactic acid; and be able to survive both acidic conditions of the stomach and alkaline conditions of the duodenum. Foods for human consumption that contain mainly LAB include fermented milk, cheeses, fruit juices, wine, and sausages. Single and mixed cultures of live microorganisms are used in probiotic preparations.

TABLE 5.3
Criteria of an Ideal Microorganism as Probiotic

1	High cell viability; thus they must be resilient to low pH and acids
2	Ability to persist in the intestine even if the probiotic strain cannot colonize the gut
3	Union to the gut epithelium to cancel the flushing effects of peristalsis
4	They should be able to interact or send signals to the immune cells associated with the gut
5	They should be of human origin
6	They should be non-pathogenic
7	They should have resistance to processing
8	They must have the capacity to influence local metabolic activity

Table 5.3 outlines the criteria for an ideal microorganism to be considered as a probiotic.

5.3.1 Health Benefits of Probiotics

The health benefits of fermented foods such as yogurt have been touted for a great number of years. However, only recently have rigorous studies explored the effects of certain bacteria that are either commensals or mutualists in the human intestine. In an effort to standardize the use of the term "probiotic." The FAO of the United Nations–WHO defines probiotics as "live microorganisms, which when administered in adequate amounts, confer a health benefit to the host." FAO–WHO guidelines published in 2002 provide specific requirements that should be met for products to meet this standard. Because these are voluntary guidelines, the consumer should be aware that some claims of probiotic activity do not meet these criteria or have not been supported by scientific, clinical studies.

Microorganisms such as *Lactobacillus* and *Bifidobacterium* are being used to develop new probiotic foods. The possible health benefits of the use of such microbial dietary adjuvants include immunomodulation, control of diarrhea, anticancer effects, and possible improvement of CD (IBD). Probiotics have become a more attractive treatment option in cases of enteric disease because the rate of antibiotic resistance among pathogens continues to climb. In addition, disease ecologists have come to recognize that some intestinal microflora can be a contributing factor to certain conditions (e.g., CD).

Acidophilus milk is produced using *L. acidophilus*. *L. acidophilus* may modify the microbial flora in the lower intestine, thus improving general health, and it is often used as a dietary adjunct, especially for lactose-intolerant persons. Many microorganisms in fermented dairy products stabilize the bowel microflora, and some appear to have antimicrobial properties. The exact nature and extent of health benefits of consuming fermented milk may involve minimizing lactose intolerance, lowering serum cholesterol, and possibly exhibiting anticancer activity. Several lactobacilli have antitumor compounds in their cell walls. Such findings suggest that diets including LAB, especially *L. acidophilus*, may contribute to the prevention of colon cancer. Another interesting group used in milk fermentations is the bifidobacteria. The genus *Bifidobacterium* contains irregular, non-sporing, gram-positive rods that may be club-shaped or forked at the end. *Bifidobacterium* is nonmotile, is anaerobic, and ferments lactose and other sugars to acetic and lactic acids. They are typical residents of the human intestinal tract, and many beneficial properties are attributed to them. Bifidobacteria are thought to help maintain the normal intestinal balance while improving lactose tolerance; to possess antitumorigenic activity; and to reduce serum cholesterol levels. In addition, some believe that they promote calcium absorption and the synthesis of B-complex vitamins. It has also been suggested that bifidobacteria reduce or prevent the excretion of rotaviruses, a cause of diarrhea among children. *Bifidobacterium*-amended fermented milk products, including yogurt, are commercially available.

5.3.2 Development of Probiotic Food

Table 5.4 exhibits the progression of probiotic food development.

Probiotics are live microbials, dietary supplements, or food ingredients that have a beneficial effect on the host by influencing the composition and/or metabolic activity of the flora of the GIT. They are opposites of antibiotics. Lilley and Stillwell (1965) coined this term to describe substances secreted by one organism that stimulate the growth of the other, although the concept evolved from the work of Metchnikoff (1908) who postulated that Balkan peasants lived very long because they consumed milk fermented with *L. delbrueckii* subspecies *bulgaricus*. According to him, this bacterium displaces the putrefactive bacteria in the GIT, thereby reducing the concentrations of toxins and improving health. It is now known that this bacterium cannot survive in the GIT and the

TABLE 5.4
The Development of Probiotic Food

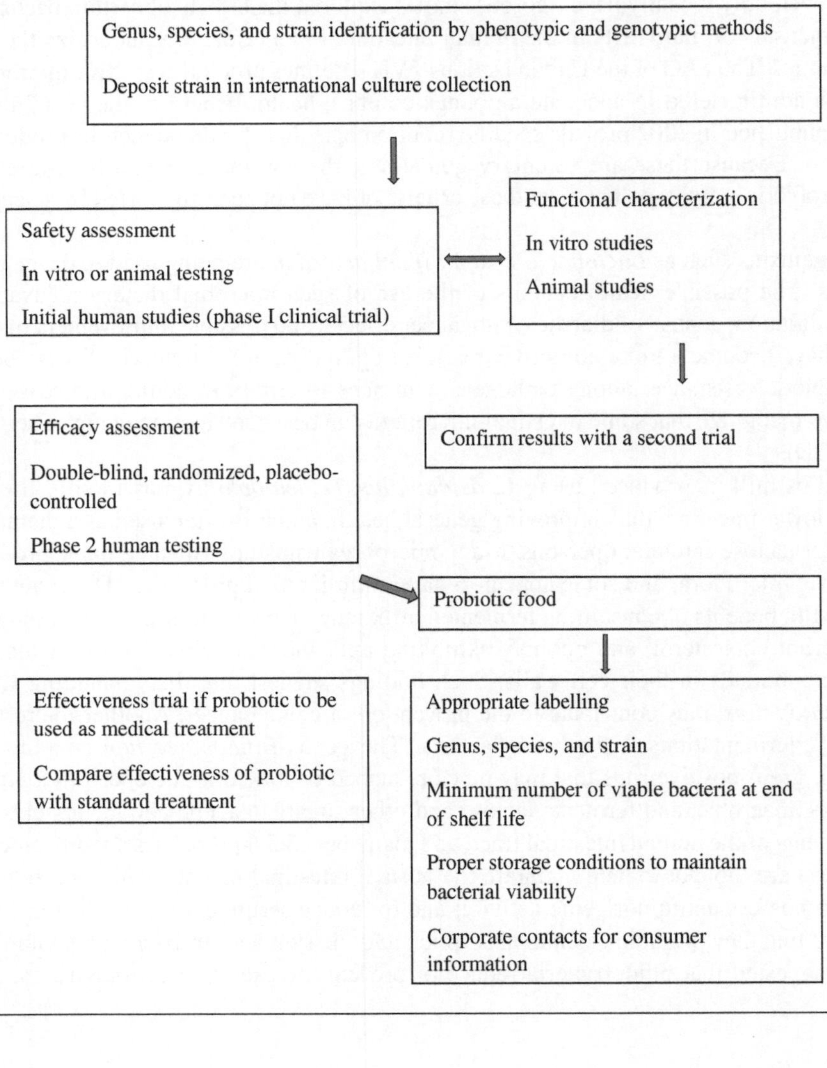

beneficial effect is probably due to its ability to allow lactose-intolerant individuals to tolerate residual lactose in fermented milk. Sperti (1971) described probiotics as tissue extracts that stimulate growth. Parker (1974) defined probiotics as organisms and substances that contribute to the balance of intestinal flora. In 1989, Fuller pronounced probiotics as a live microbial feed supplement, which beneficially affects the host animal by enhancing its intestinal microbial balance." He laid emphasis on the viability of the probiotic.

5.3.3 Metabolic Products of Probiotics

Figure 5.3 visually represents the metabolic products of probiotics.

Conventional bovine milk foods such as yogurts/curd and cheese are consumed to receive probiotic microbiome. Numerous potential advantages to the health of the receiver are credited to the ingestion of probiotic bacteria. They are assumed to boost the immunity of the host, increase resistance toward infection, and enhance the general well-being. They aid in the digestion of lactose, which results in the reduction in intestinal bloating, flatulence, and discomfort. It has also been suggested that they offer protection against *C. botulinum* spores and associated toxins (a probable reason for SID). To prevent and treat diarrheal disorder, the most acknowledged therapeutic submission is probiotics administration. The diarrhea disorders include rota virus-induced diarrhea in toddlers and old-age people. They prevent infection and traveler's diarrhea and protect against some kinds of cancer. Decrease in blood cholesterol levels and reduction in incidence of cardiovascular disease have also been attributed to probiotics. Probiotics specifically play a role in assisting and preventing the treatment of gastrointestinal diseases such as peptic ulcer disease and intractable diarrhea following treatment

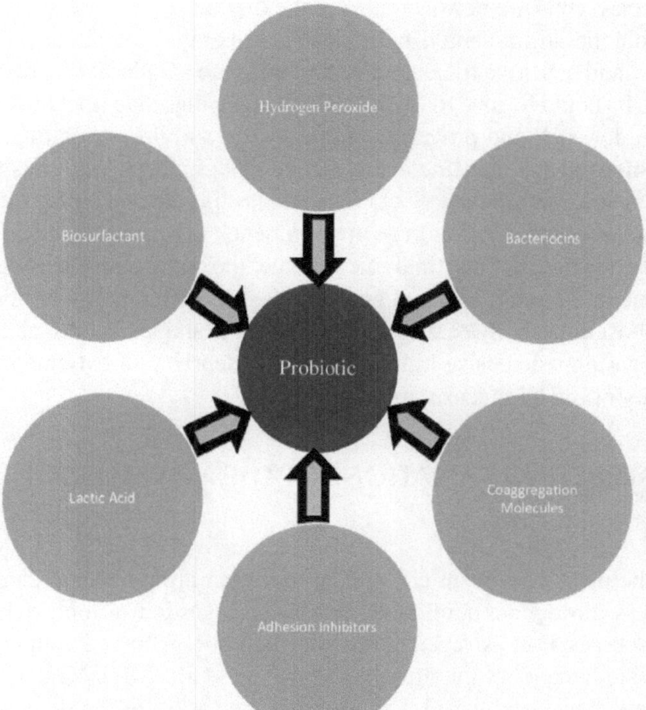

FIGURE 5.3 Metabolic products of probiotics.

with antibiotics and minimizing allergic inflammation. These beneficial effects are brought about by the alteration of the GIT microbial population, restoration of normal intestinal permeability, and increased gut barrier properties as well as intestinal immunoglobulin response. *Bifidobacterium* and *Lactobacillus* genera are the main probiotic microorganisms, but additional bacterium and fungi, e.g., *S. boulardii*, are utilized too as probiotics. *Bifidobacterium* encompasses 95% of the flora, which is the reason that breastfeeding toddlers show the minimum predominance rate of GIT species in comparison to the GIT of infants feeding on human milk, which shows some form of infections than infants fed on a cow or other formula milk. Certain particular substances in fecal matter called meconium (the sterilized liquid present in the digestive path of newborns), human colostrum, and milk known as "bifidus growth features" are responsible for the predominance of these bacteria in breast milk. These growth factors were isolated by Kuhn and his colleagues in the 1950s and consist of several large oligosaccharides or prebiotics. This term is used for undigestible food substances that possess a potential benefit for the host by purposively triggering the proliferation of anticipated anchor microorganisms in the digestive path. Prebiotic polysaccharides include a widespread group of naturally occurring carbs, such as inulin, FOSs, galacto-oligosaccharide, and lactulose that occur in plant sources having maximum congregation of inulin-provided in chicory, artichoke, onions, leeks, and garlic widely in plants.

Bifidobacterium is a gram-positive, often Y-shaped, rod-like actinomycetous bacterium. The most commonly used species of *Bifidobacterium* is *B. longum*. These bacteria produce lactase (l-isomer) and acetate from lactose but are not classified as LAB. The identifying character of this genus is the existence of fructose-6-phosphate phosphoketolase in cellular filtration. Beyond their nutritional composition (as supplying of B vitamins), probiotic microbiome fungi commonly show resistance to digestive tract passage and possess resistance to maximum antibiotics consumed. Some *Saccharomyces* species possess a protective effect, and particular activities, against different intestinal pathogens. Capsules, powders, tablets, and pellets comprising probiotic yeasts (*Saccharomyces* species) cells are now available in the market.

The potential probiotic strain should be a usual occupant of the human digestive tract, nonpathogenic in nature, and sensitive to general antibiotics, and should not be resistant to antibiotics or virulent plasmids. It should be able to live and pass via the digestive tract and should demonstrate hostility to bile salts, low pH, and proteases in preliminary in vitro screening. It should have the ability to stick to lumens of the intestine and effectively put hindrance to sites that could be overpowered by the pathogenic microbiome. Species should proliferate in an industrial environment and hold feasibility in the usual industrial storage environment.

During the proliferation of the intestinal microbiome, the connections between this microbiome with the host outcome in the progression of an exclusive and different immunity of GIT. The challenges faced by this host immune system of mucosal lining to single out both pathogenic and benign microbiomes by triggering a defensive immune response deprived of extreme inflammation which interrupts the veracity of the GI mucosal lining.

5.4 FACTORS AFFECTING VARIATIONS IN THE NORMAL GUT

5.4.1 Diet

Diet is considered the most significant constituent in determining nutrient composition, biodiversity, and exclusiveness throughout adulthood. Generally, ingestion of food rich in macronutrients containing organic sources such as vegetables, fruits, and fiber is linked with an increased amount of bulk in faces and biodiversity of gut microflora (Walker et al., 2011). Numerous humans, as well as rodent experiments, have established a substantial altercation in the digestive tract microflora over the substantial use of seaweed in the form of food supplements in the diet. In the human diet,

Gelidium seaweed supplement has impressively enhanced the expression of *Bifidobacterium* spp. bacteria without any altercations in the others (Ramani et al., 2012).

5.4.2 Age

It's a broadly accepted thought among researchers that the GIT receives its first colony of beneficial microbiomes just after parturition. New research done in the field of probiotics established that the infant GIT receives its first colony of microbiomes in the uterus itself. The intestines of normally born infants show that the infant gut microflora just after primary inoculation appears unsettled and vacant, but by the passing of time it stabilizes, settles, diversifies, and achieves the 40% to 60% resemblance same as the adult gut microflora as the infant reaches three years age (Yatsunenko et al., 2012). On the other hand, research done on the microflora of young children and adults shows that there is substantial differentiation in the ratio of *Bacteroides* and *Bifidobacterium* in comparison to men and women (Ringel-Kulka et al., 2013). Minimum functional imprints of the temporal differences in the healthy digestive tract microflora include a decreased capacity to synthesize vitamin B12, decreased actions of microbial reductases, enhanced tendency for DNA differentiation, enhanced response to stress, and immune malfunction.

5.4.3 Antibiotics

Several studies done on antibiotics have established the significant role of bactericidal and bacteriostatic activities against pathogenic foreign bodies. Experimental research established the beneficial role of antibiotics and various short- and long-term effects in the ecosystem of healthy digestive tract microflora. The most significant characteristic of normal digestive pathway microflora contrary to foreign bodies/pathogens is its capability to cause competitive exclusion. It was evident four decades ago that the use of antibiotics shows the disturbance of the competitive exclusion machinery just and when antibiotic therapy is received just after *Salmonella* infection. The damage of the broad web of interaction among the microflora was evident after the possible mechanism of this kind of interaction of *Salmonella* and the antibiotic, therefore causing the proliferation of host-derived sialic acid, which is primarily responsible for the growth of infective bacteria such as *Salmonella typhimurium* and *Clostridium difficile*. Researchers show that, after the administration of antibiotics, it was evident that there is major variation in the gut microflora that includes reduced taxonomic biodiversity and persistence of the alterations in a major ratio of individuals.

5.5 MECHANISM OF ACTION

Probiotics exert their impact through a wide variety of mechanisms initially taking place in the GIT. They promote a uniform gut microbiota and maintain a delicate uniformity of the population of the microbiome. The uniformity of the microbiome is essential for adequate digestion, followed by absorption of nutrients and protection from the adverse impact of harmful pathogens. Probiotics can also regulate the functioning of the immune system by exerting an impact on its responsiveness against foreign threats/attacks and also help in reducing inflammation. Human life is closely associated with a wide variety of microbiomes present in the derma, in the oral cavity as well, and in the gut area of the intestine. The enriched concentration of microorganisms is found in the lining of the digestive pathway, consisting of greater than 400 m^2 of surface area. The gut occupancy which works as a home for beneficial microbiome to proliferate creates the next greatest surface area in the host body just next to the surface area of the cardiopulmonary tract. A gastrointestinal pathway is a native place for affluent microflora of greater than 500 diverse bacterial strains that possess roughly significant health functions that include stimulation of immunity, defending the host from attacking pathogenic microbiome, and viruses, and helping in the digestion process to complete. The microbiome of gut microflora is established rapidly after parturition remains stable throughout the lifecycle and as well as essentially required for human equilibrium. During the development of intestinal microflora, there is interaction between the microflora with the host fallouts and in this procession, an exclusive and diverse intestinal microflora is established. The challenging feature faced by the receiver immune system of the mucosa is to differentiate both pathogenic bacteria and benign microbiome via the process of stimulating a protective immune response without additional inflammation, which possibly upset the integrity of the gastrointestinal mucosa.

The treatments such as antibiotic treatment immunosuppressive therapy and irrigation may influence alteration in the composition of microflora and ultimately affect the population of microflora. However, the additional introduction of advantageous bacterial class into the gastrointestinal path may work as a quite impressive choice for restructuring bacterial homeostasis and in the prevention of diseases.

Probiotic microbiomes have varied impacts on the receiver's cells, for example, the inhibition and therapy of a broad category of malfunctioning. The chief method of probiotic activities consists of:

1. Improvement of the epithelial barrier
2. Increased union to the mucosa of the intestine and concurrent obstruction to the union of pathogens
3. Construction of antimicrobial particles

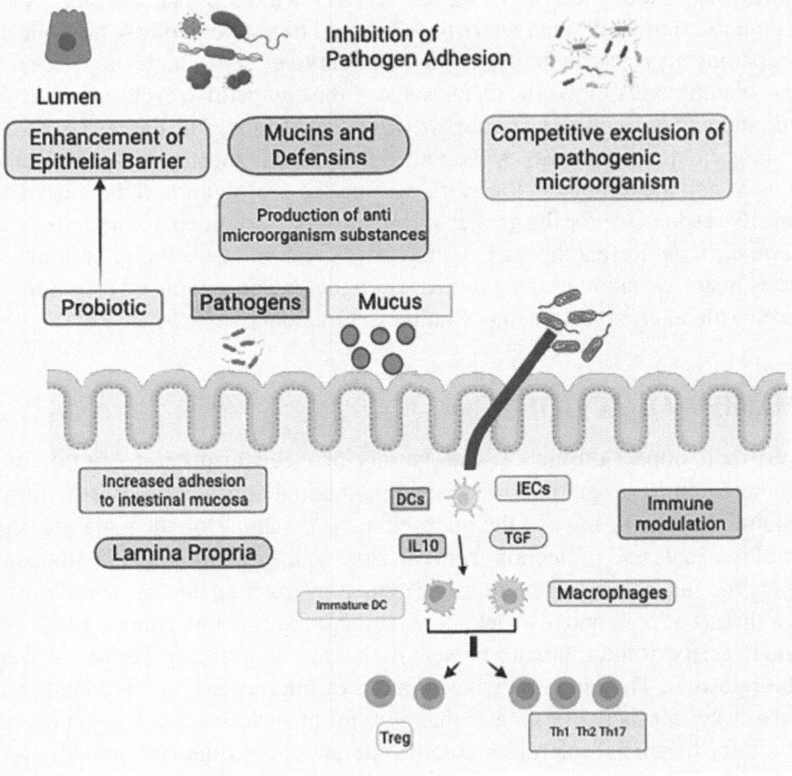

FIGURE 5.4 Mechanism of action of probiotics.

4. Modest segregation of harmful microbiome
5. Modulation of the immunity; present data display the impact of probiotics in meddling with quorum sensing

Figure 5.4 shows the mechanism of action of probiotics

5.6 PROBIOTICS: UNRAVELING THE WORLD OF BENEFICIAL MICROORGANISMS

5.6.1 Potential Health Benefits

The potential health benefits of probiotics are reaching beyond the gut. The role of the probiotic microbiome is not only related to upgraded digestion but also to relief from gastric malfunctioning like IBS and IBD. They act as an immunomodulator with the potential to minimize the severity of allergies, infections, and autoimmune diseases. Probiotics also aided in the synthesis of specific vitamins, and they also influenced metabolic processes that could impact the overall health of human beings.

5.6.2 Emerging Research Areas

Ongoing research continues to uncover novel aspects of probiotics. The gut–brain axis, a bidirectional transmission channel in both the lower intestine and the head, has garnered attention for its potential link to mental health. Recent research done in the area of probiotics suggested that probiotics also impact conditions like anxiety depression and neurological disorders, and they aid in the management of these diseases. Researchers also explore the potential use of probiotics in managing metabolic disorders like obesity and diabetes mellitus in the near future.

5.6.3 Prebiotics and Synbiotics

Probiotics often work synergistically with prebiotics, which are insoluble dietary fibers that fulfill nourishment for useful gut microbiomes. When combined, they form synbiotics, enhancing the survival and activity of probiotics in the gut. This underscores the importance of a balanced diet rich in fiber to support the growth of these beneficial microorganisms.

5.6.4 Challenges and Considerations

While the potential benefits of probiotics are compelling, several challenges must be navigated. Identifying the right strains for specific health conditions, ensuring their viability through processing and storage, and establishing appropriate dosage levels are complex tasks. Moreover, individual responses to probiotics can vary, influenced by factors such as genetics, food, and the prevailing large intestine microorganism.

5.6.5 Regulation and Commercialization

As the popularity of probiotics soars, regulation and standardization become crucial. Not all products marketed as probiotics may provide the desired benefits. It's important to choose products backed by scientific research and manufactured by reputable companies. Probiotic foods and supplements are regulated differently in various regions, further emphasizing the need for informed consumer choices.

5.7 PROBIOTIC'S CONTRIBUTION TO ENHANCING CHILDREN'S HEALTH

Probiotics play an important role in improving children's health by positively influencing their gut microbiota and overall well-being. The large intestine microbiome, a varied class of microbiota residing in the digestive path, performs a significant role in digestion, immunity development, and various aspects of well-being.

5.7.1 Digestive Health

Probiotics with the help of prebiotics support the development and proliferation of a balanced form of beneficial gut microbiota, which is required essentially for proper digestion and nutrient absorption in the human body. In infants and children, probiotics aid in reducing or minimizing common digestive disorders like diarrhea, constipation, and IBS. Probiotics also encourage the proliferation of healthy microbiomes found in the large intestine area, maintaining gut barrier function and hindering the proliferation of harmful bacteria in the gut area. Probiotics aid in maintaining a balanced gut environment, supporting efficient digestion and nutrient absorption. They can alleviate common childhood digestive issues such as constipation, diarrhea, and IBS. Probiotics promote gut barrier integrity, avoiding the translocation of damaging substances and pathogens into the bloodstream.

5.7.2 Immune System Support

As human gut is the area where the beneficial microbiota is flourishing, which is why a significant portion of the immune system has a base in the gut area. Probiotics not only aid in stimulating the proliferation of immune cells but also aid in enhancing the human body's ability to fight infections. Probiotics also help the immune system differentiate between harmful and harmless pathogens and aid in minimizing the risk of allergies and autoimmune conditions in the human body. The GALT constitutes a significant portion of the immunity. Probiotics meet with GALT, training the immunity to distinguish between harmless antigens and potential threats. This interaction contributes to immunity maturation, reducing the risk of infections, allergies, and autoimmune conditions.

5.7.3 Prevention and Management of Infections

Probiotics demonstrate to minimize the occurrence and time length of infections in children. They can help prevent and manage common childhood illnesses such as respiratory tract contaminations, ear infections, and gastrointestinal infections. Probiotics promote the production of antimicrobial substances and compete with harmful bacteria for space and nutrients in the gut. Probiotics exhibit antimicrobial properties, producing compounds that inhibit the growth of pathogens. They compete for resources and adhesion sites with harmful bacteria, reducing the risk of infections. Probiotics have demonstrated efficacy in preventing and managing infections, including respiratory tract infections, ear infections, and gastroenteritis.

5.7.4 Atopic Conditions

Probiotics may have a preventive effect on atopic conditions like eczema, allergies, and asthma. Research suggests that early exposure to certain probiotic strains can control immunity and minimize the hazard of allergic reactions and sensitivities. The development of atopic conditions, such as eczema and allergies, is influenced by the gut microbiota's composition. Probiotics, particularly certain strains of *Lactobacillus* and *Bifidobacterium*, have shown promise in reducing the risk of allergic reactions and sensitivities by modulating immune responses and maintaining gut barrier function.

5.7.5 Mood and Behavior

There is an emerging indication that the GIT–brain connection performs a role in mood regulation and behavior. Probiotics might influence this connection and potentially contribute to managing mood disorders, anxiety, and hyperactivity in children.

5.7.6 Antibiotic-Associated Issues

Antibiotic use can interrupt the natural homeostasis of the gut microbiome, leading to episodes like AAD. Probiotics can help restore a healthy gut microbiota during and after antibiotic treatment, minimizing side effects.

5.7.7 Weight Management

Some findings recommended that the digestive pathway microbiome composition in early life can influence metabolism and weight development. Probiotics might play a role in preventing childhood obesity by promoting a balanced gut microbiome.

5.7.8 Dietary and Nutritional Support

Probiotic-rich foods like yogurt and kefir can be valuable sources of nutrients, including calcium, vitamin D, and protein, contributing to children's growth and development. It's vital to note that all probiotics are different in nature, and their effects can vary based on the specific strains used.

5.8 POINTS TO CONSIDER DURING ADMINISTRATION OF PROBIOTICS FOR CHILDREN

Probiotics, established as living microbiome that provides benefits to the receiver when consumed in appropriate measures, encompass a diverse array of bacterial strains and yeast species. *Lactobacillus* and *Bifidobacterium* are among the most extensively studied genera, with individual strains demonstrating unique characteristics and potential therapeutic effects. The intricate interplay between these microorganisms and the host's physiology underscores their essential role in maintaining health. Before giving children probiotics, especially those with existing health conditions or compromised immune systems, it's advisable to consult pediatricians or healthcare professionals.

5.8.1 Appropriate Strains

Choose probiotic strains that have been well-studied and demonstrated benefits for children's health. *Lactobacillus* and *Bifidobacterium* species are generally used in children's probiotic formulations.

5.8.2 Age-Appropriate Formulations

Probiotic products are available in various forms, such as powders, capsules, and chewables. Select a formulation appropriate for your child's age and preferences.

5.8.3 Dosage and Timing

Follow the recommended dosage instructions provided by the product manufacturer or healthcare provider. Probiotics are often best taken with meals to enhance survival through stomach acid.

5.8.4 Quality and Safety

Choose reputable brands that provide high-quality, well-tested products. Look for products that are labeled as suitable for children.

5.8.5 Building a Foundation for Health

The early years of life constitute a critical period for immune system development, metabolic programming, and establishment of the digestive tract microbiota. Probiotics demonstrate a pivotal role in shaping these foundational aspects, influencing various physiological processes that impact children's health in both the short and long term.

5.8.6 Gut Microbiota Development

During infancy, the gut microbiota undergoes rapid and dynamic changes. Probiotics introduced during this period can impact the configuration and diversity of the intestine microbiota, promoting the growth of beneficial bacteria and crowding out potentially harmful pathogens. This early modulation of the microbiome is linked with reduced hazard of allergies, autoimmune disorders, and gastrointestinal issues.

5.8.7 Neurodevelopment and Behavior

The gut–brain axis, a bidirectional communication pathway between the gut and the brain, plays a role in neurodevelopment and behavior. Probiotics' impact on the gut–brain axis suggests potential benefits in managing mood disorders, anxiety, and hyperactivity in children.

5.8.8 Metabolic Health and Obesity Prevention

Emerging evidence suggests a link between the gut microbiota and metabolic health. Probiotics may play a role in preventing childhood obesity by influencing metabolism and energy balance.

5.8.9 Selecting and Administering Probiotics

When considering the use of probiotics for children, several factors should be taken into account to ensure optimal safety and effectiveness:

5.8.10 Strain Specificity

Different probiotic strains have distinct effects. Choose strains that have been well-studied and demonstrated benefits for children's health.

5.8.11 Dosage and Duration

Follow the recommended dosage provided by the product manufacturer or healthcare provider. Duration of probiotic use may vary based on the intended purpose.

5.8.12 Consultation with Healthcare Providers

Before introducing probiotics to a child's regimen, especially if the child has underlying health conditions, consult with pediatricians or healthcare professionals.

5.8.13 Evolving Landscape of Pediatric Probiotic Research

As scientific understanding evolves, ongoing research continues to unveil new insights into the potential benefits of probiotics for children's health. Researchers are exploring the intricate mechanisms through which probiotics impact various physiological processes. Additionally, studies are investigating the optimal strains, dosages, and formulations for specific health conditions.

5.9 DISEASE/DISORDERS DUE TO ALTERATION OF GUT MICROFLORA AND THEIR AMELIORATION THROUGH PROBIOTICS IN CHILDREN

5.9.1 Oral Health

To accomplish through probiotics while managing the microflora present in the oral cavity is found to be an effective method to control the oral cavity environment as the human mouth is found to be a native place of different microorganisms present in the human body like protozoa, bacteria, fungi, and viruses. The bacteria are held to be responsible for two very common diseases such as dental caries (tooth decay) and periodontal gum disorders. The presence and prevalence of pathogenic organisms found in the oral cavity cause an imbalance of all these beneficial microbiomes and ultimately cause disturbance, finally leading to different types of oral health defects such as dental caries, periodontitis, and halitosis. *Streptococcus uberis* and *Streptococcus oralis* species overpower the periodontal pathogenic bacteria. Probiotics were found to be very effective in the prevention of halitosis and also prevented the production of VOSs generated by gram-negative and gram-positive bacteria and established their colonies in periodontal pockets as well as on the dorsal surface of the tongue. The application of *L. reuter* was found to be effective in minimizing gum bleeding and gingivitis of the oral cavity (Anilkumar & Monisha, 2012).

5.9.2 Diarrhea

A number of probiotics found to be effective in the treatment of a different variety of gastrointestinal disorders. Diarrhea is considered a major global health problem showing its imprint on the millions of mortalities per annum. Probiotics are found to be effective as they help to minimize both the intensity of passing of motions and the time duration of diseased conditions.

Antibiotic-Associated Diarrhea: Once after receiving the antibiotic therapy AAD occurs and it shows that there is malfunctioning in the colony of the gut microbiome. Altercations in carbohydrate metabolism with minimization of short-chain fatty acid absorptions occur after changes in microbiota, and this results in the presence of osmotic diarrhea. When there is the proliferation of pathogenic organisms such as *Clostridium difficile* since after antibiotic therapy, it creates diarrhea. On the other hand, some bacterial strains such as *Lactobacillus rhamnosus* and *L. bulgaricus*, and yeast *Saccaromyces boulardi* are responsible for minimizing the risk of AAD. To treat and prevent the occurrence of CDI and recurrent CDI, probiotics are found to be effective. LGG has been shown to increase the expression of mucins and decline bacterial adherence (Cho & Finocchiaro, 2009). To minimize the occurrence of rotavirus infection and also in the treatment of established diseases in infants, probiotic supplementation formulas are found to be effective. To study the effectiveness of lactobacilli as a probiotic and how it minimizes the time length of occurrence of rotavirus diarrhea in infants, there were several potential mechanisms available. Treatment with *L. rhamnosus* was associated with an enhancement of IgA-specific antibody-secreting cells to rotavirus and of serum IgA antibody level during convalescence (Allen et al., 2010). Studies show that probiotics are pre-emptive and have remedial effects on different varieties of diarrhea with different etiologies. The role of different dietary probiotics has been successfully investigated under different research done on how they treat and prevent diarrhea. Probiotics were found to be effective in different clinical conditions such as infantile diarrhea, necrotizing enterocolitis, antibiotics-associated diarrhea, and recurring *C. difficle* colitis, *H. pylori* infections, IBD to cancer, female urinary genital infection, and surgical infections. Microorganisms (e.g. LGG, *L. reuteri*, certain strains of *L. casei*, *L. acidophilus*, *E. coli* strain Nissle 1917, and certain bifidobacteria and enterococci (*E. faecium* SF 68) as well as the probiotic yeast *S. boulardii*) have been examined with respect to their medicinal use, either as single strain or as mixed culture probiotics. The occurrence of AAD is still prevalent ranging from 3.2 to 29 per 100 hospitalized patients in spite of the development of newer antibiotics with a broad spectrum of activity and lesser side effects that have been generated in recent times. There were several complications occurred during the treatment of AAD including electrolyte imbalance, dehydration, toxic megacolon, and pseudo membrane colitis. The broad range of activity of antibiotics that include anaerobic bacteria, especially cephalosporin, penicillin, or clindamycin, are being linked with major rates of AAD although almost all kinds of antibiotics have been linked. A meta-analysis to evaluate the efficacy of probiotics in the prevention and treatment of AAD showed an odds ratio of 0.39 (p-value less than 0.001) in favor of active treatment over placebo with *S. boulardii*.

Rotavirus Diarrhea: To treat acute diarrhea occurring due to rotavirus infection in children, different random, **randomized double-blinded placebo control studies**, showed positive impacts while using stains such as LGG and *Bifidobacterium lactis* BB-12 for prevention.

Radiation-Induced Diarrhea: Radiation-induced diarrhea generally occurs in cancer patients. Double-blinded, placebo-controlled research investigated radiation-induced diarrhea and its effect on cancer survivors and examined the effectiveness of probiotic microbiome preparation having higher effectiveness to reduce its impact on the intensity of radiation-induced diarrhea. Further to evaluate it approximately 490 cancer patients were selected and treated with post-operative radiation therapy containing highly concentrated probiotic form formula. Research findings concluded that placebo-controlled cancer survivors suffered from grade 3 to 4 levels of diarrhea in comparison to the patients who are treated with highly concentrated probiotic microbiome preparation and thus establish the upper edge of probiotics in the treatment of radiation-induced diarrhea in cancer survivors.

Traveler's Diarrhea: A familiar well-being problem related to the GIT is traveler's diarrhea among all travelers. The range of a traveler's diarrhea is from 5% to 50% depending upon the sight of diarrhea. A meta-analysis conducted after performing randomized controlled clinical trials of travelers to India cases concluded that probiotics showing prominent impacts to prevent or minimize the effects of traveler's diarrhea include treatment with a combination of *S. boulardii*, *L. acidophilus*, and *B. bifidum*.

5.9.3 *H. pylori*

A vital reason related to chronic gastritis, peptic ulcer, and a matter of concern for digestive enmities is *H. pylori* bacteria. *H. pilori* annihilation therapy is found to be 90% effective when it is antibiotic-based. However, it's found to be expensive with possible adverse impacts and resistance to antibiotics. Research of the MEDLINE database (1966–2006) was conducted on studies that establish an association between *H. pylori* and probiotics. The findings concluded that in vitro examination of probiotics established their inhibitory effects minimized *H. pylori*-linked digestive tract inflammation in animals and enhanced *H. pylori*-linked digestive and probiotic microbiome-based therapy found to minimize the *H. pylori* therapy-associated side effects.

5.9.4 Necrotizing Enterocolitis

NE is established as one of the distressing digestive tract malfunctioning or diseases that a premature newborn might encounter in an NICU. The symptoms vary from abdominal distension, bilious vomiting, bloody diarrhea, lethargy, apnoea, and bradycardia. NE accounted for up to 25% of premature newborns admitted to NICU and may also impact one-third to one-half of all underweight newborns. The mortality rate of premature newborns ranges from 20% to 30%; premature newborns are able to live and have long-lasting consequences such as short gut syndrome, intestinal obstruction, and multi-organ failure. Cesarean section delivers low-birth-weight and preterm infants who generally require intensive care unit treatment and can be breast-feed only after several days of their birth. In these low-birth-weight preterm infants, the usual method applied to beneficial microbiomes, such as *Lactobacillus* species being ingested through a vaginal birth and proliferated by mothers' feed, does not take place. Thus, there is a greater chance that these infants may be exposed to plenty of harmful microbiomes like *Clostridium*, *Escherichia*, *Salmonella*, *Shigella*, *Campylobacter*, *Pseudomonas*, *Streptococcus*, *Enterococcus*, *Staphylococcus*, and coagulase-negative *Staphylococcus* that form their colony in the gut and upsurge the amount of NE. Also, this premature newborn got bottle feeding that ultimately resulted in fewer *Lactobacillus* and *Bifidobacterium* species in their feces in comparison to controls. Finally, the aforementioned findings concluded that there is a correlation or association between *Lactobacillus* species and NE.

5.9.5 Lactose Intolerance

The usual malfunctioning of carbohydrate metabolism is known as lactose intolerance or lactose malabsorption. The beta-galactosidase enzyme or lactase enzyme activity is compromised in the patients of lactose intolerance, thus making them unable to digest lactose completely and ultimately resulting in improper digestion of galactose in the intestine. This undigested galactose is responsible for diarrhea, vomiting, and malabsorption of other nutrients in the host body and ultimately results in malnutrition. The enzyme lactase is responsible for hydrolyzing and acts in the absorption of lactose sugar and is produced by *L. acidophilus* and *L. delbrlleckii* sp. The sign that shows bacteria responsible for metabolizing lactose in the intestine are present in the gut is the presence of hydrogen in the breath.

5.9.6 Irritable Bowel Syndrome

A multi-dimensional disease having specific signs and symptoms of blotting, diarrhea, constipation, and abdominal discomfort and pain is known as IBS. There is the possibility that gastric blotting may be produced by gut microflora, but they are also responsible for the consumption of these gases, and there is evidence this probiotic might help to minimize gas accumulation in the digestive tract and improve the homeostasis inside the bowel. A large number of scientific researchers and review studies establish the mechanism behind the working of probiotic microbiomes inside the gut and how they deliver their useful impacts on the body of the host. Some of them are a buildup of the luminal environment of the intestine, maintenance of mucosal barrier function and epithelium of the gut, and intonation of mucosal lining and immunity including both innate and adaptive immunity (Goudarzi et al., 2014).

5.9.7 Inflammatory Bowel Syndrome

CD and UC are chronic reoccurring or remitting diseases of gastrointestinal treatment with more or less common symptoms; these two diseases are collectively known as IBD. Treating the IBD using probiotics likely minimizes disease activity and increases remission through a decrease of infective microbiome proliferation while enhancing barrier function to avert or stop the attack of tight junction, minimizing gastric pH and exciting nonspecific and specific immune responses (Tiwari et al., 2012).

5.9.8 Lowering of Cholesterol Level

There have been a number of mechanisms applied to minimize cholesterol impacts of probiotics, which include the separation of bile acids through hydrolyzing enzymes of bile salt present in the probiotic microbiome; the concentration of cholesterol, which is separated by acclimatization of cholesterol through cholesterol-binding techniques of probiotics on the cell membrane of the probiotic microbiome; amalgamation of cholesterol into the cell wall of the probiotic microbiome during their proliferation; exchange of cholesterol with coprostanol; and production of SCFA during fermentation through probiotics when prebiotics are also present during the process.

5.9.9 Urogenital and Vaginal Health

Lactobacillus species were found to be effective in curing and protecting women from genital infections as a woman's vagina was declared as a native place for the most effective microbiome. Any altercations in the colony of *Lactobacillus* spp. can ultimately result in discrepancies in the vagina of a woman. *Lactobacillus* produces biosurfactants and collagen-binding proteins in the cells, which inhibit the union of pathogens in the vagina. Thus, it concluded that vaginal mucosa is subjugated by *Lactobacillus*, ultimately making it minimally friendly to the infections there. There is another mechanism called cell-to-cell communication through which probiotics trigger mucus proliferation that ultimately serves as a blockade to the pathogenic microbiome and signaling the production of the anti-inflammatory cytokine. *Lactoacidophilus* additionally produces hydrogen peroxide, which results in inhibiting the proliferation of *Candida albicans* (Daliri & Lee, 2015).

5.9.10 Food and Skin Allergy

Allergic reactions were found to be produced through small peptides and amino acids via certain bacteria. The imbalance between *Bifidobacterium* and *Clostridium* is responsible for allergies according to different research done on this. *L. casei* GG degradation produces enzymes that convert small peptides and amino acids and finally produce molecules with inhibitory impacts on lymphocyte reproduction. The usual chronic inflammatory malfunction found in newborns and children is AD. The main characteristics of AD are etching and recurrent eczematous lesions, and this condition is increasing worldwide day by day. The recent occurrence rate is 10–20% in newborns and children (Weidinger & Novak, 2016). AD is responsible for chronic psychosocial burdens on children and their families and serves as a leading nonfatal medical skin disorder (Chamlin & Chren, 2010; Silverberg, 2016; Sidbury & Khorsand, 2017). AD is also linked with a maximum risk of allergy, asthma, and cognitive health concerns (Sung et al., 2017). Tropical corticosteroids (TCS), antihistamines, and antibiotics are generally used as drug to treat infants and children with AD (Totri et al., 2017). However, these medications exert many antagonistic side impacts, and AD symptoms may occur rapidly after therapy is ended. Furthermore, long-term TCS use may stimulate fresh occurrence of AD.

Mechanisms of antiallergic probiotic bacteria include modulation of the immune system through the production of inflammatory cytokines, increasing intestinal barrier integrity, or enhancement of specific IgA responses and degradation of food antigens by means of productive enzymes of probiotics (Tiwari et al., 2012).

5.10 PROBIOTICS USED IN TREATMENT OF CHRONIC DISEASES

5.10.1 Anticarcinogenic

Lactobacillus, *Bifidobacterium*, and *E. coli* species possess anti-mutagenic activities because of their capability to metabolize and deactivate substances of mutagens. The probiotic microbiome possesses anticarcinogenic outcomes by utilizing numerous mechanisms such as inhibiting pro-carcinogen transformation into active carcinogens, deactivation of mutagenic substances, construction of anti-mutagenic substances, clampdown of the proliferation of procarcinogen microbiome, minimum absorption of mutagens from the gut, and strengthening of immune system functionality (Soccol et al., 2012).

5.10.2 HIV/AIDS

Probiotics employed in the prevention of AIDS and STDs, microbiome specifically *Lactobacillus* plays a crucial role in the regulation of the vaginal microflora. It's recommended that the production of H202 from a particular species of *Lactobacillus* is found to be crucial in the functioning of the microflora present in the vagina. This toxic molecule is the most potent local microbicide present in the human vagina. The results of experimental studies have recommended that *Lactobacillus*, given at higher potency, is viricidal for HIV-1. There exists a reverse link between vaginal lactobacilli and HIV seroconversion. Few studies recommended that *Lactobacillus* can play a role to protect women against some pathogenic microbiome present in the vagina.

5.10.2.1 Role in Infection Regulator Programs and Eradication of Multi-Drug Resistant Microbiome

The rapid rate of inappropriate use of antibiotic therapies, as well as bacterial resistance drugs, in combination with newly developed curiosity to stop pathogenic infections by adopting environment friendly methods, ultimately resulting in making of probiotic field as a field of interest for many researchers. In different recent researches, it was evident that probiotic formulas possess potential benefits against antibiotic treatment as well as pathogenic microbiomes which are responsible for deterioration of immunity of host.

Table 5.5 shows probiotics tested for use in the treatment of diarrhea in children.

Probiotics are found to be very impressive in the cure of specific illnesses in children (Fuchs-Tarlovsky et al., 2016). Live bacteria or yeast in the form of probiotics are not certainly harmless,

TABLE 5.5
Probiotics Tested for Use in the Treatment of Diarrhea in Children

Bacteria Strains	**Lactobacillus GG**
	Lactobacillus acidophilus
	Lactobacillus acidophilus LB (killed)
	Lactobacillus bulgaricus
	Bifidobacterium bifidum (now "lactis")
	Bifidobacterium breve
	Streptococcus thermophilus
	Enterococcus
	Escherichia coli
	Nissle 1917
Yeast Strains	*Saccharomyces boulardii*

but they are found to assist in giving protection to the host from pathogenic bacteria (Mizock, 2015). Administration of probiotics in specific amounts may have valuable roles not only for GIT but also found effective in the gut–brain skin axis (Ogden & Bielory, 2005; Dehingia et al., 2015; Huang et al., 2016; Huang & Hu, 2017). During the past 10 years, there have been several studies done on the benefits of probiotics in the treatment of infant AD patients. In 2000, Pessi et al. found that orally consumed probiotics supplements enhance the clinical evidence of digestive tract inflammatory markers and AD (Pessi et al., 2000). Kirjavainen et al. (2003) found minimal *Bacteroides* numbers in the fecal microflora of children with atopic eczema in comparison to healthy newborns and recommended that probiotics therapy be utilized for the treatment of AD in children (Kirjavainen et al., 2003); however, few reported contradictory inferences (Licari et al., 2015). For instance, Gruber et al. found that LGG exercised no therapeutic impacts in newborns with mild to moderate signs of AD (Gruber et al., 2007).

5.10.3 Chronic Diarrhea

The presence of diarrhea among children who are under strict medical supervision for some other reason is a well-known and exasperating reason. The reason for the spread of diarrhea is probably rotavirus infection and, to some extent, the reason behind this is *Clostridium difficile* as seen in the children. Thus, it concluded that there is a requirement for safe probiotic agents that can also be effective in minimizing these problems causing phenomena as well and it seems to be logical to choose an ideal form of probiotics to treat the children. There were conflicting results seen other than diarrhea among the infants and young children who were admitted to hospitals when the randomized controlled trials (RCTs) were evaluated for probiotics to prevent diarrhea in these hospital-admitted groups. When a group of 55 infants aged between 5 and 24 months were admitted to the hospital for chronic care treatment, they received a double-blind RCT, either a standard infant formula supplemented with *Bifidobacterium lactis* (Bb12) and *S. thermophilus* or an identical formula that do not contain probiotics. The result shows that the presence of nosocomial diarrhea was prominently reduced or minimized in children who got probiotic-supplemented formula in comparison to the placebo (7% vs. 31%, $p < 0.05$). It was also evident that the infants who received probiotics in their supplementation had a significantly lower risk of gastroenteritis. Thus, the study finally concluded that infants who received probiotics in breast formula showed a minimum duration of rotavirus shedding significantly and other important observations showed lesser contamination of rotavirus spreading in hospital settings. Further two subsequent trials were conducted in hospital settings combining LGG. In the first experimentation, a total of 81 children hospitalized between the age group of 1 and 36 months were included, and the finding shows that LGG (6×10^6 CFU) when administered orally twice per day prominently minimized the risk of nosocomial diarrhea when compared with the placebo (6.7% vs. 33.3%, $p = 0.002$). The chief etiological agent of nosocomial gastroenteritis was known as rotavirus, and its prevalence was noted predominantly between the probiotic-treated group and the control group. Surprisingly it was noted that LGG impressively minimized the occurrence of rotavirus illness in children (2.2% vs. 16.7%, $p = 0.02$). In the second experimentation including LGG in the second RCT, 220 children of the age group of 1 to 18 months were treated with LGG, and the result shows a comparative study with probiotic-treated breastfed infants and non-breastfed infants. The result shows that breastfed infants showed more resistance toward rotavirus illness in comparison to non-breastfed infants with no probiotics. However, the administration of LGG in these children at the dose of 10^{10} CFU once per day was not found to be effective in the prevention of the occurrence of nosocomial rotavirus infection when compared with placebo (25% vs. 30%, $p = 0.4$). Also, it was evident that there is no significant difference in the rates of symptomatic rotavirus enteritides when compared with placebo (13% for LGG vs. 21% in placebo; $p = 0.13$) (Guandalini et al., 2008).

The final result shows a significant contrast with the previous findings, reported while comparing children with acute watery diarrhea by the same group; LGG shows an impressive result even in the minimum dose of 60 million CFU twice per day when administered combined with the ORS. The results show minimizing the escalation of the duration of diarrhea among malnourished Indian children who already had a protected course. The experimentation was conducted in two different countries, with two different probiotic formulations on two large RCTs with a patient-level analysis of combined data evaluating outcomes in the children with age 1 month to 15 years. The study further examined the impact of both time duration and frequency of occurrence of diarrhea before and after enrollment on outcomes. There were concerns about RCTs that overlooked the benefits of probiotics as the time of administration was too late during the illness or the benefits received on the children with chronic diarrhea were minimized by children who have less acute illnesses and findings refused such assumptions.

It was also evident that no identifiable benefits of probiotic treatment were shown on eight different combinations of diarrhea having different durations and severities on any outcome explored including overall illness, severity, healthcare resource utilization, and continuing diarrhea symptoms. This further shows that initiation of probiotic therapy doesn't associate with the presence or absence of its beneficial effects on the target population as it depends on the duration of diarrhea and its frequency. It clearly stated that the effectiveness of probiotics depends more on the time when it is administered during the course of illness and provided to children with more chronic diseases. Thus, it was concluded that the duration of illness and children suffering from the more severe disease are the two essential features employed at the time of study to analyze the impact of probiotics during the course of treatment on children suffering from diarrhea. Further, when children with severe diarrhea of short duration were compared, it was evident that there was no significant difference in the number of children experiencing moderate to severe AGE or any of the other secondary outcomes between treatment groups. Earlier probiotic studies were based on the isolated outcomes of frequency of diarrhea and its duration, whereas in recent studies these outcomes establish that there are no benefits that could be attributed to probiotic treatment; otherwise, it depends on the severity and duration of diarrhea in children.

5.11 CONTRAINDICATIONS, ADVERSE EFFECTS, AND INTERACTIONS

There are no absolute contraindications to probiotics comprising *Lactobacillus* sp., *Bifidobacterium* sp., *S. thermophilus*, or *S. boulardii*. Significantly few or no adverse effects, bloating or mild gastric uneasiness, usually self-limited, are reported occasionally. Pathological infections including bacteremia were reported with probiotic species followed by oral administration. They are rare in nature, generally present in chronically ill or immunosuppressed hosts or in children with short-duration gut syndrome. It's recommended to avoid the administration of probiotics in such patients or to have knowledge about the risk of sepsis in such patients. In the review study, further examination of the safety of *L. rhamnosus* GG and *Bifidobacterium* species added that there is a minimum risk of sepsis with no further cases being reported in any of the prospective clinical trials. After the administration of probiotics, no sepsis or any other pathological colonization of harmful bacteria was reported in healthy patients. Also, no known interaction between the medications and other supplements was reported after probiotic treatment.

5.11.1 Dosages

There is a broad spectrum of studies where clinical trials were conducted on a broad range of doses of *Lactobacillus* species and other probiotics ranging from 100 million to 1.8 trillion CFUs per day with the largest dose used to minimize the risk of pouchitis relapse. A maximum number of studies examined or experimented upon the range of doses between 1 to 20 billion CFUs per day. However, the specific indication of the exact amount of doses varies within this range per day. Predominantly a high range of doses of probiotics, i.e., more than 5 billion CFUs per day for children and more than 100 billion CFUs per day for adults were found to be associated with a more important study outcome. Further, it was concluded that a higher range of doses are found to be unsafe, but they are more expensive and unnecessary. The dosages of *S. boulardii* in most studies range between 250 and 500 mg per day. The forms of probiotics generally available or sold are capsules, powder, tablets, and liquid or are sometimes incorporated with the food. Further, according to the type of the brand, the dosage of specific numbers of CFUs per serving of foods can vary. It was recommended that patients must read the label carefully before consumption to make sure that they are getting the proper amount of dose recommended.

5.12 CONCLUSION

5.12.1 Emerging Trends

The rapid rate of inappropriate use of antibiotic therapies and bacterial resistance drugs in combination with newly developed curiosity to stop pathogenic infections by adopting environment-friendly methods ultimately resulted in the making of the probiotic field, a field of interest for many researchers. In different recent research, it was evident that probiotic formulas possess potential benefits against antibiotic treatment and pathogenic microbiomes, which are responsible for the deterioration of the immunity of the host. The world of probiotics is a captivating frontier, revealing the profound impact of microorganisms on human health. From their historical roots in fermentation to their potential to address modern health challenges, probiotics offer a glimpse into the intricate symbiosis between humans and the microbial world. As scientific understanding evolves, harnessing the potential of probiotics could revolutionize healthcare, offering personalized approaches to wellness that bridge the gap between science and nature. Probiotics are live microbes, and hence they may cause an infection in the body of the host. There were different safety profiles recommended for different strains of probiotics. However, generally, it's safe for consumption as probiotic therapy. It becomes a counter-instinctive concept to consume or ingest live bacteria willingly. There are some reports that show systemic infection during the administration of *Bifidobacterium*; however, the administration of LGG or *L. casei* reported several cases of sepsis. At the time of administration of *Enterococcus* species as a probiotic, major precautions need to be taken. The potential of sepsis to be counter-checked with the risk and morbidity of sepsis-associated risk because the probiotic bacteria as found to be more pathological microbiome as well as used for microbial application. There are varied conditions such as infections, inflammation, neoplastic, and allergy, where probiotic therapy gained opposition to treat such medical conditions. There were numerous medical conditions where probiotics were willingly used to treat disorders. However, care should be taken before the administration of dosage of probiotics to any general population. Before manufacturing and administration of probiotics to the general population, standard criteria regarding quality and reliability should be checked.

5.12.2 Key Considerations and Conclusions

Further, still, there is a need for properly designed placebo-controlled studies with valid reports to ascertain the true health benefits of probiotic products in the near future. Although probiotics are found to be an effective treatment potential for certain medical conditions, for the selection of proper probiotic agents and standardization of their doses, proper knowledge about their beneficial effects and knowledge about the toxic constituents of probiotics before their administration are significant. In conclusion, probiotics offer a natural and safe way to promote children's health by positively influencing their gut microbiota and various physiological processes. While further research is ongoing, the current evidence suggests that incorporating probiotics into children's diets, under appropriate guidance, can be beneficial for their overall well-being. Probiotics, once concealed within the realms of fermentation and microbiology, have emerged as essential contributors to children's health and well-being. Their influence spans from the earliest stages of life, shaping foundational aspects of immune system development, digestion, and overall health. As research advances, harnessing the potential of probiotics in pediatric healthcare offers a promising avenue for optimizing children's growth, development, and long-term health outcomes. By nurturing the delicate symbiosis between humans and their microbial counterparts, we lay the groundwork for a healthier and more resilient generation.

BIBLIOGRAPHY

Agans, R., Rigsbee, L., Kenche, H., Michail, S., Khamis, H. J., & Paliy, O. (2011, June 1). Distal gut microbiota of adolescent children is different from that of adults. *FEMS Microbiology Ecology, 77*(2), 404–412.

Albenberg, L. G., & Wu, G. D. (2014). Diet and the intestinal microbiome: Associations, functions, and implications for health and disease. *Gastroenterology*, *146*(6), 1564–1572. https://doi.org/10.1053/j.gastro.2014.01.058

Alexander, P. E., Bonner, A. J., Agarwal, A., Li, S. A., Hariharan, A. T., Izhar, Z., Bhatnagar, N., Alba, C., Akl, E. A., Fei, Y., Guyatt, G. H., & Beyene, J. (2016). Sensitivity subgroup analysis based on single-center vs. multi-center trial status when interpreting meta-analyses pooled estimates: The logical way forward. *Journal of Clinical Epidemiology*, *74,* 80–92. https://doi.org/10.1016/j.jclinepi.2015.08.027

Allen, S. J., Martinez, E. G., Gregorio, G. V., & Dans, L. F. (2010, January 1). Probiotics for treating acute infectious diarrhoea. *The Cochrane Library*.

Amara, A. A., & Shibl, A. (2015). Role of probiotics in health improvement, infection control and disease treatment and management. *Saudi Pharmaceutical Journal*, *23*(2), 107–114. https://doi.org/10.1016/j.jsps.2013.07.001

Anandharaj, M., Sivasankari, B., & Parveen Rani, R. (2014). Effects of probiotics, prebiotics and Synbiotics on hypercholesterolemia: A review. *Chinese Journal of Biology*, *2014*, 1–7. https://doi.org/10.1155/2014/572754

Anilkumar, K., & Monisha, A. L. (2012, January 1). Role of friendly bacteria in oral health—A short review. *Oral Health & Preventive Dentistry, 10*(1).

Avershina, E., Lundgård, K., Sekelja, M., Dotterud, C., Storrø, O., Øien, T., Johnsen, R., & Rudi, K. (2016). Transition from infant- to adult-like gut microbiota. *Environmental Microbiology*, *18*(7), 2226–2236. https://doi.org/10.1111/1462-2920.13248

Behnsen, J., Deriu, E., Sassone-Corsi, M., & Raffatellu, M. (2013). Probiotics: Properties, examples, and specific applications. *Cold Spring Harbor Perspectives in Medicine*, *3*(3), a010074. https://doi.org/10.1101/cshperspect.a010074

Belkaid, Y., & Tamoutounour, S. (2016). The influence of skin microorganisms on cutaneous immunity. *Nature Reviews. Immunology*, *16*(6), 353–366. https://doi.org/10.1038/nri.2016.48

Borgeraas, H., Johnson, L. K., Skattebu, J., Hertel, J. K., & Hjelmesaeth, J. (2018). Effects of probiotics on body weight, body mass index, fat mass and fat percentage in subjects with overweight or obesity: A systematic review and meta-analysis of randomized controlled trials. *Obesity Reviews*, *19*(2), 219–232. https://doi.org/10.1111/obr.12626

Breton, A., Novikov, A., Martin, R., Tissieres, P., & Caroff, M. (2017). Structural and biological characteristics of different forms of V. filiformis lipid A: Use of MS to highlight structural discrepancies. *Journal of Lipid Research*, *58*(3), 543–552. https://doi.org/10.1194/jlr.M072900

Bron, P. A., Kleerebezem, M., Brummer, R. J., Cani, P. D., Mercenier, A., MacDonald, T. T., Garcia-Ródenas, C. L., & Wells, J. M. (2017). Can probiotics modulate human disease by impacting intestinal barrier function? *British Journal of Nutrition*, *117*(1), 93–107. https://doi.org/10.1017/S0007114516004037

Caballero, S., Carter, R., Ke, X., Sušac, B., Leiner, I. M., Kim, G. J., Miller, L., Ling, L., Manova, K., & Pamer, E. G. (2015). Distinct but spatially overlapping intestinal niches for vancomycin-resistant *Enterococcus faecium* and carbapenem-resistant Klebsiella pneumoniae. *PLOS Pathogens*, *11*(9), e1005132. https://doi.org/10.1371/journal.ppat.1005132

Cagetti, M. G., Mastroberardino, S., Milia, E., Cocco, F., Lingström, P., & Campus, G. (2013). The use of probiotic strains in caries prevention: A systematic review. *Nutrients*, *5*(7), 2530–2550. https://doi.org/10.3390/nu5072530

Cani, P. D. (2018). Human gut microbiome: Hopes, threats and promises. *Gut*, *67*(9), 1716–1725. https://doi.org/10.1136/gutjnl-2018-316723

Cani, P. D., & de Vos, W. M. (2017). Next-generation beneficial microbes: The case of Akkermansia muciniphila. *Frontiers in Microbiology*, *8*, 1765. https://doi.org/10.3389/fmicb.2017.01765

Cani, P. D., & Van Hul, M. (2015). Novel opportunities for next-generation probiotics targeting metabolic syndrome. *Current Opinion in Biotechnology*, *32*, 21–27. https://doi.org/10.1016/j.copbio.2014.10.006

Cani, P. D., Van Hul, M., Lefort, C., Depommier, C., Rastelli, M., & Everard, A. (2019). Microbial regulation of organismal energy homeostasis. *Nature Metabolism*, *1*(1), 34–46. https://doi.org/10.1038/s42255-018-0017-4

Cavaillon, J. M., & Legout, S. (2016). Centenary of the death of Elie Metchnikoff: A visionary and an outstanding team leader. *Microbes and Infection*, *18*, 577–594.

Chamlin, S. L., & Chren, M. M. (2010). Quality-of-life outcomes and measurement in childhood atopic dermatitis. *Immunology and Allergy Clinics of North America*, *30*, 281–288. 10.1016/j.iac.2010.05.004

Chang, H. Y., Chen, J. H., Chang, J. H., Lin, H. C., Lin, C. Y., & Peng, C. C. (2017). Multiple strains probiotics appear to be the most effective probiotics in the prevention of necrotizing enterocolitis and mortality: An updated meta-analysis. *PLoS One*, *12*(2), e0171579. https://doi.org/10.1371/journal.pone.0171579

Chen, Y. E., Fischbach, M. A., & Belkaid, Y. (2018). Skin microbiota-host interactions. *Nature*, *553*(7689), 427–436. https://doi.org/10.1038/nature25177

Cho, S. S., & Finocchiaro, T. (Eds.). (2009, November 19). *Handbook of prebiotics and probiotics ingredients: Health benefits and food applications*. CRC Press.

Chung, W. S., Walker, A. W., Louis, P., Parkhill, J., Vermeiren, J., Bosscher, D., Duncan, S. H., & Flint, H. J. (2016). Modulation of the human gut microbiota by dietary fibres occurs at the species level. *BMC Biology*, *14*(1), 3. https://doi.org/10.1186/s12915-015-0224-3

Cotter, P. D., Ross, R. P., & Hill, C. (2013). Bacteriocins—A viable alternative to antibiotics? *Nature Reviews Microbiology*, *11*(2), 95–105. https://doi.org/10.1038/nrmicro2937

Cresci, G. A. M., & Izzo, K. (2017). Chapter 4: Gut microbiome. In *Adult short bowel syndrome: Nutritional, medical, and surgical management, 2019* (pp. 45–54). Academic Press. https://doi.org/10.1016/B978-0-12-814330-8.00004-4

Crouzet, L., Derrien, M., Cherbuy, C., Plancade, S., Foulon, M., Chalin, B., van Hylckama Vlieg, J. E. T., Grompone, G., Rigottier-Gois, L., & Serror, P. (2018). Lactobacillus paracasei CNCM I-3689 reduces vancomycin-resistant Enterococcus persistence and promotes Bacteroidetes resilience in the gut following antibiotic challenge. *Scientific Reports*, *8*(1), 5098. https://doi.org/10.1038/s41598-018-23437-9

Crum-Cianflone, N. F., Sullivan, E., & Ballon-Landa, G. (2015). Fecal microbiota transplantation and successful resolution of multidrug-resistant-organism colonization. *Journal of Clinical Microbiology*, *53*(6), 1986–1989. https://doi.org/10.1128/JCM.00820-15

da Costa Baptista, I. P., Accioly, E., & de Carvalho Padilha, P. (2013). Effect of the use of probiotics in the treatment of children with atopic dermatitis; a literature review. *Nutricion Hospitalaria*, *28*(1), 16–26. https://doi.org/10.3305/nh.2013.28.1.6207

Daliri, E. B., & Lee, B. H. (2015). New perspectives on probiotics in health and disease. *Food Science and Human Wellness*, *4*(2), 56–65. https://doi.org/10.1016/j.fshw.2015.06.002

de Simone, C. (2019). The unregulated probiotic market. *Clinical Gastroenterology and Hepatology*, *17*(5), 809–817. https://doi.org/10.1016/j.cgh.2018.01.018

Dehingia, M., Devi, K. T., Talukdar, N. C., Talukdar, R., Reddy, N., Mande, S. S., Deka, M., & Khan, M. R. (2015). Gut bacterial diversity of the tribes of India and comparison with the worldwide data. *Scientific Reports*, *5*, 18563. https://doi.org/10.1038/srep18563

Deng, Z., Chen, M., Xie, H., Jian, D., Xu, S., Peng, Q., Sha, K., Liu, Y., Zhang, Y., Shi, W., & Li, J. (2019). Claudin reduction may relate to an impaired skin barrier in rosacea. *Journal of Dermatology*, *46*(4), 314–321. https://doi.org/10.1111/1346-8138.14792

Depommier, C., Everard, A., Druart, C., Plovier, H., Van Hul, M., Vieira-Silva, S., Falony, G., Raes, J., Maiter, D., Delzenne, N. M., de Barsy, M., Loumaye, A., Hermans, M. P., Thissen, J. P., de Vos, W. M., & Cani, P. D. (2019). Supplementation with Akkermansia muciniphila in overweight and obese human volunteers: A proof-of-concept exploratory study. *Nature Medicine*, *25*(7), 1096–1103. https://doi.org/10.1038/s41591-019-0495-2

Derrien, M., & van Hylckama Vlieg, J. E. (2015). Fate, activity, and impact of ingested bacteria within the human gut microbiota. *Trends in Microbiology*, *23*(6), 354–366. https://doi.org/10.1016/j.tim.2015.03.002

Dewulf, E. M., Cani, P. D., Claus, S. P., Fuentes, S., Puylaert, P. G., Neyrinck, A. M., Bindels, L. B., de Vos, W. M., Gibson, G. R., Thissen, J. P., & Delzenne, N. M. (2013). Insight into the prebiotic concept: Lessons from an exploratory, double blind intervention study with inulin-type fructans in obese women. *Gut*, *62*(8), 1112–1121. https://doi.org/10.1136/gutjnl-2012-303304

Di Pierro, F., Zanvit, A., Nobili, P., Risso, P., & Fornaini, C. (2015). Cariogram outcome after 90 days of oral treatment with Streptococcus Salivarius M18 in children at high risk for dental caries: Results of a randomized, controlled study. *Clinical, Cosmetic and Investigational Dentistry*, *7*, 107–113. https://doi.org/10.2147/CCIDE.S93066

Diplock, A. T., Yang, M., Collis, C. S. Kelly, M., & Rice-Evans, C. (1999). Do iron and vitamin C co-supplementation influence platelet function or LDL oxidizability in healthy volunteers? *European Journal of Clinical Nutrition, 53*, 367–374. https://www.nature.com/ejcn

Dotterud, C. K., Avershina, E., Sekelja, M., Simpson, M. R., Rudi, K., Storrø, O., Johnsen, R., & Øien, T. (2015). Does maternal perinatal probiotic supplementation alter the intestinal microbiota of mother and child? *Journal of Pediatric Gastroenterology and Nutrition*, *61*(2), 200–207. https://doi.org/10.1097/MPG.0000000000000781

Duparc, T., Plovier, H., Marrachelli, V. G., Van Hul, M., Essaghir, A., Ståhlman, M., Matamoros, S., Geurts, L., Pardo-Tendero, M. M., Druart, C., Delzenne, N. M., Demoulin, J. B., van der Merwe, S. W., van Pelt, J., Bäckhed, F., Monleon, D., Everard, A., & Cani, P. D. (2017). Hepatocyte MyD88 affects bile acids, gut microbiota and metabolome contributing to regulate glucose and lipid metabolism. *Gut*, *66*(4), 620–632. https://doi.org/10.1136/gutjnl-2015-310904

Everard, A., Belzer, C., Geurts, L., Ouwerkerk, J. P., Druart, C., Bindels, L. B., Guiot, Y., Derrien, M., Muccioli, G. G., Delzenne, N. M., de Vos, W. M., & Cani, P. D. (2013). Cross-talk between Akkermansia muciniphila and intestinal epithelium controls diet-induced obesity. *Proceedings of the National Academy of Sciences of the United States of America*, *110*(22), 9066–9071. https://doi.org/10.1073/pnas.1219451110

Everard, A., Geurts, L., Caesar, R., Van Hul, M., Matamoros, S., Duparc, T., Denis, R. G., Cochez, P., Pierard, F., Castel, J., Bindels, L. B., Plovier, H., Robine, S., Muccioli, G. G., Renauld, J. C., Dumoutier, L., Delzenne, N. M., Luquet, S., Bäckhed, F., & Cani, P. D. (2014). Intestinal epithelial MyD88 is a sensor switching host metabolism towards obesity according to nutritional status. *Nature Communications*, *5*, 5648. https://doi.org/10.1038/ncomms6648

FAO/WHO. (2001). *Evaluation of health and nutritional properties of probiotics in food including powder milk with live acid bacteria.* Report of a Joint FAO/WHO Expert Consultation, Córdoba, Argentina. http://www.who.int/foodsafety/publications/fs_management/en/probiotics.pdf?ua=1

Fuchs-Tarlovsky, V., Marquez-Barba, M. F., & Sriram, K. (2016). Probiotics in dermatologic practice. *Nutrition*, *32*(3), 289–295. https://doi.org/10.1016/j.nut.2015.09.001

Fuller, R. (1989). Probiotics in man and animals. *Journal of Applied Bacteriology*, *66*, 365–378. http://dx.doi.org/10.1111/j.1365-2672.1989.tb05105.x

Funk, A., Schnadower, D., & Freedman, S. B. (2020). Update on nonantibiotic therapies for acute gastroenteritis. *Current Opinion in Infectious Diseases*, *33*(5), 381–387. https://doi.org/10.1097/QCO.0000000000000670

Ghouri, Y. A., Richards, D. M., Rahimi, E. F., Krill, J. T., Jelinek, K. A., & DuPont, A. W. (2014). Systematic review of randomized controlled trials of probiotics, prebiotics, and Synbiotics in inflammatory bowel disease. *Clinical and Experimental Gastroenterology*, *7*, 473–487. https://doi.org/10.2147/CEG.S27530

Goldenberg, J. Z., Yap, C., Lytvyn, L., Lo, C. K., Beardsley, J., Mertz, D., & Johnston, B. C. (2017). Probiotics for the prevention of Clostridium difficile-associated diarrhea in adults and children. *Cochrane Database of Systematic Reviews*, *12*(12), CD006095. https://doi.org/10.1002/14651858.CD006095.pub4

Gomes, J. M. G., Costa, J. A., & Alfenas, R. C. G. (2017). Metabolic endotoxemia and diabetes mellitus: A systematic review. *Metabolism: Clinical and Experimental*, *68,* 133–144. https://doi.org/10.1016/j.metabol.2016.12.009

Gopalakrishnan, V., Spencer, C. N., Nezi, L., Reuben, A., Andrews, M. C., Karpinets, T. V., Prieto, P. A., Vicente, D., Hoffman, K., Wei, S. C., Cogdill, A. P., Zhao, L., Hudgens, C. W., Hutchinson, D. S., Manzo, T., Petaccia de Macedo, M., Cotechini, T., Kumar, T., Chen, W. S., . . . Wargo, J. A. (2018). Gut microbiome modulates response to anti-PD-1 immunotherapy in melanoma patients. *Science*, *359*(6371), 97–103. https://doi.org/10.1126/science.aan4236

Gordon, S. (2016). Elie Metchnikoff, the man and the myth. *Journal of Innate Immunity*, *8*(3), 223–227. https://doi.org/10.1159/000443331

Goudarzi, M., Goudarzi, H., & Rashidan, M. (2014). Probiotics: An update on mechanisms of action and clinical applications. *Novelty in Biomedicine*, *2*(1), 22–30.

Grander, C., Adolph, T. E., Wieser, V., Lowe, P., Wrzosek, L., Gyongyosi, B., Ward, D. V., Grabherr, F., Gerner, R. R., Pfister, A., Enrich, B., Ciocan, D., Macheiner, S., Mayr, L., Drach, M., Moser, P., Moschen, A. R., Perlemuter, G., Szabo, G., . . . Tilg, H. (2018). Recovery of ethanol-induced Akkermansia muciniphila depletion ameliorates alcoholic liver disease. *Gut*, *67*(5), 891–901. https://doi.org/10.1136/gutjnl-2016-313432

Groer, M. W., Luciano, A. A., Dishaw, L. J., Ashmeade, T. L., Miller, E., & Gilbert, J. A. (2014). Development of the preterm infant gut microbiome: A research priority. *Microbiome*, *2*(1), 38. https://doi.org/10.1186/2049-2618-2-38

Gruber, C., Wendt, M., Sulser, C., Lau, S., Kulig, M., Wahn, U., et al. (2007). Randomized, placebo-controlled trial of *Lactobacillus rhamnosus* GG as treatment of atopic dermatitis in infancy. *Allergy, 62*, 1270–1276. 10.1111/j.1398-9995.2007.01543.x

Guandalini, S., Pensabene, L., Zikri, M. A., et al (2008). *Lactobacillus* GG administered in oral rehydration solution to children with acute diarrhea: A multicenter European trial. *Journal of Pediatric Gastroenterology and Nutrition, 30*, 54–60.

Guarino, A., Lo Vecchio, A., Dias, J. A., Berkley, J. A., Boey, C., Bruzzese, D., Cohen, M. B., Cruchet, S., Liguoro, I., Salazar-Lindo, E., Sandhu, B., Sherman, P. M., & Shimizu, T. (2018). Universal recommendations for the management of acute diarrhea in nonmalnourished children. *Journal of Pediatric Gastroenterology and Nutrition*, *67*(5), 586–593. https://doi.org/10.1097/MPG.0000000000002053, PubMed: 29901556

Guarner, F., & Schaafsma, G. J. (1998). Probiotics. *International Journal of Food Microbiology*, *39*, 237–238. http://dx.doi.org/10.1016/S0168-1605(97)00136-0

Gueniche, A., Philippe, D., Bastien, P., Reuteler, G., Blum, S., Castiel-Higounenc, I., Breton, L., & Benyacoub, J. (2014). Randomised double-blind placebo-controlled study of the effect of Lactobacillus paracasei NCC 2461 on skin reactivity. *Beneficial Microbes*, *5*(2), 137–145. https://doi.org/10.3920/BM2013.0001

Guthrie, L., Gupta, S., Daily, J., & Kelly, L. (2017). Human microbiome signatures of differential colorectal cancer drug metabolism. *NPJ Biofilms and Microbiomes*, *3*, 27. https://doi.org/10.1038/s41522-017-0034-1

Hamasalim, H. J. (2015). The impact of some widely probiotic (Iraqi probiotic) on health and performance. *Journal of Biosciences and Medicines*, *3*(8), 25–36. https://doi.org/10.4236/jbm.2015.38003

Hamasalim, H. J. (2016). Synbiotic as feed additives relating to animal health and performance. *Advances in Microbiology*, *6*(4), 288–302. https://doi.org/10.4236/aim.2016.64028

Hänninen, A., Toivonen, R., Pöysti, S., Belzer, C., Plovier, H., Ouwerkerk, J. P., Emani, R., Cani, P. D., & De Vos, W. M. (2018). Akkermansia muciniphila induces gut microbiota remodelling and controls islet autoimmunity in NOD mice. *Gut*, *67*(8), 1445–1453. https://doi.org/10.1136/gutjnl-2017-314508

Hao, Q., Dong, B. R., & Wu, T. (2015). Probiotics for preventing acute upper respiratory tract infections. *Cochrane Database of Systematic Reviews*, *2015*(2), CD006895. https://doi.org/10.1002/14651858.CD006895.pub3

Hasslöf, P., West, C. E., Videhult, F. K., Brandelius, C., & Stecksén-Blicks, C. (2013). Early intervention with probiotic Lactobacillus paracasei F19 has no long-term effect on caries experience. *Caries Research*, *47*(6), 559–565. https://doi.org/10.1159/000350524

Havenaar, R., & Huis In't Veld, J. H. J. (1992). Probiotics; A general review. In B. Wood (Ed.), *The lactic acid bacteria in health and disease*. Elsevier. http://dx.doi.org/10.1007/978-1-4615-3522-5_6

Hedayati-Hajikand, T., Lundberg, U., Eldh, C., & Twetman, S. (2015). Effect of probiotic chewing tablets on early childhood caries—A randomized controlled trial. *BMC Oral Health*, *15*(1), 112. https://doi.org/10.1186/s12903-015-0096-5

Hiippala, K., Jouhten, H., Ronkainen, A., Hartikainen, A., Kainulainen, V., Jalanka, J., & Satokari, R. (2018). The potential of gut commensals in reinforcing intestinal barrier function and alleviating inflammation. *Nutrients*, *10*(8), E988. https://doi.org/10.3390/nu10080988

Hill, C., Guarner, F., Reid, G., Gibson, G. R., Merenstein, D. J., Pot, B., Morelli, L., Canani, R. B., Flint, H. J., Salminen, S., Calder, P. C., & Sanders, M. E. (2014). Expert consensus document: The International Scientific Association for Probiotics and Prebiotics consensus statement on the scope and appropriate use of the term probiotic. *Nature Reviews Gastroenterology and Hepatology*, *11*(8), 506–514. https://doi.org/10.1038/nrgastro.2014.66

Horton, F., Wright, J., Smith, L., Hinton, P. J., & Robertson, M. D. (2014). Increased intestinal permeability to oral chromium (51 Cr) -EDTA in human Type 2 diabetes. *Diabetic Medicine*, *31*(5), 559–563. https://doi.org/10.1111/dme.12360

Huang, R., & Hu, J. (2017). Positive effect of probiotics on constipation in children: A systematic review and meta-analysis of six randomized controlled trials. *Frontiers in Cellular and Infection Microbiology*, *7*, 153. https://doi.org/10.3389/fcimb.2017.00153

Huang, R., Wang, K., & Hu, J. (2016). Effect of probiotics on depression: A systematic review and meta-analysis of randomized controlled trials. *Nutrients*, *8*(8), E483. https://doi.org/10.3390/nu8080483

ILSI—International Life Sciences Institute, Europe Working Group. (1998). info@ilsieurope.be. ILSI Europe, Brussels, Belgium.

Jain, M., Gupta, K., & Jain, P. (2014). Significance of probiotics and prebiotics in health and nutrition. *Malaya Journal of Biosciences*, *1*(3), 181–195.

Jandhyala, S. M., Talukdar, R., Subramanyam, C., Vuyyuru, H., Sasikala, M., & Nageshwar Reddy, D. N. (2015). Role of the normal gut microbiota. *World Journal of Gastroenterology*, *21*(29), 8787–8803. https://doi.org/10.3748/wjg.v21.i29.8787

Jayashree, B., Bibin, Y. S., Prabhu, D., Shanthirani, C. S., Gokulakrishnan, K., Lakshmi, B. S., Mohan, V., & Balasubramanyam, M. (2014). Increased circulatory levels of lipopolysaccharide (LPS) and zonulin signify novel biomarkers of proinflammation in patients with type 2 diabetes. *Molecular and Cellular Biochemistry*, *388*(1–2), 203–210. https://doi.org/10.1007/s11010-013-1911-4

Kaushik, M., Kumar, S., Kapoor, R. K., & Gulati, P. (2019). Integrons and antibiotic resistance genes in water-borne pathogens: Threat detection and risk assessment. *Journal of Medical Microbiology*, *68*(5), 679–692. https://doi.org/10.1099/jmm.0.000972

Kelly, J. R., Clarke, G., Cryan, J. F., & Dinan, T. G. (2016). Brain-gut-microbiota axis: Challenges for translation in psychiatry. *Annals of Epidemiology*, *26*(5), 366–372. https://doi.org/10.1016/j.annepidem.2016.02.008

Khan, M. T., Nieuwdorp, M., & Bäckhed, F. (2014). Microbial modulation of insulin sensitivity. *Cell Metabolism*, *20*(5), 753–760. https://doi.org/10.1016/j.cmet.2014.07.006

Kim, J. K., Choi, M. S., Jeong, J. J., Lim, S. M., Kim, I. S., Yoo, H. H. et al. (2018).

Kim, S. O., Ah, Y. M., Yu, Y. M., Choi, K. H., Shin, W. G., & Lee, J. Y. (2014). Effects of probiotics for the treatment of atopic dermatitis: A meta-analysis of randomized controlled trials. *Annals of Allergy, Asthma and Immunology*, *113*(2), 217–226. https://doi.org/10.1016/j.anai.2014.05.021

Kimura, I., Inoue, D., Hirano, K., & Tsujimoto, G. (2014). The SCFA receptor GPR43 and energy metabolism. *Frontiers in Endocrinology*, *5*, 85. https://doi.org/10.3389/fendo.2014.00085

Kirjavainen, P. V., Salminen, S. J., & Isolauri, E. (2003). Probiotic bacteria in the management of atopic disease: Underscoring the importance of viability. *Journal of Pediatric Gastroenterology and Nutrition*, *36*, 223–227. 10.1097/00005176-200302000-00012

König, J., Wells, J., Cani, P. D., García-Ródenas, C. L., MacDonald, T., Mercenier, A., Whyte, J., Troost, F., & Brummer, R. J. (2016). Human intestinal barrier function in health and disease. *Clinical and Translational Gastroenterology*, *7*(10), e196. https://doi.org/10.1038/ctg.2016.54

Kootte, R. S., Levin, E., Salojärvi, J., Smits, L. P., Hartstra, A. V., Udayappan, S. D., Hermes, G., Bouter, K. E., Koopen, A. M., Holst, J. J., Knop, F. K., Blaak, E. E., Zhao, J., Smidt, H., Harms, A. C., Hankemeijer, T., Bergman, J. J. G. H. M., Romijn, H. A., Schaap, F. G., . . . Nieuwdorp, M. (2017). Improvement of insulin sensitivity after lean donor feces in metabolic syndrome is driven by baseline intestinal microbiota composition. *Cell Metabolism*, *26*(4), 611–619.e616. https://doi.org/10.1016/j.cmet.2017.09.008

Kunishima, H., Ishibashi, N., Wada, K., Oka, K., Takahashi, M., Yamasaki, Y., Aoyagi, T., Takemura, H., Kitagawa, M., & Kaku, M. (2019). The effect of gut microbiota and probiotic organisms on the properties of extended spectrum beta-lactamase producing and carbapenem resistant Enterobacteriaceae including growth, beta-lactamase activity and gene transmissibility. *Journal of Infection and Chemotherapy*, *25*(11), 894–900. https://doi.org/10.1016/j.jiac.2019.04.021

Lan, Y., Kriete, A., & Rosen, G. L. (2013). Selecting age-related functional characteristics in the human gut microbiome. *Microbiome*, *1*(1), 2. https://doi.org/10.1186/2049-2618-1-2

Laursen, M. F., Laursen, R. P., Larnkjær, A., Michaelsen, K. F., Bahl, M. I., & Licht, T. R. (2017). Administration of two probiotic strains during early childhood does not affect the endogenous gut microbiota composition despite probiotic proliferation. *BMC Microbiology*, *17*(1), 175. https://doi.org/10.1186/s12866-017-1090-7

Lee, S. M., Donaldson, G. P., Mikulski, Z., Boyajian, S., Ley, K., & Mazmanian, S. K. (2013). Bacterial colonization factors control specificity and stability of the gut microbiota. *Nature*, *501*(7467), 426–429. https://doi.org/10.1038/nature12447

Licari, A., Marseglia, A., Castellazzi, A. M., Ricci, A., Tagliacarne, C., Valsecchi, C., Castagnoli, R., & Marseglia, G. L. (2015). Atopic dermatitis: Is there a role for probiotics? *Journal of Biological Regulators and Homeostatic Agents*, *29*(suppl_1), 18–24.

Lilly, D. M., & Stillwell, R. H. (1965). Probiotics: Growth-promoting factors produced by microorganisms. *Science*, *147*, 747–748.

Liu, H. Y., Roos, S., Jonsson, H., Ahl, D., Dicksved, J., Lindberg, J. E., & Lundh, T. (2015, April 1). Effects of Lactobacillus johnsonii and Lactobacillus reuteri on gut barrier function and heat shock proteins in intestinal porcine epithelial cells. *Physiological Reports*, *3*(4). https://doi.org/10.14814/phy2.12355

Lo Vecchio, A., Dias, J. A., Berkley, J. A., Boey, C., Cohen, M. B., Cruchet, S., Liguoro, I., Salazar Lindo, E., Sandhu, B., Sherman, P., Shimizu, T., & Guarino, A. (2016). Comparison of recommendations in clinical practice guidelines for acute gastroenteritis in children. *Journal of Pediatric Gastroenterology and Nutrition*, *63*(2), 226–235. https://doi.org/10.1097/MPG.0000000000001133, PubMed: 26835905

Lopez-Lopez, A., & Camelo-Castillo, A, Ferrer, M. D., Simon-Soro, A., & Mira, A. (2017). Health- associated niche inhabitants as oral probiotics: The case of Streptococcus dentisani. *Frontiers in Microbiology*, *8*, 379.

Magalhaes, I., Pingris, K., Poitou, C., Bessoles, S., Venteclef, N., Kiaf, B., Beaudoin, L., Da Silva, J., Allatif, O., Rossjohn, J., Kjer-Nielsen, L., McCluskey, J., Ledoux, S., Genser, L., Torcivia, A., Soudais, C., Lantz, O., Boitard, C., Aron-Wisnewsky, J., . . . Lehuen, A. (2015). Mucosal-associated invariant T cell alterations in obese and type 2 diabetic patients. *Journal of Clinical Investigation*, *125*(4), 1752–1762. https://doi.org/10.1172/JCI78941

Margolis, D. J., & Mitra, N. (2017). Heterogeneity of data included in meta-analysis on persistence of atopic dermatitis changes interpretation. *Journal of the American Academy of Dermatology*, *76*(5), e181. https://doi.org/10.1016/j.jaad.2016.11.068

Marín, L., Miguélez, E. M., Villar, C. J., & Lombó, F. (2015). Bioavailability of dietary polyphenols and gut microbiota metabolism: Antimicrobial properties. *BioMed Research International*, *2015*, 905215. https://doi.org/10.1155/2015/905215

Markowiak, P., & Śliżewska, K. (2017). Effects of probiotics, prebiotics, and Synbiotics on human health. *Nutrients*, *9*(9), 1021. https://doi.org/10.3390/nu9091021

Marsh, P. D., & Zaura, E. (2017). Dental biofilm: Eco-logical interactions in health and dis- ease. *Journal of Clinical Periodontology*, *44*(suppl_18), S12–S22. https://doi.org/10.1111/jcpe.12679

Matuskova, Z., Anzenbacher, P., Vecera, R., Siller, M., Tlaskalova-Hogenova, H., Strojil, J., & Anzenbacherova, E. (2017). Effect of Lactobacillus casei on the pharmacokinetics of amiodarone in male Wistar rats. *European Journal of Drug Metabolism and Pharmacokinetics*, *42*(1), 29–36. https://doi.org/10.1007/s13318-015-0315-0

Matuskova, Z., Anzenbacherova, E., Vecera, R., Tlaskalova-Hogenova, H., Kolar, M., & Anzenbacher, P. (2014). Administration of a probiotic can change drug pharmacokinetics: Effect of E. coli Nissle 1917 on amidarone absorption in rats. *PLoS One*, *9*(2), e87150. https://doi.org/10.1371/journal.pone.0087150

Metchnikoff, É. (1907). *The prolongation of life: optimistic studies*. G.P. Putnam's Sons.

Metchnikoff, É. (1908). *L'Immunité dans les maladies infectieuses (Immunity in infectious diseases)*. Masson.

Millan, B., Park, H., Hotte, N., Mathieu, O., Burguiere, P., Tompkins, T. A., Kao, D., & Madsen, K. L. (2016). Fecal microbial transplants reduce antibiotic-resistant genes in patients with recurrent Clostridium difficile infection. *Clinical Infectious Diseases*, *62*(12), 1479–1486. https://doi.org/10.1093/cid/ciw185

Miquel, S., Martín, R., Lashermes, A., Gillet, M., Meleine, M., Gelot, A., Eschalier, A., Ardid, D., Bermúdez-Humarán, L. G., Sokol, H., Thomas, M., Theodorou, V., Langella, P., & Carvalho, F. A. (2016). Antinociceptive effect of Faecalibacterium prausnitzii in non-inflammatory IBS-like models. *Scientific Reports*, *6*, 19399. https://doi.org/10.1038/srep19399

Mizock, B. A. (2015). Probiotics. *Disease-a-Month*, *61*(7), 259–290. https://doi.org/10.1016/j.disamonth.2015.03.011

Money, N. M., Schroeder, A. R., Quinonez, R. A., Ho, T., Marin, J. R., Morgan, D. J., Dhruva, S. S., & Coon, E. R. (2020). Update on pediatric medical overuse: A systematic review. *JAMA Pediatrics*, *174*(4), 375–382. https://doi.org/10.1001/jamapediatrics.2019.5849

Monteiro-Sepulveda, M., Touch, S., Mendes-Sá, C., André, S., Poitou, C., Allatif, O., Cotillard, A., Fohrer-Ting, H., Hubert, E. L., Remark, R., Genser, L., Tordjman, J., Garbin, K., Osinski, C., Sautès-Fridman, C., Leturque, A., Clément, K., & Brot-Laroche, E. (2015). Jejunal T cell inflammation in human obesity correlates with decreased enterocyte insulin signaling. *Cell Metabolism*, *22*(1), 113–124. https://doi.org/10.1016/j.cmet.2015.05.020

Moynihan, P. (2016). Sugars and dental caries: Evidence for setting a recommended threshold for intake. *Advances in Nutrition*, *7*(1), 149–156. https://doi.org/10.3945/an.115.009365

Naidu, A. S., Bidlack, W. R., & Clemens, R. A. (1999). Probiotic spectra of lactic acid bacteria (LAB). *Critical Reviews in Food Science Nutrition*, *39*, 13–126. https://doi.org/10.1080/10408699991279187

Ng, K. M., Ferreyra, J. A., Higginbottom, S. K., Lynch, J. B., Kashyap, P. C., Gopinath, S., Naidu, N., Choudhury, B., Weimer, B. C., Monack, D. M., & Sonnenburg, J. L. (2013). Microbiota-liberated host sugars facilitate post-antibiotic expansion of enteric pathogens. *Nature*, *502*(7469), 96–99. https://doi.org/10.1038/nature12503

Nishihara, T., Suzuki, N., Yoneda, M., & Hirofuji, T. (2014). Effects of Lactobacillus salivarius- containing tablets on caries risk factors: A randomized open-label clinical trial. *BMC Oral Health*, *14*, 110. https://doi.org/10.1186/1472-6831-14-110

Nøhr, M. K., Pedersen, M. H., Gille, A., Egerod, K. L., Engelstoft, M. S., Husted, A. S., Sichlau, R. M., Grunddal, K. V., Poulsen, S. S., Han, S., Jones, R. M., Offermanns, S., & Schwartz, T. W. (2013). GPR41/FFAR3 and GPR43/FFAR2 as cosensors for short-chain fatty acids in enteroendocrine cells vs. FFAR3 in enteric neurons and FFAR2 in enteric leukocytes. *Endocrinology*, *154*(10), 3552–3564. https://doi.org/10.1210/en.2013-1142

Ogden N. S., & Bielory, L. (2005). Probiotics: A complementary approach in the treatment and prevention of pediatric atopic disease. *Current Opinion in Allergy and Clinical Immunology*, *5*, 179–184. 10.1097/01.all.0000162312.64308.fc

Ohkusa, T., Koido, S., Nishikawa, Y., & Sato, N. (2019). Gut microbiota and chronic constipation: A review and update. *Frontiers in Medicine*, *6*, 19. https://doi.org/10.3389/fmed.2019.00019

O'Toole, P. W., Marchesi, J. R., & Hill, C. (2017). Next-generation probiotics: The spectrum from probiotics to live biotherapeutics. *Nature Microbiology*, *2*, 17057. https://doi.org/10.1038/nmicrobiol.2017.57

Parker, J. B. (1974). *(MOD (PE), Aldemaston) Eight pick index of mass spectra* (2nd edn). Mass Spectroscopy Data Center.

Pessi, T., Sutas Y., Hurme M., & Isolauri E. (2000). Interleukin-10 generation in atopic children following oral *Lactobacillus rhamnosus* GG. *Clinical and Experimental Allergy, 30*, 1804–1808. 10.1046/j.1365-2222.2000.00948.x

Plovier, H., Everard, A., Druart, C., Depommier, C., Van Hul, M., Geurts, L., Chilloux, J., Ottman, N., Duparc, T., Lichtenstein, L., Myridakis, A., Delzenne, N. M., Klievink, J., Bhattacharjee, A., van der Ark, K. C., Aalvink, S., Martinez, L. O., Dumas, M. E., Maiter, D., . . . Cani, P. D. (2017). A purified membrane protein from Akkermansia muciniphila or the pasteurized bacterium improves metabolism in obese and diabetic mice. *Nature Medicine*, *23*(1), 107–113. https://doi.org/10.1038/nm.4236

Pradeep, K., Kuttappa, M. A., & Prasana, K. R. (2014). Probiotics and oral health: An update. *South African Dental Journal*, *69*(1), 20–24.

Preston, R. R., & Wilson, T. E. (2013). *Lippincott's illustrated reviews: Physiology*. Lippincott Williams & Wilkins.

Radilla-Vázquez, R. B., Parra-Rojas, I., Martínez-Hernández, N. E., Márquez-Sandoval, Y. F., Illades-Aguiar, B., & Castro-Alarcón, N. (2016). Gut microbiota and metabolic endotoxemia in young obese Mexican subjects. *Obesity Facts*, *9*(1), 1–11. https://doi.org/10.1159/000442479

Ramnani, P., Chitarrari, R., Tuohy, K., Grant, J., Hotchkiss, S., Philp, K., Campbell, R., Gill, C., & Rowland, I. (2012). In vitro fermentation and prebiotic potential of novel low molecular weight polysaccharides derived from agar and alginate seaweeds. *Anaerobe*, *18*(1), 1–6.

Rastelli, M., Cani, P. D., & Knauf, C. (2019). The gut microbiome influences host endocrine functions. *Endocrine Reviews*, *40*(5), 1271–1284. https://doi.org/10.1210/er.2018-00280

Reddy, J. J., Sampathkumar, N., & Aradhya, S. (2017, (November), 29). Probiotics in dentistry: Review of the current status. *Archives of Oral Research*, *6*(3).

Reid, G., Jass, J., Tom Sebulsky, M., & McCormick, J. K. (2003). Potential uses of probiotics in clinical practice. *Clinical Microbiol Reviews*, *16*(4), 658–672. https://doi.org/10.1128/CMR.16.4.658-672.2003

Ringel-Kulka, T., Cheng, J., Ringel, Y., Salojärvi, J., Carroll, I., Palva, A., de Vos, W. M., & Satokari, R. (2013). Intestinal microbiota in healthy US young children and adults—A high throughput microarray analysis. *PLoS One*, *8*(5), e64315. https://doi.org/10.1371/journal.pone.0064315

Rodríguez, G., Ruiz, B., Faleiros, S., Vistoso, A., Marró, M. L., Sánchez, J., Urzúa, I., & Cabello, R. (2016). Probiotic compared with standard milk for high-caries children: A cluster randomized trial. *Journal of Dental Research*, *95*(4), 402–407. https://doi.org/10.1177/0022034515623935

Romani Vestman, N., Hasslöf, P., Keller, M. K., Granström, E., Roos, S., Twetman, S., & Stecksén-Blicks, C. (2013). Lactobacillus reuteri influences regrowth of mutans streptococci after full-mouth disinfection: A double-blind, randomised controlled trial. *Caries Research*, *47*(4), 338–345. https://doi.org/10.1159/000347233

Rondanelli, M., Faliva, M. A., Perna, S., Giacosa, A., Peroni, G., & Castellazzi, A. M. (2017). Using probiotics in clinical practice: Where are we now? A review of existing meta-analyses. *Gut Microbes*, *8*(6), 521–543. https://doi.org/10.1080/19490976.2017.1345414

Routy, B., Le Chatelier, E., Derosa, L., Duong, C. P. M., Alou, M. T., Daillère, R., Fluckiger, A., Messaoudene, M., Rauber, C., Roberti, M. P., Fidelle, M., Flament, C., Poirier-Colame, V., Opolon, P., Klein, C., Iribarren, K., Mondragón, L., Jacquelot, N., Qu, B., . . . Zitvogel, L. (2018). Gut microbiome influences efficacy of PD- 1-based immunotherapy against epithelial tumors. *Science*, *359*(6371), 91–97. https://doi.org/10.1126/science.aan3706

Rutten, N. B., Gorissen, D. M., Eck, A., Niers, L. E., Vlieger, A. M., Besseling-van der Vaart, I., Budding, A. E., Savelkoul, P. H., van der Ent, C. K., & Rijkers, G. T. (2015). Long term development of gut microbiota composition in atopic children: Impact of probiotics. *PLoS One*, *10*(9), e0137681. https://doi.org/10.1371/journal.pone.0137681

Sarkar, A., Harty, S., Lehto, S. M., Moeller, A. H., Dinan, T. G., Dunbar, R. I. M., Cryan, J. F., & Burnet, P. W. J. (2018). The microbiome in psychology and cognitive neuroscience. *Trends in Cognitive Sciences*, *22*(7), 611–636. https://doi.org/10.1016/j.tics.2018.04.006

Satokari, R. (2019). Modulation of gut microbiota for health by current and next-generation probiotics. *Nutrients*, *11*(8), 1921. https://doi.org/10.3390/nu11081921

Scanlon, V. C., & Sanders, T. (2014, November 25). *Essentials of anatomy and physiology*. F. A. Davis.

Schrezenmeir, J., & de Vrese, M. (2001) Probiotics, prebiotics, and symbiotics—Approaching a definition. *American Journal of Clinical Nutrition*, *73*, 3615–3645.

Scott, K. P., Antoine, J. M., & Midtvedt, T., & van Hemert, S. (2015). Manipulating the gut micro-biota to maintain health and treat disease. *Microbial Ecology in Health and Disease*, *26*, 25877.

Seo, J. H., Shim, J. O., Choe, B. H., Moon, J. S., Kang, K. S., & Chung, J. Y. (2019). Management of acute gastroenteritis in children: A survey among members of the Korean society of pediatric, hepatology, and nutrition. *Pediatric Gastroenterology, Hepatology and Nutrition*, *22*(5), 431–440. https://doi.org/10.5223/pghn.2019.22.5.431, PubMed: 31555567

Sidbury, R., & Khorsand, K. (2017). Evolving concepts in atopic dermatitis. *Current Allergy and Asthma Reports*, *17*(7), 42. https://doi.org/10.1007/s11882-017-0710-5

Silverberg, N. B. (2016). A practical overview of pediatric atopic dermatitis, part 3: Differential diagnosis, comorbidities, and measurement of disease burden. *Cutis*, *97*(6), 408–412.

Singh, R., van Nood, E., Nieuwdorp, M., van Dam, B., ten Berge, I. J., Geerlings, S. E., & Bemelman, F. J. (2014). Donor feces infusion for eradication of extended spectrum beta-lactamase producing Escherichia coli in a patient with end stage renal disease. *Clinical Microbiology and Infection*, *20*(11), O977–O978. https://doi.org/10.1111/1469-0691.12683

Singhi, S. C., & Kumar, S. (2016). Probiotics in critically ill children. *F1000Research*, *5*, 407. https://doi.org/10.12688/f1000research.7630.1

Slavin, J. (2013). Fiber and prebiotics: Mechanisms and health benefits. *Nutrients*, *5*(4), 1417–1435. https://doi.org/10.3390/nu5041417

Soccol, C. R., de Souza Vandenberghe, L. P., Spier, M. R., Pedroni Medeiros, A. B., Yamaguishi, C. T., De Dea Lindner, J., Pandey, A., & Thomaz-Soccol, V. (2012). Probiotics, prebiotics and synbiotics, the potential of probiotics. Food Technology and Biotechnology, *48*(4), 413–434. ISSN 1330-9862.

Soltan Dallal, M. M., Davoodabadi, A., Abdi, M., Hajiabdolbaghi, M., Sharifi Yazdi, M. K., Douraghi, M., & Tabatabaei Bafghi, S. M. (2017). Inhibitory effect of Lactobacillus plantarum and Lb. fermentum isolated from the faeces of healthy infants against nonfermentative bacteria causing nosocomial infections. *New Microbes and New Infections*, *15*, 9–13. https://doi.org/10.1016/j.nmni.2016.09.003

Spanogiannopoulos, P., Bess, E. N., Carmody, R. N., & Turnbaugh, P. J. (2016). The microbial pharmacists within us: A metagenomic view of xenobiotic metabolism. *Nature Reviews Microbiology*, *14*(5), 273–287. https://doi.org/10.1038/nrmicro.2016.17

Sperti, G. S. (1971). Probiotics: 1971—cir.nii.ac.jp.

Stensson, M., Koch, G., Coric, S., Abrahamsson, T. R., Jenmalm, M. C., Birkhed, D., & Wendt, L. K. (2014). Oral administration of Lactobacillus reuteri during the first year of life reduces caries prevalence in the primary dentition at 9 years of age. *Caries Research*, *48*, 111–117.

Stripling, J., Kumar, R., Baddley, J. W., Nellore, A., Dixon, P., Howard, D., Ptacek, T., Lefkowitz, E. J., Tallaj, J. A., Benjamin, W. H., Morrow, C. D., & Rodriguez, J. M. (2015). Loss of vancomycin-resistant enterococcus fecal dominance in an organ transplant patient with Clostridium difficile colitis after fecal microbiota transplant. *Open Forum Infectious Diseases*, *2*(2), ofv078. https://doi.org/10.1093/ofid/ofv078

Sun, Y., & O'Riordan, M. X. (2013, January 1). Regulation of bacterial pathogenesis by intestinal short-chain fatty acids. *In Advances in applied microbiology* (Vol. 85, pp. 93–118). Academic Press.

Sung, M., Lee, K. S., Ha, E. G., Lee, S. J., Kim, M. A., Lee, S. W., Jee, H. M., Sheen, Y. H., Jung, Y. H., & Han, M. Y. (2017). An association of periostin levels with the severity and chronicity of atopic dermatitis in children. *Pediatric Allergy and Immunology*, *28*(6), 543–550. https://doi.org/10.1111/pai.12744 [Epub ahead of print]

Szajewska, H., Shamir, R., Turck, D., van Goudoever, J. B., Mihatsch, W. A., & Fewtrell, M. (2015). Recommendations on probiotics in allergy prevention should not be based on pooling data from different strains. *Journal of Allergy and Clinical Immunology*, *136*(5), 1422. https://doi.org/10.1016/j.jaci.2015.07.022

Taipale, T. J., Pienihäkkinen, K., Alanen, P., Jokela, J., & Söderling, E. (2013). Administration of Bifidobacterium animalis subsp. Lactis BB-12 in early childhood: A post-trial effect on caries occurrence at four years of age. *Caries Research*, *47*(5), 364–372. https://doi.org/10.1159/000348424

Taipale, T. J., Pienihäkkinen, K., Isolauri, E., Jokela, J. T., & Söderling, E. M. (2016). Bifidobacterium animalis subsp. Lactis BB-12 in reducing the risk of infections in early childhood. *Pediatric Research*, *79*(1–1), 65–69. https://doi.org/10.1038/pr.2015.174

Tannock, R., & Brown, T. E. (2000). Attention-deficit disorders with learning disorders in children and adolescents. In T. E. Brown (Ed.), *Attention-deficit disorders and comorbidities in children, adolescents, and adults* (pp. 231–295). American Psychiatric Publishing, Inc.

Teanpaisan, R., & Piwat, S. (2014). Lactobacillus paracasei SD1, a novel probiotic, reduces mutans streptococci in human volunteers: A randomized placebo-controlled trial. *Clinical Oral Investigations*, *18*(3), 857–862. https://doi.org/10.1007/s00784-013-1057-5

Thingholm, L. B., Rühlemann, M. C., Koch, M., Fuqua, B., Laucke, G., Boehm, R., Bang, C., Franzosa, E. A., Hübenthal, M., Rahnavard, A., Frost, F., Lloyd-Price, J., Schirmer, M., Lusis, A. J., Vulpe, C. D., Lerch, M. M., Homuth, G., Kacprowski, T., Schmidt, C. O., . . . Huttenhower, C. (2019). Obese individuals with and without type 2 diabetes show different gut microbial functional capacity and composition. *Cell Host and Microbe*, *26*(2), 252–264.e210. https://doi.org/10.1016/j.chom.2019.07.004

Tissier, H. (1900). *Recherches Sur La Flore Intestinale Des Nourrissons: (État Normal et Pathologique)*. G. Carré et C. Naud.

Tiwari, G., Tiwari, R., Pandey, S., & Pandey, P. (2012). Promising future of probiotics for human health: Current scenario. *Chronicles of Young Scientists*, *3*(1), 17–28.

Totri, C. R., Eichenfield, L. F., Logan, K., Proudfoot, L., Schmitt, J., Lara-Corrales, I., Sugarman, J., Tom, W., Siegfried, E., Cordoro, K., Paller, A. S., & Flohr, C. (2017). Prescribing practices for systemic agents in the treatment of severe pediatric atopic dermatitis in the US and Canada: The PeDRA TREAT survey. *Journal of the American Academy of Dermatology*, *76*(2), 281–285. https://doi.org/10.1016/j.jaad.2016.09.021

Tulini, F. L., Hymery, N., Haertlé, T., Le Blay, G., & De Martinis, E. C. (2016). Screening for antimicrobial and proteolytic activities of lactic acid bacteria isolated from cow, buffalo and goat milk and cheeses marketed in the southeast region of Brazil. *Journal of Dairy Research*, *83*(1), 115–124. https://doi.org/10.1017/S0022029915000606

Tymczyszyn, E. E., Santos, M. I., Costa, M. D., & Illanes, A., Gomez- Zavaglia, A. (2014). History, synthesis, properties, applications and regulatory issues of prebiotic oligosaccharides. *Carbohydrates Applications in Medicine*.

Ubeda, C., Bucci, V., Caballero, S., Djukovic, A., Toussaint, N. C., Equinda, M., Lipuma, L., Ling, L., Gobourne, A., Taur, Y., Jenq, R. R., van den Brink, M. R., Xavier, J. B., & Pamer, E. G. (2013). Intestinal microbiota containing Barnesiella species cures vancomycin-resistant Enterococcus faecium colonization. *Infection and Immunity*, *81*(3), 965–973. https://doi.org/10.1128/IAI.01197-12

Udayappan, S. D., Hartstra, A. V., Dallinga-Thie, G. M., & Nieuwdorp, M. (2014). Intestinal microbiota and faecal transplantation as treatment modality for insulin resistance and type 2 diabetes mellitus. *Clinical and Experimental Immunology*, *177*(1), 24–29. https://doi.org/10.1111/cei.12293

Veiga, P., Pons, N., Agrawal, A., Oozeer, R., Guyonnet, D., Brazeilles, R., Faurie, J. M., van Hylckama Vlieg, J. E., Houghton, L. A., Whorwell, P. J., Ehrlich, S. D., & Kennedy, S. P. (2014). Changes of the human gut microbiome induced by a fermented milk product. *Scientific Reports*, *4*, 6328. https://doi.org/10.1038/srep06328

Volz, T., Skabytska, Y., Guenova, E., Chen, K. M., Frick, J. S., Kirschning, C. J., Kaesler, S., Röcken, M., & Biedermann, T. (2014). Nonpathogenic bacteria alleviating atopic dermatitis inflammation induce IL-10-producing dendritic cells and regulatory Tr1 cells. *Journal of Investigative Dermatology*, *134*(1), 96–104. https://doi.org/10.1038/jid.2013.291

Walker, A. W., Ince, J., Duncan, S. H., Webster, L. M., Holtrop, G., Ze, X., Brown, D., Stares, M. D., Scott, P., Bergerat, A., & Louis, P. (2011). Dominant and diet-responsive groups of bacteria within the human colonic microbiota. *The ISME Journal*, *5*(2), 220.

Wang, I. J., & Wang, J. Y. (2015). Children with atopic dermatitis show clinical improvement after Lactobacillus exposure. *Clinical and Experimental Allergy*, *45*(4), 779–787. https://doi.org/10.1111/cea.12489

Weidinger, S., & Novak, N. (2016). Atopic dermatitis. *Lancet*, *387*(10023), 1109–1122. https://doi.org/10.1016/S0140-6736(15)00149-X

Wells, J. M., Brummer, R. J., Derrien, M., MacDonald, T. T., Troost, F., Cani, P. D., Theodorou, V., Dekker, J., Méheust, A., de Vos, W. M., Mercenier, A., Nauta, A., & Garcia-Rodenas, C. L. (2017). Homeostasis of the gut barrier and potential biomarkers. *American Journal of Physiology: Gastrointestinal and Liver Physiology*, *312*(3), G171–G193. https://doi.org/10.1152/ajpgi.00048.2015

West, C. E., Hammarström, M. L., & Hernell, O. (2013). Probiotics in primary prevention of allergic disease—Follow-up at 8–9 years of age. *Allergy*, *68*(8), 1015–1020. https://doi.org/10.1111/all.12191

West, N. P., Horn, P. L., Pyne, D. B., Gebski, V. J., Lahtinen, S. J., Fricker, P. A., & Cripps, A. W. (2014). Probiotic supplementation for respiratory and gastrointestinal illness symptoms in healthy physically active individuals. *Clinical Nutrition*, *33*(4), 581–587. https://doi.org/10.1016/j.clnu.2013.10.002

Whelan, K., & Quigley, E. M. (2013). Probiotics in the management of irritable bowel syn- drome and inflammatory bowel disease. *Current Opinion in Gastroenterology*, *29*(2), 184–189. https://doi.org/10.1097/MOG.0b013e32835d7bba

Yatsunenko, T., Rey, F. E., Manary, M. J., Trehan, I., Dominguez-Bello, M. G., Contreras, M., Magris, M., Hidalgo, G., Baldassano, R. N., Anokhin, A. P., & Heath, A. C. (2012). Human gut microbiome viewed across age and geography. *Nature*, *486*(7402), 222.

Yoon, J. H., Nam, Y., Song, E. Y., Roh, E. Y., Yoon, H. S., & Shin, S. (2015). CCL28 cannot replace IGE for severity by objective SCORAD index in atopic dermatitis in children. *Clinical Laboratory*, *61*(10), 1577–1580. https://doi.org/10.7754/Clin.Lab.2015.150311

Zhang, C., Derrien, M., Levenez, F., Brazeilles, R., Ballal, S. A., Kim, J., Degivry, M. C., Quéré, G., Garault, P., van Hylckama Vlieg, J. E., Garrett, W. S., Doré, J., & Veiga, P. (2016). Ecological robustness of the gut microbiota in response to ingestion of transient food-borne microbes. *ISME Journal*, *10*(9), 2235–2245. https://doi.org/10.1038/ismej.2016.13

Zhang, J., Guo, Z., Xue, Z., Sun, Z., Zhang, M., Wang, L., Wang, G., Wang, F., Xu, J., Cao, H., Xu, H., Lv, Q., Zhong, Z., Chen, Y., Qimuge, S., Menghe, B., Zheng, Y., Zhao, L., Chen, W., & Zhang, H. (2015). A phylo-functional core of gut microbiota in healthy young Chinese cohorts across lifestyles, geography and ethnicities. *ISME Journal*, *9*(9), 1979–1990. https://doi.org/10.1038/ismej.2015.11

Zhang, Y. J., Li, S., Gan, R. Y., Zhou, T., Xu, D. P., & Li, H. B. (2015). Impacts of gut bacteria on human health and diseases. *International Journal of Molecular Sciences, 16*(4), 7493–7519.

Zhang, Y. M., Chu, P., & Wang, W. J. (2017). PRISMA-combined alpha- blockers and antimuscarinics for ureteral stent-related symptoms: A meta-analysis. *Medicine*, *96*(7), e6098. https://doi.org/10.1097/MD.0000000000006098

Zmora, N., Zilberman-Schapira, G., Suez, J., Mor, U., Dori-Bachash, M., Bashiardes, S., Kotler, E., Zur, M., Regev-Lehavi, D., Brik, R. B., Federici, S., Cohen, Y., Linevsky, R., Rothschild, D., Moor, A. E., Ben-Moshe, S., Harmelin, A., Itzkovitz, S., Maharshak, N., . . . Elinav, E. (2018). Personalized gut mucosal colonization resistance to empiric probiotics is associated with unique host and microbiome features. *Cell, 174*(6), 1388–1405.e21. https://doi.org/10.1016/j.cell.2018.08.041

6 Probiotics in Pharmacology
Drug Delivery, Pharmacokinetics, and Mechanism Involved

Pinkal H. Patel Adarsh Jha, Janki Patel, Madan Mohan Gupta, and Deepak Sharma

6.1 BASIC ASPECTS AND PHARMACOLOGY OF PROBIOTICS

6.1.1 Introduction

Probiotics are live microorganisms that are believed to provide health benefits when consumed in adequate amounts. Probiotics are non-pathogenic microorganisms that, when consumed, exert a favorable impact on the host's biology or wellbeing. It is composed of yeasts (particularly *Saccharomyces*) and bacteria (notably *Lactobacillus* bacteria and bifidobacteria), and they are commonly found in various fermented foods and are also available in the form of supplements (Fijan, 2014). Many medical professionals had doubts about the effectiveness of randomized controlled trials before their execution. The effects and metabolism of probiotics are currently evaluated using a pharmacological approach (Gruber et al., 2013). Both differ not only between species but even between strains, and double-blind, randomized controlled experiments have demonstrated that numerous strains are productive. Here, we provide a summary of the current information, theories, and issues surrounding the pharmacokinetics, safety, and action mechanisms of probiotics in humans. Some of the key features can be summed up (Fijan & Turk, 2012; Pramanik et al., 2023) in the following subsections.

6.1.1.1 Health Benefits and Economic Value

Probiotic bacteria have been linked to various health benefits, and they are included in a wide range of foods. Probiotic supplements have gained popularity and economic value due to their association with potential health improvements.

6.1.1.2 Heterogeneous Populations

Probiotic supplements contain a significant number of different probiotic strains in each serving. These diverse populations of probiotics are believed to contribute to their potential health effects.

6.1.1.3 Antibiotic-Resistant Determinants

Some probiotic supplements carry antibiotic-resistant genes. These genes can potentially be transferred to resident gut bacteria and even opportunistic pathogens, which could pose health risks.

6.1.1.4 Safety Concerns

Despite the widely publicized health benefits, the potential health risks associated with probiotic supplements, such as antibiotic-resistant gene transfer, are not as well-researched or emphasized in scientific studies and public awareness.

6.1.1.5 Gastrointestinal Conditions

The human gut is a challenging environment for bacteria, including probiotics. The acidic environment and bile salts can potentially affect the survival and effectiveness of probiotics.

DOI: 10.1201/9781003452249-6

6.1.1.6 Tolerance to Acids and Bile Salts

The passage suggests that probiotics from supplements may have poor tolerance to the acidic environment and bile salts present in the gastrointestinal tract (GIT). This could impact their ability to confer health benefits.

6.1.1.7 Antibiotic Resistance

The study mentioned in the passage found that the probiotics tested displayed resistance to multiple antibiotics. This resistance could have implications for both their effectiveness and the potential spread of antibiotic resistance.

6.1.1.8 Adaptation and Resistance

The passage mentions that probiotics from supplements were able to adapt and gain resistance to streptomycin in a laboratory setting.

6.1.1.9 Balancing Hype and Concerns

The passage suggests that there is a need to balance the hype surrounding probiotic supplements with potential concerns, such as antibiotic resistance and poor tolerance to gastrointestinal conditions.

Probiotics, live microorganisms frequently alluded to as "good microbes," show a scope of properties that have gathered critical logical interest. These properties incorporate their capability to give medical advantages by advancing a decent stomach microbiota, supporting processing, and reinforcing the invulnerable framework. Probiotics are known for their capacity to seriously reject hurtful microbes, in this manner adding to destroy wellbeing and lessening the gamble of diseases. Besides, they assume a part in maturing non-edible dietary parts, creating short-chain unsaturated fats that benefit the digestive epithelium and by and large metabolic wellbeing. Probiotics can show strain-explicit qualities, for example, the ability to use explicit supplements and orchestrate specific nutrients. While their connection with the stomach climate is pivotal, probiotics are progressively being investigated for their capability to regulate foundational ailments past the gastrointestinal lot, including hypersensitive reactions, irritation, and, surprisingly, mental prosperity. Notwithstanding, it's vital to take note that the impacts of various probiotic strains can differ broadly, stressing the need for designated exploration to open their full remedial potential. Some of the properties of ideal probiotics can be summarized (refer to Figure 6.1) (Behnsen et al., 2013; Shi et al., 2016).

6.1.1.10 Safety

Probiotics should be safe for consumption, especially by vulnerable populations such as infants, elderly individuals, and people with compromised immune systems. They should not cause any harm or adverse effects when taken as recommended.

6.1.1.11 Viability

To be effective in their actions, probiotics must be able to survive the journey through the GIT, facing the acidic conditions of the stomach and meeting the bile salts in the small intestine, to reach the intended site of action in the gut (Aureli et al., 2011; Kardooni et al., 2023; Maia et al., 2023).

6.1.1.12 Stability

Stability during the production process, like freeze drying and encapsulation, along with the shelf life, is the major concern for probiotics (Lahtinen et al., 2005; El-Nezami et al., 1998).

6.1.1.13 Adhesion

Effective probiotics should be able to stick to the intestinal lining and colonize the gut, allowing them to interact with the host's cells and exert their beneficial effects (Monteagudo-Mera et al., 2019; Lau & Chye, 2018; Larsen et al., 2009).

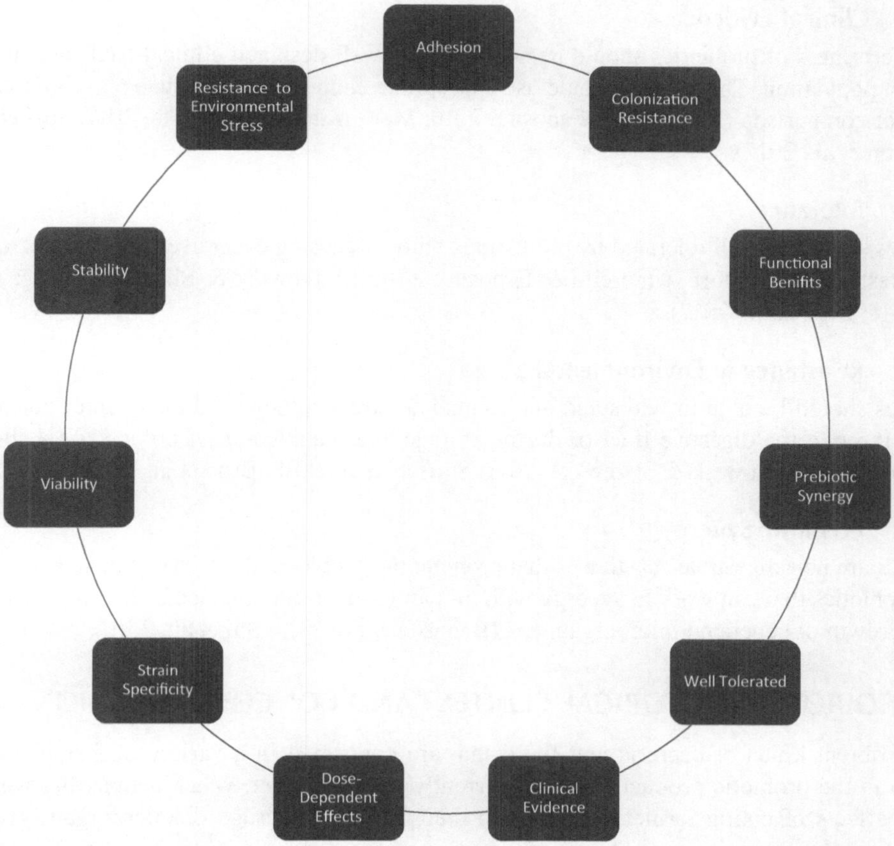

FIGURE 6.1 Properties of probiotics.

6.1.1.14 Colonization Resistance

By competing for nutrients and adhesion sites in the gut, probiotics can help prevent the growth of harmful microorganisms, thus contributing to balanced gut microbiota (Han et al., 2021; Pultz et al., 2005; Rolfe, 1984).

6.1.1.15 Functional Benefits

Probiotics should confer specific health benefits to the host. These benefits can include improving digestion, enhancing the immune system, producing beneficial compounds (such as short-chain fatty acids), and contributing to overall gut health (Aponte et al., 2020; Sarkar, 2013).

6.1.1.16 Strain Specificity

Different probiotic strains may have distinct effects. Therefore, the specific strain(s) used in a probiotic product should be well-characterized and shown to have the desired effects in scientific studies (Behnsen et al., 2013; Shi et al., 2016).

6.1.1.17 Dose-Dependent Effects

The health benefits of probiotics may be dose-dependent, meaning that a certain minimum amount of viable microorganisms needs to be consumed to achieve the desired effects (Behnsen et al., 2013; Shi et al., 2016).

6.1.1.18 Clinical Evidence

The effectiveness of probiotics should be supported by well-designed clinical trials conducted on the target population. These trials should use appropriate endpoints and include placebo-controlled groups for comparison (Umbrello & Esposito, 2016; Markowiak & Śliżewska, 2017; Sniffen et al., 2018; Bron et al., 2017).

6.1.1.19 Tolerance

Probiotics should be well tolerated by individuals without causing excessive bloating, gas, or other gastrointestinal discomfort (Umbrello & Esposito, 2016; Markowiak & Śliżewska, 2017; Sniffen et al., 2018; Bron et al., 2017).

6.1.1.20 Resistance to Environmental Stress

Probiotics should be able to withstand environmental stresses they might encounter during their passage through the digestive tract or during storage and manufacturing processes (Umbrello & Esposito, 2016; Markowiak & Śliżewska, 2017; Sniffen et al., 2018; Bron et al., 2017).

6.1.1.21 Prebiotic Synergy

Prebiotics are non-digestible substances that promote the growth and activity of beneficial gut bacteria. Probiotics that can work in synergy with prebiotics can offer enhanced benefits by encouraging the growth of beneficial microorganisms (Behnsen et al., 2013; Shi et al., 2016).

6.2 PROBIOTICS: HISTORICAL CONTEXT AND CONCEPT EVOLUTION

Many different kinds of bacteria and fungi that are consumed in a variety of formulations are included in the probiotic products that are currently on the market. When people discovered the positive effects of eating fermented foods on their health, the usage of microorganisms began (unintentionally) centuries ago. These early fermented foods are the immediate ancestors of contemporary probiotic-containing foods and goods. Yogurt and fermented milk have been consumed by humans for millennia and have played a place in both mythology and factual accounts of human history (Perles, 1997). The metabolic process known as fermentation is the way a living thing converts polysaccharides—typically starch or sugar—into an alcohol or an acid. Such physiological waste products prevent the rotting of fermented foods by lowering pH and a variety of other effects. The word "fermentation" comes from the Latin word *fermentum*, which means to boil. The name was given after it was noticed that mixes of crushed grapes held in big containers would occasionally emit bubbles as if they were boiling. While the exact beginning of human use of the fermentation process is unknown, it is generally acknowledged that it is an old method of food preservation. Dehydration is frequently cited as the only traditional method of food preservation. Strong evidence points to the vast Indus Valley civilization as the place where the technique of fermentation first emerged. Fermentation may have been used in Egypt and the Middle East as early as ancient times, according to several artifacts (McGovern, 2009). In lower Mesopotamia, between the Tigris and Euphrates rivers, in the Fertile Crescent, the first accounts of fermentation can be found as early as 6000 B.C. Laban Rayeb and Laban Khad, two traditional Egyptian fermented milk concoctions, were eaten as early as 7000 BC (Gogineni et al., 2013; Peivasteh-Roudsari et al., 2019).

Here is a step-by-step overview of the history of probiotics:

Ancient Fermented Foods (Antiquity to Middle Ages): The utilization of matured food sources traces all the way back to antiquated times. Societies all over the planet freely created strategies for aging food varieties like milk, vegetables, and grains. These cycles included the development of valuable microorganisms, possibly including lactic corrosive microbes, which unconsciously brought probiotics into the human eating routine.

The Concept of "Friendly Bacteria" (Late 19th Century): The idea of utilizing "agreeable microbes" for medical advantages began to come to fruition in the late 1900 years. Russian researcher and Nobel laureate Élie Metchnikoff proposed the possibility that specific microorganisms in yogurt could emphatically affect human wellbeing by further developing stomach capability and life span. He saw that Bulgarian laborers who consumed a lot of matured yogurt had longer life expectancies.

Identification of LAB (Early 20th Century): Scientists started distinguishing explicit types of lactic corrosive microorganisms answerable for aging in food varieties like yogurt and sauerkraut. Danish researcher Christian Hansen disengaged the bacterium answerable for yogurt maturation and named it *Lactobacillus bulgaricus*.

Introduction of Probiotic Terminology (1960s): The expression "probiotic" was first presented during the 1960s by Lilly and Stillwell, who characterized it as substances created by one microorganism that animate the development of another. This term distinguishes gainful microorganisms from pathogenic ones.

Advancements in Research and Understanding (Late 20th Century): Progressions in microbial science and innovation permitted specialists to comprehend the components of probiotics better. They started concentrating on the impacts of various stresses on stomach wellbeing, and invulnerable capability, and that's just the beginning.

Application of Probiotics in Food (the 1980s–1990s): Organizations began integrating live bacterial societies into different food items, especially dairy things like yogurt and aged milk drinks. This is obvious in the commercialization of probiotics and their combination with regular eating regimens.

Clinical Research and Health Benefits (Late 20th Century to Present): Scientists led various clinical preliminaries to investigate the potential medical advantages of probiotics. These examinations have demonstrated the way that probiotics can decidedly affect stomach-related wellbeing, resistant capability, and, surprisingly, certain circumstances like IBD and anti-microbial-related loose bowels.

Expansion of Probiotic Market (2000s to Present): The market for probiotics has developed significantly, with a wide cluster of items including supplements, practical food varieties, and refreshments. Probiotics are progressively perceived by purchasers as a method for supporting general wellbeing and prosperity.

Advancements in Microbiome Research (2010s to Present): The blast of exploration in the field of microbiome science has revealed new insight into the unpredictable connection between the stomach microbiota and human wellbeing. This has additionally highlighted the significance of probiotics in keeping a decent microbial environment.

Personalized and Precision Probiotics (Present and Beyond): Recent developments in microbiome research have led to the exploration of personalized or precision probiotics, where specific strains are chosen based on an individual's microbiome composition and health needs.

The history of probiotics reflects an evolving understanding of the benefits of beneficial microorganisms on human health, from ancient practices to modern scientific exploration. As research continues, the potential applications and benefits of probiotics are likely to expand further.

6.2.1 Selection Criteria for Probiotic Microorganisms

The precise identification and naming of the strains is the most important part of accurate probiotic characterization. Establishing that a strain belongs to a recognized, identified genus, species, and divisions for taxa in which subgroups have been classified is necessary for the recognition of probiotic bacteria. A precise strain typing is also necessary because various probiotic actions may be strain-specific. According to nomenclatural regulations, proper sample identification consists of the names of the real genus, species, and subspecies, along with an indication of the sample. The marking might contain an established culture stock's catalog identifier or an economic sample identity (Peivasteh-Roudsari et al., 2019; Binda et al., 2020).

Probiotic strains should be described in a way that supports their probiotic function. Evaluating the properties deemed essential for probiotic efficiency may reveal potential mechanisms underlying the observed clinical findings, regardless of whether clinical results are necessary to prove that probiotics work (Parker et al., 2019; Rychen et al., 2018). A few examples of such traits include the capacity to remain at essential body locations; the formation of lactate sensitivity to enzymes that break food, bile, or acid; attachment to mucus or intestinal epithelium; contact with human antibodies; exclusion from competition or production of bacteriocins or peroxides of hydrogen or other small-chain fatty acids; and antimicrobial activity via these mechanisms. Probiotic manufacturers have a fundamental duty to provide meal and nutritional supplements for users who adhere to the relevant safety standards. It is necessary to correctly identify a probiotic to the strain level as the first step in determining its safety for usage in foods and dietary supplements. This is followed by further demonstrating its safety by historical data or experiments as indicated in Figure 6.2 (Rychen et al., 2018).

6.2.2 Safety Aspects of Probiotics

Testing at the strain level and the determination of risk factors unique to a genus or species are necessary. The absence of recognized virulence factors or genes associated with acquired antimicrobial resistance is the most crucial of these. The EU's EFSA has published various norms outlining phenotypic cut-off values for resistivity and sensitivity to pertinent antibiotics as well as procedures for calculating them. The guidelines should also be used to evaluate the sensitivity of yeasts to bacteria and antimycotics. To phenotypically test possible microbial strains, standardized analytical techniques are available. If resistance is seen above cut-off levels, additional characterization is needed. The strain's whole genome sequencing will determine whether or not any identified genetic material linked to the reported sensitivity is present (Reid et al., 2019). It is advised to check for transposable elements in the region of suspected resistance genes when they are discovered. When the potential

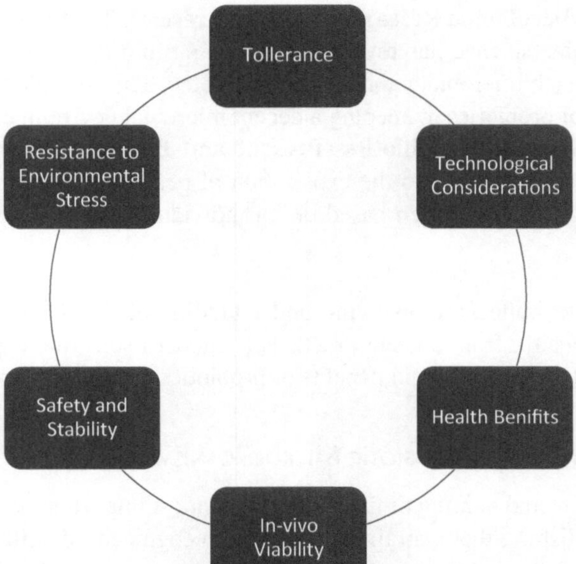

FIGURE 6.2 Selection criteria for probiotics.

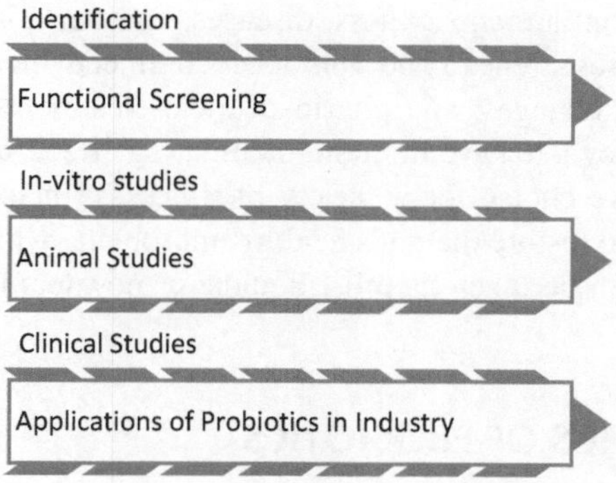

FIGURE 6.3 Safety aspects for functional probiotic food development.

that the gene responsible for resistance is transferable cannot be ruled out, it is not advised to market the strain. Otherwise, the genome sequence can be used to search at least two databases to find potential antimicrobial resistance genes. It is suggested to use a Hidden–Markov model database for microorganisms that are poorly represented in existing databases (Zheng et al., 2020).

Depending on the strain's classification and intended use, it may be necessary to examine the genetic makeup to see if any genes are present encoding for known virulence elements like toxic substances, determinants for infection, and attachment. The manufacturer must confirm that the indicated probiotic sample(s) are free of genes that can be transferred to other life forms, the antibiotic sensitivity cut-off values are undetermined, and their capacity for resistance profile is comparable with that of other individuals of the same species. In a few cases, fresh information on the taxon's sensitivity profiles may be crucial under consideration, as well as ensure that the susceptibility testing procedures are pertinent to and tailored to the physiology of the microorganisms under consideration; safety aspects are indicated in Figure 6.3 (Tegegne et al., 2022; Žuntar et al., 2020).

6.3 BENEFICIAL HEALTH PROPERTIES AND THERAPEUTIC POTENTIAL OF PROBIOTICS

Along with stomach issues, probiotics can benefit a variety of acute and chronic infectious diseases. The body's defenses can be weakened by a variety of circumstances, leading to inflammatory, viral, neoplastic, and degenerative disorders. The typical flora composition of the stomach may change as a result of other therapies such as antibiotics, radiation therapy, and immunosuppressive therapy. Probiotics and other functional food items like them aim to enhance cellular health and hasten the activation of cells' innate defensive mechanisms (Bermudez-Brito et al., 2012).

Lye Huey Shi and his co-workers indicated several beneficial effects of probiotics on the health of humans including infants, especially in the cases of post-menopausal issues, positive effects in cases of high cholesterol and high blood pressure, and lactose-intolerance patients, in addition to improving the immune system of the person concerned (Shi et al., 2016).

Malika Arora with co-investigators studied the role of probiotics for their therapeutic effects in humans. Their studies indicated the areas of urgent action, like, safety, quality, and efficacy of the probiotics for human consumption. Also, the author has indicated the regulatory aspects of the probiotics formulations (Arora et al., 2019).

J. Anita Christie and S. Geet Andrea indicated the up-to-date information on diversified probiotic products available in the market and the potential therapeutic benefits of different microbes found in this available marketed food against innumerable functional disorders along with their nutritional value (Christie & Andrea, 2021).

The impact of probiotics on human sickness, diseases, emotions, habits, and performance has been the subject of several researches. The authors recommend including probiotics and other alternative therapies, dietary changes, and pharmaceutical treatments in the treatment regimen. Since probiotics have been shown to have immune-modulating effects on the host, they are a potential therapeutic and preventive choice for a variety of illnesses, including inflammatory disease. Consuming probiotics helps to restore the gut's healthy microbiota, which helps people by boosting their immunity. Probiotics can be taken as pills, liquids, or powders (Yan & Polk, 2011; Sanders et al., 2019).

6.4 PHARMACOKINETICS OF PROBIOTICS

Adhesion to the intestinal epithelium: It has been demonstrated in numerous studies that some probiotic strains can cling to cell lines like $CaCO_2$ or HT29. These epithelial cell lines originate from the colon or the intestine. Many traits and activities of a typical cell develop the typical epithelial tissue, and the cells are polarized like those of an intestinal epithelium. As a result, it is believed that they are reliable models for predicting in vivo adhesion. It has also been suggested to use colon tissues or different cell lines (Sarem-Damerdji et al., 1995). The epithelial adhesion property varies between strains, and this property may be associated with in vivo immunomodulatory activities and competitive exclusion characteristics. Adhering strains' competitive exclusion abilities have demonstrated in vitro. A probiotic's potential to cling to the gut tissue throughout its intestinal transit must be investigated, and the in vitro models must be validated using in vivo data.

Survival of ingested probiotics to different sites of the GIT: Each genus and strain of ingested microbe has a different chance of surviving. Other microbes have a high survival rate up till excrement, whereas some are eliminated in the stomach. *Streptococcus thermophilus* and *L. bulgaricus* possess minimal intrinsic acid resistance, so they are obliterated in a matter of minutes at pH 1 and in an hour at pH. We discovered only 26% of all "ingested" *L. bulgaricus* withstood transit through the stomach when a dynamic in vitro model was employed to simulate yogurt's pH and gastric emptying (Conway et al., 1987). We demonstrated that 20% of the yogurt bacteria that have lactase remain till the very end of the small bowel and contribute to the degradation of lactose in the GIT of humans using an intestinal initiation approach. The bacteria do not even need to stay in the GIT for this action to occur; rather, they should generate lyse there and release the lactase they carry. This is a crucial point to note. Yogurt bacteria have a minimal chance of surviving in the upper gastrointestinal system; therefore, their probiotic benefits in the colon (downstream from where they survive) are irrelevant. In acidic environments, compared to *L. bulgaricus*, *L. acidophilus*, *L. reuteri*, and *L. rhamnosus* strain GG are more resilient. In various trials involving humans that used intestinal intubation procedures, it was discovered that 1–10% of *L. acidophilus* was consumed in a meal that was matured and passed to the ileum. In one of our trials, 108 CFU/ml of the Yoplait-Al strain in a cup of milk product caused 100 times more lactobacilli to pass by the ileum than a control meal did. No evidence of a permanent infestation of the small intestine was seen despite the transit lasting more than five hours. About 106 CFU/ml of *L. acidophilus*, *L. reuteri*, and *L. rhamnosus* strain GG were present in the feces, according to studies in healthy volunteers who consumed various probiotic formulations. Several investigations on humans were conducted to investigate the pharmacokinetics of the yeast *Saccharomyces boulardii*, which has been effective in lowering the incidence of *Clostridium difficile* colitis recurrence and antibiotic-associated diarrhea. The percentage of viable cells in feces was close to 0.1%, which is similar to what was found with *S. cerevisiae*, and the colon had yeast concentrations of more than 105 CFU/ml. About 60% of the consumed yeasts were found in the stool as dead cells (Pochart et al., 1989).

Colonization of the GIT by probiotics: It was demonstrated that a few patients had probiotic strains in their feces for longer periods than might be expected based on the "average endurance" of an "average human" with a "usual intestinal transit." Although it has not been verified, this may imply colonization. Probiotics are typically eliminated in feces a few days after consumption at a rate that is equal to or even faster than a transit marker. However, Johansson et al. presented intriguing results that has not to an alimentary lactobacilli colonization of the jejunal and rectal mucosa. Healthy individuals were given a soup containing 19 distinct strains of lactobacilli, and probes were used on biopsies collected 1 and 11 days after the *Lactobacillus* soup was consumed to look for colonization in the rectum and jejunum (Marteau et al., 1993). Eleven days after their consumption, two *Lactobacillus plantarum* strains were found. The other (Lp299v) initially emerged from the sourdough, while one (Lp299) was of human origin. It appears necessary to confirm this finding and test more strains using the same methods for both basic research on gut ecology and probiotic safety (Marteau et al., 2019).

6.5 TECHNIQUES USED FOR ENCAPSULATION OF PROBIOTICS

6.5.1 Conventional Approaches

A potentially sensitive microorganism is enclosed during the physiochemical or mechanical process of microencapsulation, which also creates a barrier that protects it from the outside environment. Comparing the two methods, encapsulation is different from cell immobilization. Although cells may be exposed to the outside environment while using the immobilization approach, in the encapsulation procedure, they are encased in the wall material. The bacterial cell must be kept alive during the encapsulation procedure and can range in size from 1 to 5 m. Thus, choosing the right encapsulation method is of utmost importance (Asgari et al., 2020). During industrial processing and storage, incomplete encapsulation encourages the exposure of delicate probiotics to the outside environment, breaking down cell walls and reducing nutritional qualities (Amin et al., 2021).

6.5.2 Emerging Approaches

The extrusion technique's drawback is that scaling it up is challenging, and the viability will be significantly lower after the extrusion procedure. Both from an economic and a sensory perspective, a higher core-to-wall material ratio is crucial. However, scaling up the emulsification procedure is straightforward, but the biggest issue is the dimension and structure of the enormous beads.

6.5.3 Other Emerging Techniques

The making of dried microcapsules is a substitute for the wet microcapsules made by the emulsion and extrusion processes. Additionally, spray drying might reduce the size of microcapsules, provide probiotic bacteria with a better anaerobic habitat, and improve storage capacity. Additionally, the processing of bioactive compounds like enzymes, vitamins, and other items is done via spray drying, which is a common technique in the dairy products, pharmaceuticals, and food industries. If microcapsules are in the form of dry powder, they are simple to handle and can be kept in storage for a long time (Fonseca et al., 2015). The most popular encapsulation techniques to produce dry formulations with long shelf lives include fluidized bed drying, freeze drying, spray drying, and spray-freeze drying. The most popular microencapsulation methods for probiotics are spray drying and freeze drying; hence, this review will solely cover these encapsulation methods (Anderson et al., 2010).

These emerging approaches for encapsulating probiotics aim to address challenges related to their survival, delivery, and functionality, ultimately improving their effectiveness in conferring

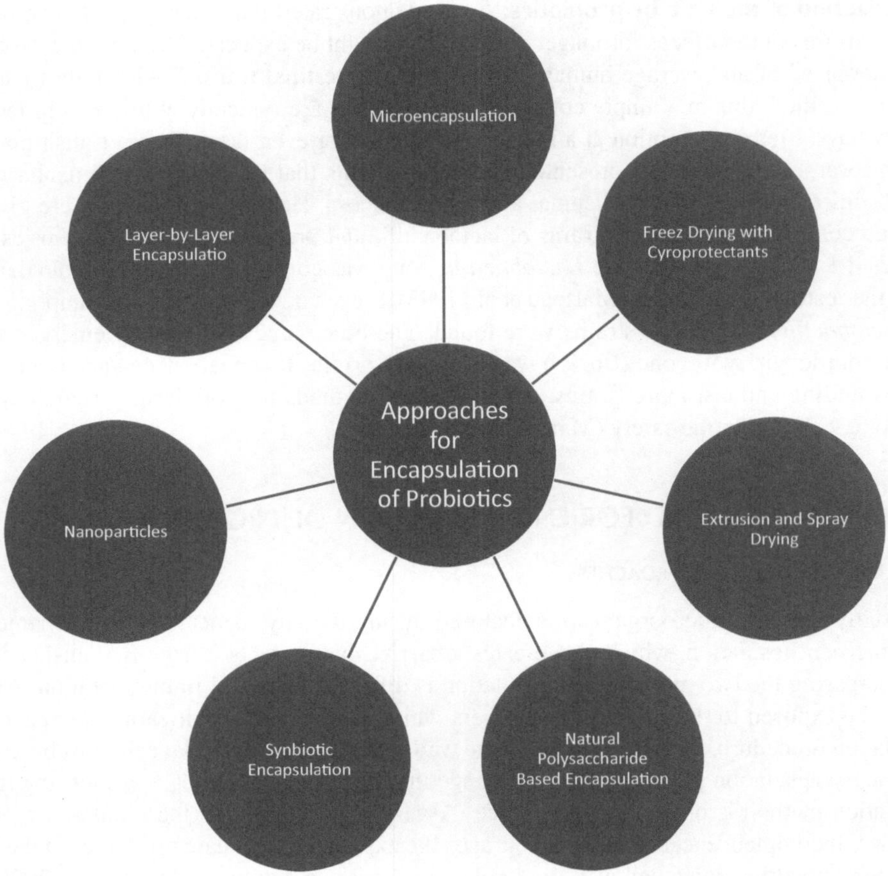

FIGURE 6.4 Emerging approaches for encapsulating probiotics.

health benefits. As technology continues to advance, these encapsulation methods are likely to contribute to the development of innovative probiotic products with enhanced stability and targeted delivery capabilities.

6.6 MECHANISM OF ACTION OF PROBIOTICS

6.6.1 Enhancement of the Epithelial Barrier

The changeable, dynamic enteric flora and luminal contents are constantly in contact with the gastric epithelial cells. An essential defense mechanism that retains the epithelium viable and protects the living from its surroundings is the intestinal barrier (Ohland & MacNaughton, 2010). The mucosa, antibacterial proteins, secretory IgA, and the junction binding complex make up the intestinal barrier's defenses. Antigens from bacteria and food can penetrate the submucosa and cause inflammatory reactions that can lead to intestinal illnesses like inflammatory bowel disease, once the operation of this barrier is disrupted. Probiotic microbes have been extensively studied for their function in this process and can assist in maintaining the intestinal barrier when consumed. Probiotics improve intestinal barrier function, although the exact processes by which they do so are not entirely understood (Hummel et al., 2012). According to several studies, one method to strengthen the integrity of activation of close junction signaling-related genome is expected to be increased by the intestinal barrier. For instance, in a T84 cell barrier model, lactobacilli altered the regulation of several genes that express sticky junction peptides, including E-cadherin and E-catenin. Additionally, the presence of PKC types like PKC and the phosphorylation of attaching juncture proteins are significantly impacted by lactobacilli in intestinal cells. It positively influences the epithelial barrier's performance (Hooper et al., 2001).

6.6.2 Increased Adhesion to Intestinal Mucosa

The relationship between probiotic bacteria and the host depends on attachment to the gut mucosa, another factor considered necessary for invasion. Probiotics' ability to adhere to the gut mucosal membrane is crucial for managing immunity and fending against infections. As a result, one of the main factors used to select new bacterial strains is adhesion, which has been associated with several beneficial probiotic outcomes. The interaction between LABs intestinal epithelial cells (IECs) and mucus is mediated by a variety of surface determinants that are present in LABs. Mucin, an intricate glycoprotein mixture that makes up a great deal of mucous and prevents dangerous microorganisms from adhering, is secreted by IECs (Castagliuolo et al., 2005). The mucous gel also contains salts, free lipids, peptides, antibodies, and others. This particular relationship has shown a potential link between probiotic bacteria's outermost proteins and the aggressive removal of germs from mucus. Bacteria contain surface adhesins that help them stick to the mucous layer, as mentioned earlier, and

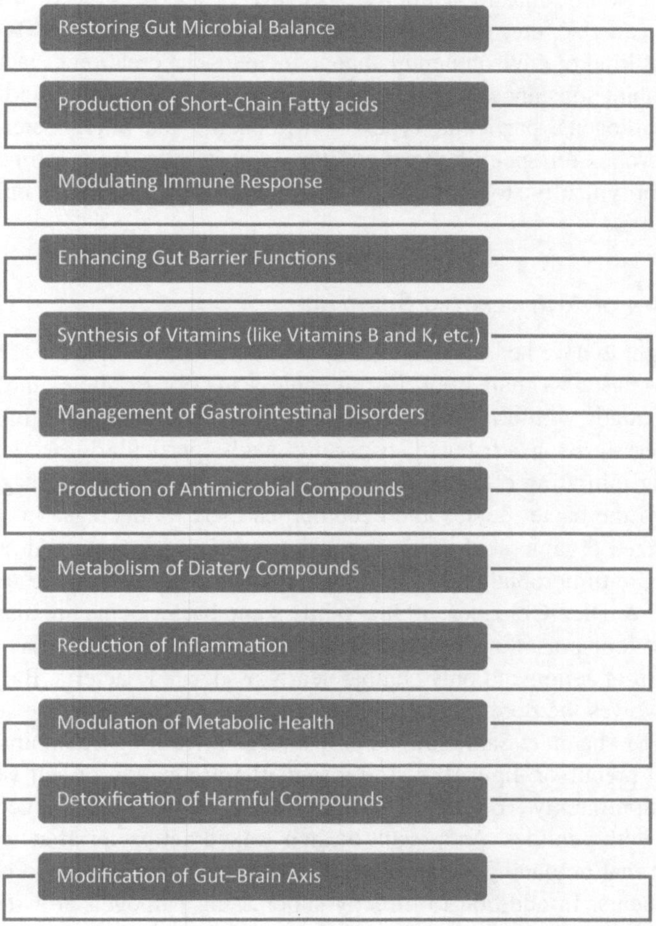

FIGURE 6.5 Mechanism of action of probiotics.

numerous *Lactobacillus* peptides have been demonstrated to enhance mucous adhesion. Proteins are the main mediators of this process, despite the involvement of saccharide groups and lipoteichoic acids (Hirano et al., 2003); refer to Figure 6.5.

6.6.3 Competitive Exclusion of Pathogenic Microorganisms

In a 1969 publication on the complete removal of *Salmonella typhimurium* from blowfly maggots, Greenberg developed the phrase "competitive exclusion" to describe the circumstance in which one species of bacteria fights more viciously than the other for locations for receptors in the intestinal system. One bacterial species may employ a variety of tactics, such as creating an unfavorable microecology, eliminating interest bacterial sites for receptors, producing and secreting antimicrobial compounds and selective metabolites, and competitively reducing essential nutrients, to stop or slow the growth of another species (Rolfe, 1991). Certain probiotic strains exhibit antagonistic effects on the adhesion of gastrointestinal pathogens. These effects produce sticky characteristics as a result of the relationship between mucins and surface peptides, which may prevent pathogenic bacteria from colonizing the probiotics. It has been discovered that lactobacilli and bifidobacteria inhibit a wide range of infections, including *E. coli*, *Salmonella*, *Helicobacter pylori*, *Listeria monocytogenes*, and rotavirus. Exclusion is the result of a variety of probiotic adhesion-inhibiting processes and characteristics, including chemical production and IEC activation (Nakamura et al., 2012). Due to a struggle for readily accessible food sources and mucosal attachment points, intestinal microbes engage in a process known to be competitive exclusion. Bacteria can also alter their habitat to make it unfavorable to rivals to obtain an edge in competition. This kind of environmental change includes the creation of lactic acid and acetic acid, two antimicrobial substances. As they correspond to carbohydrate-binding particularities with some enteropathogens, particular types of lactobacilli and bifidobacteria could compete with particular microbes for specific receptor sites on host cells. By creating steric hindrance, probiotic strains can typically stop pathogenic microbes from attaching to enterocyte pathogen receptors (Rolfe, 1991).

6.6.4 Production of Antimicrobial Substances

Probiotics are thought to have health benefits in part due to the development of LMW compounds (compounds with a mass less than 1,000 Da), organic acids, for example, and the production of bacteriostatic compounds with a mass greater than 1,000 Da. Probiotics' inhibitory impact over pathogens has generally been attributed to organic acids, particularly acetic and lactic acids, which have a strong inhibiting effect against gram-negative bacteria. The organic acid's undissociated form enters the bacteriocytes and decomposes there. A decrease in intracellular pH or the build-up of ionized organic acid inside the pathogen's cell is a potential outcome over time. Two instances of the antimicrobial peptides (AMPs) that various LABs make are bacteriocins and tiny AMPs (Russell & Diez-Gonzalez, 1998). While some bacteriocins are also effective against pathogens that cause food poisoning, bacteriocins made gram-positive bacteria (usually LAB) have a restricted spectrum of action and only combat nearly associated bacteria. Bacteriocin-mediated death frequently involves the pore-mediated destruction of target cells or the suppression of synthesis of cell walls (Bierbaum & Sahl, 2009). For instance, by forming a combination with the most significant cell wall precursor, lipid II, nisin prevents the production of cell walls in bacilli that produce spores predominantly. To form an opening in the bacterial membrane, the complex then collects and mixes with peptides. As a result of their linked antibacterial action, several investigations have shown that producing bacteriocins gives strains an advantage in challenging microbiological environments. In addition to directly suppressing pathogen growth in the intestines, the production of bacteriocins may promote the establishment and spread of producing strains (Ouwehand & Salminen, 1998).

6.6.5 Probiotics and the Immune System

Probiotic microorganisms' capacity to influence immunological function is well known. These microbes can interact with epithelial cells, lymphocytes, monocytes/macrophages, dendritic cells (DCs), and lymphocytes. The immune system is made up of both adaptive and innate immune systems. As the immune system's adaptive reaction occurs, the role of T cells and B cells, which possess a restricted focus on specific antigens, is crucial (Gómez-Llorente et al., 2010). The body's natural immune system, on the contrary, responds to identical molecular trends that are present in a broad range of illnesses, known as PAMPs, which are recognized by the body. PAMP-binding PPRs initiate the body's first resistance contrary to pathogens. The most extensively studied PPRs are toll-like receptors (TLRs). Additionally, it is known that both inside and outside of the cell NLRs and C-type lectin receptors send signals in response to bacterial interaction. IECs are the host cells that participate in the majority of probiotic interactions, as is widely recognized. DCs, which are essential for innate and adaptive immunity, can additionally come into touch with probiotics. IECs and, through their PPRs, DCs can communicate and react to gut microbial species (Lebeer et al., 2010).

6.6.6 TLRs and Probiotics

Numerous B cells, T cells, killer cells, DCs, phagocytes, fibroblasts, epithelial cells, and endothelial cells are examples of immune and non-immune cells, including transmembrane proteins known as TLRs. Eleven proteins (TLR1–TLR11) make up the TLR family in mammals. However, a stop codon in the human TLR11 gene prevents the development of human TLR11. After the ligand has been bound to extracellular leucine-rich repeats, TLRs are activated. TLR1, TLR2, TLR4, TLR5, TLR6, and TLR10 are surface-associated receptors that typically react to PAMPs associated with bacterial surfaces in humans. On the surface of endosomes, TLR3, TLR7, TLR8, and TLR9 can be found. Here, they mostly react to PAMPs made of nucleic acids produced by bacteria and viruses (Wells, 2011). On dimerizing TLR proteins containing TIR domains like MyD88, with the extremely preserved toll-interleukin-1 (IL-1) receptor (TIR) domains connector proteins, as well as TRIF, a TIR domain-containing connector protein that induces interferon (IFN), are brought in to start signaling activation. MyD88 is recruited by the TLR signaling pathway, except TLR3, and this triggers the MAPK and nuclear factor (NF)-B signaling pathways. Type 1 IFNs are expressed as a result of TLR3 through the adaptor protein TRIF. TLR-mediated signaling has also been shown to control DC maturation by upregulating several development markers, such as CD80, CD83, and CD86, and the CCR7 chemokine receptor (Vizoso Pinto et al., 2009). Additionally, by the activation of TLRs on DCs, commensal and probiotic bacteria can cause a generalized state of tolerance. Probiotics must activate TLR9 signaling to exhibit their anti-inflammatory properties. Other TLRs, like TLR3 and TLR7, have been linked to the tolerance brought on by commensal and probiotic bacteria, according to several research. After being triggered by symbiotic and probiotic microorganisms, DCs launch an appropriate response, like a transformation of Th 0 to T reg, which inhibits Th 1, Th 2, and Th 17 inflammatory responses (Vinderola et al., 2005).

6.6.7 NLRs and Probiotics

A distinct group of NLRs are bound to the membrane receptors. They are crucial in tissues and are situated beneath the cytoplasm that expresses TLRs only weakly. Although more than 20 distinct NLRs have been found, NOD1 and NOD2 are the members that have been most completely characterized. In contrast, the action of NOD2 is limited to DCs, phagocytes, Paneth cells, cells in the intestines, cells in the lungs, and buccal epithelium, other than NOD1, which is consistently used (Hakansson & Molin, 2011). Low quantities of it are also expressed in T cells. While NOD1 recognizes peptidoglycan components including meso-diaminopimelic acid, which is related to gram-negative bacteria, NOD2 recognizes muramyl dipeptide patterns that are present in a variety of microbes. In response to its agonist, NOD1, and NOD2 both self-oligomerize, attracting and stimulating adaptation protein RICK, a protein kinase that controls apoptosis caused by CD95 (Chen et al., 2009). Inflammatory mediators such as nitric oxide synthase, COX-2, cytokines, and chemotherapy attractants are produced, which are inducible and are increased as a result of this activation of NF-B and MAPKs. Several studies have looked into how probiotics affect NLR. Fernandez et al. recently showed, however, that the preventing results of *L. salivarius* Ls33 are correlated with local IL-10 manufacturing, which is eliminated in NOD2-deficient mice. In further studies, it is demonstrated that NOD2 mediates the anti-inflammatory impact of Ls33 (Bauernfeind et al., 2009).

6.7 CONCLUSION

In conclusion, this chapter highlights the promising role of probiotics in reshaping traditional pharmacological approaches. By serving as drug delivery vehicles, influencing pharmacokinetic parameters, and participating in complex host–microbe interactions, probiotics open up new avenues for enhancing drug therapies and improving patient outcomes. This chapter underscores the need for further research in this field to fully harness the potential of probiotics as a transformative force in modern pharmacology.

BIBLIOGRAPHY

Amin, T., Thakur, M., & Jain, S. C. (2021). Microencapsulation-the future of probiotic cultures. *Journal of Microbiology, Biotechnology and Food Sciences, 3,* 35–43.

Anderson, R. C., Cookson, A. L., McNabb, W. C., Park, Z., McCann, M. J., Kelly, W. J., & Roy, N. C. (2010). Lactobacillus plantarum MB452 enhances the function of the intestinal barrier by increasing the expression levels of genes involved in tight junction formation. *BMC Microbiology, 10,* 316. https://doi.org/10.1186/1471-2180-10-316

Aponte, M., Murru, N., & Shoukat, M. (2020). Therapeutic, prophylactic, and functional use of probiotics: A current perspective. *Frontiers in Microbiology, 11,* 562048. https://doi.org/10.3389/fmicb.2020.562048

Arora, M., Kaur, N., Bansal, P., & Baldi, A. (2019). Therapeutic potential of probiotics: A ray of hope or nightmare? *Applied Clinical Research, Clinical Trials and Regulatory Affairs, 6*(1), 18–33. https://doi.org/10.2174/2213476X06666190126161931

Asgari, S., Pourjavadi, A., Licht, T. R., Boisen, A., & Ajalloueian, F. (2020). Polymeric carriers for enhanced delivery of probiotics. *Advanced Drug Delivery Reviews, 161–162,* 1–21. https://doi.org/10.1016/j.addr.2020.07.014

Aureli, P., Capurso, L., Castellazzi, A. M., Clerici, M., Giovannini, M., Morelli, L., Poli, A., Pregliasco, F., Salvini, F., & Zuccotti, G. V. (2011). Probiotics and health: An evidence-based review. *Pharmacological Research, 63*(5), 366–376. https://doi.org/10.1016/j.phrs.2011.02.006

Bauernfeind, F. G., Horvath, G., Stutz, A., Alnemri, E. S., MacDonald, K., Speert, D., Fernandes-Alnemri, T., Wu, J., Monks, B. G., Fitzgerald, K. A., Hornung, V., & Latz, E. (2009). Cutting edge: NF-kappaB activating pattern recognition and cytokine receptors license NLRP3 inflammasome activation by regulating NLRP3 expression. *Journal of Immunology, 183*(2), 787–791. https://doi.org/10.4049/jimmunol.0901363

Behnsen, J., Deriu, E., Sassone-Corsi, M., & Raffatellu, M. (2013). Probiotics: Properties, examples, and specific applications. *Cold Spring Harbor Perspectives in Medicine, 3*(3), a010074. https://doi.org/10.1101/cshperspect.a010074

Bermudez-Brito, M., Plaza-Díaz, J., Muñoz-Quezada, S., Gómez-Llorente, C., & Gil, A. (2012, October 2). Probiotic mechanisms of action. *Annals of Nutrition and Metabolism, 61*(2), 160–174. https://doi.org/10.1159/000342079

Bierbaum, G., & Sahl, H. G. (2009). Lantibiotics: Mode of action, biosynthesis and bioengineering. *Current Pharmaceutical Biotechnology*, *10*(1), 2–18. https://doi.org/10.2174/138920109787048616

Binda, S., Hill, C., Johansen, E., Obis, D., Pot, B., Sanders, M. E., Tremblay, A., & Ouwehand, A. C. (2020, July 24). Criteria to qualify microorganisms as "probiotic" in foods and dietary supplements. *Frontiers in Microbiology, 11,* 1662. https://doi.org/10.3389/fmicb.2020.01662

Bron, P. A., Kleerebezem, M., Brummer, R. J., Cani, P. D., Mercenier, A., MacDonald, T. T., Garcia-Ródenas, C. L., & Wells, J. M. (2017). Can probiotics modulate human disease by impacting intestinal barrier function? *British Journal of Nutrition, 117*(1), 93–107. https://doi.org/10.1017/S0007114516004037

Castagliuolo, I., Galeazzi, F., Ferrari, S., Elli, M., Brun, P., Cavaggioni, A., Tormen, D., Sturniolo, G. C., Morelli, L., & Palù, G. (2005). Beneficial effect of auto-aggregating Lactobacillus crispatus on experimentally induced colitis in mice. *FEMS Immunology and Medical Microbiology, 43*(2), 197–204. https://doi.org/10.1016/j.femsim.2004.08.011

Chen, G., Shaw, M. H., Kim, Y. G., & Nuñez, G. (2009). NOD-like receptors: Role in innate immunity and inflammatory disease. *Annual Review of Pathology, 4,* 365–398. https://doi.org/10.1146/annurev.pathol.4.110807.092239

Anita Christie, J., & Geeta Andrea, S. (2021). Therapeutic potential of different probiotic foods. In D. Dhanasekaran & A. Sankaranarayanan (Eds.), *Advances in probiotics: Microorganisms in food and health* (pp. 449–477). Academic Press.

Conway, P. L., Gorbach, S. L., & Goldin, B. R. (1987). Survival of lactic acid bacteria in the human stomach and adhesion to intestinal cells. *Journal of Dairy Science, 70*(1), 1–12. https://doi.org/10.3168/jds.S0022-0302(87)79974-3

El-Nezami, H., Kankaanpää, P., Salminen, S., & Ahokas, J. (1998). Physicochemical alterations enhance the ability of dairy strains of lactic acid bacteria to remove aflatoxin from contaminated media. *Journal of Food Protection, 61*(4), 466–468. https://doi.org/10.4315/0362-028x-61.4.466

Fijan, S. (2014, May). Microorganisms with claimed probiotic properties: An overview of recent literature. *International Journal of Environmental Research and Public Health, 11*(5), 4745–4767. https://doi.org/10.3390/ijerph110504745

Fijan, S., & Turk, S. Š. (2012). Hospital textiles, are they a possible vehicle for healthcare-associated infections? *International Journal of Environmental Research and Public Health, 9*(9), 3330–3343. https://doi.org/10.3390/ijerph9093330

Fonseca, F., Cenard, S., & Passot, S. (2015). Freeze-drying of lactic acid bacteria. *Methods in Molecular Biology, 1257*, 477–488. https://doi.org/10.1007/978-1-4939-2193-5_24

Gogineni, V. K., Morrow, L. E., Gregory, P. J., & Malesker, M. A. (2013). Probiotics: History and evolution. *Journal of Ancient Diseases & Preventive Remedies, 1*(2), 1–7.

Gómez-Llorente, C., Muñoz, S., & Gil, A. (2010). Role of toll-like receptors in the development of immunotolerance mediated by probiotics. *Proceedings of the Nutrition Society, 69*(3), 381–389. https://doi.org/10.1017/S0029665110001527

Gruber, I., Heudorf, U., Werner, G., Pfeifer, Y., Imirzalioglu, C., Ackermann, H., Brandt, C., Besier, S., & Wichelhaus, T. A. (2013). Multidrug-resistant bacteria in geriatric clinics, nursing homes, and ambulant care-prevalence and risk factors. *International Journal of Medical Microbiology, 303*(8), 405–409. https://doi.org/10.1016/j.ijmm.2013.05.002

Hakansson, A., & Molin, G. (2011). Gut microbiota and inflammation. *Nutrients, 3*(6), 637–682. https://doi.org/10.3390/nu3060637

Han, S., Lu, Y., Xie, J., Fei, Y., Zheng, G., Wang, Z., Liu, J., Lv, L., Ling, Z., Berglund, B., & Yao, M. (2021). Probiotic gastrointestinal transit and colonization after oral administration: A long journey. *Frontiers in Cellular and Infection Microbiology, 11*, 609722. https://doi.org/10.3389/fcimb.2021.609722

Hirano, J., Yoshida, T., Sugiyama, T., Koide, N., Mori, I., & Yokochi, T. (2003). The effect of Lactobacillus rhamnosus on enterohemorrhagic Escherichia coli infection of human intestinal cells in vitro. *Microbiology and Immunology, 47*(6), 405–409. https://doi.org/10.1111/j.1348-0421.2003.tb03377.x

Hooper, L. V., Wong, M. H., Thelin, A., Hansson, L., Falk, P. G., & Gordon, J. I. (2001). Molecular analysis of commensal host-microbial relationships in the intestine. *Science, 291*(5505), 881–884. https://doi.org/10.1126/science.291.5505.881

Hummel, S., Veltman, K., Cichon, C., Sonnenborn, U., & Schmidt, M. A. (2012). Differential targeting of the E-cadherin/β-catenin complex by Gram-positive probiotic lactobacilli improves epithelial barrier function. *Applied and Environmental Microbiology, 78*(4), 1140–1147. https://doi.org/10.1128/AEM.06983-11

Lau, L. Y. J., & Chye, F. Y. (2018). Antagonistic effects of Lactobacillus plantarum 0612 on the adhesion of selected foodborne enteropathogens in various colonic environments. *Food Control, 91*, 237–247. https://doi.org/10.1016/j.foodcont.2018.04.001

Kardooni, Z., Alizadeh Behbahani, B., Jooyandeh, H., & Noshad, M. (2023). Probiotic viability, physicochemical, and sensory properties of probiotic orange juice. *Journal of Food Measurement and Characterization, 17*(2), 1817–1822. https://doi.org/10.1007/s11694-022-01771-x

Lahtinen, S. J., Gueimonde, M., Ouwehand, A. C., Reinikainen, J. P., & Salminen, S. J. (2005). Probiotic bacteria may become dormant during storage. *Applied and Environmental Microbiology, 71*(3), 1662–1663. https://doi.org/10.1128/AEM.71.3.1662-1663.2005

Larsen, N., Michaelsen, K. F., Paerregaard, A., Vogensen, F. K., & Jakobsen, M. (2009). A comparative study on adhesion and recovery of potential probiotic strains of Lactobacillus spp. By in vitro assay and analysis of human colon biopsies. *Microbial Ecology in Health and Disease, 21*, 95–99. https://doi.org/10.1080/08910600902907632

Lebeer, S., Vanderleyden, J., & De Keersmaecker, S. C. (Hosts). (2010). Host interactions of probiotic bacterial surface molecules: Comparison with commensals and pathogens. *Nature Reviews. Microbiology, 8*(3), 171–184. https://doi.org/10.1038/nrmicro2297

Maia, M. S., Domingos, M. M., & de são José, J. F. B. (2023). Viability of probiotic microorganisms and the effect of their addition to fruit and vegetable juices. *Microorganisms, 11*(5), 1335. https://doi.org/10.3390/microorganisms11051335

Markowiak, P., & Śliżewska, K. (2017). Effects of probiotics, prebiotics, and synbiotics on human health. *Nutrients, 9*(9), 1021. https://doi.org/10.3390/nu9091021

Marteau, P., Pochart, P., Bouhnik, Y., & Rambaud, J. C. (1993). Fate and effects of some transiting microorganisms in the human gastrointestinal tract. *World Review of Nutrition and Dietetics, 74,* 1–21. https://doi.org/10.1159/000422599

Marteau, P., & Vesa, T. (1998). Pharmacokinetics of probiotics and biotherapeutic agents in humans. *Bioscience and Microflora, 17*(1), 1–6. https://doi.org/10.12938/bifidus1996.17.1

McGovern, P. E. (2009). *Uncorking the past: The quest for wine, beer, and other alcoholic beverages*. University of California Press.

Monteagudo-Mera, A., Rastall, R. A., Gibson, G. R., Charalampopoulos, D., & Chatzifragkou, A. (2019, August 16). Adhesion mechanisms mediated by probiotics and prebiotics and their potential impact on human health. *Applied Microbiology and Biotechnology, 103*(16), 6463–6472. https://doi.org/10.1007/s00253-019-09978-7

Nakamura, S., Kuda, T., An, C., Kanno, T., Takahashi, H., & Kimura, B. (2012). Inhibitory effects of Leuconostoc mesenteroides 1RM3 isolated from narezushi, a fermented fish with rice, on Listeria monocytogenes infection to Caco-2 cells and A/J mice. *Anaerobe, 18*(1), 19–24. https://doi.org/10.1016/j.anaerobe.2011.11.006

Ohland, C. L., & MacNaughton, W. K. (2010). Probiotic bacteria and intestinal epithelial barrier function. *American Journal of Physiology-Gastrointestinal and Liver Physiology, 298*(6), G807–G819.

Ouwehand, A. C., & Salminen, S. J. (1998). The health effects of cultured milk products with viable and non-viable bacteria. *International Dairy Journal, 8*(9), 749–758.

Parker, C. T., Tindall, B. J., & Garrity, G. M. (2019). International code of nomenclature of prokaryotes. *International Journal of Systematic and Evolutionary Microbiology, 69*(1A), S1–S111. https://doi.org/10.1099/ijsem.0.000778

Peivasteh-Roudsari, L., Pirhadi, M., Karami, H., Tajdar-Oranj, B., Molaee-Aghaee, E., & Sadighara, P. (2019, December 31). Probiotics and food safety: An evidence-based review. *Journal of Food Safety and Hygiene, 5*(1), 1–9. https://doi.org/10.18502/jfsh.v5i1.3878

Perles, C. (1977). Le strategie alimentari nella preistoria. In J. L. Flandrin & M. Montanari (Eds.), *Storia dell'alimentazione* (pp. 12–25). Editori Laterza.

Pochart, P., Dewit, O., Desjeux, J. F., & Bourlioux, P. (1989). Viable starter culture, B-galactosidase activity and lactose in duodenum after yogurt ingestion in lactase-deficient humans. *American Journal of Clinical Nutrition, 49*(5), 828–831. https://doi.org/10.1093/ajcn/49.5.828

Pramanik, S., Venkatraman, S., Karthik, P., & Vaidyanathan, V. K. (2023). A systematic review on selection characterization and implementation of probiotics in human health. *Food Science and Biotechnology, 32*(4), 423–440. https://doi.org/10.1007/s10068-022-01210-z

Pultz, N. J., Stiefel, U., Subramanyan, S., Helfand, M. S., & Donskey, C. J. (2005). Mechanisms by which anaerobic microbiota inhibit the establishment in mice of intestinal colonization by vancomycin-resistant Enterococcus. *Journal of Infectious Diseases, 191*(6), 949–956. https://doi.org/10.1086/428090

Reid, G., Gadir, A. A., & Dhir, R. (2019, March 12). Probiotics: Reiterating what they are and what they are not. *Frontiers in Microbiology, 10,* 424. https://doi.org/10.3389/fmicb.2019.00424

Rolfe, R. D. (1984). Role of volatile fatty acids in colonization resistance to *Clostridium difficile*. *Infection and Immunity, 45*(1), 185–191. https://doi.org/10.1128/iai.45.1.185-191.1984

Rolfe, R. D. (1991). Population dynamics of the intestinal tract. In L. Blankenship (Ed.), *Colonization control of human bacterial enteropathologens in poultry* (p. 59). Elsevier.

Russell, J. B., & Diez-Gonzalez, F. (1998). The effects of fermentation acids on bacterial growth. *Advances in Microbial Physiology, 39*, 205–234. https://doi.org/10.1016/s0065-2911(08)60017-x

Rychen, G., Aquilina, G., Azimonti, G., Bampidis, V., de Lourdes Bastos, M., Bories, G., Chesson, A., Cocconcelli, P. S., Flachowsky, G., & Gropp, J. (2018). Guidance on the characterisation of microorganisms used as feed additives or as production organisms. *EFSA Journal. European Food Safety Authority, 16*(3), e05206. https://doi.org/10.2903/j.efsa.2018.5206

Sanders, M. E., Merenstein, D. J., Reid, G., Gibson, G. R., & Rastall, R. A. (2019, October). Probiotics and prebiotics in intestinal health and disease: From biology to the clinic. *Nature Reviews. Gastroenterology and Hepatology, 16*(10), 605–616. https://doi.org/10.1038/s41575-019-0173-3

Sarem-Damerdji, L. O., Sarem, F., Marchal, L., & Nicolas, J. P. (1995). In vitro colonization ability of human colon mucosa by exogenous Lactobacillus strains. *FEMS Microbiology Letters, 131*(2), 133–137. https://doi.org/10.1111/j.1574-6968.1995.tb07767.x

Sarkar, S. (2013). Probiotics as functional foods: Documented health benefits. *Nutrition and Food Science, 43*(2), 107–115. https://doi.org/10.1108/00346651311313445

Shi, L. H., Balakrishnan, K., Thiagarajah, K., Mohd Ismail, N. I., & Yin, O. S. (2016). Beneficial properties of probiotics. *Tropical Life Sciences Research, 27*(2), 73–90. https://doi.org/10.21315/tlsr2016.27.2.6

Sniffen, J. C., McFarland, L. V., Evans, C. T., & Goldstein, E. J. C. (2018). Choosing an appropriate probiotic product for your patient: An evidence-based practical guide. *PLoS One, 13*(12), e0209205. https://doi.org/10.1371/journal.pone.0209205

Tegegne, B. A., & Kebede, B. (2022, June 1). Probiotics, their prophylactic and therapeutic applications in human health development: A review of the literature. *Heliyon, 8*(6), e09725. https://doi.org/10.1016/j.heliyon.2022.e09725

Umbrello, G., & Esposito, S. (2016). Microbiota and neurologic diseases: potential effects of probiotics. *Journal of Translational Medicine, 14*(1), 1–11. https://doi.org/10.1186/s12967-016-1058-7

Vinderola, G., Matar, C., & Perdigón, G. (2005). Role of the epithelial cells in the immune effects mediated by Gram-positive probiotic bacteria. Involvement of toll-like receptors. *Clinical and Diagnostic Laboratory Immunology, 12*(9), 1075–1084. https://doi.org/10.1128/CDLI.12.9.1075-1084.2005

Vizoso Pinto, M. G., Rodríguez Gómez, M., Seifert, S., Watzl, B., Holzapfel, W. H., & Franz, C. M. (2009). Lactobacilli stimultates the innate immune response and modulate TLR expression of HT29 intestinal epithelial cells in vitro. *International Journal of Food Microbiology, 133*(1–2), 86–93. https://doi.org/10.1016/j.ijfoodmicro.2009.05.013

Wells, J. M. (2011). Immunomodulatory mechanisms of lactabacilli. *Microbial Cell Factories, 10*(suppl_1), S17. https://doi.org/10.1186/1475-2859-10-S1-S17

Yan, F., & Polk, D. B. (2011). Probiotics and immune health. *Current Opinion in Gastroenterology, 27*(6), 496–501. https://doi.org/10.1097/MOG.0b013e32834baa4d

Zheng, J., Wittouck, S., Salvetti, E., Franz, C. M. A. P., Harris, H. M. B., Mattarelli, P., O'Toole, P. W., Pot, B., Vandamme, P., Walter, J., Watanabe, K., Wuyts, S., Felis, G. E., Gänzle, M. G., & Lebeer, S. (2020, April). A taxonomic note on the genus Lactobacillus: Description of 23 novel genera, emended description of the genus Lactobacillus Beijerinck 1901, and union of Lactobacillaceae and Leuconostocaceae. *International Journal of Systematic and Evolutionary Microbiology, 70*(4), 2782–2858. https://doi.org/10.1099/ijsem.0.004107

Žuntar, I., Petric, Z., Bursać Kovačević, D., & Putnik, P. (2020, July 17). Safety of probiotics: Functional fruit beverages and nutraceuticals. *Foods, 9*(7), 947. https://doi.org/10.3390/foods9070947

7 Psychobiotics and Gut–Brain Axis—A New Paradigm for Improving Mental Health

Sunita Roy Chowdhury

7.1 INTRODUCTION

The term "psychobiotics" was coined by Professor T. Dinan of the University of College Cork, Ireland. Psychobiotics, according to him, may be referred to as "the psychological potential of the molecules synthesized by probiotic bacteria." This includes prebiotic, probiotic, symbiotic, postbiotic, and all interventions that target the gut microbiota, which has the potential to modulate microbiota–gut–brain signals and have a positive effect on the neurological functions of the host, particularly memory, cognition, mood, and anxiety (Dinan et al., 2013).

Psychobiotics have been shown to play an effective role in easing the symptoms of disorders of the CNS, such as insomnia, depression, Parkinson's disease, schizophrenia, autism, anorexia nervosa, and multiple sclerosis. According to the National Academy of Sciences' FNB, probiotics or psychobiotics are the components contained in functional foods that have health-promoting properties (Oroojzadeh et al., 2022).

However, the idea of the positive health effects of probiotics (diet) is not new. Two thousand years ago, Hippocrates, a Greek physician and the "father of medicine," suggested that "all disease begin in the gut" (Zielińska et al., 2022).

The gut (GI tract) of an adult human is an abundant ecosystem that fosters up to around 10^{13}–10^{14} microorganisms of approximately 500–1000 species of bacteria (160 per individual). There exists a perfect state of interdependence or synergy between the host and the gut microbes. Colonization of the GI system starts early in life and is fully established by 3 years of age. The early interplay between the host and the microorganisms inhabiting the GI tract is crucial for the proper development and functioning of the child's intestines, the development of its immune system, and the nervous system. The composition of the microbial community in the human gut is highly dynamic and affected by many factors; some of these are genetics, age, stress, medications, lifestyle, diet, etc. (Bermúdez-Humarán et al., 2019).

The synergy between the human host and gut microbes is mutual. The host provides an environment for the growth of the microorganisms, and the microorganisms help in the maintenance of homeostasis in the host along with aiding in the host's general well-being. The friendly gut bacteria also demonstrate antimicrobial activities. It is, therefore, logical to conclude that an unhealthy gut environment, which lacks friendly gut bacteria may weaken the mutualistic bond and also negatively affect the host health, causing diseases (Wall et al., 2014). The resident bacteria profit from the nutritionally rich and safe environment of the human gut, while they in turn provide certain benefits to the host. The benefits to the host are that the microbes make the indigestible nutrients available to the host's body, such as complex carbohydrates, certain vitamins, and by-products of metabolism. Certain bacteria also inhibit the entry of other pathogenic bacteria into the host gut and body, thereby protecting the host from many diseases (Mohajeri et al., 2018).

A unique relation between the brain of the host and the microbes residing in its GI tract has been discovered and is called the GBA (Zielińska et al., 2022). The two-way communication between the bacteria in the gut and the brain of the host involves a number of organ systems, such as the

DOI: 10.1201/9781003452249-7

GI system along with the microbes residing there, the immune system, the ENS, the ANS, and the CNS (Tremblay et al., 2021). Although the actual psychobiotic potential of these microbes is not yet fully recognized, it has, however, been established that these bacteria deliver benefits to the host through the immune response and inflammation, via the HPA axis and also through the synthesis of neuronal hormones and neuronal transmitters (Del Toro-Barbosa et al., 2020). These two-way interactions are carried out via immunological signaling, metabolic pathways, neurological connections, and hormonal messages. Any interruption in these systems can cause an alteration in behavior (Dinan et al., 2013). Through this network, the cognitive centers and the emotional centers of the brain are linked with the GI system and the resident microbes (Bermúdez-Humarán et al., 2019). Therefore, at times, it is not unusual to find intestinal and mental diseases occurring together in one person, which indicates a robust correlation between the gut, gut bacteria, and the brain (Del Toro-Barbosa et al., 2020).

The blend and behavior of the microflora present in the gut affects the entire body systems and their functioning. These microorganisms have a critical role to play in food digestion while also obtaining energy from it and in the process fermenting the undigested food. The chief energy source for these bacteria is a plant fiber, which helps the bacteria to produce certain metabolites (Hamaker & Tuncil, 2014). These microbes also synthesize some vitamins such as a few group B vitamins and also vitamin K. In the circumstances, when the equilibrium of the intestinal microflora is disrupted, it causes dysbiosis. Dysbiosis is shown to be associated not only with diseases of the digestive tract such IBDs and IBS but also with certain lifestyle disorders like diabetes type 2, obesity, and even cancer. Research in the past few years has shown that this dysbiosis also affects the brain and can cause psychological disorders such as anxiety, depression, and stress (Cichońska et al., 2023).

7.2 THE EFFECT OF NUTRITION AND THE GUT MICROFLORA ON MENTAL HEALTH

Since ancient times healthy brain function has been related to a healthy digestive system. The health of the digestive system on the other hand is dependent on the diverse microflora residing in the GI tract of the host, which impacts the host's fitness and well-being (Munawar et al., 2021). The health effects of the microflora residing in the GI tract have been studied to a great extent in recent years. Researchers have also proven that probiotics from foods have a vital role in regulating the microflora of the GI tract. Probiotics are defined as "live bacteria, which when administered in adequate amounts confer health benefits to the host." The two most common health benefits generally associated with probiotics are, first, supporting a healthy GI tract and, second, boosting the health of the body's defense system. It is also vital that these live bacteria exhibit the ability to colonize the digestive tract and ensure the safety of the host. Probiotics must be able to support healthy gut microbiota by creating a more favorable gut environment (Hill et al., 2014).

Current data suggest that the probiotics from diet provide double benefits of regulating the intestinal health of the host while simultaneously influencing the host's psychological health. The probiotics that benefit mental health are referred to as "psychobiotics" and find widespread application in psychiatric treatment. So, psychobiotics are live bacteria that are capable of delivering mental health benefits to the host (Dinan et al., 2013). Changing the composition of the gut microflora with the help of nutrition interventions (using foods containing live bacteria or those that promote the growth of these bacteria in the GI tract) has shown potential in the treatment of psychological disorders, e.g., anxiety and depression. Studies in recent years done on foods containing live bacteria have also shown that certain bacteria are more effective in influencing mental health, modulating behavior, and alleviating psychological illnesses (Cohen Kadosh et al., 2021).

The microbes in the human GI tract produce certain neuroactive substances that have an effect on neurological and psychiatric parameters, such as mood, sleep, cognition, and appetite. Imbalance in the GI microbiome or intestinal dysbacteriosis can also affect mental health negatively.

Beneficial health effects have been seen to be exerted by certain bacteria such as *Lactobacillus*, *Bifidobacterium*, and *Saccharomyces*, which they achieve through establishing the balance of gut microflora (Kali, 2016).

The composition of the GI microflora varies greatly from one human to another, although some bacterial strains commonly exist in most humans. Diet specifically has a vital role in defining the profile of the GI microflora (Leeming et al., 2019).

The effectiveness of psychobiotics (consumed in the diet) in neuropsychiatric disorders is a subject of many clinical trials and an emerging area of research. However, many meta-analyses and review studies have pointed toward the positive effects of psychobiotics on various psychological problems, for instance, depression, stress, sleep, mood, and anxiety (Tremblay et al., 2021). Nutritional therapies such as psychobiotics (including probiotics containing live bacteria and prebiotics enhancing the growth of these friendly bacteria) show promise in curing mental health problems, especially depression and anxiety. Studies so far, on the impact of psychobiotics on the neural system, have proven their ability to shape behavior and many psychological processes, thus benefiting mental health (Cohen Kadosh et al., 2021).

Bacteria are the most abundant inhabitants of the human gut. *Lactobacillus (L.)*, *Escherichia*, *Clostridium*, *Bifidobacterium (B.)*, and *Streptococcus (S)* are some of the common genres of bacteria primarily present in the gut. Additional components of the gut microflora are yeast, viruses, and fungi (Gagliardi et al., 2018).

Psychobiotics contain these live bacteria that are capable of releasing certain neuroactive substances and when ingested are capable of regulating behavior and mood. For example, a study on mice found that the ingestion of *L. brevis* helped regulate emotional behavior and the ingestion of *L. rhamnosus* helped lower stress, anxiety, and depression-linked behavior. Based on studies, it is understood that the consumption of certain species of bacteria such as *L. casei Shirtoa*, *L. helveticus*, *B. infantis*, and *L. rhamnosus* may be protective against stress, anxiety, and mood-related disorders (Cohen Kadosh et al., 2021).

Recently, prebiotics have also been included along with probiotics/psychobiotics, as they boost the progression of these beneficial GI bacteria and also aid in modifying the constitution of the gut microflora (Sarkar et al., 2016). Prebiotics may be defined as natural substances that upon absorption in the intestines produce definite modifications in GI microflora along with their activities. Prebiotics, such as oligosaccharides, stimulate the reproduction and growth of the commensal bacteria in the GI tract (Oroojzadeh et al., 2022).

Therefore, to boost the development of favorable bacteria in the GI system, it is important that prebiotics be consumed along with probiotics (Dahiya & Nigam, 2022). Synbiotics are foods that are a combination of prebiotics and probiotics. Synbiotics function through probiotics in the growth and proliferation of beneficial gut bacteria and through the prebiotics contained in them to inhibit the growth of harmful bacteria. Examples are inulin found in bananas and onions; fructo-oligosaccharides found in garlic, chicory, and asparagus; and galacto-oligosaccharides found in lentils, chickpeas, and beans. The synbiotics include strains like *Lacbobacilli*, *Bifidobacterium* spp, *S. boulardii*, and *B. coagulans* (Wasilewski et al., 2015). Examples of foods containing pre-, pro-, and post-biotics are shown in Figure 7.1.

Nutritional therapies such as psychobiotics (including probiotics containing live bacteria and prebiotics that enhance the growth of these friendly bacteria) have the capability of treating mental health problems, particularly depression and anxiety. Studies so far, on the effects of psychobiotics on the neural system, have proven their ability to shape behavior and many psychological processes, thus benefiting mental health (Cohen Kadosh et al., 2021).

7.3 THE MICROBIOTA–GUT–BRAIN AXIS

The close association of the gut and the brain is well established. The fact that this association is vital for the GI tract's proper functioning is also fully recognized. Recent research, however, has

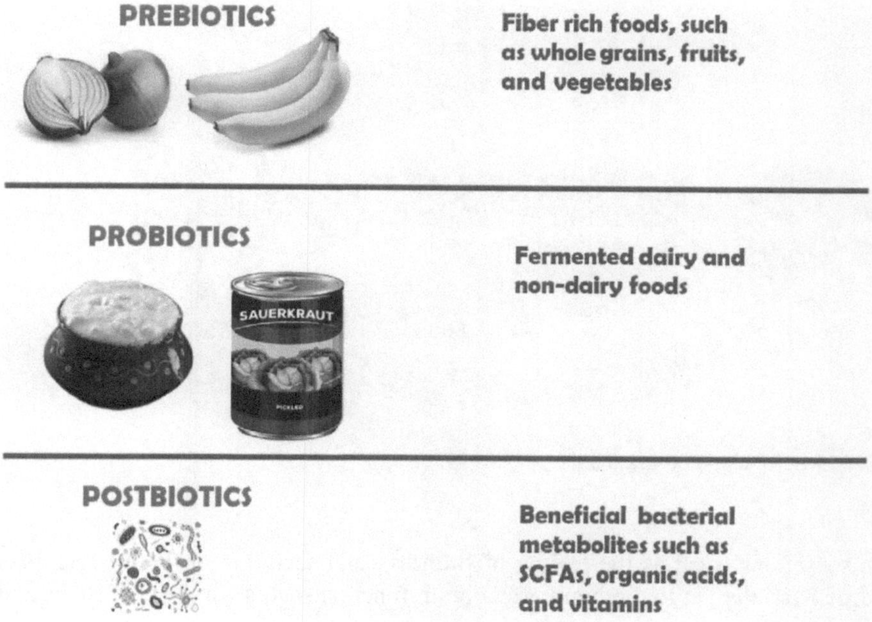

FIGURE 7.1 Foods containing psychobiotics including pre-, pro-, and post-biotics.

shown that this association is also essential for the mental well-being of the host. This depends on the two-way communication between the gut (along with its microflora) and the brain. Through research, it has also been proven that this two-way interaction between the CNS and the GI, along with its microflora, exists and is termed the GBA or the MGBA (Leung & Thuret, 2015).

In the past few years, MGBA has caught the attention of the scientific community, and researchers in this field have shown that this communication is vital not only for better learning, memory, cognition, and neurodevelopment but also for stress, anxiety, and neurodegenerative diseases (Chakrabarti et al., 2022).

Multiple overlapping pathways are involved to ensure the efficacy of this bidirectional communication network; from the host side this includes the three nervous systems, the CNS, the ANS, and the ENS, as also the immune system, and the endocrine system as depicted in Figure 7.2 (Cryan & Dinan, 2012). On the side of the microbes, the gut microbiota, which comprises bacteria, fungi, viruses, and archaea, and their metabolic by-products all participate in the bidirectional communiqué (Chakrabarti et al., 2022).

The microbes not only communicate with the cells of the intestine and with the ENS but also with the CNS directly (Carabotti et al., 2015). There are multiple mechanisms that are at play for the communications that take place between the GI microbiota and the CNS, such as neuronal, neuroendocrine, and neuroimmune pathways (Mohajeri et al., 2018). The intrinsic nervous center or the ENS regulates the overall physiology of the GI system. The enteric nerves are an integral part of the GI tract present throughout its length. The ENS is connected to the CNS via the nerves of the ANS, and this network forms the neuronal pathway of the GBA (Mittal et al., 2017).

The sympathetic and parasympathetic nerves, which are a part of the ANS, form the neuronal pathway through which the brain and the gut communicate with each other (Zhou & Foster, 2015). The two-way communiqué of the ENS, also called "the second brain" (or gut) and the CNS (or brain), also happens via the efferent and the afferent nerves (Furness, 2012). The fibers of the afferent nerves send communication to the CNS, and the CNS in turn sends a regulatory signal to the gut via the efferent nerve fibers. This two-way communication system assists in the communication from the brain to the gut to regulate the blood flow, immune system activation, muscle contractions

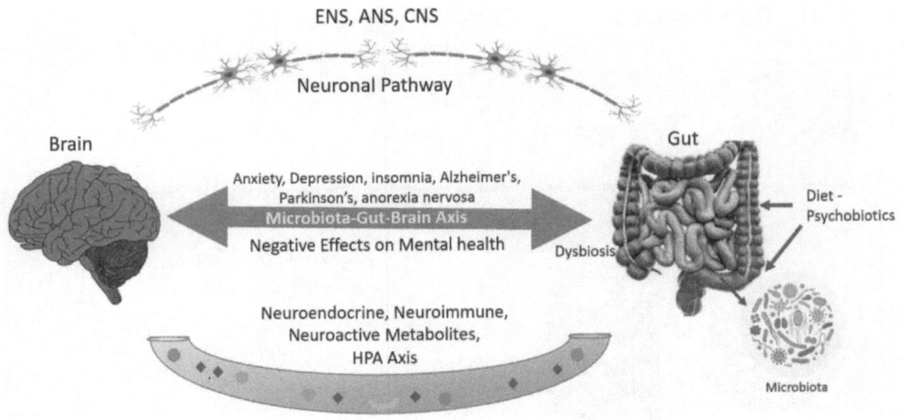

FIGURE 7.2 Microbiota–gut–brain axis.

(motility), sensations (such as the feeling of fullness), and secretion in the GI tract. Conversely, the messages from the gut to the brain affect brain function such as in areas of stress and anxiety (Dinan et al., 2013).

The vagus nerve is the other neuronal route of communication between the gut microbes and the brain (Forsythe et al., 2014), which is the X cranial nerve, originating in the medulla oblongata in the brain, which innervates the entire GI tract, heart, and the lungs. It provides involuntary muscle control in the GI tract, thereby regulating digestion, respiration, blood pressure, and heart rate (Chakrabarti et al., 2022). The vagus nerve secretions, which are a major component of the parasympathetic branch of ANS, sense the microbiota metabolites, for instance, SCFAs—acetate, butyrate, and propionate. These carry messages from the gut to the brain and trigger a response (Bonaz et al., 2018). Motor nerve signal carried by the vagus nerve, from the brain to various organs and back to the brain, is influenced by the gut microflora. The vagus nerve can also sense any variations in the gut environment (Chakrabarti et al., 2022).

The gut microflora also influences nerve functions either explicitly or implicitly and may have an effect on the pathophysiology of mental disorders. The microbes function through hormones, neurotransmitters, and neuroactive microbial metabolites (Mohajeri et al., 2018). Research conducted on germ-free animals (mostly rodents) has proven that the colonization of the GI tract, by the bacteria, is vital for the growth and maturation of both the enteral and the CNSs. In the absence of proper colonization of the gut by the microflora, alterations in the production and function of neurotransmitters, in both ENS and CNS can be seen (Carabotti et al., 2015). The connection between the enteral and the CNS also modulates host behavior. The diminished functionality of these systems has been shown to cause an increase in anxiety and stress (Vaiserman et al., 2017).

The other route of interaction between the gut and the brain is neuroendocrine or the HPA axis. This involves the interaction between three endocrine glands, namely, the hypothalamus, the pituitary, and the adrenal. This axis controls a person's response to any stressful situation and controls mood and emotional status along with digestion, energy expenditure, and storage (Mohajeri et al., 2018). Experimental studies on germ-free animals prove that the microbes in the gut impact stress reactivity and anxiety through the HPA axis (Diaz Heijtz et al., 2011).

There is growing evidence that the immune (defense) system also has a crucial role in the GBA signaling pathway (Salvo-Romero et al., 2020). Many neurological conditions have been seen to be associated with low-grade systemic inflammation, such as Parkinson's and Alzheimer's (the two leading neurodegenerative diseases) and many other cerebrovascular diseases. The inflammation could be a result of the malfunctioning of the immune response and dysbiosis in the gut (Coyle,

2011). Low-grade inflammation present in metabolic disorders is also seen to be connected to neurodegenerative and neuropsychiatric disorders. For example, studies on the role of the GI microflora that cause IBD have also shown that these are related to an increased vulnerability to Parkinson's (Fung, 2020).

Depression and anxiety are the two most common diseases that have a damaging effect on the quality and functionality of life of the individuals suffering from them. Throughout the world, there has been a steady rise in the number of individuals affected by these illnesses. Additionally, both diseases normally occur together in the same individual and are prone to recurrence (Huang & Wu, 2021). Recent studies propose that GI hormones have a role in the physiological processes that cause psychological diseases like depression and anxiety. There are also some indications that metabolic diseases like obesity coexist with mood disorders (Sun et al., 2020).

The increased focus now is on how GI microflora modify the hormones in the gut to help regulate mood. Any disturbance in the neuroendocrine system and gut microbiome has been seen to be correlated with certain metabolic disorders and also with mood disturbances. Neural messengers such as GABA, dopamine, serotonin, and noradrenaline have all been proven to be associated with the pathophysiology of the disorders of behave, or, mood, memory, emotions, attention and motivation, etc. (Huang & Wu, 2021). These neurotransmitters function like hormones. Not only are these hormones produced in the GI tract but they are also implicated in their role in the modulation of gut bacteria. Although not demonstrated in human subjects, studies on rodents suggest that the ability of microorganisms, in the GI system, to synthesize and utilize the neurotransmitters, has an effect on the host's physiology (Strandwitz, 2018).

Apart from this, microbiota and therefore probiotics have also been shown to communicate through the immune system. Bacteria in the intestines can modify the concentration of both pro-inflammatory and anti-inflammatory cytokines. These cytokines have an important role in the activation of the HPA axis and also the CNS through the vagus nerve. The activation of this hypothalamic–pituitary axis increases intestinal permeability, thereby increasing inflammation. It may also affect the tryptophan metabolism through the kyneurine pathway, leading to increased inflammation and certain neurological conditions (Wasilewski et al., 2015; Davis & Liu, 2015). Probiotic preparations containing *Lactobacillus* when given to healthy mice have been seen to improve their performance on certain tests, which were designed to provoke stress and anxiety (Romijn & Rucklidge, 2015).

SCFAs are capable of penetrating the blood–brain barrier and, therefore, can directly impact MGBA along with brain physiology. SCFAs also have a vital role in maintaining the integrity of the intestinal epithelium (Cichońska et al., 2023).

The influence that probiotics or psychobiotics have on the psychological well-being of an individual is a topic being researched to a great extent recently. Gut microflora is now believed to be a key element for proper brain programming during early life, along with genetics, and pre- and postnatal environment (Codagnone et al., 2019).

7.4 PSYCHOBIOTICS AND MENTAL HEALTH—MECHANISM OF ACTION

Research done recently proves that GI microflora not only affects the functioning of the gut and general physical well-being but also has an influence on the mental health of the host and plays a role through GBA (Liu et al., 2019). Psychobiotics are being considered as the novel approach for their effects on the MGBA. Their role was mostly being investigated on animals till now, but recently due to increasing evidence of their benefits on a number of neuropsychiatric disorders many clinical trials are being conducted. Most studies, however, have only been able to understand their efficacy on anxiety, depression, and stress (Tremblay et al., 2021).

Some specific classes of psychobiotics are capable of producing certain neuroactive substances that exert effects on the GBA, such as GABA, SCFAs, and serotonin, which are capable of affecting brain function and behavior (Oroojzadeh et al., 2022).

Certain animal trials have found that psychobiotic consumption decreases the activity of the HPA axis, which is mostly seen to be overactive during depression. Psychobiotics also promote the biosynthesis of GABA, the synthesis of which is reduced during depression. They also increase serotonin levels, the feel-happy hormone, through increased conversion from tryptophan. A meta-analysis conducted, by Ng et al., in 2017, of 10 randomized placebo-controlled, double-blind trials, concluded a statistically insignificant effect of probiotics on both healthy and depressed individuals. Significant benefits were seen only in patients with mild or moderate depression (Ng et al., 2018).

A 3-week duration study was conducted on 124 participants from both genders on the effect of fermented foods on depression. Beverages made by fermenting milk and containing psychobiotic strain *L. casei* strain Shirota were used. Half the study group received the fermented drink, and the rest of the group received a placebo. At the end of the study, the people consuming the fermented drink ranked themselves as happier compared with at the beginning, which could be ascribed to the beneficial effects of the psychobiotic strains. Both the strains used are otherwise also normally found in the human GI tract. These bacteria are important for the maintenance of gut homeostasis. They also have the ability to produce SCFAs, which have an important part to play in the communication between the brain and the gut (Takada et al., 2016).

The mechanism of action by which psychobiotics affect mental health is illustrated in Figure 7.3.

About seven studies investigated the role of live gram-positive bacteria and heat-killed bacteria of species *L. paracaesei* in rats for their effects on stress, depression, and anxiety. In most studies, it was seen that live bacteria proved to be effective in the modulation of anxiety and stress, while heat-killed bacteria did not show any effect. Similarly, treatment with psychobiotic *B. infantis* led

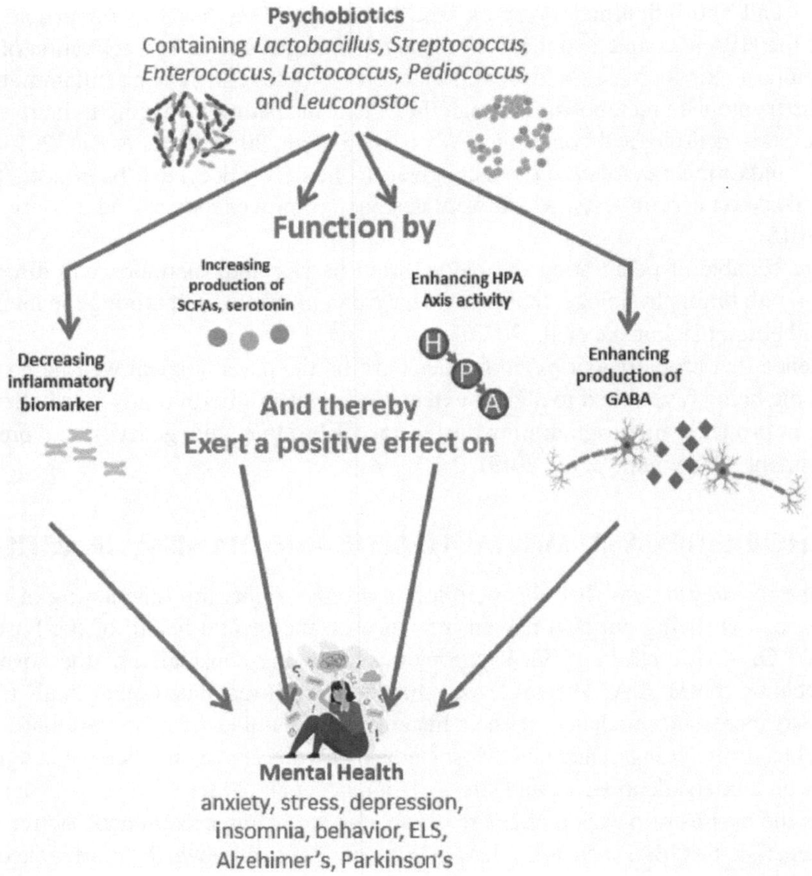

FIGURE 7.3 Psychobiotics mechanism of action.

to the reversal of the symptoms of depression. Therefore, from various studies on rodents, it was concluded that psychobiotics have a positive influence on stress, anxiety, and depression as they increase the levels of serotonin in the brain's hippocampus region (Huang & Wu, 2021).

A systemic review conducted by Wallace and Milev in 2017 concluded that psychobiotics improve symptoms associated with depression, through increased serotonin production and decreased levels of inflammatory markers. However, additional research is required to determine the dosage and psychobiotic strain effective for this treatment (Wallace & Milev, 2017).

Another meta-analysis of 28 studies by Liu et al., on the effects of psychobiotics and prebiotics on depression and anxiety, showed promising positive influence of these on anxiety and depression (Liu et al., 2019).

The effect that psychobiotics have on ELS was studied in rodents and showed that these can decrease the symptoms of ELS. The role of *L. rhamnosus* and *L. helveticus* in ELS was evident through enhanced HPA axis activity. Psychobiotics can be thought of as an innovative, effective, and noninvasive therapy for emotion-related behavior in humans as well (Cowan et al., 2016).

There is a paucity of research on the effects of psychobiotics on neurodegenerative diseases, autism, and obsessive-compulsive disorder. Also, not all psychobiotic strains share the same effects, suggesting that different responses are produced with different strains. There is still more to learn as far as the mechanism of action by which psychobiotics affect mental health. Also, how psychobiotics can help in the prevention of psychological illnesses has not yet been researched to a great extent and still needs to be explored further (Tremblay et al, 2021; Ng et al., 2019).

7.5 FUNCTIONAL FOODS RICH IN PSYCHOBIOTICS

Food these days is not only meant to satiate hunger or provide nourishment but at the same time to help in the prevention of lifestyle or metabolic disorders and to improve overall physical and psychological health (Betoret et al., 2011). Therefore, foods that provide added physiological benefits and that may decrease the threat of diseases are called functional foods. Functional foods are presently of great interest globally for health optimization. However, most foods can be described as functional to some extent because they provide taste, aroma, and nutritive value (Hasler, 2002). According to another definition, all conventional foods that possess proven physiological benefits can be defined as functional foods (Shahidi, 2012) The FAO of the United Nations defines functional food "as any food containing substances which may provide positive health effects that extend beyond its nutritional value" (Temple, 2022).

Psychobiotics through the microorganisms contained in them offer a number of psychological health benefits and are considered functional foods (Wu et al., 2021). Fermented foods are becoming popular as functional foods because of the benefits they offer for brain health. Fermented foods contain multiple microbial groups, which are capable of initiating certain biochemical reactions inside the host, thus producing several bioactive chemicals that confer health benefits on the host (Diez-Ozaeta, & Astiazaran, 2022).

Fermented foods have better nutritional quality, improved taste and texture, have a longer shelf life, and also promote food safety. All these benefits are due to the activity of the microorganisms inherent in fermented foods (Nkhata et al., 2018). Due to the presence of microbial enzymes in these foods that involve the fermentation process, anti-nutrient (phytates, tannins, etc.) activity decreases and the availability of nutrients such as saccharides, proteins, and vitamins increases (Şanlier et al., 2019). Along with providing all these benefits, fermented foods also modulate the intestinal microflora, while providing certain fermentative metabolites, such as vitamins and lactic acid. Fermentation is either spontaneous from the original ingredients or controlled by the addition of certain microbial cultures (Taylor et al., 2020).

Various species of microorganisms and basic foods are used for fermentation. Most commonly bacteria, molds, and yeasts are used due to the fact that many different kinds of fermentation are possible with them, because of the assortment of enzymes they possess (Cichońska et al., 2023).

Fermented food consumption causes the modulation of the GI microbiome that has a direct effect on mental well-being. This could be due to the synthesis of neurotransmitters—serotonin, GABA, and dopamine, by the gut microbiota, causing direct activation of the neuronal pathways or affecting the immune cells (Cenit et al., 2017). Fermented foods also enhance the neuroprotective effects of neuroactive compounds such as SCFAs, by increasing their production and bioavailability (Kumar et al., 2022).

Some psychobiotic strains have been shown to improve mood and reduce stress. In a short-term study, *Lactiplantibacillus plantarum* PS128TM strain was tested on some IT workers. It was found that this psychobiotic therapy improved sleep and self-esteem and decreased cortisol hormone (which plays a role in stress response) levels (Wu et al., 2021).

Two strains are being used all over the world to make fermented dairy products, that is, bifidobacteria and LAB. The milk products normally made by fermentation are cheese, kefir, yogurt, ice cream, etc. (Barros et al., 2020). *Lactobacillus*, *Streptococcus*, *Enterococcus*, *Lactococcus*, *Pediococcus*, and *Leuconostoc* are the bacteria included under LAB. Bifidobacteria are also anaerobic gram-positive bacteria. These are called LAB, as lactic acid, a key end product of carbohydrate metabolism. Both bifidobacteria and LAB convert pyruvic acid produced during glycolysis to lactic acid (Cichońska et al., 2023).

Although fermented dairy products provide health-promoting psychobiotic microorganisms, they may also contain allergens such as lactose and casein and may also be high in fat and cholesterol (Kumar et al., 2022).

Due to this reason, non-dairy fermented products such as vegetables, fruits, cereals, meats, and legumes are being used. These include sauerkraut, kimchi, fermented cereals, and legumes. Fermented meat and fish are also being used in traditional dishes (Tamang et al., 2016). Other products are tomato juices, blueberry pomace, apple juice, probiotic dark chocolate, apple juice, some soy products, etc. Bread is also an interesting non-dairy carrier of probiotics (Chan et al., 2021).

Figure 7.4 illustrates the psychobiotic foods that are considered functional foods.

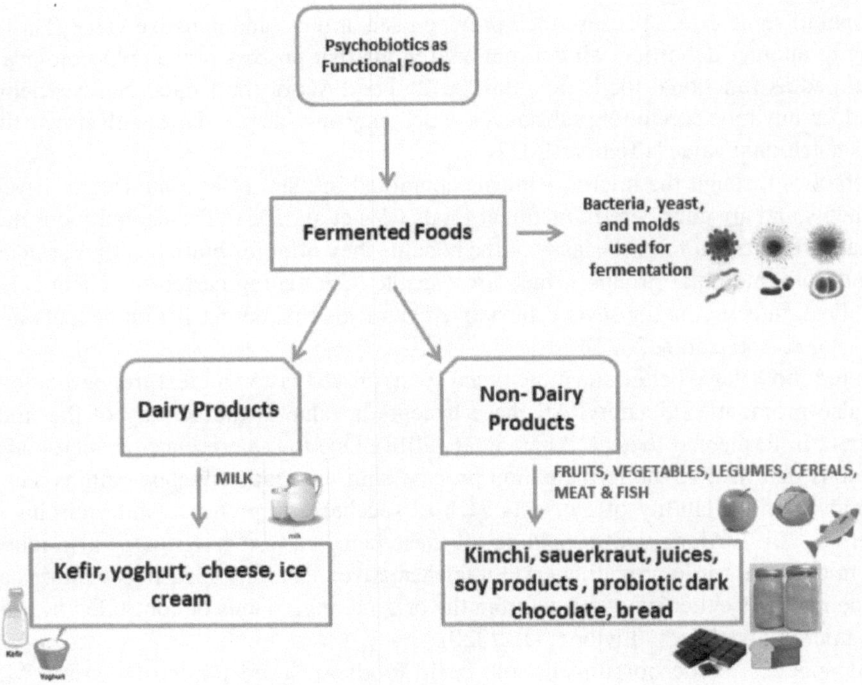

FIGURE 7.4 Psychobiotics as functional foods.

7.6 CONCLUSION

The increased prevalence of mental health-related disorders has impelled researchers to find novel ways to prevent and treat them. In this regard, a new strategy is to modulate the function of the MGB axis, through which the brain is connected to the gut via neuronal, hormonal, and immunological pathways. The indirect effect of the GI microflora in regulating actions of the neural system, synthesis of neurotransmitters, and other products of metabolism have steered the experts to investigate the aspects that have an impact on their correlation.

Most studies so far are suggestive of a close correlation between the GI microflora and intestinal symbiosis along with their connection to mental health. Research supports the fact that the treatment for mental disorders could be through interventions at the gut-microbe level. Modulating the functioning of GI microflora microbiota with psychobiotics has shown promising results so far. However, the identification of new microbial strains that may impact gut microbes thereby affecting brain activity needs to be explored.

Studies have also shown that the effect of psychobiotics in modulating behavior and brain function is regulated through the HPA axis, changes in the metabolism of neurotransmitters, and regulation of inflammatory status. Animal model studies have shown the promising potential of psychobiotics in modulating mental health, memory, and cognition. These studies also suggest that nutritional and psycho-social support needs to be part of the treatment strategy for various mental disorders. Healthy foods rich in psychobiotic strains have both preventive and curative roles in mental disorders, thereby helping to improve mental health.

Nevertheless, additional research and human clinical trials are required to understand the mechanism of the action of gut microbes on mental health and psychological conditions like depression and anxiety. More human trials are warranted to understand the therapeutic effects of psychobiotics, their action mechanism, along with the characteristics and nature of psychobiotic microorganisms that impact mental health.

BIBLIOGRAPHY

Barros, C. P., Guimarães, J. T., Esmerino, E. A., Duarte, M. C. K., Silva, M. C., Silva, R., Ferreira, B. M., Sant'Ana, A. S., Freitas, M. Q., & Cruz, A. G. (2020). Paraprobiotics and postbiotics: Concepts and potential applications in dairy products. *Current Opinion in Food Science*, *32*, 1–8. https://doi.org/10.1016/j.cofs.2019.12.003

Bermúdez-Humarán, L. G., Salinas, E., Ortiz, G. G., Ramirez-Jirano, L. J., Morales, J. A., & Bitzer-Quintero, O. K. (2019). From probiotics to psychobiotics: Live beneficial bacteria which act on the brain-gut axis. *Nutrients*, *11*(4), 890. https://doi.org/10.3390/nu11040890

Betoret, E., Betoret, N., Vidal, D., & Fito, P. (2011). Functional foods development: Trends and technologies. *Trends in Food Science and Technology*, *22*(9), 498–508. https://doi.org/10.1016/j.tifs.2011.05.004

Bonaz, B., Bazin, T., & Pellissier, S. (2018). The vagus nerve at the interface of the microbiota-gut-brain axis. *Frontiers in Neuroscience*, *12*, 49. https://doi.org/10.3389/fnins.2018.00049; PubMed: 29467611; PubMed Central: PMC5808284

Carabotti, M., Scirocco, A., Maselli, M. A., & Severi, C. (2015). The gut-brain axis: Interactions between enteric microbiota, central and enteric nervous systems. *Annals of Gastroenterology*, *28*(2), 203–209.

Cenit, M. C., Nuevo, I. C., Codoñer-Franch, P., Dinan, T. G., & Sanz, Y. (2017). Gut microbiota and attention deficit hyperactivity disorder: New perspectives for a challenging condition. *European Child and Adolescent Psychiatry*, *26*(9), 1081–1092. https://doi.org/10.1007/s00787-017-0969-z

Chakrabarti, A., Geurts, L., Hoyles, L., Iozzo, P., Kraneveld, A. D., La Fata, G., Miani, M., Patterson, E., Pot, B., Shortt, C., & Vauzour, D. (2022). The microbiota–gut–brain axis: Pathways to better brain health. Perspectives on what we know, what we need to investigate and how to put knowledge into practice. *Cellular and Molecular Life Sciences*, *79*(2), 80. https://doi.org/10.1007/s00018-021-04060-w

Chan, M. Z. A., Toh, M., & Liu, S. Q. (2021). Growth, survival, and metabolic activities of probiotics Lactobacillus rhamnosus GG and Saccharomyces cerevisiae Var. Boulardii CNCM-I745 in fermented coffee brews. *International Journal of Food Microbiology*, *350*, 109229. https://doi.org/10.1016/j.ijfoodmicro.2021.109229

Cichońska, P., Kowalska, E., & Ziarno, M. (2023). The survival of psychobiotics in fermented food and the gastrointestinal tract: A review. *Microorganisms, 11*(4), 996. https://doi.org/10.3390/microorganisms11040996

Codagnone, M. G., Spichak, S., O'Mahony, S. M., O'Leary, O. F., Clarke, G., Stanton, C., Dinan, T. G., & Cryan, J. F. (2019). Programming bugs: Microbiota and the developmental origins of brain health and disease. *Biological Psychiatry*, *85*(2), 150–163. https://doi.org/10.1016/j.biopsych.2018.06.014

Cohen Kadosh, K., Basso, M., Knytl, P., Johnstone, N., Lau, J. Y. F., & Gibson, G. R. (2021). Psychobiotic interventions for anxiety in young people: A systematic review and meta-analysis, with youth consultation. *Translational Psychiatry*, *11*(1), 352. https://doi.org/10.1038/s41398-021-01422-7

Cowan, C. S., Callaghan, B. L., & Richardson, R. (2016). The effects of a probiotic formulation (Lactobacillus rhamnosus and L. helveticus) on developmental trajectories of emotional learning in stressed infant rats. *Translational Psychiatry, 6*(5), e823. https://doi.org/10.1038/tp.2016.94

Coyle, P. K. (2011). Dissecting the immune component of neurologic disorders: A grand challenge for the 21st century. *Frontiers in Neurology, 2,* 37. https://doi.org/10.3389/fneur.2011.00037

Cryan, J. F., & Dinan, T. G. (2012). Mind-altering microorganisms: The impact of the gut microbiota on brain and behaviour. *Nature Reviews. Neuroscience*, *13*(10), 701–712. https://doi.org/10.1038/nrn3346

Dahiya, D., & Nigam, P. S. (2022). The gut microbiota influenced by the intake of probiotics and functional foods with prebiotics can sustain wellness and alleviate certain ailments like gut-inflammation and Colon-Cancer. *Microorganisms*, *10*(3), 10030665. https://doi.org/10.3390/microorganisms10030665

Davis, I., & Liu, A. (2015). What is the tryptophan kynurenine pathway and why is it important to neurotherapeutics? *Expert Review of Neurotherapeutics*, *15*(7), 719–721. https://doi.org/10.1586/14737175.2015.1049999; PubMed: 26004930; PubMed Central: PMC4482796

Del Toro-Barbosa, M., Hurtado-Romero, A., Garcia-Amezquita, L. E., & García-Cayuela, T. (2020). Psychobiotics: Mechanisms of action, evaluation methods and effectiveness in applications with food products. *Nutrients*, *12*(12), 164–174. https://doi.org/10.3390/nu12123896

Diaz Heijtz, R., Wang, S., Anuar, F., Qian, Y., Björkholm, B., Samuelsson, A., Hibberd, M. L., Forssberg, H., & Pettersson, S. (2011). Normal gut microbiota modulates brain development and behavior. *Proceedings of the National Academy of Sciences of the United States of America*, *108*(7), 3047–3052. https://doi.org/10.1073/pnas.1010529108

Diez-Ozaeta, I., & Astiazaran, O. J. (2022). Fermented foods: An update on evidence-based health benefits and future perspectives. *Food Research International*, *156,* 111133. https://doi.org/10.1016/j.foodres.2022.111133

Dinan, T. G., Stanton, C., & Cryan, J. F. (2013). Psychobiotics: A novel class of psychotropic. *Biological Psychiatry*, *74*(10), 720–726. https://doi.org/10.1016/j.biopsych.2013.05.001

Fereidoon, S. (2012). Nutraceuticals, functional foods and dietary supplements in health and disease. *Journal of Food and Drug Analysis, 20*(1), 226–230.

Forsythe, P., Bienenstock, J., & Kunze, W. A. (2014). Vagal pathways for microbiome-brain-gut axis communication. *Advances in Experimental Medicine and Biology*, *817,* 115–133. https://doi.org/10.1007/978-1-4939-0897-4_5

Fung, T. C. (2020). The microbiota-immune axis as a central mediator of gut–brain communication. *Neurobiology of Disease*, *136,* 104714. https://doi.org/10.1016/j.nbd.2019.104714

Furness, J. B. (2012). The enteric nervous system and neurogastroenterology. *Nature Reviews. Gastroenterology and Hepatology*, *9*(5), 286–294. https://doi.org/10.1038/nrgastro.2012.32

Gagliardi, A., Totino, V., Cacciotti, F., Iebba, V., Neroni, B., Bonfiglio, G., Trancassini, M., Passariello, C., Pantanella, F., & Schippa, S. (2018). Rebuilding the gut microbiota ecosystem. *International Journal of Environmental Research and Public Health, 15*(8), 1679. https://doi.org/10.3390/ijerph15081679; PubMed: 30087270; PubMed Central: PMC6121872

Hamaker, B. R., & Tuncil, Y. E. (2014). A perspective on the complexity of dietary fiber structures and their potential effect on the gut microbiota. *Journal of Molecular Biology*, *426*(23), 3838–3850. https://doi.org/10.1016/j.jmb.2014.07.028

Hasler, C. M. (2002). Functional foods: Benefits, concerns and challenges—A position paper from the American Council on Science and Health. *Journal of Nutrition, 132*(12), 3772–3781. https://doi.org/10.1093/jn/132.12.3772

Hill, C., Guarner, F., Reid, G., Gibson, G. R., Merenstein, D. J., Pot, B., Morelli, L., Canani, R. B., Flint, H. J., Salminen, S., Calder, P. C., & Sanders, M. E. (2014). Expert consensus document. The international scientific association for probiotics and prebiotics consensus statement on the scope and appropriate use of the term probiotic. *Nature Reviews. Gastroenterology and Hepatology*, *11*(8), 506–514. https://doi.org/10.1038/nrgastro.2014.66

Huang, F., & Wu, X. (2021). Brain neurotransmitter modulation by gut microbiota in anxiety and depression. *Frontiers in Cell and Developmental Biology*, *9*, 649103. https://doi.org/10.3389/fcell.2021.649103

Kali, A. (2016). Psychobiotics: An emerging probiotic in psychiatric practice. *Biomedical Journal*, *39*(3), 223–224. https://doi.org/10.1016/j.bj.2015.11.004; Epub August 9, 2016; PubMed: 27621125; PubMed Central: PMC6140288

Kumar, M. R., Azizi, N. F., Yeap, S. K., Abdullah, J. O., Khalid, M., Omar, A. R., Osman, M. A., Leow, A. T. C., Mortadza, S. A. S., & Alitheen, N. B. (2022). Clinical and preclinical studies of fermented foods and their effects on Alzheimer's disease. *Antioxidants*, *11*(5), 883. https://doi.org/10.3390/antiox11050883

Leeming, E. R., Johnson, A. J., Spector, T. D., & Le Roy, C. I. (2019). Effect of diet on the gut microbiota: Rethinking intervention duration. *Nutrients*, *11*(12), 2862. https://doi.org/10.3390/nu11122862; PubMed: 31766592; PubMed Central: PMC6950569

Leung, K., & Thuret, S. (2015). Gut microbiota: A modulator of brain plasticity and cognitive function in ageing. *Healthcare*, *3*(4), 898–916. https://doi.org/10.3390/healthcare3040898

Liu, R. T., Walsh, R. F. L., & Sheehan, A. E. (2019). Prebiotics and probiotics for depression and anxiety: A systematic review and meta-analysis of controlled clinical trials. *Neuroscience and Biobehavioral Reviews*, *102,* 13–23. https://doi.org/10.1016/j.neubiorev.2019.03.023

Mittal, R., Debs, L. H., Patel, A. P., Nguyen, D., Patel, K., O'Connor, G., Grati, M., Mittal, J., Yan, D., Eshraghi, A. A., Deo, S. K., Daunert, S., & Liu, X. Z. (2017). Neurotransmitters: The critical modulators regulating gut-brain axis. *Journal of Cellular Physiology*, *232*(9), 2359–2372. https://doi.org/10.1002/jcp.25518; Epub April 10, 2017; PubMed: 27512962; PubMed Central: PMC5772764

Mohajeri, M. H., La Fata, G., Steinert, R. E., & Weber, P. (2018). Relationship between the gut microbiome and brain function. *Nutrition Reviews, 76*(7), 481–496. https://doi.org/10.1093/nutrit/nuy009

Munawar, N., Ahsan, K., Muhammad, K., Ahmad, A., Anwar, M. A., Shah, I., Al Ameri, A. K., & Al Mughairbi, F. (2021). Hidden role of gut microbiome dysbiosis in schizophrenia: Antipsychotics or psychobiotics as therapeutics? *International Journal of Molecular Sciences*, *22*(14), 7671. https://doi.org/10.3390/ijms22147671; PubMed: 34299291; PubMed Central: PMC8307070

Ng, Q. X., Loke, W., Venkatanarayanan, N., Lim, D. Y., Soh, A. Y. S., & Yeo, W. S. (2019). A systematic review of the role of prebiotics and probiotics in autism spectrum disorders. *Medicina, 55*(5), 129. https://doi.org/10.3390/medicina55050129

Ng, Q. X., Peters, C., Ho, C. Y. X., Lim, D. Y., & Yeo, W. S. (2018). A meta-analysis of the use of probiotics to alleviate depressive symptoms. *Journal of Affective Disorders, 228,* 13–19. https://doi.org/10.1016/j.jad.2017.11.063

Nkhata, S. G., Ayua, E., Kamau, E. H., & Shingiro, J. B. (2018). Fermentation and germination improve nutritional value of cereals and legumes through activation of endogenous enzymes. *Food Science and Nutrition*, *6*(8), 2446–2458. https://doi.org/10.1002/fsn3.846

Oroojzadeh, P., Bostanabad, S. Y., & Lotfi, H. (2022). Psychobiotics: The influence of gut microbiota on the gut-brain axis in neurological disorders. *Journal of Molecular Neuroscience*, *72*(9), 1952–1964. https://doi.org/10.1007/s12031-022-02053-3; Epub July 18, 2022.

Romijn, A. R., & Rucklidge, J. J. (2015). Systematic review of evidence to support the theory of psychobiotics. *Nutrition Reviews*, *73*(10), 675–693. https://doi.org/10.1093/nutrit/nuv025

Salvo-Romero, E. S. P., Stokes, P., & Gareau, M. G. (2020). Microbiota-immune interactions: From gut to brain. *LymphoSign Journal*, *7*(1), 1–23. https://doi.org/10.14785/lymphosign-2019-0018

Şanlier, N., Gökcen, B. B., & Sezgin, A. C. (2019). Health benefits of fermented foods. *Critical Reviews in Food Science and Nutrition*, *59*(3), 506–527. https://doi.org/10.1080/10408398.2017.1383355

Sarkar, A., Lehto, S. M., Harty, S., Dinan, T. G., Cryan, J. F., & Burnet, P. W. J. (2016). Psychobiotics and the manipulation of bacteria-gut-brain signals. *Trends in Neurosciences*, *39*(11), 763–781. https://doi.org/10.1016/j.tins.2016.09.002; Epub October 25, 2016.

Shahidi, F. (2012). Nutraceuticals, functional foods and dietary supplements in health and disease. *Journal of Food and Drug Analysis*, *20*(1), 226–230.

Strandwitz, P. (2018). Neurotransmitter modulation by the gut microbiota. *Brain Research*, *1693*(B), 128–133. https://doi.org/10.1016/j.brainres.2018.03.015

Sun, L. J., Li, J. N., & Nie, Y. Z. (2020). Gut hormones in microbiota—gut–brain cross-talk. *Chinese Medical Journal*, *133*(7), 826–833. https://doi.org/10.1097/CM9.0000000000000706

Takada, M., Nishida, K., Kataoka-Kato, A., Gondo, Y., Ishikawa, H., Suda, K., Kawai, M., Hoshi, R., Watanabe, O., Igarashi, T., Kuwano, Y., Miyazaki, K., & Rokutan, K. (2016). Probiotic Lactobacillus casei Strain Shirota relieves stress-associated symptoms by modulating the gut–brain interaction in human and animal models. *Neurogastroenterology and Motility*, *28*(7), 1027–1036. https://doi.org/10.1111/nmo.12804

Tamang, J. P., Watanabe, K., & Holzapfel, W. H. (2016). Review: Diversity of microorganisms in global fermented foods and beverages. *Frontiers in Microbiology, 7,* 377. https://doi.org/10.3389/fmicb.2016.00377

Taylor, B. C., Lejzerowicz, F., Poirel, M., Shaffer, J. P., Jiang, L., Aksenov, A., Litwin, N., Humphrey, G., Martino, C., Miller-Montgomery, S., Dorrestein, P. C., Veiga, P., Song, S. J., McDonald, D., Derrien, M., & Knight, R. (2020). Consumption of fermented foods is associated with systematic differences in the gut microbiome and metabolome. *mSystems*, *5*(2), 00901–00919. https://doi.org/10.1128/mSystems.00901-19

Temple, N. J. (2022). A rational definition for functional foods: A perspective. *Frontiers in Nutrition, 9,* 957516. https://doi.org/10.3389/fnut.2022.957516

Tremblay, A., Lingrand, L., Maillard, M., Feuz, B., & Tompkins, T. A. (2021). The effects of psychobiotics on the microbiota-gut-brain axis in early-life stress and neuropsychiatric disorders. *Progress in Neuro-Psychopharmacology and Biological Psychiatry, 105,* 110142. https://doi.org/10.1016/j.pnpbp.2020.110142

Vaiserman, A. M., Koliada, A. K., & Marotta, F. (2017). Gut microbiota: A player in aging and a target for anti-aging intervention. *Ageing Research Reviews*, *35,* 36–45. https://doi.org/10.1016/j.arr.2017.01.001

Wall, R., Cryan, J. F., Ross, R. P., Fitzgerald, G. F., Dinan, T. G., & Stanton, C. (2014). Bacterial neuroactive compounds produced by psychobiotics. *Advances in Experimental Medicine and Biology*, *817,* 221–239. https://doi.org/10.1007/978-1-4939-0897-4_10

Wallace, C. J. K., & Milev, R. (2017). The effects of probiotics on depressive symptoms in humans: A systematic review. *Annals of General Psychiatry, 16*(1), 14. https://doi.org/10.1186/s12991-017-0138-2

Wasilewski, A., Zielińska, M., Storr, M., & Fichna, J. (2015). Beneficial effects of probiotics, prebiotics, synbiotics, and psychobiotics in inflammatory bowel disease. *Inflammatory Bowel Diseases, 21*(7), 1674–1682. https://doi.org/10.1097/MIB.0000000000000364

Wu, S. I., Wu, C. C., Tsai, P. J., Cheng, L. H., Hsu, C. C., Shan, I. K., Chan, P. Y., Lin, T. W., Ko, C. J., Chen, W. L., & Tsai, Y. C. (2021). Psychobiotic supplementation of PS128TM improves stress, anxiety, and insomnia in highly stressed information technology specialists: A pilot study. *Frontiers in Nutrition*, *8,* 614105. https://doi.org/10.3389/fnut.2021.614105

Zhou, L., & Foster, J. A. (2015). Psychobiotics and the gut-brain axis: In the pursuit of happiness. *Neuropsychiatric Disease and Treatment*, *11,* 715–723. https://doi.org/10.2147/NDT.S61997

Zielińska, D., Karbowiak, M., & Brzezicka, A. (2022). The role of psychobiotics to ensure mental health during the COVID-19 pandemic—A current state of knowledge. *International Journal of Environmental Research and Public Health, 19*(17), 11022. https://doi.org/10.3390/ijerph191711022

8 Probiotics in Diabetes Mellitus

Role of Probiotics in Maintaining Insulin Levels

Saliha Rizvi, Farheen Khan, Naseem Fatima, Syed Tasleem Raza, Gowhar Rashid, and Farzana Mahdi

8.1 INTRODUCTION TO DIABETES MELLITUS AND INSULIN

8.1.1 Definition and Classification of Diabetes Mellitus

DM (Gk. Diabetes = siphon—to pass through; L. mellitus = sweet) is essentially a metabolic disorder characterized inefficiency of body cells to effectively metabolize glucose due to inefficiency in insulin production or its resistance induced by hereditary/genetic and environmental factors. Increased levels of circulating glucose, due to impaired cellular ability to metabolize glucose, induce tissue damage (Sapra & Bhandari, 2023; Irfan et al., 2022). Diabetes is one of the major contributors to deaths globally, leading to 75% mortality among other categories of non-transmittable diseases like cardiovascular, lung, and cancers. IDFGD estimates show that 463 million adults (20–70 years/age group) have diabetes, which is predicted to rise to 578 crores population by 2030 (Sreepathi et al., 2022) and 700 million by 2040 globally (Irfan et al., 2022). DM is expected to affect an additional 200 million people by 2040, with the highest growth rate in populations undergoing middle-income transitions (Zheng et al., 2018).

DM is classified into type 1 diabetes (T1DM), type 2 diabetes (T2DM), MODY, gestational diabetes (GD), neonatal diabetes, and steroid-induced diabetes. The first two types are the most prevalent of all the types that occur due to insufficient insulin production (T1DM) or its inefficiency (T2DM). Type 1 usually manifests in children and adolescents whereas type 2 appears among middle- and old-age individuals with chronic hyperglycemia due to unhealthy eating habits and lifestyle. Distinct pathophysiology of T1DM and T2DM results in varying etiologies, symptoms, and therapies (Sapra & Bhandari, 2023).

T1DM is an autoimmune disorder where the beta cells of the pancreas destroy themselves, resulting in insufficient insulin production. T1DM develops gradually from infancy and then peak incidence occurs in children of the age group between 4 and 14 years (Felner et al., 2005). The prevalence rate among children below 10 years is 45% and about 2.3 cases per 1,000 adults below 20 years (Writing Group for the SEARCH for Diabetes in Youth Study Group et al., 2007). The incidence of T1DM has been growing globally, with a 2% to 5% yearly increase in Europe, Australia, and the Middle East alone (Tuomilehto, 2013).

T2DM occurs gradually due to insufficient insulin production and its resistance build-up in the body, the latter being induced by obesity and aging. T2DM generally develops during middle age but obesity in adolescents has declined the age of onset and T2DM is now increasingly diagnosed in younger age groups. The prevalence of T2DM in the US is 9% and 25% of diagnosed individuals are of age >65 years. T2DM prevalence varies greatly by ethnicity and environmental factors. It is two to six times more frequent among Native and Hispanic Americans, Blacks, and Pima Indians than in Whites in the USA. Ethnicity together with geographical region confers a greater risk of T2DM as evidenced by higher prevalence in Pima Indians living in the United States (38%) than those in Mexico (6.9%) (Sapra & Bhandari, 2023).

DOI: 10.1201/9781003452249-8

MODY is an insulin-independent autosomal dominant diabetic condition that manifests typically before the age of 25. Most MODY cases are due to genetic alterations in *HNF1A* and *GCK* genes that infer the genetic basis of this disease (Fajans et al., 2001). However, it has been observed that sometimes these genetic alterations protect the individuals from the disease. While few individuals who do not harbor the risk genotypes still develop MODY and its manifestations the justification for this finding remains unclear.

GD presents during pregnancy. Its etiology is currently unknown; however, HLA antigens (HLA DR2, 3, and 4), proinsulin and sex hormones, cortisol, prolactin, etc. are postulated to play a role by inducing non-functioning pancreatic islets and peripheral resistance to insulin (Kühl, 1998).

8.1.2 Overview of Insulin and Its Role in Glucose Metabolism

Insulin, a peptide hormone encoded by a gene located on 11p15.5, is synthesized and released by pancreatic β cells. Insulin facilitates the transport of glucose inside hepatocytes, skeletal muscle cells, and adipocytes, regulates the metabolism of lipids, protein, and carbohydrates, promotes cellular division and growth, and thus regulates blood glucose levels. Impaired insulin secretion or action leads to hyperglycemia, the defining characteristic of DM.

Hyperglycemia induces biphasic glucose-mediated insulin secretion. The transient "first phase" involves insulin release by exocytosis granules insulin secretion present in beta cells of the pancreas. In pancreatic β cells, the glucose following facilitated transport by GLUT2 is sensed by the glucose sensor GCK, which catalyzes glucose phosphorylation through glycolysis (G6P) producing ATP and prevents the release of glucose in the bloodstream (de Lonlay & Saudubray, 2000). The closing of potassium channels that utilize ATP as an energy source, causes depolarization of the cell surface resulting in the opening of calcium channels thus increasing intracellular calcium concentration and resulting in insulin secretion (Soria et al., 2004). This insulin exocytosis is facilitated by glucose-induced K+ATP-independent Ca^{2+}-dependent and independent pathway. Other agents involved in the production of insulin include protein kinase C, activated phospholipases, stimulated adenylyl cyclase activity, and activated protein kinase A in the pancreas. These pathways may be stimulated by a few hormones like pituitary adenylyl cyclase-activating peptide, vasoactive intestinal peptide, glucose-dependent insulinotropic polypeptide, and glucagon-like peptide. The aforementioned factors seem to be crucial for the continued "second phase" of insulin production (Bratanova-Tochkova et al., 2002). Insulin synthesis along with its secretion is controlled by both nutritional and non-nutrient secretagogues such as glucose and cyclic AMP, as well as environmental stimulus and the interaction of other hormones.

8.1.3 Importance of Maintaining Insulin Levels in Diabetes Management

Insulin is a 51 amino acid polypeptide produced by the pancreas, which is essential for cell development, metabolism, and glucose balance (Rahman et al., 2021). Cells such as adipocytes, skeletal muscles, and hepatocytes receive it from your blood for energy needs. Insulin regulates glucose levels in our body by causing glucose accumulation in these cells, leading to increased body weight. Additionally, insulin helps your body's other processes related to metabolism. Insulin is very important for initiation as well as persistence of numerous long-term illnesses related to glucose metabolism because it regulates a variety of physiological processes. A disturbance in hormones leads to the occurrence of diabetes.

In T2DM, the phenomenon of insulin resistance is observed where the production of insulin by the pancreas is increased but the body stops responding to insulin ultimately resulting in hyperglycemia. While glucose levels regulate both the production and secretion of insulin, the quantities needed to begin every procedure vary. While fluctuations between 2 and 4 mM stimulate insulin production, glucose amounts above 5 mM are necessary to start the process (Kaufman et al., 2015). High blood glucose levels cause a condition called hyperglycemia because research demonstrates that insulin insufficiency prevents cells from using glucose. Uncontrolled elevated glucose concentrations in the blood for a long duration can have negative effects on the neurological system, the kidneys, and the eyes in diabetic patients. Also, the inability of the body to use glucose as an energy source forces it to rely on alternative sources of energy like fats. This continual reliance on fat might result in a chronic condition known as ketoacidosis, which could result in the build-up of ketones in the bloodstream (Accili, 2018).

8.1.3.1 Effects of Hyperinsulinemia

In hyperinsulinemia, there is a greater-than-normal concentration of insulin in the blood. Inefficient signaling of insulin, alterations in mitochondrial metabolism, ER stress, changes in calcium balance and levels, dysfunctional autonomous nervous system, upregulated RAAS system, and abnormality in the generation of immunological responses are all characteristics of the hyperinsulinemic state. Heightened production of ROS, scarring of connective tissues, and cardiovascular abnormalities are the results of these pathophysiological changes (Bazotte et al., 2014).

In patients with a higher BMI than normal, hyperinsulinemia is associated heightened risk of morbidity and mortality from cardiovascular problems because it regulates insulin production, which eventually results in hyperinsulinemia (Moghetti & Tosi, 2021). Insulin insensitivity is typically responsible for hyperinsulinemia, which the pancreas responds to by manufacturing more insulin to treat. However, it can occasionally be brought on by an uncommon tumor of the pancreatic cells that produce insulin (insulinoma) or by abnormal growth or quantity of these cells (nesidioblastosis). Low blood sugar is a side effect of this illness (Coimbra et al., 2010).

8.1.3.2 Effects of Hyperglycemia

The initiation and development of hyperglycemia are influenced by inefficient islet functioning, decreased insulin production, a decline in glucose utilization, and insulin resistance observed in T2DM. Long-term hyperglycemia can also trigger additional potentially fatal side effects such as ketoacidosis and hyperglycemic hyperosmolar syndrome. Consequently, blood glucose levels are also related to the development of cardiovascular diseases (Decode Study Group, 2003). The fundamental underlying mechanism for both illnesses, despite the differences in their pathophysiology, is the reduction of insulin levels in blood accompanied by the concurrent rise of hormones such as cortisol, catecholamines, glucagon, and growth hormone which possess opposite action (Gosmanov et al., 2000).

8.1.3.3 Effect on the Liver, Skeletal Muscles, and Adipose Tissue

Endocytosis of blood glucose into hepatocytes, muscle fibers as well as adipocytes, requires insulin. Any imbalance in extrinsic sources of energy induces the lipids preserved in adipose tissue to eventually break down, resulting in hyperinsulinemia. Insulin-aided endocytosis of blood glucose in liver cells results in the production of triglycerides, glycogen, and carboxylic acids with long aliphatic chains. On the other hand, the decrease in pancreatic glucagon secretion mostly controls indirect insulin action (Ito et al., 1995), the inhibition of fat lipolysis (Sindelar et al., 1997), and the signaling pathway for insulin (Bergman, 2000), thus affecting gluconeogenesis in liver cells. Insulin endocytosis of circulating amino acids and glucose by muscle fibers utilizes it for producing proteins and production of energy via glycolysis. Apart from producing ATP, glucose is also converted into a storable form of energy as glycogen. It has been shown that reduction in muscle mass in T2DM affects the metabolism of glucose since the glucose reserves are found in skeletal muscle cells; consequently, in these patients, insulin therapy may increase optimum glucose goals (Abdulla et al., 2016).

Insulin aids in the endocytosis of free fatty acids into lipocytes which convert them into triglycerides that could be used as a form of stored energy by the cells. Alterations in glucose levels do not affect adipocytes but they are dependent on the levels of free fatty acids released by insulin in blood for utilization by cardiomyocytes (Smith, 2002). The generation of insulin is mostly influenced by the precursor triglyceride levels, and whenever insulin drives a process, that process is typically irreversible (Koyama et al., 1997).

8.2 GUT MICROBIOME AND DIABETES MELLITUS

8.2.1 Gut Microbiome Composition in Healthy Individuals vs. Individuals with Diabetes

The bacteria that live inside our bodies have a significant impact on our health. "Human microbiome" was the word initially used in 2001 by J. Lederberg. According to him, human bodies are home to an ecological ecosystem of commensal, mutually beneficial, and harmful bacteria (Lederberg & McCray, 2001). An adult human harbors more than a hundred trillion microorganisms, the majority of them residing in our gut, with the colon housing the majority of them. Bacteroidetes (23%), Firmicutes (64%), Actinobacteria (3%), and Proteobacteria (8%) constitute four primary groups contributing majorly to our intestinal microflora (Turnbaugh et al., 2007; Cunningham et al., 2021). Verrucomicrobia and Fusobacteria are two more lesser-known but important phylum (Blaut, 2013). Evidence reports that disturbance of normal intestinal microflora composition increases the incidence of disorders such as high BMI, T2DM, rheumatoid arthritis, and various malignancies (Guarner & Malagelada, 2003). It also implies that the gut microbiota might affect the healthy well-being of any individual. When it comes to phylum and class levels, the microbiome profiles of both human and animal models of T2DM showed alterations in gut microbiome profiles. However, complicating variables such as ethnicity, culture, nutrition, well-being, condition, and drug usage have made it challenging to define a "common" microbiome profile linked to T2DM. It is doubtful that a single species of microbe affects the risk of T2DM more than another (Cunningham et al., 2021).

Various studies have shown a significant decline in Clostridia and Firmicutes strains in patients suffering from diabetes while there was a significant increase in the Betaproteobacteria class of gut microbiota that was also significantly related to plasma sugar concentration in diabetics. Furthermore, the fact that T2DM is connected with the composition of intestinal microflora comes from *Bacteroidetes/Firmicutes* and *Bacteroides–Prevotella/C. coccoides–E. rectale/Firmicutes* ratios.

The gut microflora of T2DM patients vary significantly from their healthy counterparts in composition and function according to various studies. A study on 345 Chinese subjects revealed that people suffering from T2DM had mild dysbiosis, with lower levels of butyrate-secreting microbes (such as *Eubacterium rectale*, *Roseburia intestinalis*, and *Faecalibacterium prausnitzii*), while a heightened proportion of microbes such as *Bacteroides caccae*. Reportedly, there is a correlation between T2DM and the composition of gut microbes among urban Africans as well (Qin et al., 2012). *Clostridium butyricum*, *Cellulosilyticum ruminicola*, and *Clostridium paraputrificum* (butyrate producers) were found to be in lower concentrations in T2DM patients' gut microbiota, while *Desulfovibrio piger*, *Prevotella*, *Peptostreptococcus*, and *Eubacterium* were found to be more prevalent in a study from Nigerian ethnicity (Doumatey et al., 2020). Danish research found that Betaproteobacteria were much more abundant in diabetic subjects than in healthy controls and that they were positively linked with blood glucose levels (Larsen et al., 2010). In summary, a considerable shift has been observed in the ratio of intestinal microflora in diabetic subjects, which raises the need for designing novel methods and strategies to treat diabetes by controlling the gut microbiome (Du et al., 2022). We would like to highlight the fact that not all of the findings from observational studies have been reliable. For instance, one investigation using fecal samples from 18 males compared substantial variations of the microbial composition of the gut among T2DM subjects and people in good health. The overall gut microbial composition was found to be significantly associated with circulating blood glucose in diabetics showing decreased concentrations of Clostridia and increased concentrations of Bacteroidetes and Proteobacteria (Larsen et al., 2010). Three comprehensive metagenomics investigations were carried out in Europe and China, however, did not find these results (Qin et al., 2012, Karlsson et al., 2013). Prevotella gut composition was found to be comparatively low in 50 Japanese T2D patients, whereas heightened Prevotella concentration was linked with diabetes in Nigerian and Chinese studies (Huda et al., 2021)

Emphasizing diabetic complications, diabetes along with its secondary co-morbidities results in heightened inflammation throughout the body. The beginning and development of diabetic problems are associated with the decline of microbes that combat inflammation and with significantly increased inflammation-causing bacteria. Apart from diabetes gut microbes were shown to reduce inflammation in other diseases like cardiovascular disorders (*Roseburia*), stroke (*Roseburia*), and disorders of the central nervous system (*Faecalibacterium*) (Li et al., 2020).

Although preclinical trials are exciting showing the significant influence of particular microbes on the biochemical profile of diabetics, the findings in animal models are less encouraging due to a lack of clinical trials and frequently conflicting outcomes. Analyzing and testing the impact of microbial metabolites linked to T2DM, the gut microbiome, and related problems is therefore needed (Koh & Bäckhed, 2020). Thus, to identify continuous changes that occur during disease progression, it is equally crucial to look at changing shifts in microbial ratios, the functioning of intestinal microflora along with the by-products they generate during the start and progression of diabetes and its implications. The identification of bacterial profile and microbial by-products will enable the detection of the risk of disease at an earlier stage and the underlying processes, which will aid in the personalization of medical treatment based on each patient's health profile.

8.2.2 Gut Microbiota and Its Association with Insulin Resistance

Intestinal microflora makeup affects the occurrence of prediabetic disorders such as insulin resistance (Rogero & Calder, 2018). The host enzyme transforms the microbial metabolite TMA into TMAO, and increased concentrations of TMAO affect insulin resistance. A research model using microbe-free mice showed lower BMI, higher glucose tolerance, and increased insulin efficiency (Bäckhed et al., 2004). Investigations on *Akkermansia muciniphila* demonstrate that it lessens gut barrier breakdown and insulin resistance. Prediabetic individuals and those who recently suffered from T2DM were shown to have decreased concentrations of *A. muciniphila*, which may be an indicative predictor for a decline in glucose sensitivity (Zhang et al., 2013). According to various reports conducted globally, T2DM patients show less *F. prausnitzii* and *Roseburia* concentrations than controls (Jumpertz et al., 2011). The enrichment of *F. prausnitzii* has also been shown to lessen insulin resistance and inflammatory symptoms in other investigations.

Human research showed that the incorporation of BCAA in the diet increases the chances of diabetes (Asghari et al., 2018). *Prevotella copri* and *Bacteroides vulgatus* were linked with the BCAA production pathway. In further studies, mice transplanted with *P. copri* revealed elevated BCAA levels with increased resistance to insulin (Pedersen et al., 2016). It is suggested that enhanced fatty acid oxidation and phosphatidylinositol 3-kinase activation are major mechanisms by which BCAAs cause insulin resistance (Kawaguchi et al., 2011).

When the gut microbiota is altered by outside factors like nutrition, this can result in intestine microbial metabolite dysregulation and secretory alterations, which can set off a number of possible pathways that might contribute to insulin resistance and diabetes (Figure 8.1). Various studies have been conducted to decipher how microflora control insulin resistance through LPS and SCFAs as intermediates that help maintain normal glucose levels in the blood. SCFAs bind as ligands to receptors like FFAR2 and FFAR3 reducing the functioning of the histone deacetylases which reduces the risk of diabetes and insulin resistance (Gholizadeh et al., 2019). Along with SCFAs, the gut microbiota regulates LPS levels, which may affect the T2DM risk (Cani & Delzenne, 2009). LPS generated from microbes residing in the gut attaches to TLR4 receptors leading to the production of various cytokines and thus inflammation (Boutagy et al., 2016). Studies show that saturated fatty acids can activate TLR4 signaling, which causes insulin resistance and mild inflammatory response (Rogero & Calder, 2018).

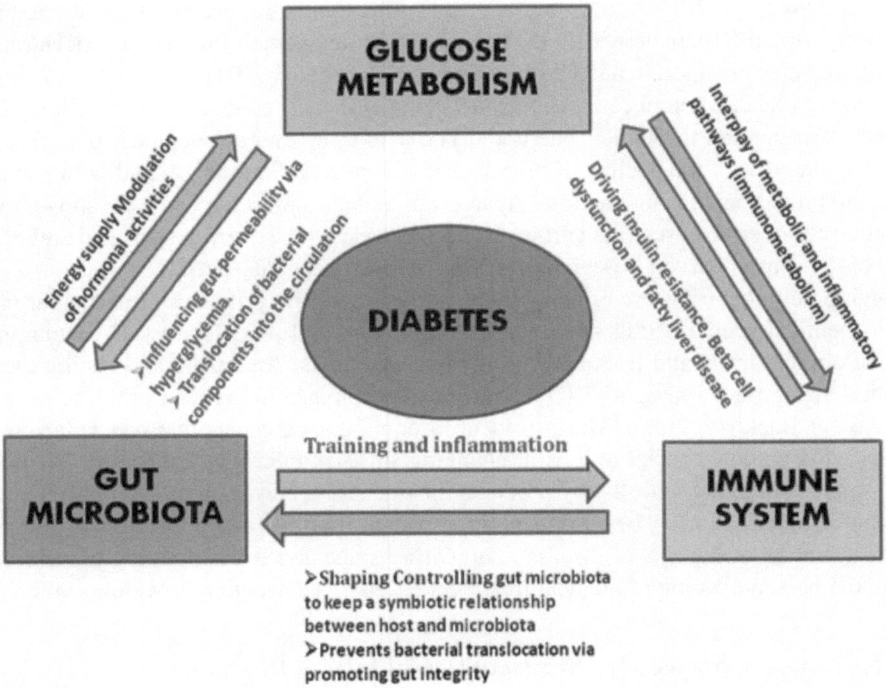

FIGURE 8.1 Interaction between gut microbiota, immune system, and glucose metabolism may drive diabetes.

8.2.3 Implications of Dysbiosis in Diabetes Development and Progression

Dysbiosis either results in an overabundance of harmful microbes and a proportional reduction of helpful microbes or an excess of pathogenic organisms. Any modification in the ratio of healthy microbiota indicates a direct relationship with T2DM (Huda et al., 2021). Dysbiosis is brought on by the interaction of the gut microbes with genes and environment that increase gut permeability and thus the movement of microbes and their secreted metabolites across it (Razmpoosh et al., 2019). Additionally, dysbiosis induces inflammation by increasing the production of ILs such as IL-6 (Hasain et al., 2020). It also results in the secretion of endotoxins in blood by the decaying microbes and the dysfunction of mitochondria in patients suffering from metabolic syndromes (Amoroso et al., 2020). Eventually, dysbiosis in intestinal microflora may increase the production of reactive species of oxygen and nitrogen like ROS and RNS by local bacteria (Hu et al., 2020).

Individuals with T2DM have significant gut microbiota dysbiosis (Zheng et al., 2022). In previous studies, it was discovered that Chinese T2DM patients have dysregulated gut microbiota (Qin et al., 2012). In particular, T2DM patients harbored increased levels of pathogenic microbes, including *E. coli*, *Cenarchaeum symbiosum*, and *Clostridium hathewayi*. Another study revealed that diabetic females in Europe had a greater abundance of Lactobacillus and a lesser abundance of *Clostridium* strains (Karlsson et al., 2013). Importantly, FBS and HbA1c were associated positively with *Lactobacillus* and negatively with *Clostridium* species, raising the possibility that they associate significantly with diabetes onset. Similarly, newly diagnosed T2DM patients had more *Lactobacillus* and fewer *Clostridium coccoides* and *Clostridium leptum* species in their gut (Chen et al., 2019). In a study by Shih et al. (2020) refractory T2DM patients in contrast to normal diabetics, had lower concentrations of *Fusobacterium* and *A. muciniphila* and greater concentrations of *B. vulgatus* and *Veillonella denticariosi* where *A. muciniphila* concentration was inversely related to HbA1c levels. Although dysbiosis of the microbiome is linked with T2DM, the exact cause behind this dysbiosis is yet to be known. The modulation of gut microbial homeostasis by a number of host chemicals is noteworthy. Sirtuin 1, a protein deacetylase, protects HFD-fed mice against metabolic problems in part by controlling the number of Firmicutes and Bacteroidetes (Caron et al., 2014). The beta cells have a transport protein for zinc ions, zinc transporter 8 (ZnT8). ZnT8 deficiency induces glucose intolerance by affecting the morphology and composition of the intestinal microbiome, resulting in increased chances of diabetes (Mao et al., 2019).

The GLP-1 secretion, insulin tolerance, and lipid profile were all improved in diabetic murine models that had a high concentration of *Acetatifactor* and *Bacteroides*, which produce lithocholic acid and prevent an increase in blood glucose levels (Pathak et al., 2018). TIMP3 alters the gut microbiome, causing inflammation by IL-6 (Mavilio et al., 2016). Overall, by altering the gut microbiota, these host proteins can reduce the risk of obesity and T2DM while improving metabolism to some extent. Instead, by causing dysbiosis in the gut microbiota, a few metabolites produced by an individual can also increase diabetes risk and the occurrence of associated co-morbidities. Inhibiting mTORC1 specifically with resveratrol reverses diabetes symptoms in mouse models, demonstrating the significance of mTORC1 in maintaining glucose homeostasis (Jung et al., 2016). Furthermore, mice fed with high-fat and fructose diets showed enhanced glucose tolerance and higher insulin levels when ANGPTL4 was lost (Janssen et al., 2018). *Adlercreutzia* and *Lactobacillus* were more prevalent in Angptl4$^{-/-}$ mice. Similar to this, the ablation of GLUT2 involved in the transport of glucose, may enhance glucose homeostasis through altering gut microbiome composition in mice models (Schmitt et al., 2017).

8.3 EFFECTS OF PROBIOTICS ON INSULIN LEVELS

8.3.1 Probiotics and Their Potential to Modulate Insulin Sensitivity

Probiotics are described as advantageous living organisms that have significant health (Hill et al., 2014). It was found to affect our immune system and the intestinal milieu apart from prevention of systemic illness and inflammation (Falcinelli et al., 2018) (Figure 8.2). The most popular probiotic bacteria are *Bifidobacterium* and *Lactobacillus* strains which constitute an integral part of probiotic supplements. The following three processes are possible for probiotics to use: Probiotics interact with gut flora to encourage the breakdown of complex sugar and fat molecules into simpler forms and regulate the synthesis of TNF-α, IL-6, etc. that cause inflammation. Their lowering can enhance insulin sensitivity and glycemic management (Han et al., 2019). Probiotics modulate key signaling processes to enhance or suppress TLRs and nucleotide-binding oligomerization domain-containing receptors (Sáez-Lara et al., 2016). Yoo and Kim showed that supplementation with healthy microbes affects the occurrence of various metabolic disorders like diabetes and maintains a healthy heart functioning by maintaining insulin levels and altering lipid profiles (Yoo & Kim, 2016). Probiotic supplementation enhanced insulin levels and reversed diabetes symptoms in pregnant ladies (Pan et al., 2021). In other trials, probiotic administration was reported to reduce the symptoms of T2DM, including better insulin response, increased intestinal integrity, and reduced ER stress (Park et al., 2015; Balakumar et al., 2018; Lim, 2016). Probiotics lower oxidative stress, decreasing intestinal permeability, and suppressing inflammation via NF-B signaling. Through a variety of possible modes of action, SCFA is essential for maintaining glucose homeostasis. SCFA's and GPCR receptors promote insulin production and lower glucagon levels resulting in suppression of hunger. Inflammation and oxidative stress can be decreased by SCFA via reducing intestinal permeability and circulating endotoxins. Apart from this SCFA also prevents the breakdown of lipid triglycerides into glycerol and free fatty acids and enhances insulin action via 5'-AMP-activated protein kinase signaling. GPR41/FFAR3 and GPR43/FFAR2 are also upregulated with SCFA in the colon which induces secretion of GLP-1 and PYY reduces glucagon production from the pancreas and promotes insulin production (Kim et al., 2018).

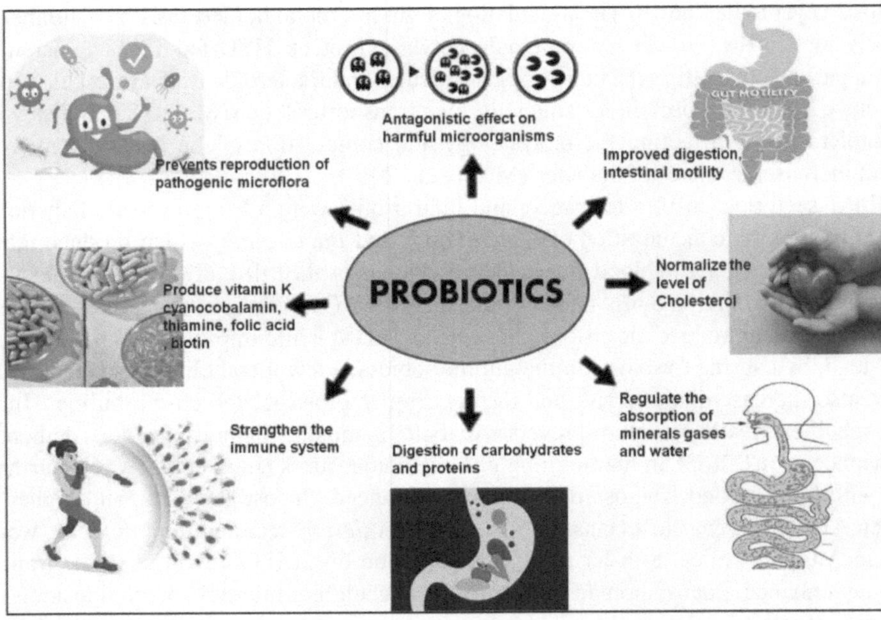

FIGURE 8.2 Biological function of probiotics.

SCFA can play significant roles in reducing inflammation and lipolysis while also controlling the production of energy (Delzenne & Cani, 2011). SCFA can suppress these inflammatory mediators and SCFAs namely acetate, propionate, and butyrate decrease nitric oxide levels in T2DM subjects (Vinolo et al., 2011). LPS-stimulated TNF-α from neutrophils was decreased by SCFA. TNF-α, IL-1, IL-6, and NO were likewise lowered in murine macrophage cells (Tedelind et al., 2007; Liu et al., 2012). SCFA reduces inflammation by suppressing NF-κB and TNF-α synthesis (Usami et al., 2008). SCFA also lowers the concentration of MCP-1, IL-10 TNF-α apart from various other cytokines involved in systemic inflammation (Cox et al., 2009). It was also shown that SCFA controls gluconeogenesis from certain non-carbohydrate carbon compounds in the gut which is one possible mechanism by which it prevents T2DM and regulates glucose homeostasis. (De Vadder et al., 2014).

8.3.2 Influence of Probiotics on Glucose Homeostasis

Keeping up the normal level of glucose is critical for reducing the onset of disorders such as T2DM and associated complications (Li et al., 2022). The exact mechanism of how these probiotic supplementations decrease the risk of diabetes remains to be fully deciphered. Early research has already concentrated on the health advantages of probiotics, which may also help to alter the gut microbiota's morphology and composition. Mostly these probiotics are composed of higher concentrations of *Enterococcus*, *Lactobacillus*, *Streptococcus*, and *Lactococcus* apart from various *Bacillus*, *E.coli*, and *Saccharomyces* species. According to certain research, Firmicutes/Bacteroidetes ratio as well as *Ruminococcus/Clostridium* and *Barnesiellaceae/E. coli/Proteobacteria* ratio increased in diabetes. However, both the proportion of *Bacteroides/Verrucomicrobiae* and the number of butyric acids synthesizing strains significantly declined (Jia et al., 2017).

After consuming probiotic-fermented milk for one and a half months glucose level was maintained in a trial on humans (Toshimitsu et al., 2019). Administration of probiotics with *Lactobacillus casei* for a month maintained levels of insulin and glucose homeostasis. Two probiotics (*Lactobacillus reuteri* ADR-1 and ADR-3) had a beneficial impact on diabetic patients (Hulston et al., 2015).

Lactobacillus plantarum OLL2712 supplementation for 3 months improved FBS, glycated albumin levels, and insulin sensitivity (Toshimitsu et al., 2019).

Paraprobiotic *Lacticaseibacillus casei 01* decreased sugar levels in non-diabetic individuals (Barros et al., 2021). A clinical trial with a 6-month multistrain administration of probiotics lowered the HOMA-IR index, secretion of endotoxin, and inflammatory mediators in residents of Arab (Sabico et al., 2019). Additionally, the beneficial results of multistrain supplementation of Symbiter included a reduction in cytokines (IL-1β, IL-6, and TNF-α) and BMI along with a reduction in the HOMA-IR index (Kobyliak et al., 2018). Another study with 8-week *L. acidophilus La5* and *Bifidobacterium lactis Bb12* supplementation resulted in a lowering of glucose concentration, increased insulin sensitivity, and better HOMA-IR index. Hsieh et al. (2018), Kobyliak et al. (2018), and Mohamadshahi et al. (2014) showed a decline in HbA1c levels after taking a probiotic preparation. Administration of *L. acidophilus* in murine models showed a significant impact on the expression of genes controlling glucose transport as well as fat metabolism (Sun et al., 2019) similar findings were also reported in another study with *L. acidophilus* administration in diabetic mice models where it modulated glucose and lipid profile and decreased diabetic symptoms.

Diabetic subjects administered with probiotic yogurt had lower FBS and HbA1c levels while much greater superoxide dismutase, glutathione peroxidase, and enhanced antioxidant profile. Pregnant women administered with *B. lactis* and *Lactobacillus rhamnosus* experienced improved glucose levels. (Laitinen et al., 2009). These probiotic strains were found to secrete two (acetate), three (propionate), and four (butyrate) carbon chain SCFAs that reverse diabetes symptoms via secretion of GLP-1 and incretin (Belenguer et al., 2006).

Other plausible probiotic effects having a significant impact on the reversal of diabetes and its symptoms include improved immune response, reduced inflammation, decreased gut permeability, and reduced ROS production (Ejtahed et al., 2012; Yadav et al., 2008). T2DM subjects administered with yogurt containing *L. acidophilus* and *B. lactis* for one and a half months showed a decline in FBS and HbA1c accompanied by an increase in antioxidant enzymes like GPx and SOD (Ejtahed et al., 2012).

In females suffering from GD supplementation of *Bifiobacterium bifidum*, *L. acidophilus*, and *L. casei* increased insulin sensitivity (Karamali et al., 2016). Moreover, oral supplementation of *L. acidophilus* alone for one month improved sensitivity to insulin without affecting the inflammatory biomarker profile (Andreasen et al., 2010).

8.3.3 Impact of Probiotics on Insulin Secretion

T2DM is linked to inflammation, which is shown by the heightened concentration of cytokines (TNF-α and IL-6) in the blood that leads to inflammation. Intriguingly, studies have shown that the administration of healthy microbes can prevent T2DM by affecting the synthesis of IL-4 and IL-10 and decreasing the concentration of TNF-α, IL-6, and CRP (Brunkwall & Orho-Melander, 2017). These pro-inflammatory substances disrupt the signaling pathway of insulin by phosphorylating IRS-1, thus reducing the efficiency of beta cells and increasing insulin tolerance (Chen et al., 2015). By enhancing or cross-feeding relationships with other potentially advantageous microorganisms, probiotics might alter normal microbiome ratios that increase the secretion of insulin leading to a decline in insulin resistance and thus reverting classical diabetes symptoms (Corb Aron et al., 2021; Gurung et al., 2020).

Probiotic supplementation is anticipated to increase glucose tolerance global data shows the positive impact of probiotic administration in preventing the degradation and inflammation of beta cells (Wang G et al., 2020; Li et al., 2016; Zhang et al., 2021). In addition, Wang L et al. (2020) showed that probiotic therapy caused enhanced secretion of insulin and pancreatic morphology. In a study on murine models, *Lactobacillus gasseri* enhanced the production of insulin by increasing the rate of transcription of Ins1, Ins2, and PDX1 genes, and reduced inflammation of beta cells by maintaining glucose homeostasis (Niibo et al., 2019). Loss of chloride ions is also related to hyperglycemia, which was found to affect insulin secretion. In a rat investigation, the administration of *L. casei* boosted the expression of chloride channel protein 2 causing higher chloride levels and enhanced insulin production (Balakumar et al., 2018).

8.4 MECHANISMS OF PROBIOTIC ACTION IN DIABETES MELLITUS

8.4.1 Modulation of Gut Microbiota by Probiotics

Probiotic-mediated modulation of intestinal microflora might exert an anti-diabetic effect via lowering oxidative damage, and inflammatory cytokines and maintaining intestinal integrity (Huda et al., 2021). Probiotics may regulate intestinal microbiome composition by inhibiting pathogenic microbial colonization by competing for colonization sites with each other and SCFAs and toxin production. Probiotics have the potential to modify human gut flora by blocking dangerous bacteria like Desulfovibrio and increasing helpful bacteria like lactic acid bacteria (Liu et al., 2021).

Evidence shows that probiotics can increase the intestinal microbial population, resulting in better T2DM management, as well as improved intestinal permeability, lower LPS in circulation, ER stress, and insulin resistance (Balakumar et al., 2018). Probiotics' effect on gut microflora has been studied and proven by preclinical trials on animal models and clinical trials on humans. Following probiotic addition, two studies discussed microbiota analysis and observed altered microbiota composition. Andreasen et al. (2010) discovered a considerable increase in the number of *L. acidophilus* species from undetectable numbers before intervention. Firouzi et al. (2017) discovered a 4.5-fold rise in the abundance of Bifidobacterium species and a two-fold rise in Lactobacillus species. Pretreatment with probiotics containing *L. acidophilus*, *Bifidobacterium infantis*, *Enterococcus faecalis*, and *Bacillus cereus* reduces the number of *Odoribacter*, *Desulfovibrio*, and *Mucispirillum*, while increasing the colonization of lactobacilli (Song et al., 2018). Yeast probiotic Saccharomyces boulardii increased the colonization of Bacteroidetes but decreased Tenericutes, Firmicutes, and Proteobacteria, which was associated with host metabolism changes indicating a role for S. boulardii in T2DM treatment (Everard et al., 2014). *B. lactis* HN019 effectively modulated microbiota since it increased bifidobacteria and lactobacilli levels considerably (Ahmed et al., 2007). These findings establish the role of probiotics in the maintenance and restoration of gut microbial balance by boosting the growth of helpful microbes while decreasing colonization of detrimental microbiota. However, the mechanism by which probiotics modulate gut microbiota is yet to be understood, probiotics may inhibit the colonization of pathogens by synthesizing SCFA and toxins, and by competing with pathogens for the site of colonization (Prabhurajeshwar & Chandrakanth, 2017; Sherman et al., 2009).

8.4.2 Probiotic Metabolites and Their Effect on Insulin-Signaling Pathways

Gut microbiota plays a critical role in the digestion and synthesizes metabolites by utilizing dietary components like lipids (linoleic acid-, berry-, ferulic acid-, catechin- and resveratrol-derived metabolites), carbohydrate (succinate, acetate, propionate, and butyrate) and protein (phenylacetic acid, hydrogen sulfide, and indole) that are associated with metabolic diseases. These probiotic metabolites directly target insulin-signaling pathways by increasing glucose influx and oxidation of lipids in muscle; decreasing the de novo synthesis of fatty acids and glucose while increasing oxidation of lipids in the hepatocytes; and improving thermogenic activity and inflammatory response in adipose tissue. As a result, gut-microbiota-synthesized metabolites, particularly SCFAs, increase the influx of glucose and oxidation of lipids in skeletal muscle, while in the hepatocytes, SCFAs decrease synthesis of fatty acids and glucose, increase oxidation of lipid via PI3K–AKT–PKB signaling pathway and AMP-activated protein kinase activation. SCFAs enhance adipocyte hyperplasia and thermogenesis, block lipolysis, and reduce the inflammatory response in adipose tissue (Figure 8.3) (Bastos & Rangel, 2022). In T2DM, receptor activation and detection by the luminal

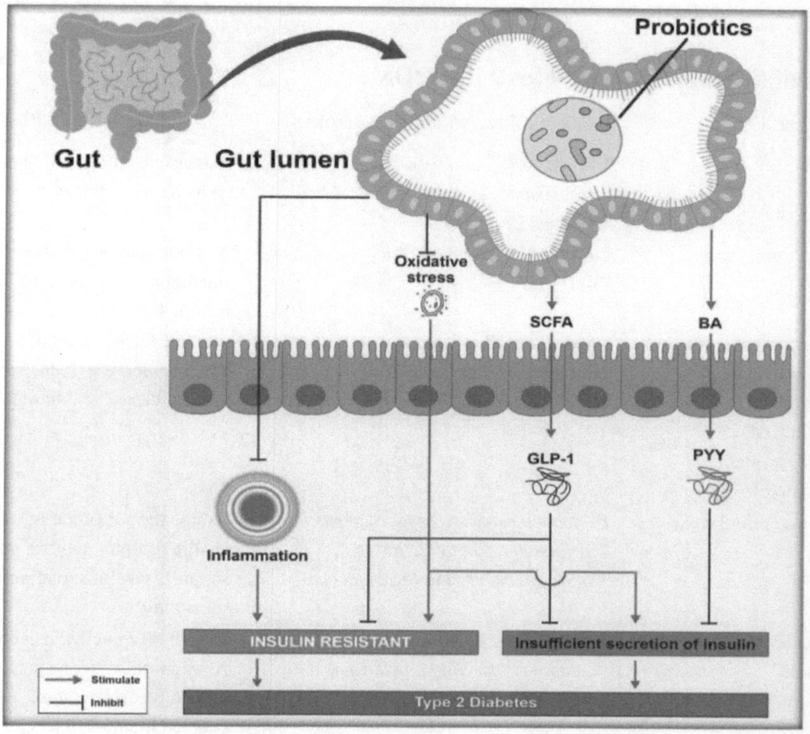

FIGURE 8.3 Molecular mechanism involved in the regulation of insulin by probiotics in type 2 diabetes.

microbiota in the intestine might phosphorylate serine residues in IRS-1, causing inflammation and lower insulin sensitivity (Gomes et al., 2014).

Important bacteria-derived metabolite and their role in T2DM is shown in Table 8.1. SCFA, an important microbiota metabolite in the colon is principally produced by *Coprococcus*, *Ruminococcus*, *Faecalibacterium*, *Megasphaera*, *Anaerostipes*, *Marvinbryantia*, *Eubacterium*, *Roseburia*, and *Blautia*. SCFA maintains blood glucose levels by stimulating the synthesis of glucagon-like peptide-1 (GLP-1) and peptide YY in the intestine increasing insulin release, delaying gastric emptying, and reducing hunger (Huda et al., 2021). Other microbiota-produced metabolites like TMA, histidine and tryptophan catabolite, bile acids, and hydrogen sulfide investigated for their role in diabetes found that they regulate host metabolic pathways, immune system, expression of genes, and integrity of intestinal epithelium (Huda et al., 2021).

8.4.3 Immunomodulatory Effects of Probiotics in Diabetes

Insulin resistance and diabetes have been linked with changes in the synthesis or activity of innate immunity proteins, inflammatory cytokines circulating in the blood, and cellular pattern-recognition receptors (Fernández-Real & Pickup, 2012). Bifidobacterium spp. Administration elevated innate immune response protein levels such as IB kinase alpha (IKK), nuclear factor kappa B inhibitor alpha (IB), protein kinase B (Akt), and extracellular-signal-regulated kinase 2 (ERK2). Akt may influence IKKα and activate IκBα, which may in turn block the action of NF-κB and, result in lower transcription of target genes encoding pro-inflammatory cytokines. ERK is an intracellular signaling enzyme involved in cellular proliferation, differentiation, and survival. Elevated ERK2 concentration in diabetic mice given *Bifidobacterium* spp. may stimulate adipocyte differentiation

TABLE 8.1
Association of Microbial Metabolites with T2DM.

Microbial Metabolite	Metabolite Producing Microbes	Association with T2DM
Trimethylamine	*Edwardsiella*, *Anaerococcus*, *Providencia*, *Desulphovibrio*, *Proteus*, *Clostridium*	Mediates hepatic insulin-signaling pathway and decreases glucose tolerance
Branched-chain amino acids	*Lactobacillus*, *Leuconostoc*, *Weissella*	Phosphorylate serine on insulin receptor substrate-1 by mTOR/S6 kinase affects insulin signaling
Tryptophan catabolites: indole; indoleacetic-, indolelactic-, indoleacrylic-, and indolepropionic acid; indolealdehyde; tryptamine; and 3-methylindole	*Clostridium*, *Ruminicoccus*, *Bacteroides*, *Lactobacillus*, *Bifidobacterium*, *Peptostreptococcus*,	Stimulate GLP-1 secretion and delay gastric emptying; reduce appetite, insulin release, and blood glucose level
Histidine catabolite: imidazole propionate	*Pectobacterium*, *Dickeya*, *Eggerthella*, *Citrobacter*, *Lactobacillus*, *Staphylococcus*, and *Streptococcus*	Mediate the activation mTORC1, inhibit insulin receptor substrates (IRS), and suppress insulin signaling and sensitivity
Bile acids: lithocholic acid and deoxycholic acid	*Eubacterium*, *Bacteroides*, *Lactobacillus*, *Bifidobacterium*, *Peptostr*, *Listeria*, *Clostridium*	Activate host nuclear receptors (famesoid X, vitamin D, pregnane X, RAR-related orphan receptor gamma, and G-protein coupled membrane receptor, membrane-type bile acid receptor) and regulate insulin sensitivity and expression of gluconeogenic genes

and increase insulin sensitivity. Furthermore, LGG therapy reduced macrophage infiltration and activation required for the onset and amplification of adipose tissue inflammation achieving the insulin-sensitizing action of LGG via inflammatory route (Miraghajani et al., 2017).

Probiotics could recognize pattern-recognition receptors (TLRs) expressed on immune cells and then regulate important signaling pathways, producing mitogen-activated protein kinases and NF-κB and communicating with the host. Furthermore, the innate immune system may be stimulated, leading to the generation of anti-inflammatory and pro-inflammatory cytokines (Liu et al., 2022). *L. rhamnosus*, *Lactobacillus helveticus*, and *Lactococcus casei* activate the innate immune system by elevating phagocytosis of macrophage, levels of ROS, NF-κB pp65, and TLR2 signaling. *Lactobacillus johnsonii* increases macrophage phagocytosis and promotes interleukin-1β (IL-1β) and Cd80 expression. *L. gasseri* orally administered boosted IgA synthesis in lamina propria and Peyer's patches by stimulating the expression of transforming growth factor β (TGF-β) and activation of TLR2 signaling (Liu et al., 2022). Stimulation of TLRs regulates anti-inflammatory cytokines and delays autoimmune disorders. TLR-regulated effects of probiotics via cytokines like TGF-β and interleukin (IL-10) and regulatory T cells protect from spontaneous diabetes (Miraghajani et al., 2017). Probiotic supplements avert and treat T2DM by reducing levels of inflammatory cytokines like TNF-α, CRP, and IL-6, and elevating levels of anti-inflammatory cytokines like interleukin-4 and 10 (Ding et al., 2021). TNF-α and serum CRP levels were significantly reduced after high dose, multistrain, probiotic powder/capsule supplement for a brief intervention period. Dysbiosis of the gut microflora may increase inflammatory biomarkers like TNF-α and CRP, resulting in abnormal activation of the immune system and persistent inflammation in T2DM patients (Ding et al., 2021). *Lactobacillus casei*'s diabetes-protective activity was associated with a low concentration of circulatory IL-6, CRP, and neutrophils, and a reduction in low-grade inflammation. *L. casei* lowers plasma glucose levels by improving aberrant post-immune responses by regulation of INF-γ and IL-2 production and decreased CD3 positive and CD4 positive T cell numbers (Miraghajani et al., 2017). *L. plantarum* treatment lowers visceral fat deposition, limits the synthesis of inflammatory adipokines, and disrupts the insulin-signaling system in peripheral tissues, and insulin sensitivity (Miraghajani et al., 2017). *L. johnsonii* promotes the innate immune response by activating membrane-bound receptors expressed on gut epithelium which stimulate type 1 INF, critical in innate immune response, resulting in a higher level of immune response avoiding diabetes. Furthermore, *L. johnsonii* regulates T-helper 17 cells (Th17) in the mesenteric lymph nodes (essential for diabetogenesis) and averts or delays type 1 diabetes (Miraghajani et al., 2017).

8.5 PRECLINICAL AND CLINICAL TRIALS ON PROBIOTICS IN DIABETES

8.5.1 Preclinical Trials on Probiotics in Diabetes

Preclinical investigation of the significance of probiotics in T2DM is extremely important given the disease's high incidence and the prospect of a novel alternative medicine to improve the quality of life. Furthermore, because probiotics are widely available and inexpensive, they may constitute an intriguing adjunct therapy option for T2DM. Recent research suggests that taking multistrain probiotics orally improves glucose tolerance, boosts antioxidant status, and reduces chronic inflammation (Singh et al., 2017). Diabetic mice treated with lactobacilli strains showed improved oxidative stress balance, notably in the liver (Dang et al., 2018).

Experimental animals used are mostly murine models as they are economical, manageable, and conveniently available, enabling researchers to employ more number of animal models in their preclinical studies, thereby generating results with high-quality evidence and more reliability. 54% of studies employed rats (*Rattus norvegicus*) as the primary animal model, while mice (*Mus musculus*) were utilized in 46% of studies; 87.5% of the animal models used in the research were males, whereas the use of female subjects was not reported. In terms of rat species, most studies chose Wistar rats (29%), followed by Sprague–Dawley rats (16%) and Goto–Kakizaki rats (4%). In terms of mouse lineages, more than 30% of the research employed C57BL/6J mice, whereas 4% used C57BL/KS/J and KKAy animals. The age of all the animals ranged from 3 to 8 weeks while the sample size ranged from 18 to 105 experimental animals. Studies show the use of male animal models over females, the reason for preference could be that female mouse models require more anti-inflammatory bacteria to maintain a healthy gut, which may increase the required probiotic dosage or the duration of probiotic administration. Given this basic difference, it becomes necessary to do research on probiotic therapy in both males and females to avoid bias in research findings (Marques et al., 2020).

The probiotic therapy duration is usually from 3 to 18 weeks. Among the probiotic strains studied, 92% of the studies used *Lactobacillus* strains singly or as mixtures with bacterial strains from genera of *Pediococcus*, *Lactococcus*, *Bifidobacterium*, *Bacillus*, *Rhizopus*, and yeasts and also *A. muciniphila* and *C. butyricum*. Regarding the mode of administration, 46% of the trials employed oral probiotic treatment, 29% used oral via gavage, and 25% administered probiotics in meals (Shubat, Tempeh, and fermented paste, juice, and milk). Irrespective of the probiotic used as a therapy for T2DM, the provided dosage varied from 10 to 10^{10} CFUs per milliliter for 4 to 18 weeks duration in the included trials.

Ninety-six percent of the preclinical research reported the concentration effect of probiotic supplements on reduction in blood glucose demonstrating the benefit of probiotic intervention for T2DM treatment however, in 4% of studies probiotics had no impact on T2DM treatment. T2DM markers improved in 22.92% of trials that employed *Lactobacillus* strains singly or as mixtures with other microorganisms as probiotics. Higher glucose tolerance, better inflammatory state, higher antioxidant activity, delayed stomach absorption of glucose, and reduced gluconeogenesis were among the underlying mechanisms (Marques et al., 2020). The effects of a few probiotic strains on T2DM in animal models are summarized in Table 8.2.

TABLE 8.2
Effects of Probiotic Strains on T2DM in Animal Models

Probiotic Species	Effects	References
Lactbacillus plantarum CCFM0236	Decreases plasma glucose level and insulin intolerance	Li et al. (2016)
L. plantarum Ln4	Decreases insulin resistance, increases insulin sensitivity	Lee et al. (2018)
L. plantarum MTCC 5690 and *Lactobacillus Fermentum* MTCC 5689	Decrease glucose level, HbA1c, plasma insulin, and HOMA-IR	Balakumar et al. (2018)
L. paracasei TD062	Decreases FBS and glucose tolerance	Dang et al. (2018)
Lactobacillus crispatus, *Lactobacillus reuteri*, and *Bacillus subtilis*	Decrease plasma glucose level and HbA1c and increase blood insulin level	Memarrast et al. (2017)
Lactobacillus kefiranofaciens, *Lactobacillus helveticus*, *L. plantarum*, *Lactococcus lactis*, and *Issatchenkia orientalis*	Decrease FBS, OGTT, HbAlc, IRI	Manaer et al. (2021)
Bifidobacterium longum	Decreases blood glucose level and renal function damage	Lin et al. (2018)
B. longum DD98 and Se–*B. longum* DD98	Decrease FBS and HbA1c	Zhao et al. (2020)
Inactivated *B. longum BR-108*	Decreases plasma glucose level	Ben Othman and Sakamoto (2020)
Bifidobacterium animalis 01	Decreases OGTT and HOMA-IR and inflammatory cytokines	Zhang et al. (2020)
L. plantarum OLL2712	Decreases plasma glucose level and IL-1β	Sakai et al. (2013)
Lactobacillus casei CCFM419	Decreases FBS, glucose intolerance, insulin intolerance, TNF-α, and IL-6 and increases GLP-1	Wang et al. (2017)
Lactobacillus rhamnosus NCDC 17	Decreases FBS, plasma insulin, and HbA1c level	Singh et al. (2017)
Lactobacillus paracasei NL41	Decreases insulin intolerance, HbA1c level, glucagon, and oxidative damage	Zeng et al. (2019)
L. rhamnosus, *Lactobacillus acidophilus*, and *Bifidobacterium bifidum*	Decrease blood glucose level, intestinal integrity, LPS translocation, and inflammation	Bagarolli et al. (2017)
Clostridium butyricum CGMCC0313.1	Decreases FBS, HbA1c, inflammatory response, and increase GLP-1	Jia et al. (2017)
Lactobacillus salivarius AP-32 and *L. reuteri* GL-104	Decrease FBS	Hsieh et al. (2020)
L. plantarum HAC01	Decreases FBS and HbA1c and increases insulin-positive β-cell	Lee et al. (2021)
Lactobacillus delbrueckii subsp. Lactis PTCC1057	Decreases FBS	Hallajzadeh et al. (2021)
Streptococcus thermophilus	Decreases FBS, glucose resistance, LPS, IL-6, and TNF-α and increase IL-10 level	Gao et al. (2019)
L. plantarum, *Lactobacillus bulgaricus*, *L. casei*, *L. acidophilus*, *Bifidobacterium infantis*, *B. longum*, *Bifidobacterium breve*	Decrease plasma glucose and increase GLP-1 and antioxidant activity	Pegah et al. (2021)

8.5.2 Clinical Trials on Probiotics in Diabetes

Clinical trials, particularly RCTs, form the basis of evidence-based therapeutics and advancement in clinical medicine. Many therapeutic alternatives established during the past 2 decades have improved the quality of life of diabetic individuals. The diversity of T2DM etiologies and consequences has made blood glucose control and complication prevention and management of diabetes challenging (Long et al., 2021). A RCT is suggested to probe the efficacy of probiotic supplements as an adjuvant treatment to improve glucose homeostasis in T2DM by modifying intestinal microbiota composition and hormone production. Probiotic supplements are thought to help blood glucose management and diabetes-associated co-morbidities in T2DM individuals. Probiotic supplements are thought to control blood glucose levels and diabetes-associated co-morbidities in people with T2DM. Clinical studies would testify to probiotic intervention as an adjuvant treatment in the treatment of T2DM. Many clinical trials have been done in recent decades to assess the anti-diabetic properties of probiotic formulations using strains belonging to genera *Lactobacillus* (*L. casei*, *L. acidophilus*, *L. reuteri*, *L. salivarius*, *Lactobacillus brevis*), *Bifidobacterium* (*B. lactis*, *B. longum*, *B. bifidum*), *Lactococcus* (*L. lactis*), *Propionibacterium*, and *Acetobacter*. The intervention time ranged from 4 to 24 weeks of administration of a single or combination of microbial species, or the flora of the intervention group's probiotic yogurt enriched with particular strains.

L. acidophilus, *L. rhamnosus*, *L. bulgaricus*, *L. casei*, *Streptococcus thermophiles*, and *B. breve*, *B. longum*, reduced FBS, increased serum insulin, and improved glycaemic status. *L. lactis*, *L. acidophilus*, *Lactococcus casei*, *B. longum*, *B. infantis*, and *B. bifidum* failed to improve HOMA-IR except for a small improvement in fasting insulin and HbA1c levels. Probiotic strains of *Lactobacillus*, *Lactococcus*, *Bifidobacterium*, *Propionibacterium*, and *Acetobacter* genera ameliorate insulin resistance. This data is summarized in Table 8.3 (Kesika et al., 2019).

For 8 weeks, a probiotic preparation containing various concentrations of *L. bulgaricus*, *L. acidophilus*, *L. rhamnosus*, *L. casei*, *S. thermophilus*, *Bifidobacterium breve*, and *B. longum* strains and also fructo-oligosaccharide (FOS) significantly lowered FBS levels in T2DM individuals compared to the control group. The probiotic and placebo groups both had higher levels of serum insulin. Furthermore, probiotic supplementation enhanced the concentration of glutathione in T2DM individuals, implying that probiotic supplements ameliorate the patient's antioxidant status and control diabetes by lowering glucose concentration in the blood (Asemi et al., 2013). A recent study reported that the same multistrain probiotic regimen, combined with FOS, improved blood glucose levels in T2DM patients. Despite the significant drop in FBS, insulin resistance or insulin levels remain unaffected. Despite the fact that supplementing a multistrain probiotic mixture with FOS increased FBS levels in T2DM individuals, further research is warranted to demonstrate the therapeutic activity of probiotic therapies (Razmpoosh et al., 2019).

For 12 weeks, a multistrain probiotic preparation (10^{10} CFU daily dose; *Lactococcus lactis*, *L. acidophilus*, *L. casei*, *B. longum*, *B. infantis*, and *B. bifidum*) intervention showed no improvement in insulin sensitivity index and HOMA-IR, except for a modest improvement in fasting plasma insulin level and HbA1c levels (Firouzi et al., 2017).

Symbiter (a mixture of varying doses of 14 probiotic strains of *Lactobacillus*, *Bifidobacterium*, *Lactococcus*, *Acetobacter*, and *Propionibacterium* genera) supplementation for eight weeks duration improved insulin sensitivity in T2DM individuals. Particularly, the HOMA-IR and HbA1c levels declined considerably in the probiotic-supplemented group as compared to the control group (Kobyliak et al., 2018).

Mirjalili et al. (2023) in the clinical trial (IRCT20220226054125N1) investigated how probiotic yogurt consumption affected plasma glucose levels in 72 T2DM individuals for 12 weeks of intervention and found no difference in FBS or HbA1c levels. After controlling for baseline covariate values, the IG had a significantly lower HbA1c than the PG but a decrease in FBS was found to be non-significant ($P > 0.05$). Probiotic yogurt eating may be beneficial for T2DM individuals. There is a need for more carefully designed clinical studies with long-term intervention.

According to these clinical trial findings, all probiotic strains have a favorable effect in modulating glycemic response. Probiotics have a good or minor impact, but no harmful effects have been seen in any trials. However, no two research with the same goal have produced the same results. Furthermore, investigations focusing on autoimmune illness and hypersensitivity in relation to probiotic administration are required. A sufficient level of immunological response induced by the ingestion of probiotics would validate the tests.

TABLE 8.3
RCT on Probiotic Intervention in T2DM Patients

Probiotic Species	Period (Weeks)	Findings	References
Lactobacillus reuteri DSM 17938	12	Improves insulin sensitivity, but HbA1c remains unaffected	Mobini et al. (2017)
Lactococcus casei, *Lactobacillus rhamnosus*, *L. acidophilus*, *Lactobacillus bulgaricus*, *Streptococcus thermophilus*, *Bifidobacterium breve*, *Bifidobacterium longum*	8	Decrease FBS, increase serum insulin, LDL level, and HOMA-IR	Asemi et al. (2013)
L. casei 431	8	Decreases FBG, insulin, and insulin resistance	Khalili et al. (2019)
L. acidophilus, *L. casei*, *L. rhamnosus*, *L. bulgaricus*, *Bifidobacterium breve*, *B. longum*, *S. thermophilus*, and FOS	6	Decrease FBS, increase HDL, but TG, TC, and insulin level remains unaffected	Razmpoosh et al. (2019)
L. acidophilus, *Bifidobacterium lactis*, *Bifidobacterium bifidum*, *B. longum*	24	Decrease FBS, HbA1c, and HOMA-IR	Kassaian et al. (2018)
Yogurt enriched with *L. acidophilus* La5 and *B. lactis* Bb-12	4	Decrease FBS, HbA1c, TG, and LDL	Rezaei et al. (2017)
Lactobacillus salivarius UBLS, *L. casei* UBLC42, *L. plantarum* UBLP40, *L. acidophilus* UBLA34, *B. breve* UBBR01, *Bacillus coagulans* UniqueIS2, and FOS	12	Decrease FBS, postprandial plasma sugar, insulin level, and HOMA-IR	Venkataraman et al. (2019)
B. bifidum W23, *B. lactis* W52, *L. acidophilus* W37, *Lactobacillus brevis* W63, *L. casei* W56, *L. salivarius* W24, *L. lactis* W19, and *L. lactis* W58	12	Decrease HOMA-IR	Sabico et al. (2017)
L. acidophilus, *L. casei*, *Lactococcus lactis*, *B. bifidum*, *B. longum*, and *Bifidobacterium infantis*	12	Decrease HbA1c and fasting insulin level	Firouzi et al. (2017)
Lactobacilli, *Bifidobacteria*, *S. thermophilus*, and FOS	9	Decrease FBS and HbA1c	Ebrahimi et al. (2017)
Symbiter containing 14 probiotic strains of lactobacilli, lactococci, bifidobacteria, propionibacteria, and *Acetobacter* genera	8	Decrease HbA1c, TNF-α, IL-1β, and HOMA-IR	Kobyliak et al. (2018)
L. reuteri ADR-1 and *L. reuteri* ADR-3	39	Decrease HbA1c	Hsieh et al. (2018)

8.6 CHALLENGES AND FUTURE DIRECTIONS

8.6.1 Limitations of Current Research on Probiotics in Diabetes Mellitus

Probiotics have a wide range of positive health advantages, but they could be beneficial only if a significant amount of live cells move to the small intestine. It has been demonstrated that many probiotic bacteria in food are destroyed by oxygen at the time of product distribution and product storage. Other factors responsible for probiotics killing are low pH and the acidic nature of the stomach (Evivie, 2013). In a study, gut microbiota was structurally modulated by using a GQD (Chinese herbal formula) in the attenuation of type-2 diabetes was reported. However, this study could not provide any clear evidence related to GQD-induced changes in the gut microbiota directly contributing to an improvement in glucose homeostasis. (Zhang et al., 2012). The gut flora was found to be responsible for insulin resistance and DM development (He & Shi, 2017). Intestinal microbiota may have an impact on metabolic diseases through a variety of potential pathways such as the control of the inflammatory response, permeability of the stomach, metabolic processes of glucose, energy use, and synthesis and oxidation of fatty acids (Gurung et al., 2020).

Gut bacteria metabolize food components to produce TMA; it is later transformed into TMAO by the liver. Studies reported that patients with T2D have increased TMAO levels. Furthermore, studies performed on mice have demonstrated that TMAO can aggravate poor glucose tolerance and increase fasting insulin levels by blocking the insulin-signaling pathway in the liver and generating inflammation in adipose tissue (Gao et al., 2014). A prospective study discovered that a higher consumption of phosphatidylcholine—the building block for the creation of TMAO—was independently associated with a higher risk of T2D (Li et al., 2015).

The current research studies using probiotics for the treatment of pre-diabetes, and DM show non-significant evidence in reference to glucose metabolism, lipid metabolism, and body composition. (Wang et al., 2021). Other challenges are inoculation, and evaluation of the viable counts of the probiotic strains, particularly when multiple probiotic strains are added. Probiotics must withstand specific technological challenges, including low pH, the presence of antimicrobial substances, high osmotic pressure, and oxygen (Antoine, 2011). Other limitations are the minimum effective dose and quantitative-effective connection of recognized beneficial probiotic strains. For example, a study was performed in which diabetes patients got 12 weeks of supplementation with one strain of *L. reuteri* DSM 17938 at two different doses (10^8 or 10^{10} CFU per day) and no improvement in HbA1c level was noted. Later the high dose of DSM 17938 supplements to the patients improved the insulin sensitivity index and serum deoxycholic acid (Mobini et al., 2017).

8.6.2 Potential Interactions and Side Effects of Probiotic Use

Presently, probiotics are frequently used as dietary supplements. They are a combination of live microorganisms that show health benefits when consumed by the human body. There is currently an enormous number of research studies being conducted with the idea "Probiotics are safe?" Probiotics are the microbes that already exist in the human body thus considered safe. Their intake may trigger some allergic reactions in the first few days after taking them. The side effects occur including mild stomach upset, flatulence, diarrhea, and bloating. Probiotics are generally safe for healthy individuals but certain people should exercise caution when utilizing probiotics supplements. The risk of infection is common in individuals who have compromised immune systems (undergoing chemo/radiotherapy), recent surgery, or any serious illness. Furthermore, in some individuals it may heighten the risk of developing infection, acquiring antibiotic resistance, or developing harmful by-products.

8.6.2.1 Potential Impact of Probiotics Usage on Medication Efficiency and Metabolism

Probiotics are found to provide positive effects in preventing and treating a wide range of diseases. Recent meta-analysis and clinical trials show the clinical utility of these probiotic microorganisms in the diagnosis, treatment, and prevention of disorders like cancer, high blood pressure, hypercholesterolemia, and type 2 DM (T2DM). Despite a large number of researches conducted on this aspect, the efficiency of probiotics in disease treatment is still not distinctly proven. The complete probiotics mode of action in the human body is also not clearly explained. Studies revealed that probiotics may enhance the efficacy of the immune system by supporting both innate and adaptive immunity. In addition, probiotics may affect the pharmacokinetics by influencing the absorption and activities of the gut microbiota's metabolism, which in turn change the drug's bioavailability. Probiotics may change the activity of intestinal transporters that transport drugs throughout the gut wall, change the composition of the gut microbiota, modify the activation or inhibition of microbial enzyme activity, or use drugs as "surrogate" substrates for its growth. Sulfasalazine is a disease-modifying anti-rheumatic drug that is widely used to treat rheumatoid arthritis and inflammatory bowel illnesses. Sulfasalazine is designed as a prodrug (azo-derivate), which the gut flora transforms into active metabolites. Sulfasalazine taken orally is absorbed in the intestine (10–30%), remaining 70% is used as a substrate by bacterial azoreductases to produce sulfapyridine and 5-aminosalicylic acid (5-ASA). Although azoreduction can also occur in the liver, colon reduction is essential for the activation of sulfasalazine. The presence of sulfapyridine in the serum appears to show adverse effects of sulfasalazine treatment resulting in nausea and abdominal discomfort. Sulfasalazine is found to be more toxic than olsalazine or balsalazide, this is because sulfasalazine azoreduction is generally much quicker than that of other prodrugs.

A common diabetes drug called gliclazide is known for its considerable interindividual variations in therapeutic response. A distinct synergistic effect was investigated between gliclazide, probiotics, and bile acids. This impact is illustrated by a decrease in the level of blood glucose and alleviation of diabetic problems. A recent in vitro study in which a probiotic combination of *L. acidophilus*, *L. rhamnosus*, and *Lactobacillus lactis* revealed that gliclazide uses passive diffusion and active transport mechanism to penetrate the probiotic bacterial membrane before being broken down by bacterial enzymes through hydroxylation and hydrolysis (Mikov et al., 2018).

8.6.2.2 Side Effects of Probiotics Use

Research studies on probiotics usage revealed health benefits in several clinical disorders but few of them show conflicting results.

- Biogenic amines are compounds that are formed due to bacterial fermentation of foods containing protein. These biogenic amines are present in some probiotic-rich food, including yogurt, sauerkraut, and kimchi. The most common amines are histamine, tyramine, tryptamine, and phenylethylamine, found in a probiotic-rich diet. Amines can stimulate the central nervous system, alter blood flow, and cause headaches in those who are sensitive to the drug (Turna et al., 2024).
- Some bacterial strains included in probiotic supplements can cause histamine production in human digestive tracts (Pugin et al., 2017). In addition, the immune system often releases the chemical histamine when it recognizes a threat. Blood arteries expand when histamine levels rise, supplying more blood to the affected area (Kyriakidis et al., 2012). Additionally, the veins become more permeable, allowing immune cells to more quickly enter the appropriate region and fight off any invaders. The affected area becomes red and swollen as a result of this process, which can also cause allergy symptoms including itching, watery eyes, a runny nose, or difficulty breathing (Kovacova-Hanuskova et al., 2015).
- Many probiotic supplements contain milk sugar, often known as lactose. There have been case reports of adverse effects of probiotics. Additionally, studies demonstrate that those with lactose sensitivity can consume up to 400 mg of lactose in medications or supplements (Montalto et al., 2008).

8.6.3 Future Directions for Research and Clinical Applications of Probiotics in Diabetes

According to the ISAPP, probiotics are bacteria that when properly provided boost the health of the host (Hill et al., 2014). Probiotics have an impact on the host through changes in intestinal permeability and mucosal immune response, alteration of appetite-regulating hormones, and regulation of the gut endocannabinoid system, which is hypothesized to be associated with inflammation and diabetes (Fatima, 2017). Probiotics have been proven to improve insulin sensitivity and reduce autoimmune responses by regulating the microflora in the gut and reducing oxidative stress and cellular immune responses. Moreover, probiotics' modulation of the intestinal microbiota regulates the host's metabolism by altering how food is broken down for energy and by biochemically transforming chemicals generated from the host or the gut microorganisms themselves. It is obvious that healthy intestinal microbiota and intestinal function are essential for maintaining good health and preventing diabetes, and it appears optimistic that diabetic illness can be treated by changes in intestinal microbiota activity and composition (He et al., 2015).

Advancements in the latest research developed powerful tools used to alter the bacterial genome, known as NGPs. Well-tolerated GRAS food-derived bacteria can synthesize or act as a delivery system for a variety of bioactive compounds. *A. muciniphila*, a member of the Akkermansiaceae family, is a common, elliptic, gram-negative bacterium and is one of the candidates for NGPs. This bacterium primarily destroys intestinal epithelial mucin after colonizing the outer mucin layer of host intestinal epithelial cells. Additionally, it enhances the release of Foxp3+, Treg, interleukin-10, and tumor growth factor; lowers islet inflammation; thickens the intestinal mucin layer; stimulates the production of new mucin proteins in intestinal epithelial cells; and delays the onset of T1D (Hänninen et al., 2018).

Recent research observed that plasma TMAO levels are not insulin resistant but found a nonlinear relationship between plasma TMAO levels and pre-diabetes prevalence. Thus, further research is needed to provide a better explanation for the developing process of the association between plasma TMAO and diabetes (Roy et al., 2020). According to available experimental and clinical studies, it was hypothesized that further research studies formulated on the alteration of intestinal flora by probiotics may be useful in the management and prevention of diabetes. The studies performed demonstrate no negative effects and intriguing results. Furthermore, the focus on how pertinent factors including the progenitor microbe, the matrix, and the fermentation conditions influence the biological impact of postbiotics will further provide clues for future research on the treatment and alleviation of DM. This innovative area of research is a wonderful opportunity for investigators, physicians, biotechnologists, and food professionals to collaborate on this idea of the alteration of gastrointestinal microbiota by probiotics as a novel therapeutic candidate for the management and treatment of DM. Furthermore, the upcoming research is likely to be based on metagenomics and metatranscriptomics, as well as metaproteomics and metabolomics/metabonomics. This will provide a possible characterization of the microbiome in great detail by studying its genetic makeup, transcription products, and metabolic processes. It will also provide clinical applications for the management and treatment of diseases including DM.

8.7 CONCLUSION

Probiotics are crucial for both good health and conditions involving the metabolism of glucose. Probiotics can affect glucose homeostasis directly or indirectly in every cell of an organism, according to various scientific studies. By raising fasting insulin levels to lower fasting glucose, and maintaining healthy lipid levels, normalizing hypertension, the administration of healthy microbial strains significantly enhances glucose homeostasis and immune response. Probiotics may help people with T2DM produce fewer inflammatory markers and regulate their glycemic state by lowering insulin resistance. Even though the majority of the claimed benefits of probiotics have been established, and favorable outcomes have been attained, there still appears to be considerable heterogeneity in outcomes, particularly between human studies, as a consequence of a number of factors that may or may not have particular impacts. Due to varying environments and geographical locations, humans are somewhat genetically unique and different from one another. They also have unique eating habits that have a big impact on their microbiota and probiotics due to various flaws like insufficient sample size, supplement preparation, intervention monitoring, sampling, inconsistent measurement, question bias, and scarcity of study protocols. However, there have only been a few studies done on humans, and it is still unclear exactly how probiotics alter the gut microbiome and affect glucose homeostasis. Before starting probiotic therapy, more thought should be paid to the condition of the microbiota, which is seen as being as distinctive as a fingerprint.

The physiology of the patient, the quantity and variety of probiotics utilized, the length of the experiment, and the follow-up period all have an impact on the results of clinical studies. It is undoubtedly possible to have substantial knowledge of the processes and their impacts by standardizing methodological techniques in in vivo investigations. Therefore, before treatment, it is important to give careful thought to determine the most suitable strain for combating a particular disease, dosages and length, sample size, age of subject, food, and potential exercise undertaken. Further assessment of other metabolic parameters influencing glycaemic control as well as potential probiotic adverse effects are currently lacking in several methodological techniques. Clinical investigations were often carried out according to a set protocol. Given the aforementioned restrictions, the investigation into mechanisms involved in such research should be the prime focus to decipher more potential functions these probiotics hold in extensive bodily processes. Therefore, more thorough research is required to comprehend the relationship between the microbiome's function, probiotics' interactions with host microbiota, and diabetes management.

BIBLIOGRAPHY

Abdulla, H., Smith, K., Atherton, P. J., & Idris, I. (2016). Role of insulin in the regulation of human skeletal muscle protein synthesis and breakdown: A systematic review and meta-analysis. *Diabetologia*, *59*(1), 44–55. https://doi.org/10.1007/s00125-015-3751-0

Accili, D. (2018). Insulin action research and the future of diabetes treatment: The 2017 Banting medal for scientific achievement lecture. *Diabetes*, *67*(9), 1701–1709. https://doi.org/10.2337/dbi18-0025

Ahmed, M., Prasad, J., Gill, H., Stevenson, L., & Gopal, P. (2007). Impact of consumption of different levels of Bifidobacterium lactis HN019 on the intestinal microflora of elderly human subjects. *Journal of Nutrition, Health and Aging*, *11*(1), 26–31. https://doi.org/10.1016/j

Amoroso, C., Perillo, F., Strati, F., Fantini, M. C., Caprioli, F., & Facciotti, F. (2020). The role of gut microbiota biomodulators on mucosal immunity and intestinal inflammation. *Cells*, *9*(5), 1234. https://doi.org/10.3390/cells9051234

Andreasen, A. S., Larsen, N., Pedersen-Skovsgaard, T., Berg, R. M., Møller, K., Svendsen, K. D., Jakobsen, M., & Pedersen, B. K. (2010). Effects of *Lactobacillus acidophilus* NCFM on insulin sensitivity and the systemic inflammatory response in human subjects. *British Journal of Nutrition*, *104*(12), 1831–1838. https://doi.org/10.1017/S0007114510002874

Antoine, J. M. (2011). Current challenges for probiotics in food. In S. Lahtinne, S. Salminen, A. Von Wright & A. Ouwehand (Eds.), *Lactic acid bacteria: Microbiological and functional aspects* (pp. 213–226). CRC Press.

Asemi, Z., Zare, Z., Shakeri, H., Sabihi, S. S., & Esmaillzadeh, A. (2013). Effect of multispecies probiotic supplements on metabolic profiles, hs-CRP, and oxidative stress in patients with type 2 diabetes. *Annals of Nutrition and Metabolism*, *63*(1–2), 1–9. https://doi.org/10.1159/000349922

Asghari, G., Farhadnejad, H., Teymoori, F., Mirmiran, P., Tohidi, M., & Azizi, F. (2018). High dietary intake of branched-chain amino acids is associated with an increased risk of insulin resistance in adults. *Journal of Diabetes*, *10*(5), 357–364. https://doi.org/10.1111/1753-0407.12639

Bäckhed, F., Ding, H., Wang, T., Hooper, L. V., Koh, G. Y., Nagy, A., Semenkovich, C. F., & Gordon, J. I. (2004). The gut microbiota as an environmental factor that regulates fat storage. *Proceedings of the National Academy of Sciences of the United States of America*, *101*(44), 15718–15723. https://doi.org/10.1073/pnas.0407076101

Bagarolli, R. A., Tobar, N., Oliveira, A. G., Araújo, T. G., Carvalho, B. M., Rocha, G. Z., Vecina, J. F., Calisto, K., Guadagnini, D., Prada, P. O., Santos, A., Saad, S. T. O., & Saad, M. J. A. (2017). Probiotics modulate gut microbiota and improve insulin sensitivity in DIO mice. *Journal of Nutritional Biochemistry*, *50*, 16–25. https://doi.org/10.1016/j.jnutbio.2017.08.006

Balakumar, M., Prabhu, D., Sathishkumar, C., Prabu, P., Rokana, N., Kumar, R., Raghavan, S., Soundarajan, A., Grover, S., Batish, V. K., Mohan, V., & Balasubramanyam, M. (2018). Improvement in glucose tolerance and insulin sensitivity by probiotic strains of Indian gut origin in high-fat diet-fed C57BL/6J mice. *European Journal of Nutrition*, *57*(1), 279–295. https://doi.org/10.1007/s00394-016-1317-7

Barros, C. P., Grom, L. C., Guimarães, J. T., Balthazar, C. F., Rocha, R. S., Silva, R., Almada, C. N., Pimentel, T. C., Venâncio, E. L., Collopy Junior, I., Maciel, P. M. C., Freitas, M. Q., Esmerino, E. A., Silva, M. C., Duarte, M. C. K. H., Sant'Ana, A. S., & Cruz, A. G. (2021). Paraprobiotic obtained by ohmic heating added in whey-grape juice drink is effective to control postprandial glycemia in healthy adults. *Food Research International*, *140*, 109905. https://doi.org/10.1016/j.foodres.2020.109905

Bastos, R. M. C., & Rangel, É. B. (2022). Gut microbiota-derived metabolites are novel targets for improving insulin resistance. *World Journal of Diabetes*, *13*(1), 65–69. https://doi.org/10.4239/wjd.v13.i1.65

Bazotte, R. B., Silva, L. G., & Schiavon, F. P. (2014). Insulin resistance in the liver: Deficiency or excess of insulin? *Cell Cycle*, *13*(16), 2494–2500. https://doi.org/10.4161/15384101.2014.947750

Belenguer, A., Duncan, S. H., Calder, A. G., Holtrop, G., Louis, P., Lobley, G. E., & Flint, H. J. (2006). Two routes of metabolic cross-feeding between *Bifidobacterium adolescentis* and butyrate-producing anaerobes from the human gut. *Applied and Environmental Microbiology*, *72*(5), 3593–3599). https://doi.org/10.1128/AEM.72.5.3593-3599.2006

Ben Othman, M., & Sakamoto, K. (2020). Effect of inactivated *Bifidobacterium longum* intake on obese diabetes model mice (TSOD). *Food Research International*, *129*, 108792. https://doi.org/10.1016/j.foodres.2019.108792

Bergman, R. N. (2000). Non-esterified fatty acids and the liver: Why is insulin secreted into the portal vein? *Diabetologia*, *43*(7), 946–952. https://doi.org/10.1007/s001250051474

Blaut, M. (2013). Ecology and physiology of the intestinal tract. *Current Topics in Microbiology and Immunology*, *358*, 247–272. https://doi.org/10.1007/82_2011_192

Boutagy, N. E., McMillan, R. P., Frisard, M. I., & Hulver, M. W. (2016). Metabolic endotoxemia with obesity: Is it real and is it relevant? *Biochimie*, *124*, 11–20. https://doi.org/10.1016/j.biochi.2015.06.020

Bratanova-Tochkova, T. K., Cheng, H., Daniel, S., Gunawardana, S., Liu, Y. J., Mulvaney-Musa, J., Schermerhorn, T., Straub, S. G., Yajima, H., & Sharp, G. W. (2002). Triggering and augmentation mechanisms, granule pools, and biphasic insulin secretion. *Diabetes*, *51* (suppl_1), S83–S90. https://doi.org/10.2337/diabetes.51.2007.s83

Brunkwall, L., & Orho-Melander, M. (2017). The gut microbiome as a target for prevention and treatment of hyperglycaemia in Type 2 diabetes: From current human evidence to future possibilities. *Diabetologia*, *60*(6), 943–951. https://doi.org/10.1007/s00125-017-4278-3

Cani, P. D., & Delzenne, N. M. (2009). The role of the gut microbiota in energy metabolism and metabolic disease. *Current Pharmaceutical Design*, *15*(13), 1546–1558. https://doi.org/10.2174/138161209788168164

Caron, A. Z., He, X., Mottawea, W., Seifert, E. L., Jardine, K., Dewar-Darch, D., Cron, G. O., Harper, M. E., Stintzi, A., & McBurney, M. W. (2014). The SIRT1 deacetylase protects mice against the symptoms of metabolic syndrome. *FASEB Journal*, *28*(3), 1306–1316. https://doi.org/10.1096/fj.13-243568

Chen, L., Chen, R., Wang, H., & Liang, F. (2015). Mechanisms linking inflammation to insulin resistance. *International Journal of Endocrinology*, *2015*, 508409–508409. https://doi.org/10.1155/2015/508409

Chen, P. C., Chien, Y. W., & Yang, S. C. (2019). The alteration of gut microbiota in newly diagnosed Type 2 diabetic patients. *Nutrition*, *63–64*, 51–56. https://doi.org/10.1016/j.nut.2018.11.019

Coimbra, S., Oliveira, H., Reis, F., Belo, L., Rocha, S., Quintanilha, A., Figueiredo, A., Teixeira, F., Castro, E., Rocha-Pereira, P., & Santos-Silva, A. (2010). Circulating adipokine levels in Portuguese patients with psoriasis vulgaris according to body mass index, severity and therapy. *Journal of the European Academy of Dermatology and Venereology*, *24*(12), 1386–1394. https://doi.org/10.1111/j.1468-3083.2010.03647.x

Corb Aron, R. A., Abid, A., Vesa, C. M., Nechifor, A. C., Behl, T., Ghitea, T. C., Munteanu, M. A., Fratila, O., Andronie-Cioara, F. L., Toma, M. M., & Bungau, S. (2021). Recognizing the benefits of pre-/probiotics in metabolic syndrome and type 2 diabetes mellitus considering the influence of Akkermansia muciniphila as a key gut Bacterium. *Microorganisms*, *9*(3), 618. https://doi.org/10.3390/microorganisms9030618

Cox, M. A., Jackson, J., Stanton, M., Rojas-Triana, A., Bober, L., Laverty, M., Yang, X., Zhu, F., Liu, J., Wang, S., Monsma, F., Vassileva, G., Maguire, M., Gustafson, E., Bayne, M., Chou, C. C., Lundell, D., & Jenh, C. H. (2009). Short-chain fatty acids act as antiinflammatory mediators by regulating prostaglandin E2 and cytokines. *World Journal of Gastroenterology*, *15*(44), 5549–5557. https://doi.org/10.3748/wjg.15.5549

Cunningham, A. L., Stephens, J. W., & Harris, D. A. (2021). Gut microbiota influence in type 2 diabetes mellitus (T2DM). *Gut Pathogens*, *13*(1), 50. https://doi.org/10.1186/s13099-021-00446-0

Dang, F., Jiang, Y., Pan, R., Zhou, Y., Wu, S., Wang, R., Zhuang, K., Zhang, W., Li, T., & Man, C. (2018). Administration of *Lactobacillus paracasei* ameliorates type 2 diabetes in mice. *Food and Function*, *9*(7), 3630–3639. https://doi.org/10.1039/c8fo00081f

de Lonlay, P., & Saudubray, J.-M. (2000). Persistent hyperinsulinaemic hypoglycaemia. In J. Fernandes, J.-M. Sudubray, & van den Berghe, P. (Eds.), *Inborn metabolic diseases: Diagnosis and treatment* (3rd ed., pp. 117–126). Springer.

De Vadder, F., Kovatcheva-Datchary, P., Goncalves, D., Vinera, J., Zitoun, C., Duchampt, A., Bäckhed, F., & Mithieux, G. (2014). Microbiota-generated metabolites promote metabolic benefits via gut–brain neural circuits. *Cell*, *156*(1–2), 84–96. https://doi.org/10.1016/j.cell.2013.12.016

DECODE Study Group, European Diabetes Epidemiology Group. (2003). Is the current definition for diabetes relevant to mortality risk from all causes and cardiovascular and noncardiovascular diseases? *Diabetes Care*, *26*(3), 688–696. https://doi.org/10.2337/diacare.26.3.688

Delzenne, N. M., & Cani, P. D. (2011). Interaction between obesity and the gut microbiota: Relevance in nutrition. *Annual Review of Nutrition*, *31*, 15–31. https://doi.org/10.1146/annurev-nutr-072610-145146

Ding, L. N., Ding, W. Y., Ning, J., Wang, Y., Yan, Y., & Wang, Z. B. (2021). Effects of probiotic supplementation on inflammatory markers and glucose homeostasis in adults with type 2 diabetes mellitus: A systematic review and meta-analysis. *Frontiers in Pharmacology*, *12*, 770861. https://doi.org/10.3389/fphar.2021.770861

Doumatey, A. P., Adeyemo, A., Zhou, J., Lei, L., Adebamowo, S. N., Adebamowo, C., & Rotimi, C. N. (2020). Gut microbiome profiles are associated with type 2 diabetes in urban Africans. *Frontiers in Cellular and Infection Microbiology*, *10*, 63. https://doi.org/10.3389/fcimb.2020.00063

Du, L., Li, Q., Yi, H., Kuang, T., Tang, Y., & Fan, G. (2022). Gut microbiota-derived metabolites as key actors in type 2 diabetes mellitus. *Biomedicine and Pharmacotherapy*, *149*, 112839. https://doi.org/10.1016/j.biopha.2022.112839; Epub March 21, 2022; PubMed: 35325852

Ebrahimi, Z. S., Nasli-Esfahani, E., Nadjarzade, A., & Mozaffari-Khosravi, H. (2017). Effect of symbiotic supplementation on glycemic control, lipid profiles and microalbuminuria in patients with non-obese type 2 diabetes: A randomized, double-blind, clinical trial. *Journal of Diabetes and Metabolic Disorders*, *16*, 23. https://doi.org/10.1186/s40200-017-0304-8

Ejtahed, H. S., Mohtadi-Nia, J., Homayouni-Rad, A., Niafar, M., Asghari-Jafarabadi, M., & Mofid, V. (2012). Probiotic yogurt improves antioxidant status in type 2 diabetic patients. *Nutrition*, *28*(5), 539–543. https://doi.org/10.1016/j.nut.2011.08.013

Everard, A., Matamoros, S., Geurts, L., Delzenne, N. M., & Cani, P. D. (2014). Saccharomyces boulardii administration changes gut microbiota and reduces hepatic steatosis, low-grade inflammation, and fat mass in obese and type 2 diabetic db/db mice. *mBio*, *5*(3), e01011–e01014. https://doi.org/10.1128/mBio.01011-14

Evivie, S. E. (2013). Preliminary studies on pharmaceutical microencapsulation for symbiotic application. *Journal of Applied and Natural Science*, *5*, 488–496.

Fajans, S. S., Bell, G. I., & Polonsky, K. S. (2001). Molecular mechanisms and clinical pathophysiology of maturity-onset diabetes of the young. *New England Journal of Medicine*, *345*(13), 971–980. https://doi.org/10.1056/NEJMra002168

Falcinelli, S., Rodiles, A., Hatef, A., Picchietti, S., Cossignani, L., & Merrifield, D. L. (2018). Influence of probiotics administration on gut microbiota core: A review on the effects on appetite control, glucose, and lipid metabolism. *Journal of Clinical Gastroenterology*, *52*(suppl_1), 50–56.

Fatima, A. (2017). Probiotics as Living Drugs to Resolve Urinary Tract Infections. *National Journal of Health Sciences*, *2*(4), 144–149. https://doi.org/10.21089/njhs.24.0144

Felner, E. I., Klitz, W., Ham, M., Lazaro, A. M., Stastny, P., Dupont, B., & White, P. C. (2005). Genetic interaction among three genomic regions creates distinct contributions to early- and late-onset type 1 diabetes mellitus. *Pediatric Diabetes*, *6*(4), 213–220. https://doi.org/10.1111/j.1399-543X.2005.00132.x

Fernández-Real, J. M., & Pickup, J. C. (2012). Innate immunity, insulin resistance and type 2 diabetes. *Diabetologia*, *55*(2), 273–278. https://doi.org/10.1007/s00125-011-2387-y

Firouzi, S., Majid, H. A., Ismail, A., Kamaruddin, N. A., & Barakatun-Nisak, M. Y. (2017). Effect of multi-strain probiotics (multi-strain microbial cell preparation) on glycemic control and other diabetes-related outcomes in people with type 2 diabetes: A randomized controlled trial. *European Journal of Nutrition*, *56*(4), 1535–1550. https://doi.org/10.1007/s00394-016-1199-8

Gao, X., Liu, X., Xu, J., Xue, C., Xue, Y., & Wang, Y. (2014). Dietary trimethylamine N-oxide exacerbates impaired glucose tolerance in mice fed a high fat diet. *Journal of Bioscience and Bioengineering*, *118*(4), 476–481. https://doi.org/10.1016/j.jbiosc.2014.03.001

Gao, X., Wang, F., Zhao, P., Zhang, R., & Zeng, Q. (2019). Effect of heat-killed Streptococcus thermophilus on type 2 diabetes rats. *PeerJ*, *7*, e7117. https://doi.org/10.7717/peerj.7117

Gholizadeh, P., Mahallei, M., Pormohammad, A., Varshochi, M., Ganbarov, K., Zeinalzadeh, E., Yousefi, B., Bastami, M., Tanomand, A., Mahmood, S. S., Yousefi, M., Asgharzadeh, M., & Kafil, H. S. (2019). Microbial balance in the intestinal microbiota and its association with diabetes, obesity and allergic disease. *Microbial Pathogenesis*, *127*, 48–55. https://doi.org/10.1016/j.micpath.2018.11.031

Gomes, A. C., Bueno, A. A., de Souza, R. G., & Mota, J. F. (2014). Gut microbiota, probiotics and diabetes. *Nutrition Journal, 13*, 60. https://doi.org/10.1186/1475-2891-13-60.

Gosmanov, A. R., Gosmanova, E. O., & Kitabchi, A. E. (2000). *Hyperglycemic crises: Diabetic ketoacidosis and hyperglycemic hyperosmolar state. Endotext*. MDText.com, Inc.

Guarner, F., & Malagelada, J. R. (2003). Gut flora in health and disease. *Lancet*, *361*(9356), 512–519. https://doi.org/10.1016/S0140-6736(03)12489-0

Gurung, M., Li, Z., You, H., Rodrigues, R., Jump, D. B., Morgun, A., & Shulzhenko, N. (2020). Role of gut microbiota in type 2 diabetes pathophysiology. *Ebiomedicine*, *51*, 102590. https://doi.org/10.1016/j.ebiom.2019.11.051

Hallajzadeh, J., Eslami, R. D., & Tanomand, A. (2021). Effect of Lactobacillus delbrueckii Subsp. Lactis PTCC1057 on serum glucose, fetuin-A, and sestrin 3 levels in streptozotocin-induced diabetic mice. *Probiotics and Antimicrobial Proteins*, *13*(2), 383–389. https://doi.org/10.1007/s12602-020-09693-0

Han, M. M., Sun, J. F., Su, X. H., Peng, Y. F., Goyal, H., Wu, C. H., Zhu, X. Y., & Li, L. (2019). Probiotics improve glucose and lipid metabolism in pregnant women: A meta-analysis. *Annals of Translational Medicine*, *7*(5), 99. https://doi.org/10.21037/atm.2019.01.61

Hänninen, A., Toivonen, R., Pöysti, S., Belzer, C., Plovier, H., Ouwerkerk, J. P., Emani, R., Cani, P. D., & De Vos, W. M. (2018). Akkermansia muciniphila induces gut microbiota remodelling and controls islet autoimmunity in NOD mice. *Gut*, *67*(8), 1445–1453. https://doi.org/10.1136/gutjnl-2017-314508

Hasain, Z., Mokhtar, N. M., Kamaruddin, N. A., Ismail, N. A. M., Razalli, N. H., Gnanou, J. V., & Ali, R. A. R. (2020). Gut microbia and gestational Daibetes mellitus: A review of host-gut microbiota interactions and their therapeutic potential. *Frontiers in Cellular and Infection Microbiology*, *10*, 188.

He, C., Shan, Y., & Song, W. (2015). Targeting gut microbiota as a possible therapy for diabetes. *Nutrition Research*, *35*(5), 361–367. https://doi.org/10.1016/j.nutres.2015.03.002

He, M., & Shi, B. (2017). Gut microbiota as a potential target of metabolic syndrome: The role of probiotics and prebiotics. *Cell and Bioscience*, *7*, 54. https://doi.org/10.1186/s13578-017-0183-1

Hill, C., Guarner, F., Reid, G., Gibson, G. R., Merenstein, D. J., Pot, B., Morelli, L., Canani, R. B., Flint, H. J., Salminen, S., & Calder, P. C. (2014). Expert consensus document. The international scientific association for probiotics and prebiotics consensus statement on the scope and appropriate use of the term probiotics. *Nature Reviews Gastroenterology and Hepatology*, *8*(506), 514.

Homayouni, A., Sahhaf, F., Hassanalilou, T., Ejtahed, H., Motayagheni, N., & Soroush, A.-R. (2016). The future of diabetes management by healthy probiotic microorganisms. *Current Diabetes Reviews*, *12*(999). https://doi.org/10.2174/1573399812666161014112515

Hsieh, M. C., Tsai, W. H., Jheng, Y. P., Su, S. L., Wang, S. Y., Lin, C. C., Chen, Y. H., & Chang, W. W. (2018). The beneficial effects of *Lactobacillus reuteri* ADR-1 or ADR-3 consumption on type 2 diabetes mellitus: A randomized, double-blinded, placebo-controlled trial. *Scientific Reports*, *8*(1), 16791. https://doi.org/10.1038/s41598-018-35014-1

Hsieh, P. S., Ho, H. H., Hsieh, S. H., Kuo, Y. W., Tseng, H. Y., Kao, H. F., & Wang, J. Y. (2020). Lactobacillus salivarius AP-32 and Lactobacillus reuteri GL-104 decrease glycemic levels and attenuate diabetes-mediated liver and kidney injury in db/db mice. *BMJ Open Diabetes Research and Care*, *8*(1), e001028. https://doi.org/10.1136/bmjdrc-2019-001028

Hu, S., Kuwabara, R., de Haan, B. J., Smink, A. M., & de Vos, P. (2020). Acetate and butyrate improve β–cell metabolism and mitochondrial respiration under oxidative stress. *International Journal of Molecular Sciences, 21*(4), 1542. https://doi.org/10.3390/ijms21041542

Huda, M. N., Kim, M., & Bennett, B. J. (2021). Modulating the microbiota as a therapeutic intervention for Type 2 diabetes. *Frontiers in Endocrinology*, *12*, 632335. https://doi.org/10.3389/fendo.2021.632335

Hulston, C. J., Churnside, A. A., & Venables, M. C. (2015). Probiotic supplementation prevents high-fat, overfeeding-induced insulin resistance in human subjects. *British Journal of Nutrition*, *113*(4), 596–602. https://doi.org/10.1017/S0007114514004097

Irfan, S., Muzaffar, H., Anwar, H., & Jabeen, F. (2022). Gut microbiota potential in type 2 diabetes [Internet]. In *Effect of microbiota on health and disease*. IntechOpen. http://doi.org/10.5772/intechopen.105616

Ito, K., Maruyama, H., Hirose, H., Kido, K., Koyama, K., Kataoka, K., & Saruta, T. (1995). Exogenous insulin dose-dependently suppresses glucopenia-induced glucagon secretion from perfused rat pancreas. *Metabolism: Clinical and Experimental*, *44*(3), 358–362. https://doi.org/10.1016/0026-0495(95)90166-3

Janssen, A. W. F., Katiraei, S., Bartosinska, B., Eberhard, D., Willems van Dijk, K., & Kersten, S. (2018). Loss of angiopoietin-like 4 (ANGPTL4) in mice with diet-induced obesity uncouples visceral obesity from glucose intolerance partly via the gut microbiota. *Diabetologia*, *61*(6), 1447–1458. https://doi.org/10.1007/s00125-018-4583-5

Jia, L., Li, D., Feng, N., Shamoon, M., Sun, Z., Ding, L., Zhang, H., Chen, W., Sun, J., & Chen, Y. Q. (2017). Anti-diabetic effects of Clostridium butyricum CGMCC0313.1 through promoting the growth of gut butyrate-producing bacteria in type 2 diabetic mice. *Scientific Reports*, *7*(1), 7046. https://doi.org/10.1038/s41598-017-07335-0

Jumpertz, R., Le, D. S., Turnbaugh, P. J., Trinidad, C., Bogardus, C., Gordon, J. I., & Krakoff, J. (2011). Energy-balance studies reveal associations between gut microbes, caloric load, and nutrient absorption in humans. *American Journal of Clinical Nutrition*, *94*(1), 58–65. https://doi.org/10.3945/ajcn.110.010132

Jung, M. J., Lee, J., Shin, N. R., Kim, M. S., Hyun, D. W., Yun, J. H., Kim, P. S., Whon, T. W., & Bae, J. W. (2016). Chronic repression of mTOR complex 2 induces changes in the gut microbiota of diet-induced obese mice. *Scientific Reports*, *6*, 30887. https://doi.org/10.1038/srep30887

Karamali, M., Dadkhah, F., Sadrkhanlou, M., Jamilian, M., Ahmadi, S., Tajabadi-Ebrahimi, M., Jafari, P., & Asemi, Z. (2016). Effects of probiotic supplementation on glycaemic control and lipid profiles in gestational diabetes: A randomized, double-blind, placebo-controlled trial. *Diabetes and Metabolism*, *42*(4), 234–241. https://doi.org/10.1016/j.diabet.2016.04.009

Karlsson, F. H., Tremaroli, V., Nookaew, I., Bergström, G., Behre, C. J., Fagerberg, B., Nielsen, J., & Bäckhed, F. (2013). Gut metagenome in European women with normal, impaired and diabetic glucose control. *Nature*, *498*(7452), 99–103. https://doi.org/10.1038/nature12198

Kassaian, N., Feizi, A., Aminorroaya, A., Jafari, P., Ebrahimi, M. T., & Amini, M. (2018). The effects of probiotics and synbiotic supplementation on glucose and insulin metabolism in adults with prediabetes: A double-blind randomized clinical trial. *Acta Diabetologica*, *55*(10), 1019–1028. https://doi.org/10.1007/s00592-018-1175-2

Kaufman, B. A., Li, C., & Soleimanpour, S. A. (2015). Mitochondrial regulation of beta-cell function: Maintaining the momentum for insulin release. *Molecular Aspects of Medicine*, *42*, 91–104. https://doi.org/10.1016/j.mam.2015.01.004

Kawaguchi, T., Izumi, N., Charlton, M. R., & Sata, M. (2011). Branched-chain amino acids as pharmacological nutrients in chronic liver disease. *Hepatology*, *54*(3), 1063–1070. https://doi.org/10.1002/hep.24412

Kesika, P., Sivamaruthi, B. S., & Chaiyasut, C. (2019). Do probiotics improve the health status of individuals with diabetes mellitus? A review on outcomes of clinical trials. *BioMed Research International, 2019*, 1531567. https://doi.org/10.1155/2019/1531567

Khalili, L., Alipour, B., Asghari Jafar-Abadi, M., Faraji, I., Hassanalilou, T., Mesgari Abbasi, M., Vaghef-Mehrabany, E., & Alizadeh Sani, M. (2019). The effects of Lactobacillus casei on glycemic response, serum sirtuin1 and fetuin-A levels in patients with type 2 diabetes mellitus: A randomized controlled trial. *Iranian Biomedical Journal*, *23*(1), 68–77. https://doi.org/10.29252/.23.1.68

Kim, Y. A., Keogh, J. B., & Clifton, P. M. (2018). Probiotics, prebiotics, synbiotics and insulin sensitivity. *Nutrition Research Reviews*, *31*(1), 35–51. https://doi.org/10.1017/S095442241700018X

Kobyliak, N., Falalyeyeva, T., Mykhalchyshyn, G., Kyriienko, D., & Komissarenko, I. (2018). Effect of alive probiotic on insulin resistance in type 2 diabetes patients: Randomized clinical trial. *Diabetes and Metabolic Syndrome*, *12*(5), 617–624. https://doi.org/10.1016/j.dsx.2018.04.015

Koh, A., & Bäckhed, F. (2020). From association to causality: The role of the gut microbiota and its functional products on host metabolism. *Molecular Cell*, *78*(4), 584–596. https://doi.org/10.1016/j.molcel.2020.03.005

Kovacova-Hanuskova, E., Buday, T., Gavliakova, S., & Plevkova, J. (2015). Histamine, histamine intoxication and intolerance. *Allergologia et Immunopathologia (Madr)*, *43*(5), 498–506. https://doi.org/10.1016/j.aller.2015.05.001

Koyama, K., Chen, G., Lee, Y., & Unger, R. H. (1997). Tissue triglycerides, insulin resistance, and insulin production: Implications for hyperinsulinemia of obesity. *American Journal of Physiology*, *273*(4), E708–E713. https://doi.org/10.1152/ajpendo.1997.273.4.E708

Kühl, C. (1998). Etiology and pathogenesis of gestational diabetes. *Diabetes Care*, 21(suppl_2), B19–B26.

Kyriakidis, D. A., Theodorou, M. C., & Tiligada, E. (2012). Histamine in two component system-mediated bacterial signaling. *Frontiers in Bioscience (Landmark Edition)*, *17*(3), 1108–1119. https://doi.org/10.2741/3976

Laitinen, K., Poussa, T., Isolauri, E., & Nutrition, Allergy, Mucosal Immunology and Intestinal Microbiota Group. (2009). Probiotics and dietary counselling contribute to glucose regulation during and after pregnancy: A randomised controlled trial. *British Journal of Nutrition*, *101*(11), 1679–1687. https://doi.org/10.1017/S0007114508111461

Larsen, N., Vogensen, F. K., van den Berg, F. W., Nielsen, D. S., Andreasen, A. S., Pedersen, B. K., Al-Soud, W. A., Sørensen, S. J., Hansen, L. H., & Jakobsen, M. (2010). Gut microbiota in human adults with type 2 diabetes differs from non-diabetic adults. *PLoS One*, *5*(2), e9085. https://doi.org/10.1371/journal.pone.0009085

Lederberg, J., & McCray, A. (2001). Ome sweet omics—A genealogical treasury of words. *Scientist*, *15*(7), 8.

Lee, E., Jung, S. R., Lee, S. Y., Lee, N. K., Paik, H. D., & Lim, S. I. (2018). *Lactobacillus plantarum* Strain Ln4 attenuates diet-induced obesity, insulin resistance, and changes in hepatic mRNA levels associated with glucose and lipid metabolism. *Nutrients*, *10*(5), 643. https://doi.org/10.3390/nu10050643

Lee, Y. S., Lee, D., Park, G. S., Ko, S. H., Park, J., Lee, Y. K., & Kang, J. (2021). Lactobacillus plantarum HAC01 ameliorates type 2 diabetes in high-fat diet and streptozotocin-induced diabetic mice in association with modulating the gut microbiota. *Food and Function*, *12*(14), 6363–6373. https://doi.org/10.1039/D1FO00698C

Li, W. Z., Stirling, K., Yang, J. J., & Zhang, L. (2020). Gut microbiota and diabetes: From correlation to causality and mechanism. *World Journal of Diabetes*, *11*(7), 293–308. https://doi.org/10.4239/wjd.v11.i7.293

Li, X., Wang, N., Yin, B., Fang, D., Jiang, T., Fang, S., Zhao, J., Zhang, H., Wang, G., & Chen, W. (2016). Effects of Lactobacillus plantarum CCFM0236 on hyperglycaemia and insulin resistance in high-fat and streptozotocin-induced type 2 diabetic mice. *Journal of Applied Microbiology*, *121*(6), 1727–1736. https://doi.org/10.1111/jam.13276

Li, Y., Wang, D. D., Chiuve, S. E., Manson, J. E., Willett, W. C., Hu, F. B., & Qi, L. (2015). Dietary phosphatidylcholine intake and type 2 diabetes in men and women. *Diabetes Care*, *38*(2), e13–e14. https://doi.org/10.2337/dc14-2093

Li, Y., Wu, Y., Wu, L., Qin, L., & Liu, T. (2022). The effects of probiotic administration on patients with prediabetes: A meta-analysis and systematic review. *Journal of Translational Medicine*, *20*(1), 498. https://doi.org/10.1186/s12967-022-03695-y

Lim, S. M. (2016). Lactobacillus sakei OK67 ameliorates high-fat diet-induced blood glucose intolerance and obesity in mice by inhibiting gut microbiota lipopolysaccharide production and inducing colon tight junction protein expression. *Nutrition Research*, *36*(4), 337–348.

Lin, Y., Ren, Y., Zhang, Y., Zhou, J., Zhou, F., Zhao, Q., Xu, G., & Hua, Z. (2018). Protective role of nanoselenium-enriched *Bifidobacterium longum* in delaying the onset of streptozotocin-induced diabetes. *Royal Society Open Science*, *5*(12), 181156. https://doi.org/10.1098/rsos.181156

Liu, T., Li, J., Liu, Y., Xiao, N., Suo, H., Xie, K., Yang, C., & Wu, C. (2012). Short-chain fatty acids suppress lipopolysaccharide-induced production of nitric oxide and proinflammatory cytokines through inhibition of NF-κB pathway in RAW264.7 cells. *Inflammation*, *35*(5), 1676–1684. https://doi.org/10.1007/s10753-012-9484-z

Liu, Y., Wang, J., & Wu, C. (2021). Modulation of gut microbiota and immune system by probiotics, prebiotics, and post-biotics. *Frontiers in Nutrition*, *8*, 634897. https://doi.org/10.3389/fnut.2021.634897

Long, J., Liang, R., Zheng, Q., Yuan, G., Xin, Z., Chen, X., Lai, F., & Liu, Y. (2021). Overview of clinical trials on type 2 diabetes mellitus: A comprehensive analysis of the ClinicalTrials.gov database. *Diabetes, Metabolic Syndrome and Obesity: Targets and Therapy*, *14*, 367–377. https://doi.org/10.2147/DMSO.S288065

Manaer, T., Yu, L., Nabi, X. H., Dilidaxi, D., Liu, L., & Sailike, J. (2021). The beneficial effects of the composite probiotics from camel milk on glucose and lipid metabolism, liver and renal function and gut microbiota in db/db mice. *BMC Complementary Medicine and Therapies*, *21*(1), 127. https://doi.org/10.1186/s12906-021-03303-4

Mao, Z., Lin, H., Su, W., Li, J., Zhou, M., Li, Z., Zhou, B., Yang, Q., Zhou, M., Pan, K., He, J., & Zhang, W. (2019). Deficiency of ZnT8 promotes adiposity and metabolic dysfunction by increasing peripheral serotonin production. *Diabetes*, *68*(6), 1197–1209. https://doi.org/10.2337/db18-1321

Marques, A. M., Sarandy, M. M., Novaes, R. D., Gonçalves, R. V., & Freitas, M. B. (2020). Preclinical relevance of probiotics in type 2 diabetes: A systematic review. *International Journal of Experimental Pathology*, *101*(3–4), 68–79. https://doi.org/10.1111/iep.12359

Mavilio, M., Marchetti, V., Fabrizi, M., Stöhr, R., Marino, A., Casagrande, V., Fiorentino, L., Cardellini, M., Kappel, B., Monteleone, I., Garret, C., Mauriello, A., Monteleone, G., Farcomeni, A., Burcelin, R., Menghini, R., & Federici, M. (2016). A role for Timp3 in microbiota-driven hepatic steatosis and metabolic dysfunction. *Cell Reports*, *16*(3), 731–743. https://doi.org/10.1016/j.celrep.2016.06.027

Memarrast, F., Ghafouri-Fard, S., Kolivand, S., Nodooshan, S. J., Neyazi, N., Sadroddiny, E., & Motevaseli, E. (2017). Comparative evaluation of probiotics effects on plasma glucose, lipid, and insulin levels in streptozotocin-induced diabetic rats. *Diabetes/Metabolism Research and Reviews*, *33*(7), e2912. https://doi.org/10.1002/dmrr.2912

Mikov, M., Đanić, M., Pavlović, N., Stanimirov, B., Goločorbin-Kon, S., Stankov, K., & Al-Salami, H. (2018). Potential applications of gliclazide in treating type 1 diabetes mellitus: Formulation with bile acids and probiotics. *European Journal of Drug Metabolism and Pharmacokinetics*, *43*(3), 269–280. https://doi.org/10.1007/s13318-017-0441-y

Miraghajani, M., Dehsoukhteh, S. S., Rafie, N., Hamedani, S. G., Sabihi, S., & Ghiasvand, R. (2017). Potential mechanisms linking probiotics to diabetes: A narrative review of the literature. *São Paulo Medical Journal*, *135*(2), 169–178. https://doi.org/10.1590/1516-3180.2016.0311271216

Mirjalili, M., Salari Sharif, A., Sangouni, A. A., Emtiazi, H., & Mozaffari-Khosravi, H. (2023). Effect of probiotic yogurt consumption on glycemic control and lipid profile in patients with type 2 diabetes mellitus: A randomized controlled trial. *Clinical Nutrition ESPEN*, *54*, 144–149. https://doi.org/10.1016/j.clnesp.2023.01.014

Mobini, R., Tremaroli, V., Ståhlman, M., Karlsson, F., Levin, M., Ljungberg, M., Sohlin, M., Bertéus Forslund, H., Perkins, R., Bäckhed, F., & Jansson, P. A. (2017). Metabolic effects of *Lactobacillus reuteri* DSM 17938 in people with type 2 diabetes: A randomized controlled trial. *Diabetes, Obesity and Metabolism*, *19*(4), 579–589. https://doi.org/10.1111/dom.12861

Moghetti, P., & Tosi, F. (2021). Insulin resistance and PCOS: Chicken or egg? *Journal of Endocrinological Investigation*, *44*(2), 233–244. https://doi.org/10.1007/s40618-020-01351-0

Mohamadshahi, M., Veissi, M., Haidari, F., Javid, A. Z., Mohammadi, F., & Shirbeigi, E. (2014). Effects of probiotic yogurt consumption on lipid profile in type 2 diabetic patients: A randomized controlled clinical trial. *Journal of Research in Medical Sciences*, *19*(6), 531–536.

Montalto, M., Gallo, A., Santoro, L., D'Onofrio, F., Curigliano, V., Covino, M., Cammarota, G., Grieco, A., Gasbarrini, A., & Gasbarrini, G. (2008). Low-dose lactose in drugs neither increases breath hydrogen excretion nor causes gastrointestinal symptoms. *Alimentary Pharmacology and Therapeutics*, *28*(8), 1003–1012. https://doi.org/10.1111/j.1365-2036.2008.03815.x

Niibo, M., Shirouchi, B., Umegatani, M., Morita, Y., Ogawa, A., Sakai, F., Kadooka, Y., & Sato, M. (2019). Probiotic Lactobacillus gasseri SBT2055 improves insulin secretion in a diabetic rat model. *Journal of Dairy Science*, *102*(2), 997–1006. https://doi.org/10.3168/jds.2018-15203

Pan, Y. Q., Zheng, Q. X., Jiang, X. M., Chen, X. Q., Zhang, X. Y., & Wu, J. L. (2021). Probiotic supplements improve blood glucose and insulin resistance/sensitivity among healthy and GDM pregnant women: A systematic review and meta-analysis of randomized controlled trials. *Evidence-Based Complementary and Alternative Medicine: eCAM*, *2021*, 9830200. https://doi.org/10.1155/2021/9830200

Park, K. Y., Kim B., & Hyun C. K. (2015). Lactobacillus rhamnosus GG improves glucose tolerance through alleviating er stress and suppressing macrophage activation in db/db mice. *Journal of Clinical Biochemistry and Nutrition*, *56*(3), 240–246.

Pathak, P., Xie, C., Nichols, R. G., Ferrell, J. M., Boehme, S., Krausz, K. W., Patterson, A. D., Gonzalez, F. J., & Chiang, J. Y. L. (2018). Intestine farnesoid X receptor agonist and the gut microbiota activate G-protein bile acid receptor-1 signaling to improve metabolism. *Hepatology*, *68*(4), 1574–1588. https://doi.org/10.1002/hep.29857

Pedersen, H. K., Gudmundsdottir, V., Nielsen, H. B., Hyotylainen, T., Nielsen, T., Jensen, B. A., Forslund, K., Hildebrand, F., Prifti, E., Falony, G., Le Chatelier, E., Levenez, F., Doré, J., Mattila, I., Plichta, D. R., Pöhö, P., Hellgren, L. I., Arumugam, M., Sunagawa, S., . . . Pedersen, O. (2016). Human gut microbes impact host serum metabolome and insulin sensitivity. *Nature*, *535*(7612), 376–381. https://doi.org/10.1038/nature18646

Pegah, A., Abbasi-Oshaghi, E., Khodadadi, I., Mirzaei, F., & Tayebinai, H. (2021). Probiotic and resveratrol normalize GLP-1 levels and oxidative stress in the intestine of diabetic rats. *Metabolism Open*, *10*, 100093. https://doi.org/10.1016/j.metop.2021.100093

Prabhurajeshwar, C., & Chandrakanth, R. K. (2017). Probiotic potential of Lactobacilli with antagonistic activity against pathogenic strains: An in vitro validation for the production of inhibitory substances. *Biomedical journal*, *40*(5), 270–283. https://doi.org/10.1016/j.bj.2017.06.008

Pugin, B., Barcik, W., Westermann, P., Heider, A., Wawrzyniak, M., Hellings, P., Akdis, C. A., & O'Mahony, L. (2017). A wide diversity of bacteria from the human gut produces and degrades biogenic amines. *Microbial Ecology in Health and Disease*, *28*(1), 1353881. https://doi.org/10.1080/16512235.2017.1353881

Qin, J. J., Li, Y. R., Cai, Z. M., Li, S. H., Zhu, J. F., Zhang, F., Liang, S., Zhang, W., Guan, Y., Shen, D., Peng, Y., Zhang, D., Jie, Z., Wu, W., Qin, Y., Xue, W., Li, J., Han, L., Lu, D., . . . Wang, J. (2012). A metagenome-wide association study of gut microbiota in type 2 diabetes. *Nature*, *490*(7418), 55–60. https://doi.org/10.1038/nature11450

Rahman, M. S., Hossain, K. S., Das, S., Kundu, S., Adegoke, E. O., Rahman, M. A., Hannan, M. A., Uddin, M. J., & Pang, M. G. (2021). Role of insulin in health and disease: An update. *International Journal of Molecular Sciences*, *22*(12), 6403. https://doi.org/10.3390/ijms22126403

Razmpoosh, E., Javadi, A., Ejtahed, H. S., Mirmiran, P., Javadi, M., & Yousefinejad, A. (2019). The effect of probiotic supplementation on glycemic control and lipid profile in patients with type 2 diabetes: A randomized placebo controlled trial. *Diabetes and Metabolic Syndrome*, *13*(1), 175–182. https://doi.org/10.1016/j.dsx.2018.08.008

Rezaei, M., Sanagoo, A., Jouybari, L., Behnampoo, N., & Kavosi, A. (2017). The effect of probiotic yogurt on blood glucose and cardiovascular biomarkers in patients with type II diabetes: A randomized controlled trial. *Evidence Based Care Journal*, *6*(4), 26–35.

Rogero, M. M., & Calder, P. C. (2018). Obesity, inflammation, toll-like receptor 4 and fatty acids. *Nutrients*, *10*(4). https://doi.org/10.3390/nu10040432

Roy, S., Yuzefpolskaya, M., Nandakumar, R., Colombo, P. C., & Demmer, R. T. (2020). Plasma trimethylamine-N-oxide and impaired glucose regulation: Results from the oral infections, glucose intolerance and insulin resistance study (ORIGINS). *PLoS One*, *15*(1), e0227482. https://doi.org/10.1371/journal.pone.0227482

Sabico, S., Al-Mashharawi, A., Al-Daghri, N. M., Wani, K., Amer, O. E., Hussain, D. S., Ahmed Ansari, M. G., Masoud, M. S., Alokail, M. S., & McTernan, P. G. (2019). Effects of a 6-month multi-strain probiotics supplementation in endotoxemic, inflammatory and cardiometabolic status of T2DM patients: A randomized, double-blind, placebo-controlled trial. *Clinical Nutrition*, *38*(4), 1561–1569. https://doi.org/10.1016/j.clnu.2018.08.009

Sabico, S., Al-Mashharawi, A., Al-Daghri, N. M., Yakout, S., Alnaami, A. M., Alokail, M. S., & McTernan, P. G. (2017). Effects of a multi-strain probiotic supplement for 12 weeks in circulating endotoxin levels and cardiometabolic profiles of medication naïve T2DM patients: A randomized clinical trial. *Journal of Translational Medicine*, *15*(1), 249. https://doi.org/10.1186/s12967-017-1354-x

Sáez-Lara, M. J., Robles-Sanchez, C., Ruiz-Ojeda, F. J., Plaza-Diaz, J., & Gil, A. (2016). Effects of probiotics and Synbiotics on obesity, insulin resistance syndrome, Type 2 diabetes and non-alcoholic fatty liver disease: A review of human clinical trials. *International Journal of Molecular Sciences*, *17*(6), 928. https://doi.org/10.3390/ijms17060928

Sakai, T., Taki, T., Nakamoto, A., Shuto, E., Tsutsumi, R., Toshimitsu, T., Makino, S., & Ikegami, S. (2013). *Lactobacillus plantarum* OLL2712 regulates glucose metabolism in C57BL/6 mice fed a high-fat diet. *Journal of Nutritional Science and Vitaminology*, *59*(2), 144–147. https://doi.org/10.3177/jnsv.59.144

Sapra, A., & Bhandari, P. (2023). Diabetes. In *StatPearls [Internet]*. StatPearls Publishing. https://www.ncbi.nlm.nih.gov/books/NBK551501/

Schmitt, C. C., Aranias, T., Viel, T., Chateau, D., Le Gall, M., Waligora-Dupriet, A. J., Melchior, C., Rouxel, O., Kapel, N., Gourcerol, G., Tavitian, B., Lehuen, A., Brot-Laroche, E., Leturque, A., Serradas, P., & Grosfeld, A. (2017). Intestinal invalidation of the glucose transporter GLUT2 delays tissue distribution of glucose and reveals an unexpected role in gut homeostasis. *Molecular Metabolism*, *6*(1), 61–72. https://doi.org/10.1016/j.molmet.2016.10.008

Sherman, P. M., Ossa, J. C., Johnson-Henry, K. (2009). Unraveling Mechanisms of Action of Probiotics. *Nutrition in Clinical Practice*, *24*(1), 10–14. https://doi.org/10.1177/0884533608329231

Shih, C. T., Yeh, Y. T., Lin, C. C., Yang, L. Y., & Chiang, C. P. (2020). Akkermansia muciniphila is negatively correlated with hemoglobin A1c in refractory diabetes. *Microorganisms*, *8*(9), 1360. https://doi.org/10.3390/microorganisms8091360

Sindelar, D. K., Chu, C. A., Rohlie, M., Neal, D. W., Swift, L. L., & Cherrington, A. D. (1997). The role of fatty acids in mediating the effects of peripheral insulin on hepatic glucose production in the conscious dog. *Diabetes*, *46*(2), 187–196. https://doi.org/10.2337/diab.46.2.187

Singh, S., Sharma, R. K., Malhotra, S., Pothuraju, R., & Shandilya, U. K. (2017). *Lactobacillus rhamnosus* NCDC17 ameliorates type-2 diabetes by improving gut function, oxidative stress and inflammation in high-fat-diet fed and streptozotocintreated rats. *Beneficial Microbes*, *8*(2), 243–255. https://doi.org/10.3920/BM2016.0090

Smith, U. (2002). Impaired ('diabetic') insulin signaling and action occur in fat cells long before glucose intolerance—Is insulin resistance initiated in the adipose tissue? *International Journal of Obesity and Related Metabolic Disorders*, *26*(7), 897–904. https://doi.org/10.1038/sj.ijo.0802028

Song, H., Wang, W., Shen, B., Jia, H., Hou, Z., Chen, P., & Sun, Y. (2018). Pretreatment with probiotic bifico ameliorates colitis-associated cancer in mice: Transcriptome and gut flora profiling. *Cancer Science*, *109*(3), 666–677. https://doi.org/10.1111/cas.13497

Soria, B., Quesada, I., Ropero, A. B., Pertusa, J. A., Martín, F., & Nadal, A. (2004). Novel players in pancreatic islet signaling: From membrane receptors to nuclear channels. *Diabetes*, *53* (suppl_1), S86–S91. https://doi.org/10.2337/diabetes.53.2007.s86

Sreepathi, N., Jayanthi, M. K., Chandra, S. J., Bajpe, S. N., & Ramu, R. (2022). Probiotic intervention in the treatment of diabetes mellitus: A review. *Journal of Pure and Applied Microbiology*, *16*(3), 1519–1529. https://doi.org/10.22207/JPAM.16.3.25

Sun, Q., Zhang, Y., Li, Z., Yan, H., Li, J., & Wan, X. (2019). Mechanism analysis of improved glucose homeostasis and cholesterol metabolism in high-fat-induced obese mice treated with *La*-SJLH001 *via* transcriptomics and culturomics. *Food and Function*, *10*(6), 3556–3566. https://doi.org/10.1039/C9FO00205G

Tedelind, S., Westberg, F., Kjerrulf, M., & Vidal, A. (2007). Anti-inflammatory properties of the short-chain fatty acids acetate and propionate: A study with relevance to inflammatory bowel disease. *World Journal of Gastroenterology*, *13*(20), 2826–2832. https://doi.org/10.3748/wjg.v13.i20.2826

Toshimitsu, T., Gotou, A., Furuichi, K., Hachimura, S., & Asami, Y. (2019). Effects of 12-wk Lactobacillus plantarum OLL2712 treatment on glucose metabolism and chronic inflammation in prediabetic individuals: A single-arm pilot study. *Nutrition*, *58*, 175–180. https://doi.org/10.1016/j.nut.2018.07.116

Tuomilehto, J. (2013). The emerging global epidemic of type 1 diabetes. *Current Diabetes Reports*, *13*(6), 795–804. https://doi.org/10.1007/s11892-013-0433-5

Turna, N. S., Chung, R., & McIntyre, L. (2024). A review of biogenic amines in fermented foods: Occurrence and health effects. *Heliyon*, *10*(2), e24501. https://doi.org/10.1016/j.heliyon.2024.e24501

Turnbaugh, P. J., Ley, R. E., Hamady, M., Fraser-Liggett, C. M., Knight, R., & Gordon, J. I. (2007). The human microbiome project. *Nature*, *449*(7164), 804–810. https://doi.org/10.1038/nature06244

Usami, M., Kishimoto, K., Ohata, A., Miyoshi, M., Aoyama, M., Fueda, Y., & Kotani, J. (2008). Butyrate and trichostatin A attenuate nuclear factor κB activation and tumor necrosis factor α secretion and increase prostaglandin E2 secretion in human peripheral blood mononuclear cells. *Nutrition Research*, *28*(5), 321–328. https://doi.org/10.1016/j.nutres.2008.02.012

Venkataraman, R., Jose, P., & Jose, J. (2019). Impact of probiotics on health-related quality of life in type II diabetes mellitus: A randomized single-blind, placebo-controlled study. *Journal of Natural Science, Biology and Medicine*, *10*(1), 2–7. https://doi.org/10.4103/jnsbm.JNSBM_31_18

Vinolo, M. A., Rodrigues, H. G., Hatanaka, E., Sato, F. T., Sampaio, S. C., & Curi, R. (2011). Suppressive effect of short-chain fatty acids on production of proinflammatory mediators by neutrophils. *Journal of Nutritional Biochemistry*, *22*(9), 849–855. https://doi.org/10.1016/j.jnutbio.2010.07.009

Wang, G., Li, X., Zhao, J., Zhang, H., & Chen, W. (2017). *Lactobacillus casei* CCFM419 attenuates type 2 diabetes via a gut microbiota dependent mechanism. *Food and Function*, *8*(9), 3155–3164. https://doi.org/10.1039/C7FO00593H

Wang, G., Si, Q., Yang, S., Jiao, T., Zhu, H., Tian, P., Wang, L., Li, X., Gong, L., Zhao, J., Zhang, H., & Chen, W. (2020). Lactic acid bacteria reduce diabetes symptoms in mice by alleviating gut microbiota dysbiosis and inflammation in different manners. *Food and Function*, *11*(7), 5898–5914. https://doi.org/10.1039/c9fo02761k

Wang, L., Shang, Q., Guo, W., Wu, X., Wu, L., Wu, L., & Chen, T. (2020). Evaluation of the hypoglycemic effect of probiotics via directly consuming glucose in intestines of STZ-induced diabetic mice and glucose water-induced diabetic mice. *Journal of Functional Foods*, *64*, 103614. https://doi.org/10.1016/j.jff.2019.103614

Wang, X., Yang, J., Qiu, X., Wen, Q., Liu, M., Zhou, D., & Chen, Q. (2021). Probiotics, pre-biotics and synbiotics in the treatment of pre-diabetes: A systematic review of randomized controlled trials. *Frontiers in Public Health*, *9*, 645035. https://doi.org/10.3389/fpubh.2021.645035

Writing Group for the SEARCH for Diabetes in Youth Study Group, Dabelea, D., Bell, R. A., D'Agostino, R. B., Imperatore, G., Johansen, J. M., Linder, B., Liu, L. L., Loots, B., Marcovina, S., Mayer-Davis, E. J., Pettitt, D. J., & Waitzfelder, B. (2007). Incidence of diabetes in youth in the United States. *JAMA*, *297*(24), 2716–2724. https://doi.org/10.1001/jama.297.24.2716

Yadav, H., Jain, S., & Sinha, P. R. (2008). Oral administration of dahi containing probiotic *Lactobacillus acidophilus* and *Lactobacillus casei* delayed the progression of streptozotocin-induced diabetes in rats. *Journal of Dairy Research*, *75*(2), 189–195. https://doi.org/10.1017/S0022029908003129

Yan, F., Li, N., Shi, J., Li, H., Yue, Y., Jiao, W., Wang, N., Song, Y., Huo, G., & Li, B. (2019). Lactobacillus acidophilus alleviates type 2 diabetes by regulating hepatic glucose, lipid metabolism and gut microbiota in mice. *Food and Function*, *10*(9), 5804–5815. https://doi.org/10.1039/C9FO01062A

Yoo, J. Y., & Kim, S. S. (2016). Probiotics and prebiotics: Present status and future perspectives on metabolic disorders. *Nutrients*, *8*(3), 173. https://doi.org/10.3390/nu8030173

Zeng, Z., Yuan, Q., Yu, R., Zhang, J., Ma, H., & Chen, S. (2019). Ameliorative effects of probiotic *Lactobacillus paracasei* NL41 on insulin sensitivity, oxidative stress, and beta-cell function in a type 2 diabetes mellitus rat model. *Molecular Nutrition and Food Research*, *63*(22), e1900457. https://doi.org/10.1002/mnfr.201900457

Zhang, J., Wang, S., Zeng, Z., Qin, Y., Shen, Q., & Li, P. (2020). Anti-diabetic effects of *Bifidobacterium animalis* 01 through improving hepatic insulin sensitivity in type 2 diabetic rat model. *Journal of Functional Foods*, *67*, 103843. https://doi.org/10.1016/j.jff.2020.103843

Zhang, X., Shen, D., Fang, Z., Jie, Z., Qiu, X., Zhang, C., Chen, Y., & Ji, L. (2013). Human gut microbiota changes reveal the progression of glucose intolerance. *PLoS One*, *8*(8), e71108. https://doi.org/10.1371/journal.pone.0071108

Zhang, X., Zhao, Y., Zhang, M., Pang, X., Xu, J., Kang, C., Li, M., Zhang, C., Zhang, Z., Zhang, Y., Li, X., Ning, G., & Zhao, L. (2012). Structural changes of gut microbiota during berberine-mediated prevention of obesity and insulin resistance in high-fat diet-fed rats. *PLoS One*, *7*(8), e42529. https://doi.org/10.1371/journal.pone.0042529

Zhang, Y., Wu, T., Li, W., Zhao, Y., Long, H., Liu, R., Sui, W., & Zhang, M. (2021). Lactobacillus casei LC89 exerts antidiabetic effects through regulating hepatic glucagon response and gut microbiota in type 2 diabetic mice. *Food and Function*, *12*(18), 8288–8299. https://doi.org/10.1039/d1fo00882j

Zhao, D., Zhu, H., Gao, F., Qian, Z., Mao, W., Yin, Y., Tan, J., & Chen, D. (2020). Antidiabetic effects of selenium-enriched *Bifidobacterium longum* DD98 in type 2 diabetes model of mice. *Food and Function*, *11*(7), 6528–6541. https://doi.org/10.1039/D0FO00180E

Zheng, Y., Ley, S. H., & Hu, F. B. (2018). Global aetiology and epidemiology of type 2 diabetes mellitus and its complications. *Nature Reviews. Endocrinology*, *14*(2), 88–98. https://doi.org/10.1038/nrendo.2017.151

Zheng, Z., Sun, B., Dongsheng, Y., & Zhu, C. (2022). Sec. Microbiome in Health and Disease. Gut microbiota: An important player in type 2 diabetes mellitus. *Frontiers in Cellular and Infection Microbiology*, *2022*, 12.

9 Probiotics and Gastro-Intestinal Disorders

Augmentation, Enhancement, and Strengthening of Epithelial Lining

Reza Karimi and Dorsa Hosseinzadeh

9.1 INTRODUCTION

Probiotics are live organisms with a beneficial effect on the host if consumed in sufficient quantities. They have indicated critical potential as restorative alternatives for an assortment of diseases. In addition, they are highly effective at preventing infections and treating numerous gastro-intestinal diseases. Probiotics can ameliorate or prevent diseases including antibiotic-associated diarrhea, *Clostridium difficile* infections, *Helicobacter pylori* infections, inflammatory bowel diseases (including Crohn's disease and ulcerative colitis), necrotizing enterocolitis, and irritable bowel syndrome. The most important criteria for probiotics are their toleration level to acid and bile in gastro-intestinal conditions, bile salt hydrolyzing activity, capacity to stick to gastro-intestinal mucosa, deprivation, and competitive adhesion to mucosal and epithelial surfaces, antimicrobial action, and inhibition of pathogenic microorganisms. The protective influence of probiotics relies on their adhesion to epithelial cell layers. To function properly, it is necessary to attach and establish a proper link between the probiotics and the epithelium. Hence, adhesion capacity has influences on a wide range of diseases (Javanshir et al., 2021). Other important attributes of probiotics are improvement of barrier functionality, regulation of intestinal epithelial permeability, modification of intestinal microbiota, competitive adhesion to the epithelial surfaces, anti-inflammatory and antioxidant activities, suppression of the growth of pathogens, production of antimicrobial substances, and immunomodulation (Ohland & MacNaughton, 2010). All probiotics do not have equal attributes, and their benefits are strain and dose-dependent. Hence, it would be unreasonable to assume that the effects of a particular strain can be generalized to other variations of the same strain (Szajewska et al., 2010). In this chapter, the most important discussed issues are about how the probiotics affect the epithelial lining and their effectiveness in gastro-intestinal disorders.

9.2 BARRIER FUNCTIONS OF THE INTESTINAL EPITHELIAL LINING

The gastro-intestinal barrier consists of four main components including the beneficial bacteria, the mucus layer containing molecules of IgA and antimicrobial components, the single layer of epithelial cells, and the gut-related lymphoid tissue (Dempsey & Corr, 2022). The lining of the intestines is continuously exposed to the contents within the intestines and the diverse and ever-changing microorganisms present in the digestive system. Compared to the areas close to the beginning of the digestive tract, bacteria populations gradually increase in the lower small gut tract, cecum, and colon, reaching levels of 10^{10} to 10^{12} CFU per gram of intestinal material in the colon. The gut microflora is believed to consist of over 500 primarily anaerobic bacterial species (Preidis & Versalovic, 2009). Regardless of fundamental microbial species that are basic in each human, the microbiota of every person has a particular bacterial unique finger impression. In other words, it has a layout of its own species which is not the same as others. The epithelium is more than just

 DOI: 10.1201/9781003452249-9

a physical barrier which includes different epithelial cells with multiple functions. It has a critical role in nutrient intake regulations, critical role in homeostasis, vital regulation of antigen sensitization, and interaction with the microbiota (Ali et al., 2020). It also continuously varies due to interaction with the dynamic luminal. The role of epithelial barrier function is crucial in protecting against infection and inflammation. To prevent excessive inflammatory reactions, the epithelium has evolved strategies to restrict the growth of bacteria, minimize direct interaction with them, and hinder the spread of bacteria into the underlying tissue. Disturbance of the protective barrier of epithelium can result in an improper inflammatory reaction, believed to be a contributing factor in some disorders such as inflammatory bowel diseases, Crohn's disease, and ulcerative colitis. There are several aspects to the protective function of the intestinal barrier, such as the mucosal layer's role, the generation of antibacterial peptides, the release of IgA antibodies, adhesion mechanisms, the binding of probiotics in the gut to the epithelial layer, the creation of epithelial binding complex (Wang et al., 2018), and dynamic junctional complexes (Ohland & MacNaughton, 2010).

The mucus is a crucial layer of physical defense. It has a considerable role in decreasing adherence to pathogens. On the other hand, it provides materials for slow-growing commensal anaerobic microorganisms. It also protects the host from microbial penetration and different digestive enzymes. Releasing of mucus by goblet cells leads to the renewal of the mucus layer. Goblet cells are present alongside enterocytes throughout the digestive tract and are covered with mucin. These cells produce elongated mucin molecules that are heavily glycosylated. The mucins are either positioned on the cell surface or released into the lumen to create the protective mucus layer. Out of the various types of mucin glycoproteins present in humans, MUC2 stands as the most prevalent glycoprotein in the mucus of both the small and large intestines. While the amine and carboxyl termini do not undergo glycosylation to an equal degree, they contain a substantial amount of cysteine residues, which participate in the creation of disulfide bonds within and between molecules. These glycan groups provide protection against proteolytic enzymes and contribute to the hydrophilic properties of mucins. In addition, the connections formed by disulfide bonds create a network of glycoproteins that act as the foundation of the mucus membrane (Kelsall, 2008). Mucins create defense by safeguarding the epithelium against potentially harmful substances and molecules, simultaneously functioning as a lubricant to facilitate the movement of the intestines. Additionally, they are able to attach to carbohydrates on the surface of epithelial cells, creating the lower layer that securely binds to the mucosa, while the upper layer remains loosely attached (Phillipson et al., 2008). Another physical barrier function is referred to as the underlying layer of intestinal epithelial cells. It is facilitated by intercellular tight junctions, which comprise desmosomes, gap junctions, and adherent junctions. These components are based on different integral proteins including occludins, zonula occludens, and claudins. These proteins work to sustain the integrity of the cellular lining's barrier function via the paracellular transport regulation of different items such as ions, metabolites, and macromolecules. A cluster of enduring stem cells situated at the bottom of the crypt replenishes every few days. They are responsible for the constant regeneration of tube-like structures with crypts and lining epithelial cells (Clevers, 2013). The aforementioned stem cells generate progenitors and various differentiated epithelial cell types as they move up the crypt-villus axis through division before they undergo programmed cell death (apoptosis) and shedding into the lumen of the small and large intestines. The differentiated epithelial cell subtypes encompass absorptive cells (colonocytes, enterocytes), Paneth cells (found in the small intestine), enteroendocrine cells, tuft cells, goblet cells, and M cells. Each of these cell types plays an important role in the digestive, neuroendocrine, and immune functions of the barrier (Clevers, 2013). As previously mentioned, the epithelium and its related mucus layer are the primary defense against bacteria, acting as the first line of protection. Also, they perform a crucial role in establishing tolerance toward commensal members of the microbiota, ensuring a balanced and harmonious relationship with beneficial microorganisms. To achieve this goal, the barrier maintains a state of reduced responsiveness to microbial ligands, which is quite different from the immune-stromal-rich layer beneath it known as the lamina propria. Within the lamina propria, inborn and accommodative immune cells reside, exhibiting significantly higher reactivity toward both commensal and pathogenic microbial ligands. This contrast ensures that the barrier can appropriately respond to potential threats while fostering tolerance toward the beneficial members of the microbiota. The damage to the protective barrier of the gut is frequently connected to some intestinal diseases and various inflammatory conditions, both locally within the gut and systemically throughout the body. For instance, a reduced expression of proteins that contribute to the tight junction results in an increase in intestinal permeability. This increased permeability is linked to the development of local intestinal food allergies and can also contribute to systemic allergic conditions like asthma (Chen et al., 2014). It can lead to an inflammatory response if the integrity of the epithelial barrier is compromised, potentially leading to intestinal disorders. This is caused by the entry of pathogens and food allergens into the intestinal mucosa (Geirnaert et al., 2017). Generally, particular elements associated with the host and the microbiota can cause vulnerability in the epithelial barrier. Host factors encompass genetic or epigenetic modifications that affect protein expression, leading to changes in the epithelial barrier. These alterations can be either intrinsically programmed within the intestinal epithelial cells or extrinsically regulated by external factors. The host factors are crucial determinants in the modulation of the epithelial barrier in the intestines. These factors can be grouped into two categories: Genetic or epigenetic modifications and external factors. Genetic or epigenetic modifications refer to changes in the genetic code or modifications of the gene expression patterns. These alterations can occur within the intestinal epithelial cells themselves, giving rise to variations in protein expression. As a result, the barrier function of the epithelial cells may be influenced. On the other hand, external factors can also influence the epithelial barrier function. These factors can include various environmental cues, such as dietary components, gut microbiota, and immune response. Therefore, understanding the relationship between the intestinal microbiota and the epithelium is important, as the microbiome can serve as a pathway for changes influenced by various external environmental factors, including diet.

9.3 ROLE OF PROBIOTICS IN IMPROVING THE INTESTINAL EPITHELIAL BARRIER FUNCTION

Probiotics can be used to re-establish the function of the intestinal barrier. While the mechanisms of improvement of intestinal barrier function by probiotics have not been extensively explored, there are indications that upregulation of genes involved in cell signaling might be one of the potential ways they enhance the unity of the intestine (Anderson et al., 2010). The epithelial cells respond strongly to microbial signals, leading to local inflammation that can damage the intestinal epithelial barrier (Boonma et al., 2014). Strong activation of epithelial cells by microbial ligands leads to local inflammatory reactions that can cause the destruction of the intestinal epithelial barrier. The impact of the chemokine response varies across different probiotic strains. Additionally, a single probiotic strain has the ability to either increase or decrease the expression of specific chemokines. It has been reported that *Bifidobacterium bifidum* PRL2010 stimulates the production of CCL19 cytokine while suppressing the production of CCL22. This finding suggests that probiotics can elicit unique responses in terms of chemokine production, depending on the specific strain used (Turroni et al., 2014).

One of the important issues is apoptosis. Apoptosis is a natural phenomenon of programmed cell death that occurs in multicellular organisms and plays a key role in maintaining tissue homeostasis and eliminating damaged or unwanted cells. During apoptosis, cells undergo structural changes and DNA fragmentation and eventually break down into smaller apoptotic bodies. According to reports *Lactobacillus rhamnosus* GG can inhibit apoptosis induced by cytokines in epithelial cell models by preventing tumor necrosis factor (TNF) (Yan & Polk, 2006). In a study on mice, *L. rhamnosus* GG prevented programmed cell death and inflammation of the epithelial cells (Gaudier et al., 2005). Another mechanism in this regard is autophagy which is a cellular process in which cells break down and recycle their own components and plays a key role in achieving cellular health and preventing the accumulation of damaged components. It can be viewed as a crucial adaptive response to stress, as it aids in promoting cell survival, and it is essential for maintaining the integrity of the epithelial barrier. Certain *Bifidobacterium* strains have been discovered in an intestinal cell line, and they appear to promote autophagy in these cells (Lin et al., 2014). Studies indicate that autophagy plays a significant role in maintaining optimal intestinal function, and when this process is impaired, it can disrupt the balance and stability of the intestines. Gram-negative bacterial lipopolysaccharide is a major contributor to the development of pathogenic autophagy, which can result in the cytotoxicity of intestinal epithelial cells. Utilizing probiotics to induce autophagy is a potential strategy to prevent the harmful effects on epithelial cells and offer a novel means of protection (Han et al., 2016).

Increasing mucin is also another considerable issue. Probiotics can enhance the in vitro mucin expression and production of mucus as a potential way to enhance barrier function and prevent the entry of harmful microorganisms. In other in vitro studies, it has been indicated that *Lactobacillus* species can increase the expression of mucin in human epithelial cells, resulting in blockage invasion and attachment of pathogenic *Escherichia coli* (Mack et al., 2003). Another study showed that this probiotic had mitogenic effects and increased mucosal regeneration (Caballero-Franco et al., 2007). It has been reported that p40 *Lactobacillus* GG is able to activate the epidermal growth factor receptors, leading to an increase in the mucin production (Wang et al., 2014). Various types of *Lactobacillus* strains raised mucin production via upregulation of MUC-2 mucin gene expression in human intestinal cell lines Caco-2 (Mattar et al., 2002) and HT29 (MUC3) (Mack et al., 2003), thereby hindering the invasion and attachment of some pathogens such as *E. coli*. Also, the cell extract from *L. acidophilus* A4 was capable of raising MUC2 expression in HT29 cells (Kim et al., 2008). Generally, probiotics might enhance mucus production in vivo, but additional research is required to arrive at a definite conclusion.

One of the protective barrier mechanisms in epithelial cells involves producing and releasing antimicrobial substances. Beneficial microorganisms are crucial for maintaining healthy gut functions. Due to the close connection between the beneficial microbiota and the balance of the host's mucosal environment, the substances released by these beneficial bacteria can be viewed as a fundamental component of the intestinal defense. This is particularly true where these substances have a part to play in the prevention or elimination of harmful pathogens. When assessing the function of the gut barrier, it is important to take into account both these bacteria and the substances they produce. Aside from changing the levels at which host cell-generated antimicrobial peptides (AMPs) are expressed, probiotics also show the ability of harmful microorganisms elimination. They achieve this by generating antimicrobial substances such as SCFAs, bacteriocins, or microcins. Some of the released AMPs in epithelial cells are defensin and cathelicidin. These peptides help combat microbial threats and maintain the cell's defense against infections. Probiotics take a part in controlling the expression and secretion of defensin, and this regulation is influenced by local inflammatory mediators (Habil et al., 2014). In vitro studies have revealed that some strains of *Lactobacillus* such as *L. casei* (DN-114001), *L. casei* Shirota (YIT9029), *L. rhamnosus* (GG), *L. rhamnosus* (GR1) and *L. johnsonii* (La1) (Fayol-Messaoudi et al., 2005) and *Bifidobacterium* such as *B. thermophilum* RBL67 (Tanner et al., 2016) have the ability to eliminate or clear *Salmonella enterica* serovar *typhimurium*. The growth of pathogens, such as enterohemorrhagic *E. coli*, can be hindered by probiotic bacteria because of the formation of acetic and lactic acids, resulting in a decrease in the luminal pH (Dempsey & Corr, 2022).

Another mechanism that can be related to barrier functioning is secretory immunoglobulins. In cases of infection, probiotics have been observed to enhance overall levels of secretory immunoglobulin A (sIgA), including those targeted against specific pathogens, without typically triggering the production of sIgA specific to the probiotics themselves. Probiotics also exert a range of other immune-modulating impacts within the human intestines, such as encouraging the evolution of regulatory T cells and tolerogenic dendritic cells and suppressing the production of inflammatory cytokines.

One of the most crucial protective barrier mechanisms is tight junctions, which are comprised of multiple proteins. They play a vital role in achieving the unity of this barrier by securely binding the cells together. The disruption of tight junction proteins, which results in breaking the gastrointestinal barrier, has been seen in infection caused by pathogenic bacteria including *E. coli*, *C. difficile*, *C. rodentium*, *Vibrio cholera*, and *S. Typhimurium* (Ulluwishewa et al., 2011). In some cell barrier models, *Lactobacillus* strains have been seen to exert a regulatory influence on various genes encoding binding proteins, including Cadherin and β-catenin. In other words, these strains stabilize adherens junctions through two mechanisms including boosting the levels of E-cadherin expression and reinforcing the E-cadherin/β-catenin complex through an increased phosphorylation of β-catenin. On the other hand, the presence of *Lactobacillus* strains during the incubation with intestinal cells significantly impacts the phosphorylation of binding proteins (Hummel et al., 2012). A clinical investigation focusing on small intestine barrier function revealed that *L. plantarum* strains (WCFS1 and CIP104448, TIFN101) influenced the upregulation of gene expression related to tight junction and adherens junction proteins (Mujagic et al., 2017). It has been shown that *L. rhamnosus* GG ATCC 53103 increases the expression of ZO-1, claudin, and occludin in Caco-2 cells (Orlando et al., 2014). The same strain has been found to boost the expression of ZO-1 and improve the distribution of protein claudin-1. This is an important defense mechanism for *E. coli* O157:H7 infection (Johnson-Henry et al., 2008). Different strains of *L. plantarum* have also caused enhanced expression of ZO and occluding (Anderson et al., 2010; Qin et al., 2009). The application of *L. plantarum* into the duodenum led to an enhancement in ZO-1 and occludin staining near the tight junctions through the activation of TLR-2 (Karczewski et al., 2010). It has been speculated that the enhancement of barrier unity is achieved by modifying the structure and arrangement of proteins involved in tight junctions rather than simply increasing the abundance of these proteins (Dempsey & Corr, 2022). Regardless of probiotics, some prebiotics include inulin

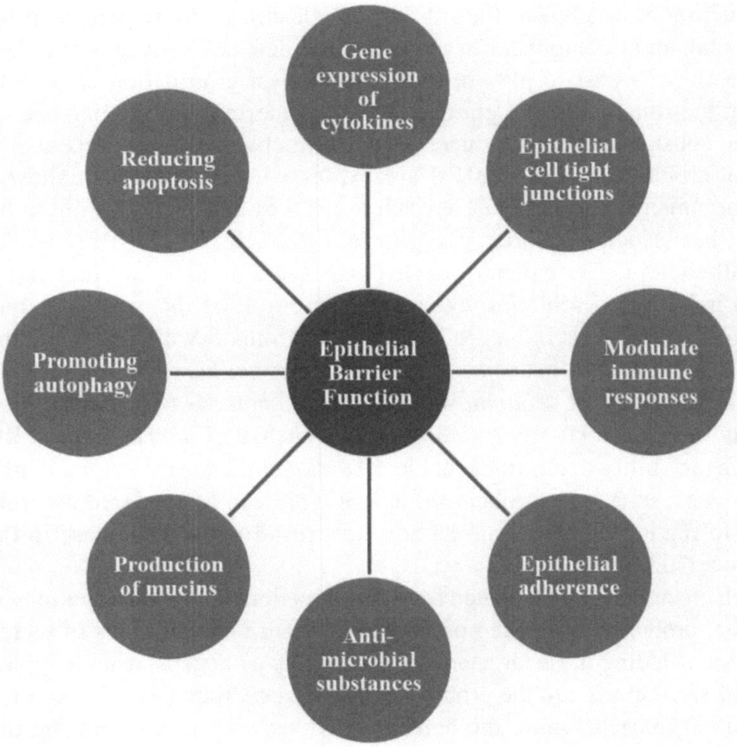

FIGURE 9.1 Classified mechanisms of probiotics in intestinal epithelial barrier functions.

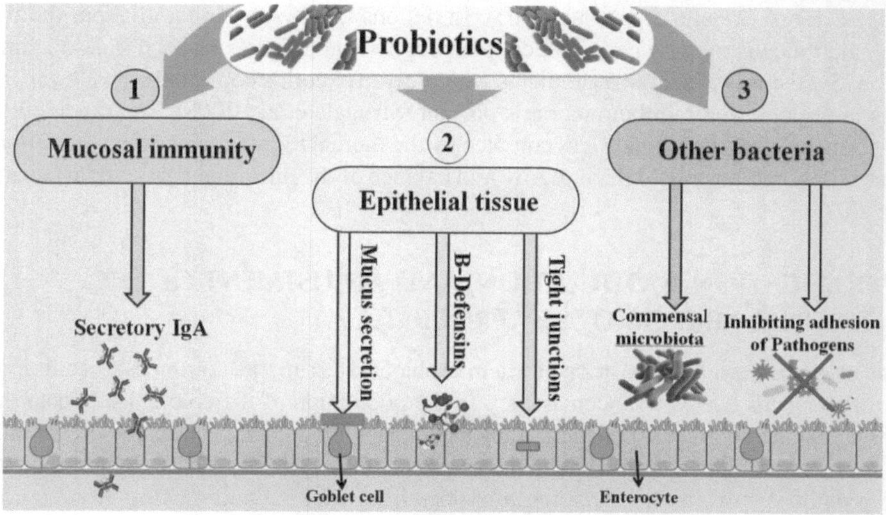

FIGURE 9.2 Pathways of probiotics in improving the intestinal epithelial barrier functions.

and fructo-oligosaccharide (Johnson-Henry et al., 2014) as well as other metabolites produced from fermentation such as short-chain fatty acids (SCFAs) (Jiang et al., 2013) have the ability to control the release of proinflammatory substances, the generation of AMPs, and the functioning of the epithelial barrier. Some studies have suggested that prebiotics may take a part in influencing the behavior of B cells, NKT cells, effector T cells, and Tregs (Nakamura et al., 2012). Functions of probiotics in strengthening the intestinal epithelial barrier have been briefly classified and visualized in Figures 9.1 and 9.2, respectively.

9.4 EFFECT OF PROBIOTICS ON EPITHELIAL OBSTRUCTION AND REGULATION OF INTESTINAL EPITHELIAL PERMEABILITY

Dynamic junctional complexes regulate permeability between intestinal epithelial cells. Different parameters such as intestinal problems and diseases determine the association between different amounts of proinflammatory cytokines and intestinal penetrability. The breakdown of gut barrier integrity has been identified as an initial occurrence in the development of several gastro-intestinal conditions such as celiac disease, multiple sclerosis, inflammatory bowel disease, obesity, and type 1 diabetes (Vancamelbeke & Vermeire, 2017). In addition, the intake of non-pathogenic bacteria may help to strengthen barrier functions by reducing cell permeability, offering natural protection against harmful agents, and strengthening the physical barrier of the mucus layer. This could play a role in safeguarding against infections, averting chronic inflammation, and upholding the integrity of the mucosal lining (Boirivant & Strober, 2007). The thickness of mucus can range between 50 and 800 micrometers; however, the region closest to the epithelium, measuring around 30 micrometers, is typically devoid of bacteria in individuals with good health (Swidsinski et al., 2007). The mucus serves as the initial obstacle encountered by intestinal bacteria, and in the case of an infection, pathogens must breach this barrier to access the epithelial cells. Microbes have evolved various strategies to break down mucus, enabling them to invade or acquire nutrients from the mucus. Some microorganisms such as *H. pylori* are capable of reducing the disulfide bonds within mucin. Some others such as *Pseudomonas aeruginosa* (Aristoteli & Willcox, 2003), *Candida albicans* (De Repentigny et al., 2000), and *Entamoeba histolytica* (Moncada et al., 2000) exhibit protease activity. Also, certain microorganisms including mixed oral and intestinal microbial communities have glycosidase activity (Macfarlane et al., 2005). In regions affected by inflammation, the thickness of the colonic mucous membrane is reduced, leading to higher levels of bacterial attachment and penetration (Swidsinski et al., 2007). Patients with ulcerative colitis commonly have thinner mucus, especially in regions where inflammation is present (Strugala et al., 2008). The modulation of the partially permeable barrier is made less complex by the mutual regulation between the different elements that collaborate to uphold the integrity and balance of the intestinal barrier (Vancamelbeke & Vermeire, 2017).

9.5 MODIFICATION, MODULATION, AND ADJUSTMENT OF THE INTESTINAL MICROBIOTA BY PROBIOTICS

Variations in the bacterial composition of gut microbiota interrupt the commensal relationship with the host that happens due to an inconsistency in the population of the commensal bacteria. When pathogens substitute commensal bacteria, they can occupy the intestinal wall and create inflammation and promote carcinogenic metabolites and signals (Wang & Li, 2022). Some proposed ways in which probiotics work are by stopping microbes from sticking and moving around, creating a less hospitable environment inside the gut (e.g., by changing the pH), making particular proteins that can kill bacteria such as bacteriocins, or triggering the body's own defenses like activating human defensins (Cammarota et al., 2014). The bacteria that are ingested make their way to the gut environment and start producing lipopolysaccharides to colonize. This activates dendritic cells, which trigger T-cell activation and B-cell differentiation. These B cells then release IgA, which helps eliminate pathogens. Additionally, the bacteria generate bacteriocins, which are AMPs that kill pathogens. They also decrease the luminal pH by producing organic acids, creating conditions that prevent the growth of pathogens. These bacteria generate growth factors such as vitamins and EPSs that support growth and metabolic reactions in the intestinal environment. The immune system responds to the presence of acetate, butyrate, and propionate by activating defense mechanisms (Indira et al., 2019). Maintaining a healthy balance in the GIT is crucial for preventing various diseases. The gastro-intestinal epithelium is the primary point of contact between the host and microorganisms. Any pathogen that invades the intestinal mucosa can trigger an immune response. Alterations in the microflora's composition and diversity are linked to many gastro-intestinal disorders, including inflammatory bowel disease, colorectal cancer, and irritable bowel syndrome. Additionally, these changes are associated with parenteral disorders such as cystic fibrosis, allergies, and bronchial asthma. Studies suggest that probiotics may help regulate and restore balance in the gut microbiota. This is achieved by improving the growth and activity of probiotics while suppressing pathogens. Although the exact mechanism of how probiotics achieve this is still unclear, it has commonly been assumed that they can prevent the growth of pathogens by producing SCFAs and toxins and competing for the same colonization sites (Liu et al., 2021). Probiotics can promote the production of β-defensin and IgA antibodies and manipulate the intestinal microbiome by suppressing the growth of pathogens. They also can strengthen the intestinal barrier by inducing mucin production (Hemarajata & Versalovic, 2013). For example, *E. coli* Nissle 1917 promotes β-defensin-2 upregulation in Caco-2 cells (Giorgetti et al., 2015). Mice that were given a diet high in fat had noticeable changes in the bacteria in their intestines that are linked to various illnesses. When probiotics were given to obese animals through injections, it was found that the type of bacteria called Firmicutes in their intestines decreased, while another type called Actinobacteria increased. Using probiotics can help fix imbalances in gut microbiota and reduce inflammation in mice. Therefore, gut flora plays a significant role in the treatment of diseases that cause inflammation (Wang et al., 2021). Probiotics aid in the production of vitamins and enzymes, which play a part in regulating biochemical reactions. B-complex vitamins (especially vitamin B_{12}) and vitamin K are produced by probiotics and help the growth of useful bacteria in the gut environment. Pyridoxine (vitamin B_6) helps the initial development of the nervous system. *Bifidobacterium* species are the main pyridoxine producers. Thiamine, also known as vitamin B_1, is another B-complex vitamin

TABLE 9.1
Effects of Probiotics on Signaling Pathways

Probiotic	Mechanism of Action	Results	References
Lactobacillus plantarum	Prevents the p38 and ERK1/2 MAPK signaling pathways activation	Controlling the innate immune response caused by ETEC K88 and inhibiting the excessive respond	Yang et al. (2021)
Lactobacillus delbrueckii CIDCA 133	Modulates TLR2/4/Myd88/NF-κB inflammatory signaling pathway	Enhancing 5-fluorouracil chemotherapy-induced mucositis	Barroso et al. (2022)
Lactobacillus rhamnosus	Promotes GALT to produce immune factors, induces an immune response, and is resistant to pathogen invasion	Mediating the regulation of NF-κB, MAPK, and ERK signaling pathways by surface-layer protein and EPSs for regulating intestinal cytokines	Geng et al. (2021)
Bacillus	Modulates TLR2/4/Myd88/NF-κB signaling pathway	Improvement of intestinal immune function	Du et al. (2018)

that is important for making fatty acids, aromatic amino acids, and other important substances that are needed for the brain. Researchers found that *Bifidobacterium* species are the main thiamine producers. *Propionibacterium shermani*, *L. reuteri*, and *S. typhinurium* are also the main producers of Vitamin B_{12} (Indira et al., 2019). Probiotics help improve the intestine lining by activating TLR specifically TLR2. Also, they can increase the immunity of the intestine by cytokines of TLR-like receptors. Other signaling pathways related to the MyD88 factor, NF-κB, MAPK, PKC, PI3K, STAT, p38, and ERK1/2 are known to be important for intestinal barrier function, and the combination of cellular signaling pathways methods can be affected by the use of probiotics (Gou et al., 2022). Table 9.1 mentions some probiotics and their effects on signaling pathways.

Certain types of helpful bacteria can control mucus production, which affects the characteristics of the protective layer in the intestine and indirectly influences the immune system. *L. plantarum* increases the expression of MUC2 and MUC3 genes in HT-29 and stimulates epithelial cells to secrete mucin and reduces the attachment of pathogens to the epithelium. Also, *E. coli* Nissle 1917 enhanced the expression of some genes including MUC2, MUC3, MUC5A, and MUC5AC (La Fata et al., 2018).

9.6 COMPETITIVE ADHESION AND ATTACHMENT OF PROBIOTICS TO INTESTINAL EPITHELIAL SURFACES

Adhesion ability is the initial condition for the effective performance of probiotics. The strains that settle and colonize in the intestinal mucosa are recognized faster by the host due to better interaction with the host's digestive system and cause immune responses in the host's body. Also, the adhesion of probiotics to the mucosa prevents pathogenic microorganisms from attaching to the intestinal cells (van Zyl et al., 2020). One of the mechanisms of probiotics is the probiotic's antagonism against pathogens. The main requirement for selecting the right strain is adhesion ability, which varies from strain to strain. Probiotic strains with high adhesion capacity can block pathogen binding by competing for host binding sites (Monteagudo-mera et al., 2019). In recent years, scientists have been using human intestinal cell lines such as HT-29 and Caco2 cells to choose beneficial strains in vitro. The human gut is usually studied using HT-29 and Caco-2 cells (Radhamanalan & Dharumadurai, 2022). In general, bacteria have a tendency to attach to surfaces for survival, which helps bacteria to remain present in the gut microbiota for several days. In this regard, the hydrophobicity of the bacterial surface is one of the most considerable factors governing the mechanism of bacterial adhesion to surfaces. Adhesion of bacteria to the intestinal surface can be established initially by nonspecific physical hydrophobic binding, followed by a second adhesion step by specific components of the cellular wall (Haddaji et al., 2015).

The surface structures of probiotics that help them attach to surfaces are also called adhesins or ligands. Different surface proteins, pili, and EPSs are the most important examples of surface structures (Gorreja & Walker, 2022). Surface proteins are mainly multifunctional cytoplasmic proteins that apply moonlighting functions as cell wall-anchored proteins (Muscariello et al., 2020). Mucus-binding proteins, which include Mub (mucus-binding protein) and MucBP (mucin-binding protein) domains, can bind to the peptidoglycan cell wall with a C-terminal motif, LPXTG (Monteagudo-Mera et al., 2019). *L. reuter* Mub take an important part in mucosal adhesion in *Lactobacillus* strains. *B. animalis* subsp. *Lactis* and *B. bifidum* also bind to plasminogen or human enterocytes through these surface proteins (Javanshir et al., 2021). *L. plantarum*, *L. acidophilus*, *L. fermentum*, and *L. johnsonii* also use mucus-binding protein adhesins that attach to the mucosal layer (Muscariello et al., 2020). Pre-treatment of cell lines Caco-2 and HT-29 with purified Mubs5s6 prevented enteropathogenic *E. coli* from attaching. This process happened because Mubs5s6 attached to Hsp90, cytokeratins, and laminin, which are three infection-related ligands in the host mucosa (Singh et al., 2018). There are six mucus-binding domains in The Mub of *L. plantarum* 91 and the last two domains are thought to be involved in exhibiting high adhesiveness in human gastrointestinal tissue. We can purify and utilize Mub from *L. plantarum* 91 in other species (Gorreja & Walker, 2022).

Mucus adhesion-promoting proteins (MapAs) are also one of the important cell surface proteins in lactobacilli species that strengthen their attachment to GIT mucosa. Also, AP48-MapAs are parts of MapAs in the structure of *L. reuteri* LA92 that have AMP properties. While Mub and MapA function is not clarified yet DSM17938, it seems that their existence is beneficial for multiple *L. reuteri* strains. It has been demonstrated that MapA genes in the eight *L. reuteri* tested, significantly increased when co-cultured with Caco-2 cells as a model for barrier function intestinal tract. The existence of Mud and MapS proposes openings to present modern strains of *L. reuteri* as potential probiotics (Singh et al., 2021). This protein is similar to a protein called CnBP, found in *L. crispatus*. It can attach to Caco-2 cells and collagen (Muscariello et al., 2020). Due to the multifunctional nature of these proteins, they take a part in regulating the gut microbiota. Some strains of *L. reuteri* (104 R and LA92) are not usually in clinical use, but some strains such as *L. reuteri* DSM17938 are used to treat infant diseases. According to meta-analysis there is still no agreement on whether this type of bacteria is really helpful, especially for infants with colic (Gorreja & Walker, 2022).

Gram-positive probiotic bacteria have an external layer made of proteins called a surface layer. This special paracrystalline structure is made by a protein called surface-layer-protein (SLP) that assembles itself (do Carmo et al., 2018). The surface-layer proteins of probiotic bacteria are different in each strain. They can interact with receptors in the intestine cells, which triggers immune responses and helps regulate the immune system (Malanovic & Lohner, 2016). The SLPs that play the role of scaffolding for the cell surface proteins are called SLAPs. *Levilactobacillus brevis* is a lactic acid bacterium that can inhibit bacterial infection and modulate the immune system. This microorganism exists in dairy products such as milk and cheese, fermented products, and the intestinal tract of humans and animals (Mazzeo et al., 2022). For example, the fibronectin-binding protein of *L. acidophilus* is an SLAP. SlpAs are formed by lactobacilli bacteria and are specifically assigned to *L. acidophilus* group A. Bacteria containing these proteins include; *L. acidophilus*, *L. gallinarum*, *L. crispatus*, *L. amylophilus*, *L. jensenii*, *L. kefiranofaciens*, *L. helveticus*, and *L. amylovorus* (Sanders et al., 2018). The ability of *Ligilactobacillus salivarius* REN to adhere to intestinal cells is controlled by choline-binding protein A (CbpA). The research showed that there is a receptor called enolase on HT-29 cells that can recognize CbpA (Wang et al., 2017). *L. acidophilus* SlpAs can prevent infection by blocking the receptor DC-SIGN and murine hydrolase activity (Acosta et al., 2016).

Collagen-binding protein (Cbp) can bind to components of the GIT extracellular collagen and is a bacterial cell surface protein. *Lactiplantibacillus plantarum* LM3, 91, and W2 from *Lactobacillus* strains have the ability to bind to collagen. At first collagen binding was seen to be a pathogenic factor due to its ability to promote the colonization of pathogens, but probiotics could mirror the same process without causing injury (Gorreja & Walker, 2022). The Cbp protein is the major influencing factor in preventing the adhesion of *E. coli* to constituents of the extracellular matrix (ECM). Fibronectin acts as a goal for bacterial adhesins in the GIT and has been recognized in bacteria associated with a host. In pathogens, some FnBPs can cause virulence through adhesion, invasion, and interference with signal transmission. Despite the fact that FnBPs in probiotic strains are essential for attachment to their ecological sites, they are not sufficient to cause harmfulness (Hymes & Klaenhammer, 2016). Addition of the Cbp gene from *L. reuteri* Pg4 species to *L. casei* ATCC 393 bacteria, which has low adhesion ability, resulted in higher competitiveness against pathogenic microorganisms in Caco-2 cells (Monteagudo-Mera et al., 2019).

Sortase-dependent proteins or LPXTG-containing proteins are a group of surficial proteins that attach to the cell wall by forming strong chemical covalent bonds after going through the membrane via the sec pathway. Sortase is a membrane-related transpeptidase that exist in gram-positive bacteria. Sortases are accountable for binding a major group of released proteins to the cell surface by identification of a motif (LPXTG) preserved in these proteins. In simple words, the two-arginine or sec pathway is used for most proteins that have to be transferred outside of cells. The latter recognizes unfolded proteins that own a special tag called signal peptide at the start of their chain. This tag is made up of three parts: a hydrophobic H region, a basic N region, and a C region that owns a specific site where it can be cut by a special enzyme called signal peptidase (Javanshir et al., 2021).

Aggregating factors are high molecular weight molecules that contain large amounts of threonine and lysine. They are part of the large family of snow-fake forming collagen-binding aggregation factors proteins. *L. reuteri* RC-14 and *L. rhamnosus* GR-1 from lactobacilli strains can apply positive effects on our wellbeing by auto-aggregation and co-aggregation ability and preventing the colonization of *C. glabrata*. AggLb or auto-aggregation promoting protein is the biggest protein of cell surface found in lactobacilli (Miljkovic et al., 2019).

Fimbriae or pili help bacteria move and stick to surfaces. Type IV pili in gram-negative bacteria have been extensively studied. They help bacteria to attach and colonize in mucosal membrane. Some studies have indicated that gram-positive bacteria such as *Bifidobacterium* can also express this kind of pili. Furthermore, certain types of *Lactobacillus* bacteria have the ability to create SpaCBA pili. The remarkable ability of *L. rhamnosus* LGG to bind to the gastro-intestinal layer is due to the presence of SpaC at the tip of the pili, which is actually a mucus-binding protein (Monteagudo-Mera et al., 2019). In some lactobacilli (such as *L. rhamnosus* and *L. ruminus*) and bifidobacteria (*lactis*, *bifidum*, *longum*, *adolescentis*, and *dentium*), certain kinds of pili that depend on sortase and are found on the outer surface of cells have been identified. These pilin-like appendages often have a close connection with the inside lining of the intestines and they have the ability to attach to mucin. Mucin binding through Mub and pili is identified as the main mechanisms of probiotic activity that help them stay in the GIT and competitive exclusion of pathogens (Sanders et al., 2018).

EPSs authorize the connection between GIT cells and probiotics, they also help probiotic survival by adhering to the gastro-intestinal mucosal epithelium. EPS is present in a wide range of bacteria, such as the *Lactobacillus* and *Bifidobacterium* genera. The probiotic LGG appears to use EPSs to prevent pathogens from sticking to surfaces. This effect is stronger with higher doses of EPS. *B. animals* IPLA-R1 and *B. animalis* subsp. *Lactis* are being studied. The study found that EPSs or biofilm formation can interfere with other bacteria (pathogens and probiotics) (Gorreja &

Walker, 2022). The EPS obtained from *L. plantarum* WLPL04 revealed a strong capability to block the formation of biofilms by harmful bacteria like *E. coli* O157:H7, *P. aeruginosa* CMCC10104, *S. Typhimurium* ATCC13311, and *Staphylococcus aureus* CMCC26003 In addition, the EPS strongly stopped the HT-29 cells from proliferation (Liu et al., 2017).

9.7 ANTI-INFLAMMATORY AND ANTIOXIDANT ACTIVITY OF PROBIOTICS IN THE INTESTINAL EPITHELIUM

9.7.1 Anti-Inflammatory Activity

Probiotics in the gut lumen can connect to lamina propria by dendrites and be imported into the lumen by M-cells transcytosis. Probiotics can affect the immune system in two ways: By producing TNF-α, IL-1β, and IL-12 and activating the signals of the immune system or operating tolerance signaling by encouraging anti-inflammatory cytokines such as TGF-β and IL-10. Macrophages and dendritic cells can induce the production of regulatory T cells (iTregs) in a TGF-β/IL-10 rich environment. The iTregs take a part in peripheral immune tolerance. A standard mixture of *L. casei* and *L. acidophilus*, *L. reuteri*, *B. bifidum*, and *Streptococcus thermophilus* upregulates the iTregs population. Atopic dermatitis, colitis, and rheumatoid arthritis (auto-immune disorders) are hyper-immune disorders that develop due to an uncontrolled immune response (Kang & Im, 2015). In simple terms, probiotics can help reduce inflammation in four different ways: help reduce inflammation by producing more butyrate, tolerance induction by increasing the cytokines ratio, lowering the number of eosinophils in serum, and expression of a protein called metalloproteinase-9. Proinflammatory responses are reduced by NF-κB regulation by *Lactobacillus*. In addition, probiotics regulate dendritic cell's maturation into anti-inflammatory cytokines for example IL-10.

Probiotics release a lot of SCFAs while they ferment food fibers. Acetate is one of these SCFAs that help in decreasing the inflammation in diseases such as colitis and asthma in animal models. Neutrophils stop inflammation by attaching G protein-coupled receptors (GPR 41, 43) to SCFAs (Eslami et al., 2020). One of the SCFAs, known as butyric acid, is the most effective in reducing inflammation. Inflammation of the intestinal lining is often linked to various diseases and is caused by lack of energy. Butyric acid is one of the sources of energy for the intestinal cells and has an advantageous effect on the immune system of both the intestinal and other mucosal cells. Butyric acid also regulates gene expression by influencing both stimulants and inhibitors that control gene expression. A few of these pathways are associated with histone hyperacetylation because of the prevention of the histone deacetylase enzyme activity (Markowiak-Kopeć & Śliżewska, 2020). The application of probiotics caused changes in the composition of gut bacteria, favoring the growth of beneficial types such as *Prevotella* and *Oscillibacter* that produce substances that reduce inflammation, resulting in the promotion of anti-inflammatory Treg/Type 1 regulatory T cells in the gut (Li et al., 2016).

9.7.2 Antioxidant Activity

9.7.2.1 Controlling the Enzymes that Produce Reactive Oxygen Species

The NADPH oxidase (NOX) complex makes a significant amount of reactive oxygen species. There are seven types of NOX in humans that produce ROS for different purposes like protecting the body and signaling. *Bacillus amyloliquefaciens* SC06 helps to decrease the function of NOX and p47phox expression, which is caused by H_2O_2 in IPEC-1, also *L. coryniformis* CECT5711, *L. fermentum* CECT5716, and *L. gasseri* CECT5714 were able to reduce the activity and gene expressions of NOX-1 and NOX-4 in rats with high blood pressure (Wang et al., 2017). When cytochrome P450 (CYP) enzymes don't work properly, they can cause the production of ROS and oxidative stress because CYP enzymes are responsible for xenobiotic substance metabolism. A few probiotics diminish the expression of (CYP). For example, *L. casei* can decrease the production of CYP1A1 in the intestines of male rats (Heydari et al., 2022).

9.7.2.2 Ability to Chelate Metal Ions

Transition metal ions can cause hydrogen peroxide to break down into peroxyl and alkoxy radicals. They can also start lipid peroxidation, which increases oxidative stress (Hoffmann et al., 2021). Ions Fe^{2+} and Cu^{2+} are produced in free-radical reactions. The Fe^{2+} creates a substance called HO· through the Fenton reaction. Additionally, Cu^{2+} that is released from chromatin can also aid in the formation of HO·. Many types of lactic acid bacteria strains have been discovered to have significant chelating ability for both Cu^{2+} and Fe^{2+} (Feng & Wang, 2020). It may be the chelators found in probiotic intracellular extracts that make this bacteria's chelation ability possible (Wang et al., 2017). DPPH free-radical scavenging property of probiotics Analysis shows that the most significant Fe^{+2} chelation activity was recorded for *S. salivarius* ST62HK with 98.2%. *S. salivarius* ST59HK shows the highest DPPH free-radical scavenging was 85.24% (Rwubuzizi et al., 2023). *L. rhamnosus* GG's ability of iron chelating and superoxide radical scavenging inhibits lipid peroxidation. Since probiotics live in the colon, it's possible that they protect the body by doing certain things in the intestines, like producing enzymes and substances like SOD, inducing the production of antioxidants and chelating activities (Faraki & Rahmani, 2021).

9.7.2.3 Antioxidant Metabolites

Metabolites produce by probiotics include folate, glutathione (GSH), and butyrate. GSH is a cellular non-enzymatic cellular antioxidant that removes hydroxyl, peroxynitrite, and hydrogen peroxides radicals mainly by cooperating with selenium-dependent glutathione peroxidase (Wang et al., 2017). Folate is a type of vitamin that helps in different chemical reactions in our body by receiving one-carbon units from other molecules (Chugh & Kamal-Eldin, 2020). Folate is a group of chemicals that are similar to folic acid. Lactobacilli and bifidobacteria strains can produce naturally folate-enriched products (Andlid et al., 2018). Butyrate shows a wide extent of activities, including counting, metabolic pathways controller, and anti-inflammatory, antioxidant, anti-obesity, and anti-angiogenesis activities (Amiri et al., 2021). *C. butyricum* strain MIYAIRI 588 is a butyrate-generating probiotic. The antioxidant properties have been revealed in rats with non-alcoholic fatty liver disease against oxidative stress in the liver (Endo et al., 2013).

9.7.2.4 Antioxidant Enzymes System

Superoxide is a common type of ROS made by the mitochondria. However, an enzyme called SOD can convert superoxide into safer substances like hydrogen peroxide and water. Bacteria can use Fe-SOD and Mn-SOD (Wang et al., 2017). Lactic acid bacteria own their special antioxidant enzymatic system and a wide range of them can produce antioxidant enzymes that break down free radicals into O_2 and H_2O_2. Scientists have found that SOD activity can be found in cell-free extracts from certain types of bacteria called *Lactococcus* and *S. thermophilus*, however, *Lactococcus* shows more significant SOD activity than *S. thermophiles* (Feng & Wang, 2020). Also, an enzyme called catalase (CAT) helps protect cells from damage by breaking down hydrogen peroxide, which stops the formation of harmful hydroxyl radicals by the Fenton reaction (Tomusiak-Plebanek et al., 2018). *Lactobacillus* with higher levels of catalase were better at reducing inflammation in mice with inflammatory bowel disease compared to strains of the same bacteria that produce SOD (Tomusiak-Plebanek et al., 2018).

9.7.2.5 Antioxidant Communication Pathway Controlled by Probiotics

The transcription factor NF-κB mediates inflammatory cytokines expression in inflammatory conditions. ROS activates NF-κB which is the initial transcription factor that reacts to oxidative stress. The *Bacillus* strain LBP32 extracellular polysaccharide inhibits NF-κB and ROS production and inhibits LPS-related inflammation in some macrophages called RAW 264.7 (Heydari et al., 2022).

For example, the VSL#3 mixture of probiotics could block NF-κB (Diao et al., 2014). Activation of Nrf2 upregulates numerous genes such as genes involved in xenobiotics, and ROS detoxification that endures oxidative and environmental stressors. Probiotics can effectively apply their antioxidant effects by regulating the Nrf2-Keap1-ARE pathway (Wang et al., 2017). Also, researchers found new evidence that showed how a probiotic called *B. amyloliquefaciens* SC06 helps reduce oxidative stress caused by H_2O_2 in IPEC-1 cells by lowering levels of ROS and regulating Nrf2 expressions (Wang et al., 2017). PKC is responsible for controlling the phosphorylation of hydroxyls on serine and threonine remaining parts in proteins. MAPKs, including ERK, JNK, and p38-MAPK, are involved in multiple signaling pathways (Feng & Wang, 2020).

9.7.2.6 Exopolysaccharides

The properties of EPS natural compounds synthesized by specific bacteria like *L. plantarum*, *L. gasseri*, *L. acidophilus*, and *L. rhamnosus* are believed to have the potential to combat tumors and safeguard against ROS (Angelin & Kavitha, 2020). EPS (partly purified) of *L. plantarum* YML009 has antioxidant activities such as modulating antioxidant activities and ROS scavenging (Seo et al., 2015).

9.8 INHIBITION OF THE GROWTH OF PATHOGENS BY PROBIOTICS

There are various ways in which probiotic bacteria can suppress the growth of pathogens. These methods include competing against pathogens for adhesion to the epithelial barrier's binding sites, competing for nutrients, producing antimicrobial substances, and preventing the expression of virulence factors. As mentioned in detail earlier, competitive exclusion (CE) is a special probiotic strategy that includes the addition of probiotics to the GIT to reduce the colonization of pathogens in the gut. In this situation, one exclusive species of bacteria in the gut microbiota competes for binding sites in the intestine more strongly than other species. Fighting over nutrition sources, decreasing the pH level, and creating substances such as bacteriocins are some of the main ways that pathogens are kept out by competition. The term "colonization resistance" means using probiotics to stop or control infections in the intestines (Plaza-Diaz et al., 2019).

When present in the human colon, probiotics can ferment non-digestible carbohydrates and produce SCFAs like butyrate, acetate, and propionate (Figure 9.3) (Chang et al., 2021). Toxicity caused by SCFA can lead to growth inhibition due to various defects in cellular processes. These defects can vary depending on the pathway, organism, and environmental conditions. For instance, in *E. coli*, propionate has a greater impact on the synthesis of DNA compared to the synthesis of proteins, RNA, lipids, or cell walls. Similarly, *B. subtilis* experienced inhibited amino acid uptake after being exposed to acetate and propionate. The SCFA not only affects the functions of the host but also acts as a source of carbon for the microbiota within the body. However, at high concentrations, they can have toxic effects on bacteria. Many in vitro studies have demonstrated that the toxicity can be attributed to the non-ionized forms of these acids, which are more prominent at low pH levels (Sun & O'Riordan, 2013). The release of SCFAs can lower the pH of the hindgut by releasing H^+ ions, which helps to prevent pathogen invasion and colonization. The consumption of luminal oxygen by SCFAs, particularly butyrate, creates an anaerobic condition that reduces the growth of aerobic pathogens such as *Salmonella* in the gut lumen (Liu et al., 2021). The addition of butyrate or propionate can decrease the expression of invasion genes in Wildtype (WT) *S. enterica typhimurium*, while acetate does not have the same effect. The molecular processes of inhibition have been extensively studied, and SCFA metabolism has been found to be significant. This involves the conversion of acetate and propionate into acetyl-phosphate and propionyl-CoA, respectively that take a part in controlling the expression of virulence genes (Sun & O'Riordan, 2013). Butyrate inhibits the bacterial growth of *L. monocytogenes* by altering its carbon metabolism. It also affects the generation of the virulence factor, called listeriolysin O (Rinehart et al., 2018). Propionate inhibits the growth of *S. typhimurium* by producing toxic products and disrupting intracellular pH homeostasis (Jacobson et al., 2018).

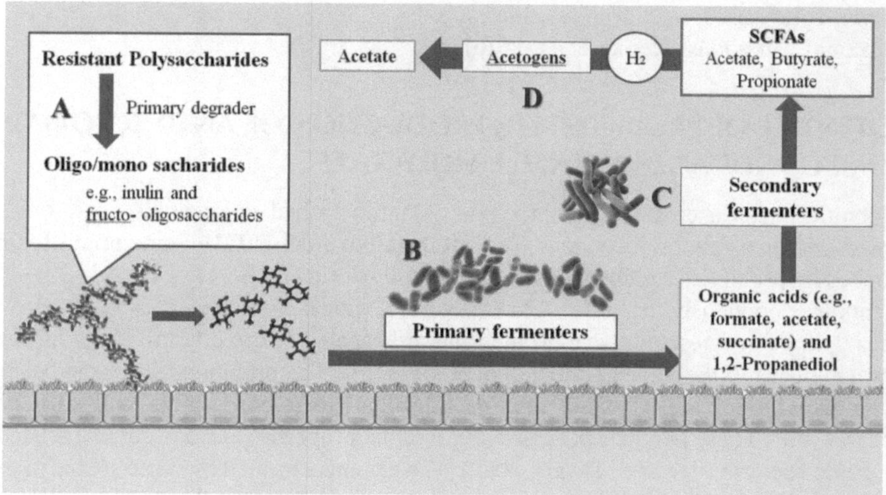

FIGURE 9.3 An overview of SCFAs production steps in GIT. (A) In the first step, polysaccharides are hydrolyzed and converted into oligo/monosaccharides. (B) Primary fermenters such as *Bacteroides* utilize oligo/monosaccharides to produce organic acids and alcohols such as 1,2-propanediol. (C) Secondary fermenters use these metabolites to generate SCFAs. (D) Finally, H_2 serves as an electron donor for acetogen and produces acetate.

Certain types of bacteria, specifically lactobacilli and bifidobacteria, have the ability to create peptides called bacteriocins. These bacteriocins have antimicrobial properties, meaning they can inhibit the growth of pathogens in the gastro-intestinal (Plaza-Diaz et al., 2019). Bacteriocins, peptides manufactured by bacteria, are small and able to withstand high temperatures, and they exhibit the capacity to eliminate other bacteria. They are membrane-active peptides whose presence is particularly prominent in gram-positive bacteria and eliminate the target bacteria by causing a disturbance on their cell wall. Due to these features, bacteriocins help the CE of pathogens, and interference competition amid the host's microbiota and improve the colonization of probiotics (Umu et al., 2017). Most bacteriocins of lactic acid bacteria can be divided into two classes. Class I are known as "lanthionine-containing bacteriocins" that involve nisin, linaridin, lasso peptide, azoline, glycocin, cyanobactin, sactiobiotic, and thiopeptide. Bacteriocins of Class II are called "non-lanthionine-containing bacteriocins" and are grouped into four categories based on their size (Lopetuso et al., 2019). Class Iia bacteriocins are a certain type of bacteriocins that are similar to pediocin. They usually work well against *Listeria* bacteria, but they can also affect other types of bacteria like *Enterococcus*, *Lactobacillus*, *Leuconostoc*, *Pediococcus*, and *Clostridium*. Subclass b consists of plantaricins E, F, J, and K. Class IIc bacteriocins, such as garvacin ML, are circular in shape due to their connected starting and ending points. Class IId comprises all bacteriocins that do not fall under the previously mentioned groups, including enterocin Q and linear bacteriocins (Lopetuso et al., 2019; Umu et al., 2017).

Enterococcus faecalis produce bactofencin A or bacteriocin 21 that can kill bacteria that are resistant to multiple drugs. It also helps to control the competition between different types of bacteria in the intestines (Kommineni et al., 2015). Bacteriocins help specific communities in the GIT to survive by choosing strains that can resist changes caused by the diet, neutralizing natural defenses, bile salts, and harmful factors, and stopping other species from colonizing. This causes the improvement of the gut barrier function and the immune response (Lopetuso et al., 2019). Bacteriocins of lactic acid bacteria are effective against *S. aureus*, *S. enteritidis*, *L. monocytogenes* (Umu et al., 2017), and vancomycin-resistant *enterococci* (Kommineni et al., 2015). Certain metabolites produced by *L. acidophilus* and *L. plantarum* have been found to prevent the growth of *C. difficile*,

Helicobacter, rotaviruses, and drug-resistant strains of *Shigella* species and *E. coli* in specific gastro-intestinal conditions (Kumar et al., 2016).

9.9 POTENTIAL OF PROBIOTICS IN PRODUCTION OF ANTIMICROBIAL COMPOUNDS AND DEFENSIVE MOLECULES

Many probiotic bacteria create different types of antimicrobial compounds, including SCFAs, organic acids, ethanol, bacteriocins, and H_2O_2 (Rabetafika et al., 2023). Some important metabolites produced by probiotics are shown in Figure 9.4.

As mentioned previously, bacterial AMPs are also known as bacteriocins. They are a group of peptides that are synthesized by ribosomes and are capable of directly killing or inhibiting the growth of pathogens in the lumen (Rabetafika et al., 2023). The probiotic lactic acid bacteria produce bacteriocins, which are typically small peptides that create pores on the cell wall of bacteria and kill target cells. These peptides possess antimicrobial properties and can combat related strains and pathogenic bacteria (Pawar & Tiwari, 2022). The channels formed by bacteriocins in the target cell membrane cause the leakage of small ions, which results in the collapse of the proton-motive force (Abanoz & Kunduhoglu, 2018).

The microbiota in the colon produces SCFAs via the anaerobic fermentation of indigestible carbohydrates such as resistant starch and dietary fiber. These SCFAs are the main metabolites and can directly or indirectly affect gut–brain communication and brain function (Silva et al., 2020). The proximal colon contains the highest levels of SCFAs, which can either be used by enterocytes in that area or transported into the bloodstream via the gut epithelium. There are two main signaling mechanisms involving SCFAs: inhibition of histone deacetylases and activation of G-protein-coupled receptors. The histone deacetylases play a crucial role in regulating gene expression, so inhibiting them can lead to a wide range of effects downstream (Tan et al., 2014). The SCFAs play a vital role in creating an acidic environment in the intestines. This helps to fight against pathogenic microorganisms that thrive in weak alkaline environments (Mirzaei et al., 2022). Butyrate is a type of SCFA that has therapeutic benefits for several diseases. These include antibiotic-associated diarrhea, inflammatory bowel disease,

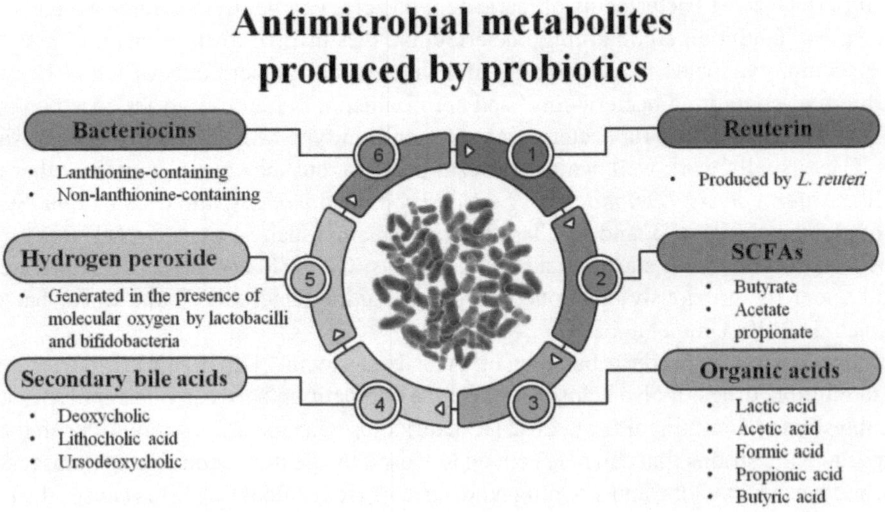

FIGURE 9.4 Some important metabolites produced by probiotics that affect an extensive range of gram-positive/gram-negative bacteria and suppress the growth and colonization of pathogens in the gastro-intestinal tract.

heart disease, and colon cancer. It is interesting to learn that 10% of our daily caloric needs as humans are fulfilled by SCFAs produced in the large intestine. Even more fascinating is the fact that among these acids, butyrate, produced in colonocytes, gives us 60-70% of our energy (Indira et al., 2019).

Organic acids (e.g., citric acid, lactic acid, and acetic acid) also possess antimicrobial characteristics based on their capability to penetrate cell membranes, due to their lipophilic nature in their undissociated structure, to alter the concentrations of protons and associated anions in the cytoplasm (Gómez-García et al., 2019). Organic acids have the ability to decrease the intracellular pH, which stops the active transport of excess internal protons and requires the use of cellular adenosine triphosphate (ATP), leading to cell depletion. These organic acids target various aspects of bacteria, including cell walls, cytoplasmic membranes, and specific metabolism, which ultimately results in the elimination and demise of harmful microorganisms (Bangar et al., 2022). Lactic acid bacteria use conjugated linoleic acid (CLA) as a way to detoxify unsaturated fatty acids and convert them to saturated fatty acids. This is done through the biohydrogenation pathway, with linoleate isomerase being the enzyme that facilitates the conversion of linoleic acid (LA) to CLA (Shaikh et al., 2018). The main producers of LA are *Lactobacillus*, *Bifidobacterium*, and *Lactococcus*. CLA was capable of preventing the growth of pathogenic bacteria such as *S. typhimurium* and EHEC by downregulating the bacterial virulence gene expression (Peng et al., 2018). Research has shown that CLA has the ability to change the physiochemical characteristics of certain pathogens. This includes altering their surface hydrophobicity, auto-aggregation, and morphology. The CLA achieves this by linking with the cytoplasmic membrane and interrupting the phospholipid or extracellular polysaccharides biosynthesis (Peng & Biswas, 2017).

Reuterin (β-hydroxypropionaldehyde) is a natural antimicrobial compound that is resistant to proteolytic and lipolytic enzymes. It is produced by the *L. reuteri* INIA P579 strain and has been found to be effective against several foodborne pathogens such as *Clostridium* species, *E. coli*, *L. monocytogenes*, *Salmonella* species, and *Shigella* species (Mogoşanu et al., 2017). Research has shown that reuterin has the ability to effectively hinder the growth of *H. pylori* and diminish the expression of its virulence genes such as *vacA*, *flaA*, and *luxS*. This indicates that reuterin may play a crucial role in achieving a healthy gastro-intestinal microbiota by preventing the proliferation of other commensal and harmful microorganisms including *H. pylori* (Urrutia-Baca et al., 2018). In addition, multiple studies have discovered that solutions containing reuterin possess antimicrobial properties that can fight off a wide range of bacteria, including both gram-negative and gram-positive types, as well as molds, yeasts, and protozoa. Reuterin unequivocally depletes free thiol groups in glutathione (GSH) and other proteins including enzymes, which causes a lack of harmony in the cellular redox status that causes the inevitable death of bacterial cells. The antimicrobial effects of reuterin are primarily attributed to acrolein (Asare et al., 2020).

Certain types of bacteria, such as lactobacilli and bifidobacteria, produce hydrogen peroxide (H_2O_2) when exposed to molecular oxygen. However, the specific enzymes responsible for this process are not well understood. In *L. johnsonii* NCC533, the primary source of H_2O_2 is NADH-dependent flavin reductase (nfr), and removing this gene leads to a decrease in H_2O_2 production when oxygen is present (Singh et al., 2018). The process of oxygen-dependent lactate utilization involves three reactions that can produce H_2O_2. These reactions are (i) oxidation of pyruvate and are catalyzed by the Pox enzyme; (ii) oxidation of lactate, being catalyzed by the Lox enzyme; and (iii) oxidation of NADH and being catalyzed by the NOX enzyme (Hertzberger et al., 2014). H_2O_2 production is not affected by the predicted genes that encode pyruvate oxidase, lactate oxidase, or NADH oxidase. In lactic acid bacteria, the primary factor contributing to H_2O_2 production is the lactate usage mechanism that depends on oxygen. This pathway oxidizes lactate through acetyl-phosphate and pyruvate to acetate, producing H_2O_2, CO_2, NADH, and ATP (Hertzberger et al., 2014).

9.10 THERAPEUTIC PERFORMANCE OF PROBIOTICS IN THE PREVENTION AND TREATMENT OF DAMAGE IN EPITHELIAL INJURY AND WOUND HEALING

One of the functions of probiotics is to facilitate the restoration of epithelial barriers after injury. It has been reported that *E. coli* Nissle EcN1917 counteracts the intestinal mucosal barrier dysfunction induced by enteropathogenic *E. coli* and aids in the restoration of T84 and Caco-2 mucosal cells. In this regard, the binding proteins ZO-2 and the expression of PKC protein kinase play a role in promoting this influence, contributing to the regeneration of a robust binding complex (Fábrega et al., 2017). Similar mechanisms have been reported for *L. casei* DN-114001 and VSL3 which can preserve intestinal barrier function (Merenstein et al., 2010). Also, *L. casei* VSL3 has shown protection of the epithelial barrier (Javanshir et al., 2021). In an animal study on rats that were orally fed *Bacillus* SC06 for 24 days, it has been shown that this probiotic resulted in significant intestinal tissue repair and mitigated apoptosis by controlling the expression of Bcl2, Bax, and cleaved caspase-3. This strain also activates autophagy via upregulation of LC3 and Beclin1 and the degradation of p62 which occurs in IEC-6 cells and rat jejunum. It has also been revealed that p38 MAPK is involved in this autophagy. Totally, it was found that *Bacillus* SC06 can mitigate oxidative stress-induced diseases and apoptosis by p38-mediated autophagy and regulation of the extracellular kinases by enhancing the strong-binding protein expression (Wu et al., 2019).

Probiotics can also protect and prevent cytokines-induced epithelial damage (Shida et al., 2011). Disruption of epithelial integrity results in apoptosis of epithelial cells. Apoptosis and elevated levels of inflammatory cytokines are two primary pathological factors that characterize some diseases such as inflammatory bowel diseases. It has been indicated that *L. rhamnosus* GG generates P40 and p75, which are soluble proteins. These proteins improve intestinal epithelial cell homeostasis and inhibit cell apoptosis caused by cytokines in the intestinal epithelium in animal and human studies (Yan et al., 2007). In addition, they regulate the level of a growth-promoting signal in the outer layer of cells via activating the epidermal growth factor receptor. In mouse epithelial cells, the aforementioned pathway reduces cell death triggered by cytokines and encourages the development of IgA antibodies. Another way in which these two proteins enhance the growth and survival of intestinal epithelial cells is by stimulating the generation of heat shock proteins (Hsp72 and Hsp25) in the cells. These heat shock proteins play a part in safeguarding important binding proteins. They have the ability to protect against colitis and hinder the breakdown of tight junctions caused by hydrogen peroxide through a mechanism dependent on protein kinase C. In vivo studies have shown that the colonic goblet cells co-express intestinal trefoil factor 3 (TFF3) along with MUC2, and it is proposed to facilitate the process of wound healing (Kalabis et al., 2006). In a study on rats fed with VSL#3 containing *L. plantarum*, *L. casei*, *L. acidophilus*, *L. bulgaricus*, *B. longum*, *B. breve*, and *B. infantis*, no increase has been seen in the expression of colonic TFF3 (Caballero-Franco et al., 2007). Some studies have demonstrated that probiotics are not able to strengthen barrier function through the upregulation of TFF3; also they do not exhibit effectiveness in healing existing inflammation. Indeed, the effectiveness of probiotics is limited to the prevention of inflammation (Boirivant & Strober, 2007).

9.11 CLINICAL APPLICATIONS OF PROBIOTICS IN GASTRO-INTESTINAL DISEASES

9.11.1 Effects of Probiotics on Antibiotic-Associated Diarrhea

Probiotics and antibiotics are considered for the prevention of diarrhea associated with antibiotics. The main variations in the intestinal microflora with antibiotics are a decrease in total population and diversity of *Bacteroides* and *Bifiobacterium* species. These reductions are related to the decrease of amylolytic attributes and improve the growth of facultative anaerobic microorganisms including *Clostridia*, *Eubacteria*, and *Fusobacteria* species (Mueller et al., 2006). *Saccharomyces boulardii* is in clinical use for the prevention of antibiotic-associated diarrhea (Can et al., 2006; Kotowska et al., 2005; Szajewska et al., 2006). A meta-analysis of randomized controlled trials indicated that *S. boulardii* is protective against antibiotic-associated diarrhea in adults (McFarland, 2010). Another meta-analysis of randomized controlled trials revealed a significant protective effect of *S. boulardii* for antibiotic-associated diarrhea (Szajewska & Mrukowicz, 2005). In an animal study, following the administration of antibiotics, the mice that were given this probiotic yeast (*S. boulardii*) were able to restore their typical microbiota at a faster rate when compared with mice in the control group. This suggests that *S. boulardii* has the potential to promote the restoration of a healthy microbiota because it remains unaffected by the use of antibiotics (Barc et al., 2008). Other randomized controlled trials have also reported efficacy for *L. rhamnosus* GG in the prevention of antibiotic-associated diarrhea (Wenus et al., 2008).

9.11.2 Effects of Probiotics on *Clostridium Difficile* Infections

C. difficile as a spore-forming and anaerobic bacterium causes gastro-intestinal infection with diarrhea and colitis. It has been shown that *S. boulardii* can produce proteases that degrade *C. difficile* toxins and its colonic receptor site directly (Pothoulakis, 2009). This probiotic yeast can also enhance anti-toxin secretory IgA amounts in the intestinal environment (Qamar et al., 2001). A significant decrease has been seen in *C. difficile* infections with the use of a mixed probiotic milkshake (Hickson et al., 2007). *S. boulardii* is even effective in recurrent *C. difficile* infections. Practicing probiotics along with antibiotics such as vancomycin or metronidazole has been increased for recurrent *C. difficile* infections (Gogineni et al., 2013).

9.11.3 Effects of Probiotics on *Helicobacter Pylori* Infections

H. pylori is a small rod-shaped bacterium. It causes duodenal peptic ulceration and it can be the most important factor in some disorders such as gastric cancer, chronic gastritis, and other gastric disorders. In vitro studies have indicated that probiotics have a direct antimicrobial effect, by competition with *H. pylori*, prevention of adherence, and generation of antimicrobial metabolites. In randomized, double-blind, placebo-controlled trials, patients received antibiotics and *Lactobacillus* GG. It was shown that the probiotic significantly improved nausea, taste disturbance, and diarrhea. It is necessary to mention that eradication rates and epigastric pain did not improve during the treatment (Armuzzi et al., 2001). In another randomized double-blind placebo-controlled study, four groups of probiotics including *Lactobacillus* GG, *S. boulardii*, *L. acidophilus*, and *B. lactis* were received by *H. pylori*-positive patients. Probiotics significantly improved diarrhea and taste disturbance. However, they did not significantly improve epigastric pain and nausea. There was no significant difference in eradication rates among different probiotics groups (Cremonini et al., 2002). In a double-blind placebo with randomized controlled trials study, milk-based fruit drinks incorporated with *Lactobacillus GG*, *Propionibacterium*, *Bifidobacterium* were used. The probiotics did not improve diarrhea, taste disturbance epigastric pain and nausea. No significant difference was seen in eradication rates between the probiotic groups (Myllyluoma et al., 2005). Another meta-analysis reported that *S. boulardii* significantly raised the eradication rate and diminished the risk of *H. Pylori* therapy-related diarrhea (Szajewska et al., 2010).

9.11.4 Effects of Probiotics on Inflammatory Bowel Diseases

Inflammatory bowel disease is a chronic idiopathic inflammatory disease of the gut with a relapsing and remitting course (Herlihy & Feakins, 2022). It comprises Crohn's disease and ulcerative colitis, which are the most common entities of this disease (Shao et al., 2021). A decrease in the population of bifidobacteria (Macfarlane et al., 2005) and lactobacilli (Macfarlane et al., 2005) has been seen in patients with ulcerative colitis. It has been reported that a symbiotic formulation containing *L. paracasei* has diminished the plasma and lymphocyte levels of proinflammatory cytokines in ulcerative colitis patients (Federico et al., 2009). In some randomized double-blind placebo-controlled trials, *L. rhamnosus* GG did not have any positive effect on patients with Crohn's disease (Bousvaros et al., 2005). In a randomized double-blind placebo-controlled trial, *L. johnsonii* LA1 had no significant decrease in endoscopic recurrence after 6 months (Marteau et al., 2006). In some cases, it has been reported that administering probiotics did not influence the maintenance of remission in patients with inflammatory bowel disease (Mallon et al., 2007). In certain studies involving cases of Crohn's disease, *Lactobacillus* species were demonstrated to induce negative effects such as vomiting, nausea, epigastric pain, or constipation (Rolfe et al., 2006).

9.11.5 Effects of Probiotics and Irritable Bowel Syndrome

Various animal and human studies have shown the effects of changes in the intestinal microbiota composition on intestinal physiological functions and irritable bowel syndrome. Different studies have also reported that gastroenteritis can be a trigger for this syndrome. The enhanced risk of developing irritable bowel syndrome following gastroenteritis and dysbiosis reveals that the gastrointestinal microbiota can be a therapeutic goal in irritable bowel syndrome. Some reviews have considered the effectiveness of probiotics in the treatment of irritable bowel syndrome (Moayyedi et al., 2010). A systematic review of different probiotics evaluated for the treatment of irritable bowel syndrome showed that *B. infantis* 35624 was the only strain that caused considerable improvements in irritable bowel syndrome symptoms (Brenner et al., 2009).

9.11.6 Effects of Probiotics on Necrotizing Enterocolitis

Necrotizing enterocolitis is identified by severe intestinal inflammation and necrosis (Meister et al., 2020). This disease occurs primarily in preterm infants and is inversely related to gestational age and birth weight. Bacterial colonization pattern is crucial in the pathogenesis of necrotizing enterocolitis. Meta-analysis studies have reported that the use of prophylactic probiotics reduced rates of necrotizing enterocolitis, mortality, and relative risk of necrotizing enterocolitis. The best results have been seen with probiotics based on mixed probiotic species and/or with a combination of *L. acidophilus* and *Bifidobacterium* species (Guthmann et al., 2010). In a multicenter randomized controlled trial, probiotics, in the form of *B. bifidum* and *L. acidophilus*, fed enterally to very low birth weight premature infants for six weeks reduced the incidence of necrotizing enterocolitis or death (Lin et al., 2008). Generally, changing the strain specificity, dosage, and duration of clinical trials leads to evolve the advantages of probiotics in certain gastro-intestinal diseases.

9.12 CONCLUSION

Different probiotic products vary in doses and combinations. All of the probiotic products are not created equal. The benefits of probiotics depend on the strain, dosage, duration of treatment, counts of bacteria per serving (CFUs), and matrices of formulations. Some product formulations may have different combinations of probiotic strains. The selection of probiotics depends on the intended health benefit for special applications. The health benefits of probiotic strains need to be supported by clinical-based evidence. Recognition of clinical properties of effective probiotic strains in different probiotic-based trials and their functional mechanisms clarify the real beneficial effect of probiotics in gastro-intestinal disorders. Different mechanisms of probiotics in strengthening the intestinal epithelial barrier are reducing apoptosis of intestinal cells, promoting autophagy, enhanced production of mucin, effects on host cell AMPs, antimicrobial factors, epithelial adherence, immunomodulatory effects, and epithelial cell tight junctions. It is required to get stronger evidence from complementary studies of different probiotic species and strains. Undoubtedly, it is difficult to compare similar effects by a probiotic strain in different contexts such as laboratory, animal studies, and human trials. Some discrepancies among in vitro and in vivo findings can be referred to genetic factors, diverse foundation of immune system capabilities, microbiota diversity, diet, stress, etc. These variations make interpretation of the available results difficult. Particular attention is paid to the impact of different strains and metabolites that affect epithelial lining in terms of prevention/treatment of gastro-intestinal disorders and diseases. Probiotics do not act through the same mechanisms. Therefore, any extrapolation of positive/negative effects between probiotic species/strains or products/supplements should be avoided. More scientific evidence is needed to fully establish the effectiveness of probiotics in promoting health and to determine optimal probiotic species, doses, and formulations.

BIBLIOGRAPHY

Abanoz, H. S., & Kunduhoglu, B. (2018). Antimicrobial activity of a bacteriocin Produced by Enterococcus faecalis KT11 against Some Pathogens and Antibiotic-Resistant Bacteria. *Korean Journal for Food Science of Animal Resources, 38*(5), 1064–1079. https://doi.org/10.5851/kosfa.2018.e40

Acosta, M. P., Ruzal, S. M., & Cordo, S. M. (2016). S-layer proteins from *Lactobacillus* sp. Inhibit bacterial infection by blockage of DC-SIGN cell receptor. *International Journal of Biological Macromolecules, 92,* 998–1005. https://doi.org/10.1016/j.ijbiomac.2016.07.096

Ali, A., Tan, H., & Kaiko, G. E. (2020). Role of the intestinal epithelium and its interaction with the microbiota in food allergy. *Frontiers in Immunology, 11*, 604054. https://doi.org/10.3389/fimmu.2020.604054

Amiri, P., Hosseini, S. A., Ghaffari, S., Tutunchi, H., Ghaffari, S., Mosharkesh, E., Asghari, S., & Roshanravan, N. (2021). Role of butyrate, a Gut microbiota Derived Metabolite, in cardiovascular diseases: A comprehensive narrative review. *Frontiers in Pharmacology, 12,* 837509. https://doi.org/10.3389/fphar.2021.837509

Anderson, R. C., Cookson, A. L., McNabb, W. C., Park, Z., McCann, M. J., Kelly, W. J., & Roy, N. C. (2010). *Lactobacillus plantarum* MB452 enhances the function of the intestinal barrier by increasing the expression levels of genes involved in tight junction formation. *BMC Microbiology, 10,* 316. https://doi.org/10.1186/1471-2180-10-316

Andlid, T. A., D'Aimmo, M. R., & Jastrebova, J. (2018). Folate and bifidobacteria. In P. Mattarelli, B. Biavati, W. H. Holzapfel & B. J. B. Wood (Eds.), *The bifidobacteria and related organisms. Biology, taxonomy, applications* (pp. 195–212). Academic Press.

Angelin, J., & Kavitha, M. (2020). Exopolysaccharides from probiotic bacteria and their health potential. *International Journal of Biological Macromolecules, 162,* 853–865. https://doi.org/10.1016/j.ijbiomac.2020.06.190

Aristoteli, L. P., & Willcox, M. D. P. (2003). Mucin degradation mechanisms by distinct *Pseudomonas aeruginosa* isolates *in vitro. Infection and Immunity, 71*(10), 5565–5575. https://doi.org/10.1128/IAI.71.10.5565-5575.2003

Armuzzi, A., Cremonini, F., Bartolozzi, F., Canducci, F., Candelli, M., Ojetti, V., Cammarota, G., Anti, M., De Lorenzo, A., Pola, P., Gasbarrini, G., & Gasbarrini, A. (2001). The effect of oral administration of *Lactobacillus* GG on antibiotic-associated gastrointestinal side-effects during *Helicobacter pylori* eradication therapy. *Alimentary Pharmacology and Therapeutics, 15*(2), 163–169. https://doi.org/10.1046/j.1365-2036.2001.00923.x

Asare, P. T., Zurfluh, K., Greppi, A., Lynch, D., Schwab, C., Stephan, R., & Lacroix, C. (2020). Reuterin demonstrates potent antimicrobial activity against a broad panel of human and poultry meat *Campylobacter* spp. isolates. *Microorganisms, 8*(1), 78. https://doi.org/10.3390/microorganisms8010078

Bangar, S. P., Suri, S., Trif, M., & Ozogul, F. (2022). Organic acids production from lactic acid bacteria: A preservation approach. *Food Bioscience, 46,* 101615. https://doi.org/10.1016/j.fbio.2022.101615

Barc, M. C., Charrin-Sarnel, C., Rochet, V., Bourlioux, F., Sandré, C., Boureau, H., Doré, J., & Collignon, A. (2008). Molecular analysis of the digestive microbiota in a gnotobiotic mouse model during antibiotic treatment: Influence of Saccharomyces boulardii. *Anaerobe, 14*(4), 229–233. https://doi.org/10.1016/j.anaerobe.2008.04.003

Barroso, F. A. L., de Jesus, L. C. L., da Silva, T. F., Batista, V. L., Laguna, J., Coelho-Rocha, N. D., Vital, K. D., Fernandes, S. O. A., Cardoso, V. N., Ferreira, E., Martins, F. S., Drumond, M. M., Mancha-Agresti, P., Birbrair, A., Barh, D., & Azevedo, V. (2022). *Lactobacillus delbrueckii* CIDCA 133 ameliorates chemotherapy-induced mucositis by modulating epithelial barrier and TLR2/4/Myd88/NF-κB signaling pathway. *Frontiers in Microbiology, 13,* 858036. https://doi.org/10.3389/fmicb.2022.858036

Boirivant, M., & Strober, W. (2007). The mechanism of action of probiotics. *Current Opinion in Gastroenterology, 23*(6), 679–692. https://doi.org/10.1097/MOG.0b013e3282f0cffc

Boonma, P., Spinler, J. K., Venable, S. F., Versalovic, J., & Tumwasorn, S. (2014). *Lactobacillus rhamnosus* L34 and *Lactobacillus casei* L39 suppress *Clostridium difficile*-induced IL-8 production by colonic epithelial cells. *BMC Microbiology, 14,* 177. https://doi.org/10.1186/1471-2180-14-177

Bousvaros, A., Guandalini, S., Baldassano, R. N., Botelho, C., Evans, J., Ferry, G. D., Goldin, B., Hartigan, L., Kugathasan, S., Levy, J., Murray, K. F., Oliva-Hemker, M., Rosh, J. R., Tolia, V., Zholudev, A., Vanderhoof, J. A., & Hibberd, P. L. (2005). A randomized, double-blind trial of *Lactobacillus* GG versus placebo in addition to standard maintenance therapy for children with Crohn's disease. *Inflammatory Bowel Diseases, 11*(9), 833–839. https://doi.org/10.1097/01.mib.0000175905.00212.2c

Caballero-Franco, C., Keller, K., De Simone, C., & Chadee, K. (2007). The VSL#3 probiotic formula induces mucin gene expression and secretion in colonic epithelial cells. *American Journal of Physiology. Gastrointestinal and Liver Physiology, 292*(1), G315–G322. https://doi.org/10.1152/ajpgi.00265.2006

Cammarota, G., Ianiro, G., Bibbò, S., & Gasbarrini, A. (2014). Gut microbiota modulation: Probiotics, antibiotics or fecal microbiota transplantation? *Internal and Emergency Medicine, 9*(4), 365–373. https://doi.org/10.1007/s11739-014-1069-4

Can, M., Beşirbellioglu, B. A., Avci, I. Y., Beker, C. M., & Pahsa, A. (2006). Prophylactic *Saccharomyces boulardii* in the prevention of antibiotic-associated diarrhea: A prospective study. *Medical Science Monitor, 12*(4), PI19–PI22.

Chang, Y. H., Jeong, C. H., Cheng, W. N., Choi, Y., Shin, D. M., Lee, S., & Han, S. G. (2021). Quality characteristics of yogurts fermented with short-chain fatty acid-producing probiotics and their effects on mucin production and probiotic adhesion onto human colon epithelial cells. *Journal of Dairy Science, 104*(7), 7415–7425. https://doi.org/10.3168/jds.2020-19820

Chen, T., Liu, X., Ma, L., He, W., Li, W., Cao, Y., & Liu, Z. (2014). Food allergens affect the intestinal tight junction permeability in inducing intestinal food allergy in rats. *Asian Pacific Journal of Allergy and Immunology, 32*(4), 345–353. https://doi.org/10.12932/AP0443.32.4.2014

Chugh, B., & Kamal-Eldin, A. (2020). Bioactive compounds produced by probiotics in food products. *Current Opinion in Food Science, 32,* 76–82. https://doi.org/10.1016/j.cofs.2020.02.003

Clevers, H. (2013). The intestinal crypt, a prototype stem cell compartment. *Cell, 154*(2), 274–284. https://doi.org/10.1016/j.cell.2013.07.004

Cremonini, F., Di Caro, S., Covino, M., Armuzzi, A., Gabrielli, M., Santarelli, L., Nista, E. C., Cammarota, G., Gasbarrini, G., & Gasbarrini, A. (2002). Effect of different probiotic preparations on anti-helicobacter pylori therapy-related side effects: A parallel group, triple blind, placebo-controlled study. *American Journal of Gastroenterology, 97*(11), 2744–2749. https://doi.org/10.1111/j.1572-0241.2002.07063.x

De Repentigny, L., Aumont, F., Bernard, K., & Belhumeur, P. (2000). Characterization of binding of *Candida albicans* to small intestinal mucin and its role in adherence to mucosal epithelial cells. *Infection and Immunity, 68*(6), 3172–3179. https://doi.org/10.1128/IAI.68.6.3172-3179.2000

Dempsey, E., & Corr, S. C. (2022). *Lactobacillus* spp. For gastrointestinal health: Current and future perspectives. *Frontiers in Immunology, 13,* 840245. https://doi.org/10.3389/fimmu.2022.840245

Diao, Y., Xin, Y., Zhou, Y., Li, N., Pan, X., Qi, S., Qi, Z., Xu, Y., Luo, L., Wan, H., Lan, L., & Yin, Z. (2014). Extracellular polysaccharide from *Bacillus* sp. Strain LBP32 prevents LPS-induced inflammation in RAW 264.7 macrophages by inhibiting NF-κB and MAPKs activation and ROS production. *International Immunopharmacology, 18*(1), 12–19. https://doi.org/10.1016/j.intimp.2013.10.021

do Carmo, F. L. R., Rabah, H., De Oliveira Carvalho, R. D. O., Gaucher, F., Cordeiro, B. F., da Silva, S. H., Le Loir, Y., Azevedo, V., & Jan, G. (2018). Extractable bacterial surface proteins in probiotic–host interaction. *Frontiers in Microbiology, 9,* 645. https://doi.org/10.3389/fmicb.2018.00645

Du, W., Xu, H., Mei, X., Cao, X., Gong, L., Wu, Y., Li, Y., Yu, D., Liu, S., Wang, Y., & Li, W. (2018). Probiotic *Bacillus* enhance the intestinal epithelial cell barrier and immune function of piglets. *Beneficial Microbes, 9*(5), 743–754. https://doi.org/10.3920/BM2017.0142

Endo, H., Niioka, M., Kobayashi, N., Tanaka, M., & Watanabe, T. (2013). Butyrate-producing probiotics reduce nonalcoholic fatty liver disease progression in rats: New insight into the probiotics for the gut-liver axis. *PLoS One, 8*(5), e63388. https://doi.org/10.1371/journal.pone.0063388

Eslami, M., Bahar, A., Keikha, M., Karbalaei, M., Kobyliak, N. M., & Yousefi, B. (2020). Probiotics function and modulation of the immune system in allergic diseases. *Allergologia et Immunopathologia, 48*(6), 771–788. https://doi.org/10.1016/j.aller.2020.04.005

Fábrega, M. J., Rodríguez-Nogales, A., Garrido-Mesa, J., Algieri, F., Badía, J., Giménez, R., Gálvez, J., & Baldomà, L. (2017). Intestinal anti-inflammatory effects of outer membrane vesicles from Escherichia coli Nissle 1917 in DSS-experimental colitis in mice. *Frontiers in Microbiology, 8,* 1274. https://doi.org/10.3389/fmicb.2017.01274

Faraki, A., & Rahmani, F. (2021). The antioxidant activity of lactic acid bacteria and probiotics: A review. *Journal of Food Safety and Hygiene, 6,* 168–182. https://doi.org/10.18502/jfsh.v6i4.7563

Fayol-Messaoudi, D., Berger, C. N., Coconnier-Polter, M. H., Liévin-Le Moal, V. L.-L., & Servin, A. L. (2005). pH-, lactic acid-, and non-lactic acid-dependent activities of probiotic Lactobacilli against *Salmonella enterica* serovar Typhimurium. *Applied and Environmental Microbiology, 71*(10), 6008–6013. https://doi.org/10.1128/AEM.71.10.6008-6013.2005

Federico, A., Tuccillo, C., Grossi, E., Abbiati, R., Garbagna, N., Romano, M., Tiso, A., Blanco, Cdel, V., & Loguercio, C. (2009). The effect of a new symbiotic formulation on plasma levels and peripheral blood mononuclear cell expression of some pro-inflammatory cytokines in patients with ulcerative colitis: A pilot study. *European Review for Medical and Pharmacological Sciences, 13*(4), 285–293.

Feng, T., & Wang, J. (2020). Oxidative stress tolerance and antioxidant capacity of lactic acid bacteria as probiotic: A systematic review. *Gut Microbes, 12*(1), 1801944. https://doi.org/10.1080/19490976.2020.1801944

Gaudier, E., Michel, C., Segain, J. P., Cherbut, C., & Hoebler, C. (2005). The VSL# 3 probiotic mixture modifies microflora but does not heal chronic dextran-sodium sulfate-induced colitis or reinforce the mucus barrier in mice. *Journal of Nutrition, 135*(12), 2753–2761. https://doi.org/10.1093/jn/135.12.2753

Geirnaert, A., Calatayud, M., Grootaert, C., Laukens, D., Devriese, S., Smagghe, G., Takumi, T., Hashimoto, R., Otani, H., Pazour, G. J., Hsu, V. W., & de Wiele, T. V. (2017). Butyrate-producing bacteria supplemented *in vitro* to Crohn's disease patient microbiota increased butyrate production and enhanced intestinal epithelial barrier integrity. *Scientific Reports, 7,* 1.

Geng, T., He, F., Su, S., Sun, K., Zhao, L., Zhao, Y., Bao, N., Pan, L., & Sun, H. (2021). Probiotics *Lactobacillus rhamnosus* GG ATCC53103 and *Lactobacillus plantarum* JL01 induce cytokine alterations by the production of TCDA, DHA, and succinic and palmitic acids, and enhance immunity of weaned piglets. *Research in Veterinary Science, 137,* 56–67. https://doi.org/10.1016/j.rvsc.2021.04.011

Giorgetti, G., Brandimarte, G., Fabiocchi, F., Ricci, S., Flamini, P., Sandri, G., Trotta, M. C., Elisei, W., Penna, A., Lecca, P. G., Picchio, M., & Tursi, A. (2015). Interactions between innate immunity, microbiota, and probiotics. *Journal of Immunology Research, 2015,* 501361. https://doi.org/10.1155/2015/501361

Gogineni, V. K., Morrow, L. E., & Malesker, M. A. (2013). Probiotics: Mechanisms of action and clinical applications. *Journal of Probiotics and Health, 1,* 101. https://doi.org/10.4172/jph.1000101

Gómez-García, M., Sol, C., de Nova, P. J. G., Puyalto, M., Mesas, L., Puente, H., Mencía-Ares, Ó., Miranda, R., Argüello, H., Rubio, P., & Carvajal, A. (2019). Antimicrobial activity of a selection of organic acids, their salts and essential oils against swine enteropathogenic bacteria. *Porcine Health Management, 5,* 32. https://doi.org/10.1186/s40813-019-0139-4

Gorreja, F., & Walker, W. A. (2022). The potential role of adherence factors in probiotic function in the gastrointestinal tract of adults and pediatrics: A narrative review of experimental and human studies. *Gut Microbes, 14*(1), 2149214. https://doi.org/10.1080/19490976.2022.2149214

Gou, H. Z., Zhang, Y. L., Ren, L. F., Li, Z. J., & Zhang, L. (2022). How do intestinal probiotics restore the intestinal barrier? *Frontiers in Microbiology, 13,* 929346. https://doi.org/10.3389/fmicb.2022.929346

Guthmann, F., Kluthe, C., & Bührer, C. (2010). Probiotics for prevention of necrotising enterocolitis: An updated meta-analysis. *Klinische Padiatrie, 222*(5), 284–290. https://doi.org/10.1055/s-0030-1254113

Habil, N., Abate, W., Beal, J., & Foey, A. D. (2014). Heat-killed probiotic bacteria differentially regulate colonic epithelial cell production of human β-defensin-2: Dependence on inflammatory cytokines. *Beneficial Microbes, 5*(4), 483–495. https://doi.org/10.3920/BM2013.0061

Haddaji, N., Mahdhi, A. K., Krifi, B., Ismail, M. B., & Bakhrouf, A. (2015). Change in cell surface properties of *Lactobacillus casei* under heat shock treatment. *FEMS Microbiology Letters, 362*(9), fnv047. https://doi.org/10.1093/femsle/fnv047

Han, C., Ding, Z., Shi, H., Qian, W., Hou, X., & Lin, R. (2016). The role of probiotics in lipopolysaccharide-induced autophagy in intestinal epithelial cells. *Cellular Physiology and Biochemistry, 38*(6), 2464–2478. https://doi.org/10.1159/000445597

Hemarajata, P., & Versalovic, J. (2013). Effects of probiotics on gut microbiota: Mechanisms of intestinal immunomodulation and neuromodulation. *Therapeutic Advances in Gastroenterology, 6*(1), 39–51. https://doi.org/10.1177/1756283X12459294

Herlihy, N., & Feakins, R. (2022). Gut inflammation induced by drugs: Can pathology help to differentiate from inflammatory bowel disease? *United European Gastroenterology Journal, 10*(5), 451–464. https://doi.org/10.1002/ueg2.12242

Hertzberger, R., Arents, J., Dekker, H. L., Pridmore, R. D., Gysler, C., Kleerebezem, M., & de Mattos, M. J. T. (2014). H_2O_2 production in species of the *Lactobacillus acidophilus* group: A central role for a novel NADH-dependent flavin reductase. *Applied and Environmental Microbiology, 80*(7), 2229–2239. https://doi.org/10.1128/AEM.04272-13

Heydari, A., Parvini, F., & Allahyari-Fard, N. (2022). Functional foods and antioxidant effects: Emphasizing the role of probiotics. In N. Shiomi & A. Savitskaya (Eds.), *Current topics in functional food*. IntechOpen.

Hickson, M., D'Souza, A. L., Muthu, N., Rogers, T. R., Want, S., Rajkumar, C., & Bulpitt, C. J. (2007). Use of probiotic *Lactobacillus* preparation to prevent diarrhoea associated with antibiotics: Randomised double blind placebo controlled trial. *BMJ, 335*(7610), 80. https://doi.org/10.1136/bmj.39231.599815.55

Hoffmann, A., Kleniewska, P., & Pawliczak, R. (2021). Antioxidative activity of probiotics. *Archives of Medical Science, 17*(3), 792–804. https://doi.org/10.5114/aoms.2019.89894

Hummel, S., Veltman, K., Cichon, C., Sonnenborn, U., & Schmidt, M. A. (2012). Differential targeting of the E-cadherin/β-catenin complex by gram-positive probiotic lactobacilli improves epithelial barrier function. *Applied and Environmental Microbiology, 78*(4), 1140–1147. https://doi.org/10.1128/AEM.06983-11

Hymes, J. P., & Klaenhammer, T. R. (2016). Stuck in the middle: Fibronectin-binding proteins in gram-positive bacteria. *Frontiers in Microbiology, 7,* 1504. https://doi.org/10.3389/fmicb.2016.01504

Indira, M., Venkateswarulu, T. C., Abraham Peele, K., Nazneen Bobby, M., & Krupanidhi, S. (2019). Bioactive molecules of probiotic bacteria and their mechanism of action: A review. *3 Biotech, 9*(8), 306. https://doi.org/10.1007/s13205-019-1841-2

Jacobson, A., Lam, L., Rajendram, M., Tamburini, F., Honeycutt, J., Pham, T., Van Treuren, W., Pruss, K., Stabler, S. R., Lugo, K., Bouley, D. M., Vilches-Moure, J. G., Smith, M., Sonnenburg, J. L., Bhatt, A. S., Huang, K. C., & Monack, D. (2018). A gut commensal-produced metabolite mediates colonization resistance to *salmonella* infection. *Cell Host and Microbe, 24*(2), 296–307.e7. https://doi.org/10.1016/j.chom.2018.07.002

Javanshir, N., Hosseini, G. N. G., Sadeghi, M., Esmaeili, R., Satarikia, F., Ahmadian, G., & Allahyari, N. (2021). Evaluation of the function of probiotics, emphasizing the role of their binding to the intestinal epithelium in the stability and their effects on the immune system. *Biological Procedures Online, 23*(1), 23. https://doi.org/10.1186/s12575-021-00160-w

Jiang, W., Sunkara, L. T., Zeng, X., Deng, Z., Myers, S. M., & Zhang, G. (2013). Differential regulation of human cathelicidin LL-37 by free fatty acids and their analogs. *Peptides, 50,* 129–138. https://doi.org/10.1016/j.peptides.2013.10.008

Johnson-Henry, K. C., Donato, K. A., Shen-Tu, G., Gordanpour, M., & Sherman, P. M. (2008). *Lactobacillus rhamnosus* Strain GG prevents enterohemorrhagic Escherichia coli O157:H7-induced changes in epithelial barrier function. *Infection and Immunity, 76*(4), 1340–1348. https://doi.org/10.1128/IAI.00778-07

Johnson-Henry, K. C., Pinnell, L. J., Waskow, A. M., Irrazabal, T., Martin, A., Hausner, M., & Sherman, P. M. (2014). Short-chain fructo-oligosaccharide and inulin modulate inflammatory responses and microbial communities in Caco2-bbe cells and in a mouse model of intestinal injury. *Journal of Nutrition, 144*(11), 1725–1733. https://doi.org/10.3945/jn.114.195081

Kalabis, J., Rosenberg, I., & Podolsky, D. K. (2006). Vangl1 protein acts as a downstream effector of intestinal trefoil factor (ITF)/TFF3 signaling and regulates wound healing of intestinal epithelium. *Journal of Biological Chemistry, 281*(10), 6434–6441. https://doi.org/10.1074/jbc.M512905200

Kang, H. J., & Im, S. H. (2015). Probiotics as an immune modulator. *Journal of Nutritional Science and Vitaminology, 61*(suppl), S103–S105. https://doi.org/10.3177/jnsv.61.S103

Karczewski, J., Troost, F. J., Konings, I., Dekker, J., Kleerebezem, M., Brummer, R. J., & Wells, J. M. (2010). Regulation of human epithelial tight junction proteins by *Lactobacillus plantarum* in vivo and protective effects on the epithelial barrier. *American Journal of Physiology. Gastrointestinal and Liver Physiology, 298*(6), G851–G859. https://doi.org/10.1152/ajpgi.00327.2009

Kelsall, B. L. (2008). Innate and adaptive mechanisms to control pathological intestinal inflammation. *Journal of Pathology, 214*(2), 242–259. https://doi.org/10.1002/path.2286

Kim, Y., Kim, S. H., Whang, K. Y., Kim, Y. J., & Oh, S. (2008). Inhibition of *Escherichia coli* O157:H7 attachment by interactions between lactic acid bacteria and intestinal epithelial cells. *Journal of Microbiology and Biotechnology, 18*(7), 1278–1285.

Kommineni, S., Bretl, D. J., Lam, V., Chakraborty, R., Hayward, M., Simpson, P., Cao, Y., Bousounis, P., Kristich, C. J., & Salzman, N. H. (2015). Bacteriocin production augments niche competition by enterococci in the mammalian gastrointestinal tract. *Nature, 526*(7575), 719–722. https://doi.org/10.1038/nature15524

Kotowska, M., Albrecht, P., & Szajewska, H. (2005). *Saccharomyces boulardii* in the prevention of antibiotic-associated diarrhoea in children: A randomized doubleblind placebo-controlled trial. *Alimentary Pharmacology and Therapeutics, 21*(5), 583–590. https://doi.org/10.1111/j.1365-2036.2005.02356.x

Kumar, M., Dhaka, P., Vijay, D., Vergis, J., Mohan, V., Kumar, A., Kurkure, N. V., Barbuddhe, S. B., Malik, S. V., & Rawool, D. B. (2016). Antimicrobial effects of *Lactobacillus plantarum* and *Lactobacillus acidophilus* against multidrug-resistant enteroaggregative *Escherichia coli. International Journal of Antimicrobial Agents, 48*(3), 265–270. https://doi.org/10.1016/j.ijantimicag.2016.05.014

La Fata, G., Weber, P., & Mohajeri, M. H. (2018). Probiotics and the gut immune system: Indirect regulation. *Probiotics and Antimicrobial Proteins, 10*(1), 11–21. https://doi.org/10.1007/s12602-017-9322-6

Lau, L. Y. J., & Chye, F. Y. (2018). Antagonistic effects of *Lactobacillus plantarum* 0612 on the adhesion of selected foodborne enteropathogens in various colonic environments. *Food Control, 91,* 237–247. https://doi.org/10.1016/j.foodcont.2018.04.001

Li, J., Sung, C. Y. J., Lee, N., Ni, Y., Pihlajamäki, J., Panagiotou, G., & El-Nezami, H. (2016). Probiotics modulated gut microbiota suppresses hepatocellular carcinoma growth in mice. *Proceedings of the National Academy of Sciences of the United States of America, 113*(9), E1306–E1315. https://doi.org/10.1073/pnas.1518189113

Lin, H. C., Hsu, C. H., Chen, H. L., Chung, M. Y., Hsu, J. F., Lien, R. I., Tsao, L. Y., Chen, C. H., & Su, B. H. (2008). Oral probiotics prevent necrotizing enterocolitis in very low birth weight preterm infants: A multicenter, randomized, controlled trial. *Pediatrics, 122*(4), 693–700. https://doi.org/10.1542/peds.2007-3007

Lin, R., Jiang, Y., Zhao, X. Y., Guan, Y., Qian, W., Fu, X. C., Ren, H. Y., & Hou, X. H. (2014). Four types of bifidobacteria trigger autophagy response in intestinal epithelial cells. *Journal of Digestive Diseases, 15*(11), 597–605. https://doi.org/10.1111/1751-2980.12179

Liu, L., Li, Q., Yang, Y., & Guo, A. (2021). Biological function of short-chain fatty acids and its regulation on intestinal health of poultry. *Frontiers in Veterinary Science, 8,* 736739. https://doi.org/10.3389/fvets.2021.736739

Liu, Z., Zhang, Z., Qiu, L., Zhang, F., Xu, X., Wei, H., & Tao, X. (2017). Characterization and bioactivities of the exopolysaccharide from a probiotic strain of *Lactobacillus plantarum* WLPL04. *Journal of Dairy Science, 100*(9), 6895–6905. https://doi.org/10.3168/jds.2016-11944

Lopetuso, L. R., Giorgio, M. E., Saviano, A., Scaldaferri, F., Gasbarrini, A., & Cammarota, G. (2019). Bacteriocins and bacteriophages: Therapeutic weapons for gastrointestinal diseases? *International Journal of Molecular Sciences, 20*(1), 183. https://doi.org/10.3390/ijms20010183

Macfarlane, S., Furrie, E., Kennedy, A., Cummings, J. H., & Macfarlane, G. T. (2005). Mucosal bacteria in ulcerative colitis. *British Journal of Nutrition, 93*(suppl_1), S67–S72. https://doi.org/10.1079/bjn20041347

Macfarlane, S., Woodmansey, E. J., & Macfarlane, G. T. (2005) Colonization of mucin by human intestinal bacteria and establishment of biofilm communities in a two-stage continuous culture system. *Applied and Environmental Microbiology, 71*(11), 7483–7492. https://doi.org/10.1128/AEM.71.11.7483-7492.2005

Mack, D. R., Ahrne, S., Hyde, L., Wei, S., & Hollingsworth, M. A. (2003). Extracellular MUC3 mucin secretion follows adherence of *Lactobacillus* strains to intestinal epithelial cells *in vitro. Gut, 52*(6), 827–833. https://doi.org/10.1136/gut.52.6.827

Malanovic, N., & Lohner, K. (2016). Gram-positive bacterial cell envelopes: The impact on the activity of antimicrobial peptides. BBA—Biomembranes. *Biochimica et Biophysica Acta, 1858*(5), 936–946. https://doi.org/10.1016/j.bbamem.2015.11.004

Mallon, P., McKay, D., Kirk, S., & Gardiner, K. (2007). Probiotics for induction of remission in ulcerative colitis. *Cochrane Database of Systematic Reviews, 17*(4), CD005573. https://doi.org/10.1002/14651858.CD005573.pub2

Markowiak-Kopeć, P., & Śliżewska, K. (2020). The effect of probiotics on the production of short-chain fatty acids by human intestinal microbiome. *Nutrients, 12*(4), 1107. https://doi.org/10.3390/nu12041107

Marteau, P., Lémann, M., Seksik, P., Laharie, D., Colombel, J. F., Bouhnik, Y., Cadiot, G., Soulé, J. C., Bourreille, A., Metman, E., Lerebours, E., Carbonnel, F., Dupas, J. L., Veyrac, M., Coffin, B., Moreau, J., Abitbol, V., Blum-Sperisen, S., & Mary, J. Y. (2006). Ineffectiveness of *Lactobacillus johnsonii* LA1 for prophylaxis of postoperative recurrence in Crohn's disease: A randomised, double blind, placebo controlled GETAID trial. *Gut, 55*(6), 842–847. https://doi.org/10.1136/gut.2005.076604

Mattar, A. F., Teitelbaum, D. H., Drongowski, R. A., Yongyi, F., Harmon, C. M., & Coran, A. G. (2002). Probiotics up-regulate MUC-2 mucin gene expression in a Caco-2 cellculture model. *Pediatric Surgery International, 18*(7), 586–590. https://doi.org/10.1007/s00383-002-0855-7

Mazzeo, M. F., Reale, A., Di Renzo, T., & Siciliano, R. A. (2022). Surface layer protein pattern of *Levilactobacillus brevis* Strains investigated by proteomics. *Nutrients, 14*(18), 3679. https://doi.org/10.3390/nu14183679

McFarland, L. V. (2010). Systematic review and meta-analysis of *Saccharomyces boulardii* in adult patients. *World Journal of Gastroenterology, 16*(18), 2202–2222. https://doi.org/10.3748/wjg.v16.i18.2202

Meister, A. L., Doheny, K. K., & Travagli, R. A. (2020). Necrotizing enterocolitis: It's not all in the gut. *Experimental Biology and Medicine, 245*(2), 85–95. https://doi.org/10.1177/1535370219891971

Merenstein, D., Murphy, M., Fokar, A., Hernandez, R. K., Park, H., Nsouli, H., Sanders, M. E., Davis, B. A., Niborski, V., Tondu, F., & Shara, N. M. (2010). Use of a fermented dairy probiotic drink containing *Lactobacillus casei* (DN-114 001) to decrease the rate of illness in kids: The DRINK study a patient-oriented, double-blind, cluster-randomized, placebocontrolled, clinical trial. *European Journal of Clinical Nutrition, 64*(7), 669–677. https://doi.org/10.1038/ejcn.2010.65

Miljkovic, M., Thomas, M., Serror, P., Rigottier-Gois, L., & Kojic, M. (2019). Binding activity to intestinal cells and transient colonization in mice of two *Lactobacillus paracasei* subsp. *Paracasei* strains with high aggregation potential. *World Journal of Microbiology and Biotechnology, 35*(6), 85. https://doi.org/10.1007/s11274-019-2663-4

Mirzaei, R., Dehkhodaie, E., Bouzari, B., Rahimi, M., Gholestani, A., Hosseini-Fard, S. R., Keyvani, H., Teimoori, A., & Karampoor, S. (2022). Dual role of microbiota-derived short-chain fatty acids on host and pathogen. *Biomedicine and Pharmacotherapy, 145,* 112352. https://doi.org/10.1016/j.biopha.2021.112352

Moayyedi, P., Ford, A. C., Talley, N. J., Cremonini, F., Foxx-Orenstein, A. E., Brandt, L. J., & Quigley, E. M. M. (2010). The efficacy of probiotics in the treatment of irritable bowel syndrome: A systematic review. *Gut, 59*(3), 325–332. https://doi.org/10.1136/gut.2008.167270

Mogoşanu, G. D., Grumezescu, A. M., Bejenaru, C., & Bejenaru, L. E. (2017). Natural products used for food preservation. In A. M. Grumezescu (Ed.), *Nanotechnology in the agri-food industry, food preservation* (pp. 365–411). Academic Press.

Moncada, D., Yu, Y., Keller, K., & Chadee, K. (2000). *Entamoeba histolytica* cysteine proteinases degrade human colonic mucin and alter its function. *Archives of Medical Research, 31*(suppl_4), S224–S225. https://doi.org/10.1016/s0188-4409(00)00227-7

Monteagudo-Mera, A., Rastall, R. A., Gibson, G. R., Charalampopoulos, D., & Chatzifragkou, A. (2019). Adhesion mechanisms mediated by probiotics and prebiotics and their potential impact on human health. *Applied Microbiology and Biotechnology, 103*(16), 6463–6472. https://doi.org/10.1007/s00253-019-09978-7

Mueller, S., Saunier, K., Hanisch, C., Norin, E., Alm, L., Midtvedt, T., Cresci, A., Silvi, S., Orpianesi, C., Verdenelli, M. C., Clavel, T., Koebnick, C., Zunft, H. J., Doré, J., & Blaut, M. (2006). Differences in fecal microbiota in different European study populations in relation to age, gender, and country: A cross-sectional study. *Applied and Environmental Microbiology, 72*(2), 1027–1033. https://doi.org/10.1128/AEM.72.2.1027-1033.2006

Mujagic, Z., de Vos, P., Boekschoten, M. V., Govers, C., Pieters, H.-J. H. M., de Wit, N. J. W., Bron, P. A., Masclee, A. A., & Troost, F. J. (2017). The effects of *Lactobacillus plantarum* on small intestinal barrier function and mucosal gene transcription; a randomized double-blind placebo controlled trial. *Scientific Reports, 7,* 40128. https://doi.org/10.1038/srep40128

Muscariello, L., De Siena, B., & Marasco, R. (2020). *Lactobacillus* cell surface proteins involved in interaction with mucus and extracellular matrix components. *Current Microbiology, 77*(12), 3831–3841. https://doi.org/10.1007/s00284-020-02243-5

Myllyluoma, E., Veijola, L., Ahlroos, T., Tynkkynen, S., Kankuri, E., Vapaatalo, H., Rautelin, H., & Korpela, R. (2005). Probiotic supplementation improves tolerance to *Helicobacter pylori* eradication therapy—A placebo-controlled, double-blind randomized pilot study. *Alimentary Pharmacology and Therapeutics, 21*(10), 1263–1272. https://doi.org/10.1111/j.1365-2036.2005.02448.x

Nakamura, S., Kuda, T., An, C., Kanno, T., Takahashi, H., & Kimura, B. (2012). Inhibitory effects of *Leuconostoc mesenteroides* 1RM3 isolated from narezushi, a fermented fish with rice, on *Listeria monocytogenes* infection to Caco-2 cells and A/J mice. *Anaerobe, 18*(1), 19–24. https://doi.org/10.1016/j.anaerobe.2011.11.006

Ohland, C. L., & MacNaughton, W. K. (2010). Probiotic bacteria and intestinal epithelial barrier function. *American Journal of Physiology. Gastrointestinal and Liver Physiology, 298*(6), G807–G819. https://doi.org/10.1152/ajpgi.00243.2009

Orlando, A., Linsalata, M., Notarnicola, M., Tutino, V., & Russo, F. (2014). *Lactobacillus* GG restoration of the gliadin induced epithelial barrier disruption: The role of cellular polyamines. *BMC Microbiology, 14,* 19. https://doi.org/10.1186/1471-2180-14-19

Pawar, A., & Tiwari, S. K. (2022). Bacteriocin-producing probiotic lactic acid bacteria in controlling dysbiosis of the gut microbiota. *Frontiers in Cellular and Infection Microbiology, 12,* 851140. https://doi.org/10.3389/fcimb.2022.851140

Peng, M., & Biswas, D. (2017). Short chain and polyunsaturated fatty acids in host gut health and food-borne bacterial pathogen inhibition. *Critical Reviews in Food Science and Nutrition, 57*(18), 3987–4002. https://doi.org/10.1080/10408398.2016.1203286

Peng, M., Tabashsum, Z., Patel, P., Bernhardt, C., & Biswas, D. (2018). Linoleic Acids Overproducing *Lactobacillus casei* Limits Growth, Survival, and Virulence of *Salmonella Typhimurium* and enterohaemorrhagic Escherichia coli. *Frontiers in Microbiology, 9*, 2663. https://doi.org/10.3389/fmicb.2018.02663

Phillipson, M., Johansson, M. E. V., Henriksnäs, J., Petersson, J., Gendler, S. J., Sandler, S., Persson, A. E., Hansson, G. C., & Holm, L. (2008). The gastric mucus layers: Constituents and regulation of accumulation. *American Journal of Physiology: Gastrointestinal and Liver Physiology, 295*(4), G806–G812. https://doi.org/10.1152/ajpgi.90252.2008

Plaza-Diaz, J., Ruiz-Ojeda, F. J., Gil-Campos, M., & Gil, A. (2019). Mechanisms of action of probiotics. *Advances in Nutrition, 10*(suppl_1), S49–S66. https://doi.org/10.1093/advances/nmy063

Pothoulakis, C. (2009). Review article: Anti-inflammatory mechanisms of action of *Saccharomyces boulardii. Alimentary Pharmacology and Therapeutics, 30*(8), 826–833. https://doi.org/10.1111/j.1365-2036.2009.04102.x

Preidis, G. A., & Versalovic, J. (2009). Targeting the human microbiome with antibiotics, probiotics, and prebiotics: Gastroenterology enters the metagenomics era. *Gastroenterology, 136*(6), 2015–2031. https://doi.org/10.1053/j.gastro.2009.01.072

Qamar, A., Aboudola, S., Warny, M., Michetti, P., Pothoulakis, C., LaMont, J. T., & Kelly, C. P. (2001). *Saccharomyces boulardii* stimulates intestinal immunoglobulin A immune response to Clostridium difficile toxin A in mice. *Infection and Immunity, 69*(4), 2762–2765. https://doi.org/10.1128/IAI.69.4.2762-2765.2001

Qin, H., Zhang, Z., Hang, X., & Jiang, Y. L. (2009). *Plantarum* prevents enteroinvasive. *BMC Microbiology, 9,* 63. https://doi.org/10.1186/1471-2180-9-63

Rabetafika, H. N., Razafindralambo, A., Ebenso, B., & Razafindralambo, H. L. (2023). Probiotics as antibiotic alternatives for human and animal applications. *Encyclopedia, 3*(2), 561–581. https://doi.org/10.3390/encyclopedia3020040

Radhamanalan, G., & Dharumadurai, D. (2022). Assessment of probiotics adhesion to mammalian cells. In M. K. Dwivedi, N. Amaresan, A. Sankaranarayanan, & R. Begum (Eds.), *Biosafety assessment of probiotic potential. Methods and protocols in food science* (pp. 179–183). Humana Press. https://doi.org/10.1007/978-1-0716-2509-5_20

Rinehart, E., Newton, E., Marasco, M. A., Beemiller, K., Zani, A., Muratore, M. K., Weis, J., Steinbicker, N., Wallace, N., & Sun, Y. (2018). *Listeria monocytogenes* response to propionate is differentially modulated by anaerobicity. *Pathogens, 7*(3), 60. https://doi.org/10.3390/pathogens7030060

Rolfe, V. E., Fortun, P. J., Hawkey, C. J., & Bath-Hextall, F. (2006). Probiotics for maintenance of remission in Crohn's disease. *Cochrane Database of Systematic Reviews, 18*(4), CD004826. https://doi.org/10.1002/14651858.CD004826.pub2

Rwubuzizi, R., Kim, H., Holzapfel, W. H., & Todorov, S. D. (2023). Beneficial, safety, and antioxidant properties of lactic acid bacteria: A next step in their evaluation as potential probiotics. *Heliyon, 9*(4), e15610. https://doi.org/10.1016/j.heliyon.2023.e15610

Sanders, M. E., Benson, A., Lebeer, S., Merenstein, D. J., & Klaenhammer, T. R. (2018). Shared mechanisms among probiotic taxa: Implications for general probiotic claims. *Current Opinion in Biotechnology, 49,* 207–216. https://doi.org/10.1016/j.copbio.2017.09.007

Seo, B.-J., Bajpai, V. K., Rather, I. A., & Park, Y.-H. (2015). Partially purified exopolysaccharide from *Lactobacillus plantarum* YML009 with total phenolic content, antioxidant and free radical scavenging efficacy. *Indian Journal of Pharmaceutical Education and Research, 49*(4), 282–292. https://doi.org/10.5530/ijper.49.4.6

Shaikh, A. E., Pawar, A., Parmar, H., N Vadgama, R., M Lali, A., & A Odaneth, A. (2018). Conjugated linoleic acid production by lactic acid bacteria: A bio-transformation study in media with oil hydrolysates. *Journal of Applied Biotechnology and Bioengineering, 5*(5), 321–327. https://doi.org/10.15406/jabb.2018.05.00158

Shao, B. Z., Yao, Y., Zhai, J. S., Zhu, J. H., Li, J. P., & Wu, K. (2021). The role of autophagy in inflammatory bowel disease. *Frontiers in Physiology, 12*, 621132. https://doi.org/10.3389/fphys.2021.621132

Shida, K., Nanno, M., & Nagata, S. (2011). Flexible cytokine production by macrophages and T cells in response to probiotic bacteria: A possible mechanism by which probiotics exert multifunctional immune regulatory activities. *Gut Microbes, 2*(2), 109–114. https://doi.org/10.4161/gmic.2.2.15661

Silva, Y. P., Bernardi, A., & Frozza, R. L. (2020). The role of short-chain fatty acids from gut microbiota in gut-brain communication. *Frontiers in Endocrinology, 11,* 25. https://doi.org/10.3389/fendo.2020.00025

Singh, A. K., Hertzberger, R. Y., & Knaus, U. G. (2018). Hydrogen peroxide production by lactobacilli promotes epithelial restitution during colitis. *Redox Biology, 16,* 11–20. https://doi.org/10.1016/j.redox.2018.02.003

Singh, T. P., Tehri, N., Kaur, G., & Malik, R. K. (2021). Cell surface and extracellular proteins of potentially probiotic *Lactobacillus reuteri* as an effective mediator to regulate intestinal epithelial barrier function. *Archives of Microbiology, 203*(6), 3219–3228. https://doi.org/10.1007/s00203-021-02318-2

Strugala, V., Dettmar, P. W., & Pearson, J. P. (2008). Thickness and continuity of the adherent colonic mucus barrier in active and quiescent ulcerative colitis and Crohn's disease. *International Journal of Clinical Practice, 62*(5), 762–769. https://doi.org/10.1111/j.1742-1241.2007.01665.x

Sun, Y., & O'Riordan, M. X. D. (2013). Regulation of bacterial pathogenesis by intestinal short-chain fatty acids. *Advances in Applied Microbiology, 85,* 93–118. https://doi.org/10.1016/B978-0-12-407672-3.00003-4

Swidsinski, A., Loening-Baucke, V., Theissig, F., Engelhardt, H., Bengmark, S., Koch, S., Lochs, H., & Dörffel, Y. (2007). Comparative study of the intestinal mucus barrier in normal and inflamed colon. *Gut, 56*(3), 343–350. https://doi.org/10.1136/gut.2006.098160

Szajewska, H., Horvath, A., & Piwowarczyk, A. (2010). Meta-analysis: The effects of Saccharomyces boulardii supplementation on Helicobacter pylori eradication rates and side effects during treatment. *Alimentary Pharmacology and Therapeutics, 32*(9), 1069–1079. https://doi.org/10.1111/j.1365-2036.2010.04457.x

Szajewska, H., & Mrukowicz, J. (2005). Meta-analysis: Non-pathogenic yeast *Saccharomyces boulardii* in the prevention of antibiotic-associated diarrhoea. *Alimentary Pharmacology and Therapeutics, 22*(5), 365–372. https://doi.org/10.1111/j.1365-2036.2005.02624.x

Szajewska, H., Ruszczyński, M., & Radzikowski, A. (2006). Probiotics in the prevention of antibiotic-associated diarrhea in children: A meta-analysis of randomized controlled trials. *Journal of Pediatrics, 149*(3), 367–372. https://doi.org/10.1016/j.jpeds.2006.04.053

Tan, J., McKenzie, C., Potamitis, M., Thorburn, A. N., Mackay, C. R., & Macia, L. (2014). The role of short-chain fatty acids in health and disease. In F. W. Alt (Ed.), *Advances in immunology* (Vol. 121, pp. 91–119). Academic Press.

Tanner, S. A., Chassard, C., Rigozzi, E., Lacroix, C., & Stevens, M. J. A. (2016). *Bifidobacterium thermophilum* RBL67 impacts on growth and virulence gene expression of *Salmonella enterica* subsp. *Enterica* serovar Typhimurium. *BMC Microbiology, 16,* 46. https://doi.org/10.1186/s12866-016-0659-x

Tomusiak-Plebanek, A., Heczko, P., Skowron, B., Baranowska, A., Okoń, K., Thor, P. J., & Strus, M. (2018). Lactobacilli with superoxide dismutase-like or catalase activity are more effective in alleviating inflammation in an inflammatory bowel disease mouse model. *Drug Design, Development and Therapy, 12,* 3221–3233. https://doi.org/10.2147/DDDT.S164559

Turroni, F., Taverniti, V., Ruas-Madiedo, P., Duranti, S., Guglielmetti, S., Lugli, G. A., Gioiosa, L., Palanza, P., Margolles, A., van Sinderen, D., & Ventura, M. (2014). *Bifidobacterium bifidum* PRL2010 modulates the host innate immune response. *Applied and Environmental Microbiology, 80*(2), 730–740. https://doi.org/10.1128/AEM.03313-13

Ulluwishewa, D., Anderson, R. C., McNabb, W. C., Moughan, P. J., Wells, J. M., & Roy, N. C. (2011). Regulation of tight junction permeability by intestinal bacteria and dietary components. *Journal of Nutrition, 141*(5), 769–776. https://doi.org/10.3945/jn.110.135657

Umu, Ö. C. O., Rudi, K., & Diep, D. B. (2017). Modulation of the gut microbiota by prebiotic fibres and bacteriocins. *Microbial Ecology in Health and Disease, 28*(1), 1348886. https://doi.org/10.1080/16512235.2017.1348886

Urrutia-Baca, V. H., Escamilla-García, E., de la Garza-Ramos, M. A., Tamez-Guerra, P., Gomez-Flores, R., & Urbina-Ríos, C. S. (2018). *In vitro* antimicrobial activity and downregulation of virulence gene expression on *Helicobacter pylori* by reuterin. *Probiotics and Antimicrobial Proteins, 10*(2), 168–175. https://doi.org/10.1007/s12602-017-9342-2

van Zyl, W. F., Deane, S. M., & Dicks, L. M. T. (2020). Molecular insights into probiotic mechanisms of action employed against intestinal pathogenic bacteria. *Gut Microbes, 12*(1), 1831339. https://doi.org/10.1080/19490976.2020.1831339

Vancamelbeke, M., & Vermeire, S. (2017). The intestinal barrier: A fundamental role in health and disease. *Expert Review of Gastroenterology and Hepatology, 11*(9), 821–834. https://doi.org/10.1080/17474124.2017.1343143

Wang, J., Ji, H., Wang, S., Liu, H., Zhang, W., Zhang, D., & Wang, Y. (2018). Probiotic *Lactobacillus plantarum* promotes intestinal barrier function by strengthening the epithelium and modulating gut microbiota. *Frontiers in Microbiology, 9*, 1953. https://doi.org/10.3389/fmicb.2018.01953

Wang, L., Cao, H., Liu, L., Wang, B., Walker, W. A., Acra, S. A., & Yan, F. (2014). Activation of epidermal growth factor receptor mediates mucin production stimulated by p40, a *Lactobacillus rhamnosus* GG-derived protein. *Journal of Biological Chemistry, 289*(29), 20234–20244–22044. https://doi.org/10.1074/jbc.M114.553800

Wang, R., Jiang, L., Zhang, M., Zhao, L., Hao, Y., Guo, H., Sang, Y., Zhang, H., & Ren, F. (2017). The adhesion of *Lactobacillus salivarius* REN to a human intestinal epithelial cell line requires S-layer proteins. *Scientific Reports, 7,* 44029. https://doi.org/10.1038/srep44029

Wang, X., Zhang, P., & Zhang, X. (2021). Probiotics regulate gut microbiota: An effective method to improve immunity. *Molecules, 26*(19), 6076. https://doi.org/10.3390/molecules26196076

Wang, Y., & Li, H. (2022). Gut microbiota modulation: A tool for the management of colorectal cancer. *Journal of Translational Medicine, 20*(1), 178. https://doi.org/10.1186/s12967-022-03378-8

Wang, Y., Wu, Y., Wang, Y., Fu, A., Gong, L., Li, W., & Li, Y. (2017). *Bacillus amyloliquefaciens* SC06 alleviates the oxidative stress of IPEC-1 via modulating Nrf2/Keap1 signaling pathway and decreasing ROS production. *Applied Microbiology and Biotechnology, 101*(7), 3015–3026. https://doi.org/10.1007/s00253-016-8032-4

Wang, Y., Wu, Y., Wang, Y., Xu, H., Mei, X., Yu, D., Wang, Y., & Li, W. (2017). Antioxidant properties of probiotic bacteria. *Nutrients, 9*(5), 521. https://doi.org/10.3390/nu9050521

Wenus, C., Goll, R., Loken, E. B., Biong, A. S., Halvorsen, D. S., & Florholmen, J. (2008). Prevention of antibiotic-associated diarrhoea by a fermented probiotic milk drink. *European Journal of Clinical Nutrition, 62*(2), 299–301. https://doi.org/10.1038/sj.ejcn.1602718

Wu, Y., Wang, B., Xu, H., Tang, L., Li, Y., Gong, L., Wang, Y., & Li, W. (2019). Probiotic *Bacillus* attenuates oxidative stress-induced intestinal injury via p38-mediated autophagy. *Frontiers in Microbiology, 10,* 2185. https://doi.org/10.3389/fmicb.2019.02185

Yan, F., Cao, H., Cover, T. L., Whitehead, R., Washington, M. K., & Polk, D. B. (2007). Soluble proteins produced by probiotic bacteria regulate intestinal epithelial cell survival and growth. *Gastroenterology, 132*(2), 562–575. https://doi.org/10.1053/j.gastro.2006.11.022

Yan, F., & Polk, D. B. (2006). Probiotics as functional food in the treatment of diarrhea. *Current Opinion in Clinical Nutrition and Metabolic Care, 9*(6), 717–721. https://doi.org/10.1097/01.mco.0000247477.02650.51

Yang, K. M., Zhu, C., Wang, L., Cao, S. T., Yang, X. F., Gao, K. G., & Jiang, Z. Y. (2021). Early supplementation with *Lactobacillus plantarum* in liquid diet modulates intestinal innate immunity through toll-like receptor 4-mediated mitogen-activated protein kinase signaling pathways in young piglets challenged with *Escherichia coli* K88. *Journal of Animal Science, 99*(6), skab128. https://doi.org/10.1093/jas/skab128

10 Probiotics and Cancer
Role in Chemoprevention

Akanksha Yadav, Luxita Sharma, and Debasrita Banerjee

10.1 INTRODUCTION

The term "chemoprevention" encompasses the utilization of various natural or chemical compounds to prevent cancer progression and reverse it (Steward & Brown, 2013). Cancer is a deadly malignancy and one of the major reasons of death and morbidity globally. Cancer is an unmanageable cell division and is normally recognized at the advanced phase of development. Insufficient DNA repair or mutations during DNA replication can cause this. The main risk factors are UV radiation, genetics, unhealthy lifestyle, infectious agents, and polluted environment exposure. The most common types of cancer that cause increases in the number of deaths are gastric, colorectal, bladder, prostate, lung, liver, ovarian, and breast cancers (Ferlay et al., 2015). The incidences of cancer disease have been gradually developing throughout the world (WHO, 2020).

Probiotic is a phrase of the current era that refers to "for life" and friendly bacterial relations with favorable effects on human health (Bagchi, 2014). The term "probiotic" refers to live non-pathogenic healthy microbes that are used as food supplements, nutraceuticals, and biotherapeutic agents that provide host well-being (Salminen et al., 2021). Probiotics are considered functional foods due to one of the main mechanisms providing beneficial health effects. Over the fermentation process, nutrients are broken down by yeast, fungi, or bacteria into simpler metabolites; hence, fermented probiotic foods may help enhance the bioavailability of nutrients like vitamins, fats, proteins, carbohydrates, and minerals (Shah et al., 2023). Probiotics possess antioxidant activity, provide defense against peroxidation of fatty acids, and reduce oxidative stress. The activity of the intestinal microbiota plays an essential role in providing energy and defense against chronic diseases (Wang et al., 2017). Dietary probiotic functional food is mainly associated with meat products, plant-based foods, dairy products, and non-dairy fermented food products that may fulfill our daily nutritional needs for healthy living (Dahiya & Nigam, 2022). Probiotics have major functional qualities that display a positive prevention response against health disorders, like gastrointestinal problems, diabetes, obesity, and various types of cancer (Tegegne & Kebede, 2022). Lactic acid bacteria can produce natural antioxidants like bioactive peptides such as glutathione, GPX, and CAT to help suppress cancer cells. The gut microbiota plays a significant role in the maintenance of human health. Healthy strains of probiotics such as *Bifidobacterium*, *Lactobacillus casei*, *Bacillus coagulans*, *Lactobacillus rhamnosus*, and *Lactococcus lactis* are used in the pharmaceutical and food industry as shown in Figure 10.1. They play a significant role in enzyme production, bioavailability of nutrients, and immunomodulation by decreasing inflammation, lowering cholesterol, and alleviating cancer disease (Zheng et al., 2020). The unique qualities of probiotics are resistance to the action of acid, tolerance of bile antimicrobial activity, antagonistic activity against pathogens, and mutagenic and bile salt hydrolase potential (Hassan, 2019). Angiogenesis functions of probiotics may include the alteration of provocative cytokine profiles, management of the mechanism of strain-related problems, the enhancement of nutrient absorption, the reduction of hypersensitivity reactions, stress response, and invasion of pathogenic bacteria (Plaza-Diaz et al., 2019). Probiotic metabolites such as lipopolysaccharides, exopolysaccharides, and SCFAs have immune-modulatory activity that can help prevent various types of cancer and promote a healthy life. SCFAs are byproducts of probiotics that may lower luminal pH, enhance the absorption of macro and micronutrients,

 DOI: 10.1201/9781003452249-10

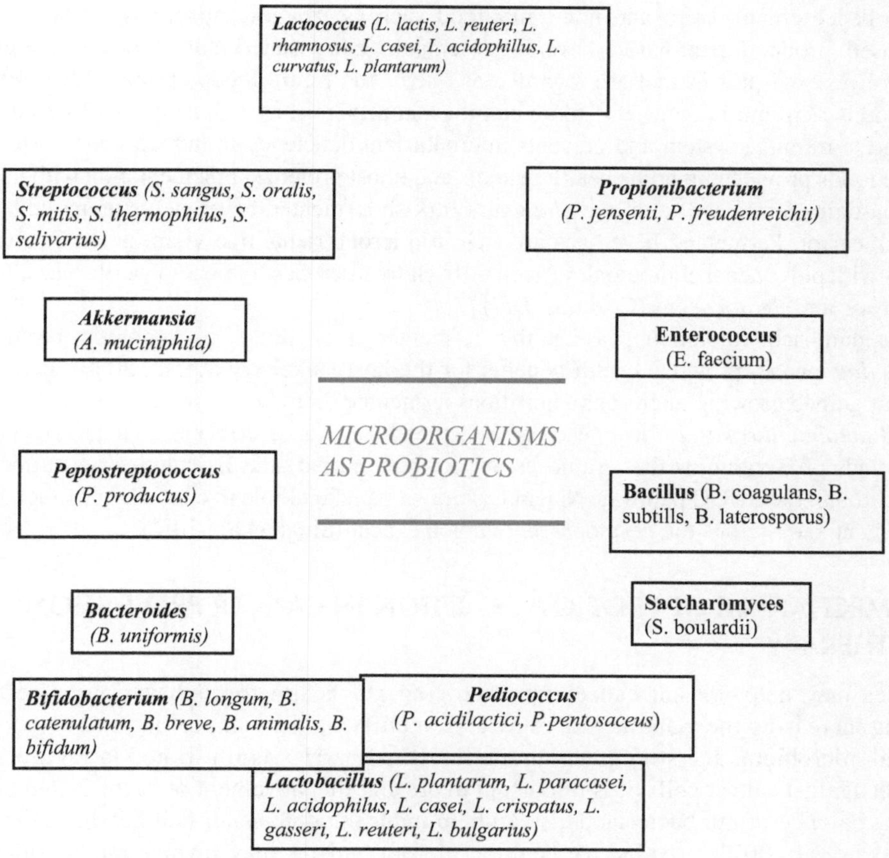
Lactococcus (L. lactis, L. reuteri, L. rhamnosus, L. casei, L. acidophillus, L. curvatus, L. plantarum)
Streptococcus (S. sangus, S. oralis, S. mitis, S. thermophilus, S. salivarius)
Propionibacterium (P. jensenii, P. freudenreichii)
Akkermansia (A. muciniphila)
Enterococcus (E. faecium)
MICROORGANISMS AS PROBIOTICS
Peptostreptococcus (P. productus)
Bacillus (B. coagulans, B. subtills, B. laterosporus)
Bacteroides (B. uniformis)
Saccharomyces (S. boulardii)
Bifidobacterium (B. longum, B. catenulatum, B. breve, B. animalis, B. bifidum)
Pediococcus (P. acidilactici, P.pentosaceus)
Lactobacillus (L. plantarum, L. paracasei, L. acidophilus, L. casei, L. crispatus, L. gasseri, L. reuteri, L. bulgarius)

FIGURE 10.1 Healthy microorganisms as probiotics.

promote constituents of gut microbiota, suppress the growth of infective microbes like food-borne unhealthy bacteria, provide energy to colonocytes, and have an antitumor effect through promoting apoptosis mechanism as well (Portincasa et al., 2022). Dysbiosis of the gut microbiome helps boost the vulnerability of the host regarding colonization by pathobionts (Carding et al., 2015). The anti-pathogenic activity of probiotics reduces the risk of non-communicable diseases and boosts the absorption of essential nutrients. The anti-inflammatory properties of probiotics can prevent cancer cell growth by numerous distinct pathways, like boosting the production of immunoglobulin A levels, management of cyclooxygenase-2, and regulation of NF-kB and IFN-γ. Probiotics are potentially beneficial and affect the metabolism of the gut microbiota during chemotherapy and radiotherapy, thereby decreasing their toxic side effects in cancer prevention and GRAS. Based on recent studies, the healthy live microorganism may annihilate carcinogen toxicity in the human body (Shamekhi et al., 2020).

10.2 PROBIOTICS-BASED FOOD PRODUCTS AND NUTRITIONAL BENEFITS

Lactic acid bacteria have the maximum attraction due to their nutritional and therapeutic benefits along with probiotic attributes, having especially GRAS status (Zhang et al., 2020). Probiotic-based food companies have introduced their dietary supplement products with a minimum standard dose of microbes, that is, 10^6–10^7 CFU/g probiotic culture (Neffe-Skocińska et al., 2018). Probiotic-rich foods are categorized as fermented dairy food like yogurt, cheese, cultured flavored buttermilk, acidic milk ice cream, kefir, and non-dairy food such as Japanese miso, soy cereals, legumes, millet-based product, fruit-based beverages, tempeh, beer, sauerkraut, chocolate, sourdough, kimchi, olives, and pickles that are regarded as one of the future foods (Tomar, 2019). Probitics-based food is rich in micronutrients like vitamins and minerals, as well as it has proven a positive effect on the immune system and prevents micronutrient deficiency in human health. Meat-based probiotic foods provide numerous health benefits and boost protein supplementation with good bacteria. Non-dairy fermented food like *Shalgam* (Turkish fermented beverage) is prepared by turnip and black carrot. Fermented beverages are rich in micronutrients like vitamins A, B, and C and minerals with polyphenol compounds as well as friendly microbes like Lactobacillaceae along with *Leuconostoc* and *Pediococcus* (Coskun, 2017).

Antioxidant-rich *Kombucha*, a healthy fermented tea source of probiotic bacteria like *Lactobacillus genus*, provides health benefits for the host (Jakubczyk et al., 2020). Ready-to-eat *Yakult* has gained growing interest as a nutritious fermented dairy beverage that contains probiotics, namely, *Lactobacillus casei shirota* used all over the globe (Katan, 2012). Gut bacteria can produce several kinds of B vitamins that are necessary for humankind, and B vitamins will affect tumor genesis through the SGOC pathway. Niacin has drawn beneficial role in colitis by prostaglandin D2 enhancement and inhibits the development of colon cancer (Singh et al., 2014).

10.3 MECHANISM OF PROBIOTICS ACTION IN CANCER PREVENTION THERAPY

Probiotics may help prevent cancer by improving gut health through various mechanisms, including increasing the manufacture of SCFAs, modifying the composition and activity of the intestinal microbiota, and strengthening the intestinal barrier as illustrated in Figure 10.2. To help fight against cancer cells, it is important to prevent the movement of bacteria and maintain a healthy balance of gut bacteria. This can help induce apoptosis, or cell death, in the tumors (Śliżewska et al., 2021). Live active healthy microorganisms may involve modulation of certain enzymes associated with the cellular detox process, involving preventing the activity of free radicals, affecting the other mutagenic and carcinogenic substances as well as stimulating immune function through an immunomodulation mechanism and modulating the intestinal microflora. They have antioxidant properties, anti-inflammatory effects, antiproliferative activity, and anti-metastatic properties, which also helpful in the inhibition of various types of cancer (Noor et al., 2023).

10.4 CANCER-INHIBITING BACTERIA

Trillions of microbes, such as *Lactobacillus*, *Bifidobacterium*, *Faecalibaculum rodentium*, and *Streptococcus thermophilus*, in the human intestinal tract may help prevent cancer by having an immunomodulatory effect and positive impact on the gut microbiome. Healthy live bacteria *Lactobacillus* spp. are generally used as a nutraceutical against cancer disease. Lactic acid bacteria may help reduce the growth and development of CRC as an inflammatory effect is also beneficial to gut health (Zhang et al., 2022). *Bifidobacterium bifidum* is a genus of gram-positive specialized anaerobic bacteria that exhibit antitumor effects on cancer cells. The isolated *Bifidobacterium* spp. were particularly administered in the tumors of mice suffering from breast cancer and were found to have remarkably prevented tumor growth with no side effects like weight reduction and kidney and liver failure. It can be a potential carrier of anticancer proteins against malignant tumors and also regulates intestinal homeostasis and controls the initiation of cancer (Verma et al., 2018). *F. rodentium* and *Holdemanella biformis* may produce SCFAs that prevent the growth of tumor cells and acetylation of protein by the inhibition of calcineurin and NFATc3 activation, and they may be used as cancer protection therapy (Zagato et al., 2020). *S. thermophilus* is a probiotic that promotes digestive and immune health and can also release folate to reduce tumor growth. Dietary nutrient

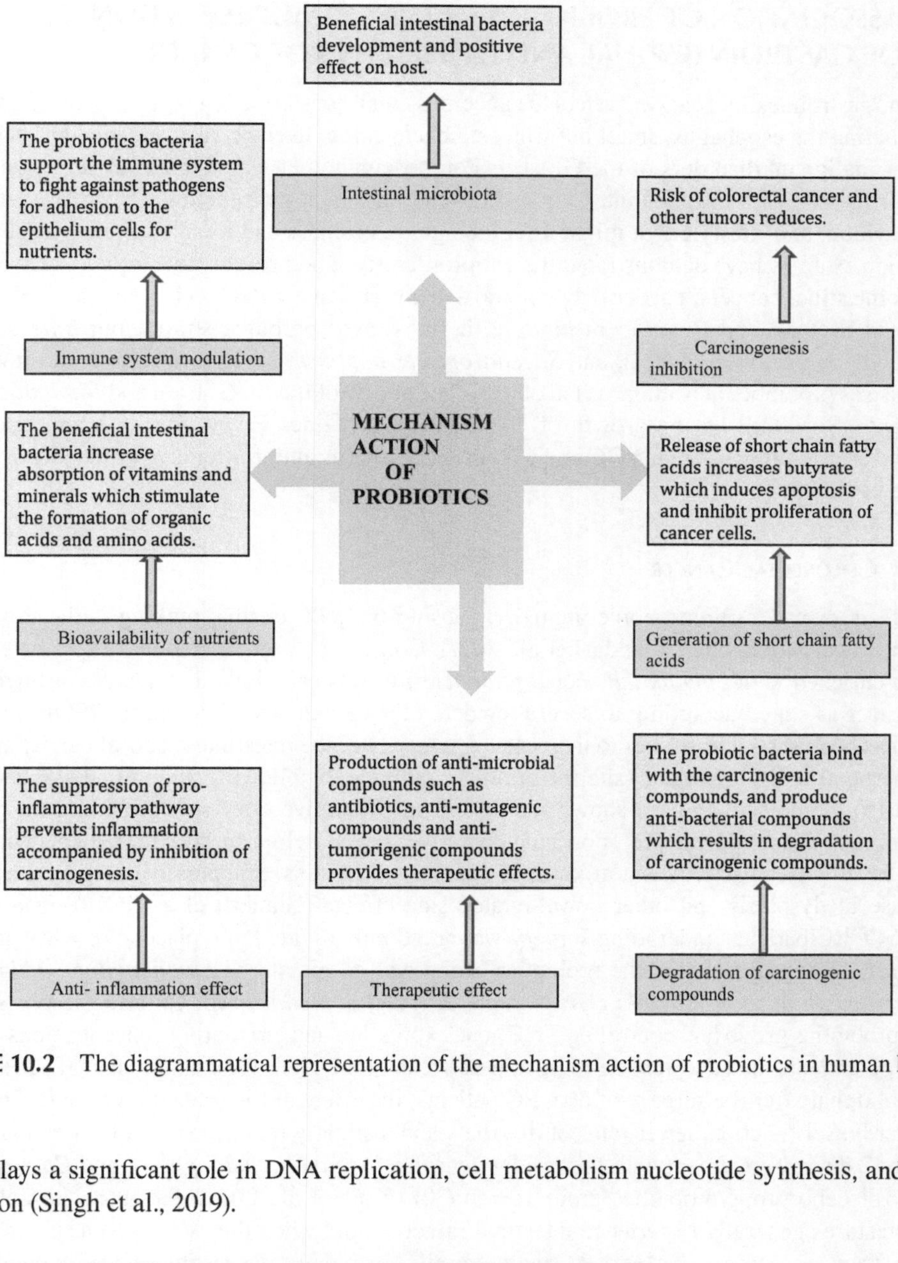

FIGURE 10.2 The diagrammatical representation of the mechanism action of probiotics in human health.

folate plays a significant role in DNA replication, cell metabolism nucleotide synthesis, and tumor inhibition (Singh et al., 2019).

10.5 GUT MICROBIOTA AND ANTICANCER THERAPY

The gut microbiota, observed as "the second genome" of humankind, may exhibit a positive effect by the inhibition of pathogen infection and modulation of cancer therapy by enhancing chemotherapy, radiotherapy, and surgery (Kunika et al., 2023). The gut microbiota is importantly proven to have an effective role by inducing the host immune responses and supporting homeostasis in the human body. After treatment with cyclophosphamide, there is an increase in IFN-γ and CD8+ T cells due to the translocation of *Enterococcus hirae* and the accumulation of *Barnesiella intestinihominis*. It can promote the growth of reactive oxygen species that are responsible for increasing drug efficacy. Gut microbiota's microbial metabolites boost immunity, provide antioxidant and antitumor effects, and mitigate therapy-induced adverse effects on human health (Li et al., 2021).

10.6 ASSOCIATION OF PROBIOTICS IN THE CHEMOPREVENTION OF GASTROINTESTINAL AND OTHER TYPES OF CANCER

The term "gastrointestinal cancer" refers to cancerous conditions affecting organs involved in digestion, including the esophagus, small intestine, stomach, colon, liver, rectum, gallbladder, pancreas, and other malignant disorders of the GI tract (Pourhoseingholi et al., 2015). They are regarded as complex illnesses with intricate interactions between immunology, genetics, epigenetics, environment, nutrition, and lifestyle that might affect the gut microbiota and its role in tumor genesis and progression. Studies have demonstrated the antiproliferative and pro-apoptotic effects of probiotics on gastrointestinal cancers, particularly colonic and gastric cancer (GC) cells (Kumar et al., 2010). Lactic acid bacteria and *Bifidobacterium* are the most used probiotic strains, but *Enterococcus*, *Escherichia coli*, *S. thermophilus*, and *Saccharomyces boulardii* species are also under investigation for use as probiotics (Javanmard et al., 2018). The ability of the *LGG* strain and *Bifidobacterium adolescentis* SPM0212 on the growth of colon cancer cell lines HT29, SW 480, and Caco-2 to inhibit the proliferation of human GC and colon cancer cells as antiproliferative products is reported (Orlando et al., 2012).

10.6.1 Colorectal Cancer

CRC affects over 1 million people annually, causing 500,000 deaths, making it the third-most common cancer worldwide (Bhandari et al., 2017). Consuming a good amount of fermented milk products enriched with *Lactobacillus* or *Bifidobacterium* has been linked to a lesser occurrence of colon cancer as stated according to several epidemiological studies (Geier et al., 2006). Probiotic therapy has been shown in studies to increase the integrity of the intestinal mucosal barrier and prevent superficial incision surgical-site infections in individuals following abdominal surgery (Aisu et al., 2015). Some studies have shown the beneficial preventive effects of probiotics on patients with colorectal cancer during pre-, post, and operative stages. Before surgery for patients with CRC who get healthy live bacteria as a mixture of one or more strains, preoperative surgery may cause a decrease in dysbiosis and other bowel-related side effects (Gianotti et al., 2010). In a certain study, 164 CRC patients undergoing surgery were randomly divided into placebo (n = 80) and probiotics (n = 84) groups, where the probiotics group was administered *Lactobacillus acidophilus*, *Lactobacillus plantarum*, *Bifidobacterium lactis BB*, and *S. boulardii* for 15 days. Results showed that the probiotics group had controlled TNF gene expression and circulating concentrations of IL-6 via SOCS3 and also had a lower rate of postoperative complications (Kotzampassi et al., 2015). The study found that after the surgery of 60 CRC patients, the effect of the probiotic group had resulted in quicker bowel function, fewer rates of diarrhea, and a slightly reduced rate of bacteremia recovery after 12 days of treatment with the *Bifidobacterium longum*, *L. acidophilus*, and *Enterococcus faecalis* (placebo group/probiotics group n = 30/30) (Yang et al., 2016). Patients with colorectal liver metastases generally experience intestinal infection and when they were given the probiotics (*L. plantarum*, *L. acidophilus*, and *B. longum*) orally for 6 days, the results showed a decrease in serum zonulin level and the rate of liver barrier from metastasis (Liu et al., 2015).

10.6.2 Gastric Cancer

GC is the leading cause of cancer-related deaths across the globe (Zhu et al., 2018). In patients with GC after surgery, taking probiotics and fiber reduces the occurrence of diarrhea, improves bowel movement, and reduces bowel problems (Zhao et al., 2017). In animal models, probiotics such as *B. bifidum*, *L. acidophilus*, *L. rhamnosus*, and *Lactobacillus salivarius* have been shown to have positive inhibitory effects on eradicating *Helicobacter pylori* infection (Zhu & Liu, 2017). A recent meta-analysis found that utilizing probiotics as a complement to antibiotic therapy is very effective in eliminating *H. pylori* (Losurdo et al., 2018).

10.6.3 Bladder Cancer

LGG may prevent bladder cancer just as successfully as BCG. In a certain study, it was found that the treatment of mice with LGG enhanced the preventive response, restored the levels of XCL1 in the bladders, and attracted a significant number of macrophages and neutrophils to the tumor site. They may perform a significant role in BCG immunotherapy in the treatment of bladder cancer (Seow et al., 2010). Another study found that probiotics enhanced dendritic cell activity, which in turn activated natural killer cells, which had a significant effect on immunological manipulation (Feyisetan et al., 2012).

10.6.4 Prostate Cancer

A study found that treatment with *Lactobacillus* improved the natural killer activity of PBMC against prostate cancer. The study's findings indicated that *Lactobacillus* produced tumor necrosis factor-related apoptosis-inducing ligand (TNFAIL), which helped the natural killer activity and raised the possibility that a new TNFAIL-based therapy approach for cancerous tumors might be developed (Horinaka et al., 2010).

10.6.5 Other Types of Cancers

Studies have been carried out to support the connection between probiotics and other kinds of GI cancer, such as pancreatic, esophageal, and liver cancers; however, these studies are less numerous than those on CRC and GC (Richman et al., 2017). Probiotics have been shown to prevent pancreatic cancer through a variety of pathways, including the regulation of diseases like liver, diabetes, pancreatic necrosis, and obesity. Probiotics were found to slow the progression of HCC in mice models and also modify the microbiota's composition and decrease the size of liver tumors. Additionally, the study demonstrated that probiotic supplementation could control angiogenic variables (Li et al., 2016).

Skin cancer: Skin cancer is the most prevalent type of cancer worldwide. The study investigated how probiotics and their metabolites may prevent skin cancer, and lipoteichoic acids from LGG were used orally in hairless mice. More IFN, TH, and CTL cells were produced by the T cells of the treated participants, and the appearance of the tumor is delayed (Weill et al., 2013). A study found that kefir significantly reduced intracellular reactive oxygen species and suppressed morphological alterations caused by UVC exposure in skin cancer (Nagira et al., 2002).

Cervical cancer: Recent studies observed that probiotics have potential to the suppress cervical cancer by improving, modulating, or reducing apoptosis, proliferation, and inflammation and inhibiting metastasis (Jahanshahi et al., 2020).

Head and neck cancer: The study investigated how *L. acidophilus* affected tongue cancer where probiotics were cultured with cancer cells for 48 hours, and it was observed that doing so significantly reduced the multiplication of malignant cells (Xiaoyan et al., 2012).

Breast cancer: Probiotics, as functional food, may be fighting against breast cancer, by enhancing immunity, as proven by the cell-based and animal model study. It has been discovered that *Bacillus subtilis* product surfactin has an anticancer effect on breast cancer cells, and it is said to have a dose-dependent impact that slows cell growth by about 10 ng/mL throughout 24 hours (Lee et al., 2012). Consuming *L. casei shirota* and isoflavones frequently since adolescence can decrease the risk of breast cancer in women, as shown by a study. Consuming *L. casei shirota* and isoflavones frequently since adolescence can decrease the risk of breast cancer in women, as shown by a study. There may be a biological interaction between *Lactobacillus* and isoflavones (Toi et al., 2013).

10.6.6 Leukemia

A study used PFT to test the apoptotic effect of a kefir grain product (Lactobacillus) on MDR leukemia cells. PFT has been demonstrated to promote cancer cell apoptosis in a dose-dependent way and suggested that PFT may hold potential as a therapeutic for the management of MDR leukemia (Ghoneum & Gimzewski, 2014). In leukemia, kefir drinking reduces cell proliferation and boosts apoptosis (Jalali et al., 2016).

10.7 APPLICATION OF PROBIOTICS METABOLITES FOR THE PREVENTION OF CANCER

Functional metabolites obtained from live healthy probiotics may play a significant role in the inhibition of tumor development through the modulation of host immunity. Extracts from lactobacilli induce cancer cell apoptosis through the development of SCFAs, conjugated linoleic acid, and other anti-carcinogenic metabolites. Lipopolysaccharides produced by bacteria also activate toll-like receptor 4, stimulating T cell–mediated immune response against tumor cells (Paulos et al., 2007).

SCFAs, such as acetic acid, butyric acid, and propionic acid, are crucial in carbohydrate metabolism. Over the building of SCFAs and the growth of butyrate due to the anaerobic respiration of wheat grains, maltodextrin reduces the growth of malignant cells (He et al., 2020). It has antioxidant effects and anti-inflammatory properties that help prevent the proliferation of cancer cells and regulate immunological function. Probiotics *L. salivarius* FP35, *Pediococcus pentosaceus* FP3, *L. salivarius* FP25, and *Enterococcus faecium* FP51 also suppress the rapid production of colon cancer cells by the secretion of butyric and propionic acids (Thirabunyanon & Hongwittayakorn, 2013). Particularly, metabolites like conjugated linoleic acids used as dietary supplements composed of probiotic bacteria can prevent colorectal cancer in a recent study on mice models (Ewaschuk et al., 2006). The p8 protein derived from probiotics has anti-colorectal cancer effects by halting the cell cycle induction. This protein has been isolated from bacterial probiotics and has shown anticancer activity in humans, making it a potential candidate for biopharmaceutical protein (An et al., 2019). Exopolysaccharide extracted from probiotics plays a key role in the suppression of cancer. Various recent studies observed that lactic acid bacteria present in the gut help in the suppression of tumors by immunomodulation therapy and also activate phagocytes to reduce harmful cancer cells (Górska et al., 2019).

10.8 CONCLUSION

In conclusion, probiotics have excellent nutritional and therapeutic potential against cancer. Supplementation of fermented dairy and dairy probiotic-rich foods has many medical significance like regulating the intestinal microflora, reducing gastrointestinal problems, and suppressing carcinogenesis in the gut. They have important nutraceutical properties that can protect against different types of cancer and minimize the side effects of therapies like chemotherapy, radiation, and surgery. Gut microbiota helps enhance the effectiveness of immunotherapy as well as regulate metabolism and hematopoiesis, inhibiting inflammation and pathogen infection. Functional metabolite products such as SCFAs, conjugated linoleic acid, inhibitory proteins, tryptophan, polysaccharides, siderophores, and nucleic acids may act as anticancer agents in human health.

Finally, many challenges remain for now to minimize adverse effects related to probiotics and to find a comprehensive way that encompasses microbial regulation remedies for recent cancer management systems.

BIBLIOGRAPHY

Abdul Rahim, M. B. H., Chilloux, J., Martinez-Gili, L., Neves, A. L., Myridakis, A., Gooderham, N., & Dumas, M. E. (2019). Diet-induced metabolic changes of the human gut microbiome: Importance of short-chain fatty acids, methylamines and indoles. *Acta Diabetologica, 56*(5), 493–500. https://doi.org/10.1007/s00592-019-01312-x

Aisu, N., Tanimura, S. H. U., Yamashita, Y., Yamashita, K., Maki, K., Yoshida, Y., Sasaki, T., Takeno, S., & Hoshino, S. (2015). Impact of perioperative probiotic treatment for surgical site infections in patients with colorectal cancer. *Experimental and Therapeutic Medicine, 10*(3), 966–972. https://doi.org/10.3892/etm.2015.2640

An, B. C., Hong, S., Park, H. J., Kim, B. K., Ahn, J. Y., Ryu, Y., An, J. H., & Chung, M. J. (2019). Anti-colorectal cancer effects of probiotic-derived p8 protein. *Genes, 10*(8), 624. https://doi.org/10.3390/genes10080624

Bagchi, T. (2014). Traditional food and modern lifestyle: Impact of probiotics. *Indian Journal of Medical Research, 140*(3), 333–335.

Bhandari, A., Woodhouse, M., & Gupta, S. (2017). Colorectal cancer is a leading cause of cancer incidence and mortality among adults younger than 50 years in the USA: A SEER-based analysis with comparison to other young-onset cancers. *Journal of Investigative Medicine, 65*(2), 311–315. https://doi.org/10.1136/jim-2016-000229

Carding, S., Verbeke, K., Vipond, D. T., Corfe, B. M., & Owen, L. J. (2015). Dysbiosis of the gut microbiota in disease. *Microbial Ecology in Health and Disease, 26*(1), 26191. https://doi.org/10.3402/mehd.v26.26191

Coskun, F. (2017). A traditional Turkish fermented nonalcoholic beverage. *Beverages, 3*(4), 49. https://doi.org/10.3390/beverages3040049

Cremon, C., Barbaro, M. R., Ventura, M., & Barbara, G. (2018). Pre-and probiotic overview. *Current Opinion in Pharmacology, 43,* 87–92. https://doi.org/10.1016/j.coph.2018.08.010

Dahiya, D., & Nigam, P. S. (2022). Nutrition and health through the use of probiotic strains in fermentation to produce non-dairy functional beverage products supporting gut microbiota. *Foods, 11*(18), 2760. https://doi.org/10.3390/foods11182760

Ewaschuk, J. B., Walker, J. W., Diaz, H., & Madsen, K. L. (2006). Bioproduction of conjugated linoleic acid by probiotic bacteria occurs in vitro and in vivo in mice. *The Journal of Nutrition, 136*(6), 1483–1487. https://doi.org/10.1093/jn/136.6.1483

Ferlay, J., Soerjomataram, I., Dikshit, R., Eser, S., Mathers, C., Rebelo, M., Parkin, D. M., Forman, D., & Bray, F. (2015). Cancer incidence and mortality worldwide: Sources, methods and major patterns in GLOBOCAN 2012. *International Journal of Cancer, 136*(5), E359–E386. https://doi.org/10.1002/ijc.29210

Feyisetan, O., Tracey, C., & Hellawell, G. O. (2012). Probiotics, dendritic cells and bladder cancer. *BJU International, 109*(11), 1594–1597. https://doi.org/10.1111/j.1464-410X.2011.10749.x

Fitzmaurice, C., Allen, C., Barber, R. M., Barregard, L., Bhutta, Z. A., Brenner, H., & Satpathy, M. (2017). Global, regional, and national cancer incidence, mortality, years of life lost, years lived with disability, and disability-adjusted life-years for 32 cancer groups, 1990 to 2015: A systematic analysis for the global burden of disease study. *JAMA Oncology, 3*(4), 524–548. https://doi.org/10.1001/jamaoncol.2016.5688

Geier, M. S., Butler, R. N., & Howarth, G. S. (2006). Probiotics, prebiotics and Synbiotics: A role in chemoprevention for colorectal cancer? *Cancer Biology and Therapy, 5*(10), 1265–1269. https://doi.org/10.4161/cbt.5.10.3296

Ghoneum, M., & Gimzewski, J. (2014). Apoptotic effect of a novel kefir product, PFT, on multidrug-resistant myeloid leukemia cells via a hole-piercing mechanism. *International Journal of Oncology, 44*(3), 830–837. https://doi.org/10.3892/ijo.2014.2258

Gianotti, L., Morelli, L., Galbiati, F., Rocchetti, S., Coppola, S., Beneduce, A., Gilardini, C., Zonenschain, D., Nespoli, A., & Braga, M. (2010). A randomized double-blind trial on perioperative administration of probiotics in colorectal cancer patients. *World Journal of Gastroenterology, 16*(2), 167–175. https://doi.org/10.3748/wjg.v16.i2.167

Górska, A., Przystupski, D., Niemczura, M. J., & Kulbacka, J. (2019). Probiotic bacteria: A promising tool in cancer prevention and therapy. *Current Microbiology, 76*(8), 939–949. https://doi.org/10.1007/s00284-019-01679-8

Hassan, Z. (2019). Anti-cancer and biotherapeutic potentials of probiotic bacteria. *Journal of Cancer Science and Therapy, 11*(1), 009–013. https://doi.org/10.4172/1948-5956.1000575

He, J., Zhang, P., Shen, L., Niu, L., Tan, Y., Chen, L., Zhao, Y., Bai, L., Hao, X., Li, X., Zhang, S., & Zhu, L. (2020). Short-chain fatty acids and their association with signalling pathways in inflammation, glucose and lipid metabolism. *International Journal of Molecular Sciences, 21*(17), 6356. https://doi.org/10.3390/ijms21176356

Horinaka, M., Yoshida, T., Kishi, A., Akatani, K., Yasuda, T., Kouhara, J., Wakada, M., & Sakai, T. (2010). Lactobacillus strains induce TRAIL production and facilitate natural killer activity against cancer cells. *FEBS Letters, 584*(3), 577–582. https://doi.org/10.1016/j.febslet.2009.12.004

Jahanshahi, M., Maleki Dana, P., Badehnoosh, B., Asemi, Z., Hallajzadeh, J., Mansournia, M. A., Yousefi, B., Moazzami, B., & Chaichian, S. (2020). Anti-tumor activities of probiotics in cervical cancer. *Journal of Ovarian Research, 13*(1), 68. https://doi.org/10.1186/s13048-020-00668-x

Jakubczyk, K., Kałduńska, J., Kochman, J., & Janda, K. (2020). Chemical profile and antioxidant activity of the kombucha beverage derived from white, green, black and red tea. *Antioxidants, 9*(5), 447. https://doi.org/10.3390/antiox9050447

Jalali, F., Sharifi, M., & Salehi, R. (2016). Kefir induces apoptosis and inhibits cell proliferation in human acute erythroleukemia. *Medical Oncology, 33*(1), 7. https://doi.org/10.1007/s12032-015-0722-8

Javanmard, A., Ashtari, S., Sabet, B., Davoodi, S. H., Rostami-Nejad, M., Esmaeil Akbari, M. E., Niaz, A., & Mortazavian, A. M. (2018). Probiotics and their role in gastrointestinal cancers prevention and treatment; an overview. *Gastroenterology and Hepatology from Bed to Bench, 11*(4), 284–295.

Katan, M. B. (2012). Why the European Food Safety Authority was right to reject health claims for probiotics. *Beneficial Microbes, 3*(2), 85–89. https://doi.org/10.3920/BM2012.0008

Kotzampassi, K., Stavrou, G., Damoraki, G., Georgitsi, M., Basdanis, G., Tsaousi, G., & Giamarellos-Bourboulis, E. J. (2015). A four-probiotics regimen reduces postoperative complications after colorectal surgery: A randomized, double-blind, placebo-controlled study. *World Journal of Surgery, 39*(11), 2776–2783. https://doi.org/10.1007/s00268-015-3071-z

Kumar, M., Kumar, A., Nagpal, R., Mohania, D., Behare, P., Verma, V., Kumar, P., Poddar, D., Aggarwal, P. K., Henry, C. J., Jain, S., & Yadav, H. (2010). Cancer-preventing attributes of probiotics: An update. *International Journal of Food Sciences and Nutrition, 61*(5), 473–496. https://doi.org/10.3109/09637480903455971

Kunika, Frey, N., & Rangrez, A. Y. (2023). Exploring the involvement of gut microbiota in cancer therapy-induced cardiotoxicity. *International Journal of Molecular Sciences, 24*(8), 7261. https://doi.org/10.3390/ijms24087261

Lee, J. H., Nam, S. H., Seo, W. T., Yun, H. D., Hong, S. Y., Kim, M. K., & Cho, K. M. (2012). The production of surfactin during the fermentation of cheonggukjang by potential probiotic Bacillus subtilis CSY191 and the resultant growth suppression of MCF-7 human breast cancer cells. *Food Chemistry, 131*(4), 1347–1354. https://doi.org/10.1016/j.foodchem.2011.09.133

Li, J., Sung, C. Y. J., Lee, N., Ni, Y., Pihlajamäki, J., Panagiotou, G., & El-Nezami, H. (2016). Probiotics modulated gut microbiota suppresses hepatocellular carcinoma growth in mice. *Proceedings of the National Academy of Sciences of the United States of America, 113*(9), E1306–E1315. https://doi.org/10.1073/pnas.1518189113

Liu, Z., Li, C., Huang, M., Tong, C., Zhang, X., Wang, L., Peng, H., Lan, P., Zhang, P., Huang, N., Peng, J., Wu, X., Luo, Y., Qin, H., Kang, L., & Wang, J. (2015). Positive regulatory effects of perioperative probiotic treatment on postoperative liver complications after colorectal liver metastases surgery: A double-center and double-blind randomized clinical trial. *BMC Gastroenterology, 15,* 34. https://doi.org/10.1186/s12876-015-0260-z

Li, W., Deng, X., & Chen, T. (2021). Exploring the Modulatory Effects of Gut Microbiota in Anti-Cancer Therapy. *Frontiers in oncology*, *11*, 644454. https://doi.org/10.3389/fonc.2021.644454

Losurdo, G., Cubisino, R., Barone, M., Principi, M., Leandro, G., Ierardi, E., & Di Leo, A. (2018). Probiotic monotherapy and Helicobacter pylori eradication: A systematic review with pooled-data analysis. *World Journal of Gastroenterology, 24*(1), 139–149. https://doi.org/10.3748/wjg.v24.i1.139

Mattila-Sandholm, T., Myllärinen, P., Crittenden, R., Mogensen, G., Fondén, R., & Saarela, M. (2002). Technological challenges for future probiotic foods. *International Dairy Journal, 12*(2–3), 173–182. https://doi.org/10.1016/S0958-6946(01)00099-1

Nagira, T., Narisawa, J., Teruya, K., Katakura, Y., Shim, S. Y., Kusumoto, K., Tokumaru, S., Tokumaru, K., Barnes, D. W., & Shirahata, S. (2002). Suppression of UVC-induced cell damage and enhancement of DNA repair by the fermented milk, Kefir. *Cytotechnology*, *40*(1-3), 125–137. https://doi.org/10.1023/A:1023984304610

Neffe-Skocińska, K., Rzepkowska, A., Szydłowska, A., & Kołożyn-Krajewska, D. (2018). Trends and possibilities of the use of probiotics in food production. In A. M. Holban & A. M. Grumezescu (Eds.), *Alternative and replacement foods* (Vol. 17, pp. 65–94). Academic Press.

Noor, S., Ali, S., Riaz, S., Sardar, I., Farooq, M. A., & Sajjad, A. (2023). Chemopreventive role of probiotics against cancer: A comprehensive mechanistic review. *Molecular Biology Reports, 50*(1), 799–814. https://doi.org/10.1007/s11033-022-08023-7

Orlando, A., Refolo, M. G., Messa, C., Amati, L., Lavermicocca, P., Guerra, V., & Russo, F. (2012). Antiproliferative and proapoptotic effects of viable or heat-killed Lactobacillus paracasei IMPC2. 1 and Lactobacillus rhamnosus GG in HGC-27 gastric and DLD-1 colon cell lines. *Nutrition and Cancer, 64*(7), 1103–1111. https://doi.org/10.1080/01635581.2012.717676

Paulos, C. M., Wrzesinski, C., Kaiser, A., Hinrichs, C. S., Chieppa, M., Cassard, L., Palmer, D. C., Boni, A., Muranski, P., Yu, Z., Gattinoni, L., Antony, P. A., Rosenberg, S. A., & Restifo, N. P. (2007). Microbial translocation augments the function of adoptively transferred self/tumor-specific CD8+ T cells via TLR4 signaling. *Journal of Clinical Investigation, 117*(8), 2197–2204. https://doi.org/10.1172/JCI32205

Plaza-Diaz, J., Ruiz-Ojeda, F. J., Gil-Campos, M., & Gil, A. (2019). Mechanisms of action of probiotics. *Advances in Nutrition, 10*(suppl_1), S49–S66. https://doi.org/10.1093/advances/nmy063

Portincasa, P., Bonfrate, L., Vacca, M., De Angelis, M., Farella, I., Lanza, E., Khalil, M., Wang, D. Q., Sperandio, M., & Di Ciaula, A. (2022). Gut microbiota and short chain fatty acids: Implications in glucose homeostasis. *International Journal of Molecular Sciences, 23*(3), 1105. https://doi.org/10.3390/ijms23031105

Pourhoseingholi, M. A., Vahedi, M., & Baghestani, A. R. (2015). Burden of gastrointestinal cancer in Asia; an overview. *Gastroenterology and Hepatology from Bed to Bench, 8*(1), 19–27.

Raman, M., Ambalam, P., Kondepudi, K. K., Pithva, S., Kothari, C., Patel, A. T., Purama, R. K., Dave, J. M., & Vyas, B. R. M. (2013). Potential of probiotics, prebiotics and Synbiotics for management of colorectal cancer. *Gut Microbes, 4*(3), 181–192. https://doi.org/10.4161/gmic.23919

Richman, D. M., Tirumani, S. H., Hornick, J. L., Fuchs, C. S., Howard, S., Krajewski, K., Ramaiya, N., & Rosenthal, M. (2017). Beyond gastric adenocarcinoma: Multimodality assessment of common and uncommon gastric neoplasms. *Abdominal Radiology, 42*(1), 124–140. https://doi.org/10.1007/s00261-016-0901-x

Salminen, S., Collado, M. C., Endo, A., Hill, C., Lebeer, S., Quigley, E. M. M., Sanders, M. E., Shamir, R., Swann, J. R., Szajewska, H., & Vinderola, G. (2021). The international scientific association of probiotics and prebiotics (ISAPP) consensus statement on the definition and scope of postbiotics. *Nature Reviews. Gastroenterology and Hepatology, 18*(9), 649–667. https://doi.org/10.1038/s41575-021-00440-6

Şanlier, N., Gökcen, B. B., & Sezgin, A. C. (2019). Health benefits of fermented foods. *Critical Reviews in Food Science and Nutrition, 59*(3), 506–527. https://doi.org/10.1080/10408398.2017.1383355

Şener, D., Bulut, H. N., & Güneş Bayir, A. G. (2021). Probiotics and relationship between probiotics and cancer types. *Bezmiâlem Science, 9*(4), 490–497. https://doi.org/10.14235/bas.galenos.2021.5375

Seow, S. W., Cai, S., Rahmat, J. N., Bay, B. H., Lee, Y. K., Chan, Y. H., & Mahendran, R. (2010). Lactobacillus rhamnosus GG induces tumor regression in mice bearing orthotopic bladder tumors. *Cancer Science, 101*(3), 751–758. https://doi.org/10.1111/j.1349-7006.2009.01426.x

Serban, D. E. (2014). Gastrointestinal cancers: Influence of gut microbiota, probiotics and prebiotics. *Cancer Letters, 345*(2), 258–270. https://doi.org/10.1016/j.canlet.2013.08.013

Shah, A. M., Tarfeen, N., Mohamed, H., & Song, Y. (2023). Fermented foods: Their health-promoting components and potential effects on gut microbiota. *Fermentation, 9*(2), 118. https://doi.org/10.3390/fermentation9020118

Shamekhi, S., Lotfi, H., Abdolalizadeh, J., Bonabi, E., & Zarghami, N. (2020). An overview of yeast probiotics as cancer biotherapeutics: Possible clinical application in colorectal cancer. *Clinical and Translational Oncology, 22*(8), 1227–1239. https://doi.org/10.1007/s12094-019-02270-0

Singh, N., Gurav, A., Sivaprakasam, S., Brady, E., Padia, R., Shi, H., Thangaraju, M., Prasad, P. D., Manicassamy, S., Munn, D. H., Lee, J. R., Offermanns, S., & Ganapathy, V. (2014). Activation of Gpr109a, receptor for niacin and the commensal metabolite butyrate, suppresses colonic inflammation and carcinogenesis. *Immunity, 40*(1), 128–139. https://doi.org/10.1016/j.immuni.2013.12.007

Singh, R., Chandrashekharappa, S., Bodduluri, S. R., Baby, B. V., Hegde, B., Kotla, N. G., Hiwale, A. A., Saiyed, T., Patel, P., Vijay-Kumar, M., Langille, M. G. I., Douglas, G. M., Cheng, X., Rouchka, E. C., Waigel, S. J., Dryden, G. W., Alatassi, H., Zhang, H. G., Haribabu, B., . . . & Jala, V. R. (2019). Enhancement of the gut barrier integrity by a microbial metabolite through the Nrf2 pathway. *Nature Communications, 10*(1), 89. https://doi.org/10.1038/s41467-018-07859-7

Śliżewska, K., Markowiak-Kopeć, P., & Śliżewska, W. (2021). The role of probiotics in cancer prevention. *Cancers, 13*(1), 20. https://doi.org/10.3390/cancers13010020

So, S. S., Wan, M. L., & El-Nezami, H. (2017). Probiotics-mediated suppression of cancer. *Current Opinion in Oncology, 29*(1), 62–72. https://doi.org/10.1097/CCO.0000000000000342

Steward, W. P., & Brown, K. (2013). Cancer chemoprevention: a rapidly evolving field. *British journal of cancer*, *109*(1), 1–7. https://doi.org/10.1038/bjc.2013.280

Tegegne, B. A., & Kebede, B. (2022). Probiotics, their prophylactic and therapeutic applications in human health development: A review of the literature. *Heliyon*, *8*(6), e09725. https://doi.org/10.1016/j.heliyon.2022.e09725

Thirabunyanon, M., & Hongwittayakorn, P. (2013). Potential probiotic lactic acid bacteria of human origin induce antiproliferation of colon cancer cells via synergic actions in adhesion to cancer cells and short-chain fatty acid bioproduction. *Applied Biochemistry and Biotechnology, 169*(2), 511–525. https://doi.org/10.1007/s12010-012-9995-y

Toi, M., Hirota, S., Tomotaki, A., Sato, N., Hozumi, Y., Anan, K., Nagashima, T., Tokuda, Y., Masuda, N., Ohsumi, S., Ohno, S., Takahashi, M., Hayashi, H., Yamamoto, S., & Ohashi, Y. (2013). Probiotic beverage with soy isoflavone consumption for breast cancer prevention: A case-control study. *Current Nutrition and Food Science, 9*(3), 194–200. https://doi.org/10.2174/1573401311309990001

Tomar, O. (2019). The effects of probiotic cultures on the organic acid content, texture profile and sensory attributes of Tulum cheese. *International Journal of Dairy Technology, 72*(2), 218–228. https://doi.org/10.1111/1471-0307.12574

Verma, R., Lee, C., Jeun, E. J., Yi, J., Kim, K. S., Ghosh, A., Byun, S. H., Lee, C. G., Kang, H. J., Kim, G. C., Jun, C. D., Jan, G., Suh, C. H., Jung, J. Y., Sprent, J., Rudra, D., De Castro, C., Molinaro, A., Surh, C. D., & Im, S. H. (2018). Cell surface polysaccharides of Bifidobacterium bifidum induce the generation of Foxp3+ regulatory T cells. *Science Immunology, 3*(28), eaat6975. https://doi.org/10.1126/sciimmunol.aat6975

Wang, Y., Wu, Y., Wang, Y., Xu, H., Mei, X., Yu, D., Wang, Y., & Li, W. (2017). Antioxidant properties of probiotic bacteria. *Nutrients, 9*(5), 521. https://doi.org/10.3390/nu9050521

Weill, F. S., Cela, E. M., Paz, M. L., Ferrari, A., Leoni, J., & González Maglio, D. H. G. (2013). Lipoteichoic acid from Lactobacillus rhamnosus GG as an oral photoprotective agent against UV-induced carcinogenesis. *British Journal of Nutrition, 109*(3), 457–466. https://doi.org/10.1017/S0007114512001225

World Health Organization. (2020). *WHO report on cancer: Setting priorities, investing wisely and providing care for all*. WHO.

Xiaoyan, S., Jun, C., Tuanjie, C., Decheng, B., & Xiangyi, H. (2012). A study on human tongue cancer cells' proliferation affected by Lactobacillus acidophilus. *West China Journal of Stomatology, 30*(1).

Yang, Y., Xia, Y., Chen, H., Hong, L., Feng, J., Yang, J., Yang, Z., Shi, C., Wu, W., Gao, R., Wei, Q., Qin, H., & Ma, Y. (2016). The effect of perioperative probiotics treatment for colorectal cancer: Short-term outcomes of a randomized controlled trial. *Oncotarget, 7*(7), 8432–8440. https://doi.org/10.18632/oncotarget.7045

Zagato, E., Pozzi, C., Bertocchi, A., Schioppa, T., Saccheri, F., Guglietta, S., Fosso, B., Melocchi, L., Nizzoli, G., Troisi, J., Marzano, M., Oresta, B., Spadoni, I., Atarashi, K., Carloni, S., Arioli, S., Fornasa, G., Asnicar, F., Segata, N., . . . & Rescigno, M. (2020). Endogenous murine microbiota member Faecalibaculum rodentium and its human homologue protect from intestinal tumour growth. *Nature Microbiology, 5*(3), 511–524. https://doi.org/10.1038/s41564-019-0649-5

Zhang, S. L., Han, B., Mao, Y. Q., Zhang, Z. Y., Li, Z. M., Kong, C. Y., Wu, Y., Chen, G. Q., & Wang, L. S. (2022). Lacticaseibacillus paracasei sh2020 induced antitumor immunity and synergized with anti-programmed cell death 1 to reduce tumor burden in mice. *Gut Microbes, 14*(1), 2046246. https://doi.org/10.1080/19490976.2022.2046246

Zhang, X., Esmail, G. A., Alzeer, A. F., Arasu, M. V., Vijayaraghavan, P., Choi, K. C., & Al-Dhabi, N. A. (2020). Probiotic characteristics of Lactobacillus strains isolated from cheese and their antibacterial properties against gastrointestinal tract pathogens. *Saudi Journal of Biological Sciences, 27*(12), 3505–3513. https://doi.org/10.1016/j.sjbs.2020.10.022

Zhao, R., Wang, Y., Huang, Y., Cui, Y., Xia, L., Rao, Z., Zhou, Y., & Wu, X. (2017). Effects of fiber and probiotics on diarrhea associated with enteral nutrition in gastric cancer patients: A prospective randomized and controlled trial. *Medicine, 96*(43), e8418. https://doi.org/10.1097/MD.0000000000008418

Zheng, J., Wittouck, S., Salvetti, E., Franz, C. M. A. P., Harris, H. M. B., Mattarelli, P., O'Toole, P. W., Pot, B., Vandamme, P., Walter, J., Watanabe, K., Wuyts, S., Felis, G. E., Gänzle, M. G., & Lebeer, S. (2020). A taxonomic note on the genus Lactobacillus: Description of 23 novel genera, emended description of the genus Lactobacillus Beijerinck 1901, and union of Lactobacillaceae and Leuconostocaceae. *International Journal of Systematic and Evolutionary Microbiology, 70*(4), 2782–2858. https://doi.org/10.1099/ijsem.0.004107

Zhu, L. N., Zhan, Y., Zhang, J., Chen, L., & Wu, X. (2018). Effects of probiotics combined with enteral nutrition on gastrointestinal function of postoperative patients with esophageal cancer. Zhongguo Weishengtaxixue Zazhi. *Chinese Journal of Microecology, 30*(8), 924–927.

Zhu, X. Y., & Liu, F. (2017). Probiotics as an adjuvant treatment in Helicobacter pylori eradication therapy. *Journal of Digestive Diseases, 18*(4), 195–202. https://doi.org/10.1111/1751-2980.12466

11 Probiotics
Unleashing the Regenerative Potential for Neuronal Health in Neurodegenerative Diseases

Shrimanti Das, Atharva A. Mahajan, Anuvab Dey, Akanksha Bhattacharya, Suryakshi Bhunia, Renesa Dasgupta, Madhurima Majumdar, Neelparna Indu, Anirban Hait, and Subhrojyoti Ghosh

11.1 INTRODUCTION

11.1.1 Neurodegenerative Diseases: An Escalating Public Health Concern

In the last decade, there has been a significant increase in attention focused on well-being and disorders related to neurodegeneration. Neurodegenerative diseases (NDs) refer to a collection of disorders that impact the nerve cells in the brain and spinal cord. These conditions prompt the gradual decline of these nerve cells, ultimately resulting in the impairment and eventual cessation of function in the regions they control (Ojha et al., 2023). In recent neurological and psychiatric research, significant attention has been directed toward investigating the disruption in gut microbial populations, commonly known as gut dysbiosis. Notably, this line of research has underscored the exploration of imbalances that favor a pathogenic condition.

11.1.2 The Gut–Brain Axis: Linking the Microbiota and Neurodegeneration

The gut microbiota is a diverse and constantly evolving community of microorganisms in the digestive system. This complex ecosystem plays a substantial role in influencing the health and susceptibility to diseases in the host. Intriguingly, there exists a multifaceted and mutually influential connection between the gut microbiota and the brain, which scientists refer to as the GBA. This axis creates links between the operational functions of the digestive system and the emotional and cognitive regions of the brain. These connections rely on intricate interactions that encompass the brain and nervous system, immunological players, and endocrine systems.

The changes in composition of the mentioned microbiota not only contribute to gastrointestinal disturbances but also extend their influence on the brain, potentially triggering maladies. Among these conditions, Alzheimer's disease emerges as a prevalent form of dementia that predominantly affects older individuals.

Through a plethora of experimental and clinical investigations, insights have emerged highlighting the function of gut microbiota in shaping the cognitive faculties of the host. Dysbiosis, characterized by an uneven distribution of gut microbes commonly linked with the aging process, has been implicated in the advancement of neurodegenerative conditions. Dysbiosis triggers the release of substances such as amyloid and LPSs, which can compromise both the structure of the gastrointestinal and blood–brain barriers. These disruptions serve as a catalyst for inflammatory signaling

DOI: 10.1201/9781003452249-11

pathways, thus fostering neuroinflammation and consequent neuronal damage, ultimately culminating in neuronal demise as observed in Alzheimer's disease (Kesika et al., 2021).

Moreover, the composition and variety of gut microbiota play a crucial role in influencing the quantities of metabolites, neurotransmitters, and SCFAs (such as butyrate, propionate, and acetate) generated by the microbiota. These substances are significant outcomes of microbial fermentation in the gut and are influenced by factors like diet. These compounds are important byproducts of microbial fermentation in the gut and are subject to influence from factors such as dietary choices (Gubert et al., 2020).

The ANS delivers the most immediate neurological response to the gut, inducing swift alterations in gut physiology. This is achieved by directly innervating the target organ, a phenomenon observed in both normal and pathological states. For instance, this process is evident in the context of the pain response and stress (Dinan & Cryan, 2012).

11.1.3 Rationale for Exploring Probiotics as a Regenerative Therapy

Probiotics refer to viable microorganisms that, upon administration in appropriate quantities, confer prospective physiological advantages to the host organism through their constructive modulation of gut microbiota equilibrium, subsequently enhancing holistic physiological welfare. Probiotic entities are acknowledged for their capacity to foster health via the activation of endogenous gut microbiota, modulation of host immune responses, mitigation of cholesterol levels, and multifarious physiological functions. Concurrently, the metabolic byproducts produced by these microorganisms, encompassing bacteriocins, lactic acid, and hydrogen peroxide—collectively termed postbiotics—emanate as significant agents with antimicrobial properties, exhibiting efficacy across an extensive spectrum of pathogenic bacterial strains, as elucidated by Silva et al. in 2020. Elie Metchnikoff postulated the potential enhancement of well-being through orchestrated gut microbiome manipulation using beneficial bacterial strains inherent in yogurt. This conceptual framework subsequently crystallized into the medical (Ojha et al., 2023) recognized as probiotics, as expounded by Mackowiak in 2013 (Yadav et al., 2022). Probiotics have the ability to modify the makeup of the gut microbiota, which may result in reduced inflammation and potentially offer relief from neuroinflammatory processes. Studies on probiotics suggest that when administered, they can enhance the diversity of the gut microbiota, leading to regulatory effects on inflammation and providing resistance against the colonization of external harmful microorganisms. Specific gut bacteria have the ability to synthesize neurotransmitters like serotonin and dopamine, which have essential roles in regulating mood and cognitive functions. Disruptions in the balance of these neurotransmitters are linked to neurodegenerative conditions. Probiotics with the ability to regulate neurotransmitter production could potentially impact disease progression. The rationale for exploring probiotics as a regenerative modality for neurodegenerative disorders is rooted in the intricate association between gut microbiota and brain fitness.

11.2 INTERRELATION

11.2.1 Bidirectional Communication: Gut Microbiota and the Brain

The microorganisms present in the intestinal tract, often called the gut microbiome, encompass a diverse population of microorganisms, such as bacteria, viruses, fungi, and various other microbes, residing in the gastrointestinal tract of both humans and other animals. These microorganisms have a significant impact on multiple aspects of well-being, including digestive processes, metabolic functions, immune responses, and even neurological health (Jandhyala et al., 2015). The diversity of the human gut microbes is remarkable, consisting of trillions of microbial cells representing numerous distinct species. The composition of the gut microbiota can vary considerably among

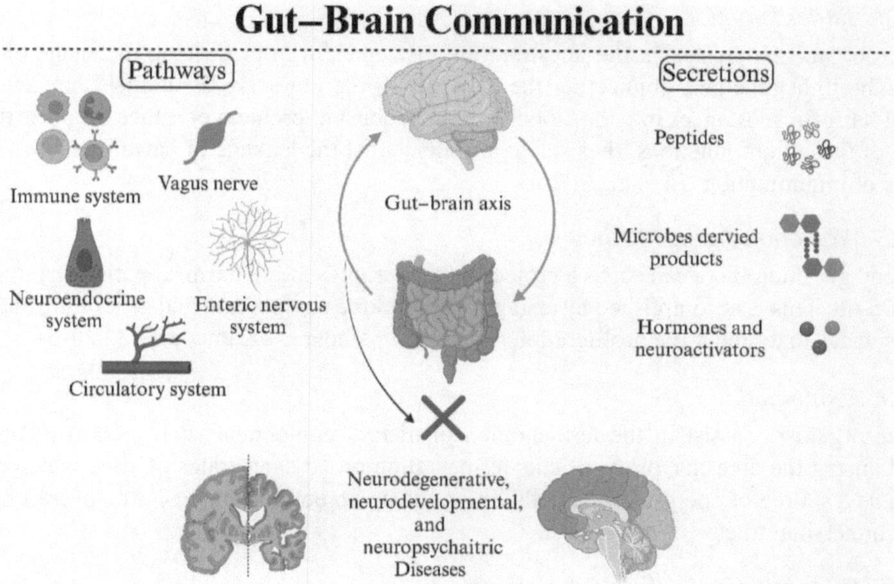

FIGURE 11.1 Gut–brain communication. The communication leads to the activation of pathways such as the immune system, neuroendocrine system, enteric nervous system, and circulatory system. This, in turn, leads to the secretion of peptides, neuro-activators, and hormones. Disruption of this axis leads to neurological disorders.

individuals, and it is influenced by a range of factors, including genetics, dietary preferences, age, environment, and medical history. The balance and diversity of these microorganisms are believed to be important for maintaining optimal health (see Figure 11.1) (Thursby & Juge, 2017).

11.2.1.1 Functions and Roles of Gut Microbiota

11.2.1.1.1 Digestion and Nutrient Absorption

The gut microbiota has a crucial role in breaking down intricate carbohydrates and fibers. These microorganisms possess enzymes capable of transforming these usually indigestible compounds into simpler substances, like SCFAs, which the body can absorb and utilize for energy. Furthermore, they aid in the decomposition of specific plant-based compounds, making nutrients accessible that would otherwise remain out of reach (Jandhyala et al., 2015).

11.2.1.1.2 Metabolism

Certain gut microorganisms participate in metabolic activities, including the fermentation of dietary fibers, resulting in the production of SCFAs such as butyrate, acetate, and propionate. These compounds not only serve as a source of energy for the cells lining the gastrointestinal tract but also have broader effects that extend beyond the gut, influencing metabolism, inflammation, and even appetite regulation.

11.2.1.1.3 Immune System Modulation

The gut microbiota plays a critical role in training the immune system. They help educate immune cells to distinguish between harmless substances (like food particles) and harmful pathogens. This interaction prevents the immune system from overreacting to harmless stimuli and helps maintain a balanced immune response (Bengmark, 2013).

11.2.1.1.4 Barrier Function

The microorganisms present in the intestinal are instrumental in preserving the shape of the gut barrier. The tight junctions connecting the cells lining the gut serve as a shield, preventing the access of harmful substances into the bloodstream. A robust microbiota presence supports the preservation of these tight junctions, thus safeguarding against the leakage of harmful substances and the onset of inflammation (Li et al., 2020).

11.2.1.1.5 Protection Against Pathogens

A balanced gut microbiota can act as a protective barrier, preventing harmful pathogens from colonizing the gut. This is accomplished by engaging in resource competition and generating antimicrobial substances that hinder the proliferation of harmful pathogens (Kamada et al., 2013).

11.2.1.1.6 Fermentation

Gut microorganisms assist in the fermentation of dietary components that remain incompletely digested during the digestive process. This fermentation process generates SCFAs, which not only function as a source of energy for the cells lining the colon but also enhance the overall health of the gastrointestinal tract.

11.2.1.1.7 Synthesis of Bioactive Compounds

Some gut bacteria have the ability to produce bioactive compounds, such as secondary bile acids. These compounds have been linked to various health effects, including the regulation of lipid metabolism and blood pressure (O'Shea et al., 2012).

The two-way exchange of information between the gut microbiota and the brain is referred to as the GBA. This axis represents a complex and intricate connection through which the gut and the brain influence each other's functions and activities. This interaction takes place through diverse routes, encompassing neural, endocrine (hormonal), and immune signaling pathways. The GBA is of paramount importance in not only overseeing gastrointestinal operations but also in shaping emotional and cognitive functions. A key contributor to this axis is the vagus nerve, which comprises sensory and motor fibers, establishing connections from the brainstem to multiple organs, including the gastrointestinal tract. This nerve facilitates a two-way exchange of information between the gut and the brain, with signals from the gut traveling along the vagus nerve to impact functions such as appetite, feelings of fullness, and the digestive process. Conversely, the brain can send signals down the vagus nerve to regulate gut functions, such as controlling the rate of gastric emptying and promoting coordinated contractions for digestion. The microorganisms in the gut can manufacture neurotransmitters, which are molecules that act as messengers transmitting signals among nerve cells within the brain. For example, certain gut bacteria produce serotonin, a neurotransmitter known for its role in mood regulation. Alterations in serotonin levels are linked to mood disorders like depression. By producing neurotransmitters, gut bacteria can directly impact brain function and emotional states (Strandwitz, 2018). The microbes present in the intestine have the ability to influence the production and release of hormones responsible for regulating appetite, metabolism, and responses to stress. One example is the impact of gut bacteria on hormones like ghrelin and leptin, which play crucial roles in controlling appetite and maintaining energy balance (Martin et al., 2019). Moreover, a significant proportion of the body's immune cells resides in the gut, and microbes present in the intestine have an important function in the maturation of the immune system. A well-balanced microbiota helps prevent unwarranted immune reactions to harmless substances. Dysbiosis can lead to inflammation, which can have implications for both gut and brain health. Chronic inflammation is increasingly recognized as contributing to various neurological disorders (Salzman, 2011). The GBA has significant ramifications for mental well-being and behavioral patterns.

Research in animal models and some human studies suggests that an imbalanced gut microbiota may contribute to anxiety, depression, and neurodevelopmental disorders. The exact mechanisms remain partially elucidated, but it is hypothesized that the gut microbiota possesses the ability to regulate inflammation, neurotransmitter production, and hormonal signaling, all of which exert an influence on the well-being of the brain. The relationship between the GBA and the body's response to stress is highly intertwined. Stress has the potential to induce changes in the gut microbiota's composition, thereby influencing the diversity and balance of bacteria present. Conversely, the microbes present in the gut can shape the body's reaction to stress by controlling the release of stress hormones such as cortisol. This mutually influential relationship between stress and the gut microbiota carries implications for disorders associated with stress.(Dinan & Cryan, 2012).

Because of the bidirectional communication between the microbes in the gut and the brain, researchers are exploring interventions designed to alter the gut microbiota to improve mental health and well-being. Probiotics, which are live microorganisms that are beneficial, and prebiotics, which are fibers that nourish beneficial gut bacteria, are being investigated for their potential to alleviate symptoms of anxiety, depression, and stress. As the understanding of the GBA grows, the concept of personalized medicine is gaining traction. Customizing interventions based on an individual's distinct microbes present in the intestine makeup and health characteristics has the potential to result in more efficient approaches to treating mental health conditions.

11.2.2 Disruptions in Gut–Brain Communication in Neurodegenerative Diseases

Irregularities in the communication between the gut and the brain have been linked to several NDs. These are progressive conditions marked by the gradual deterioration of nerve cells (neurons) in the brain and, in some instances, the spinal cord. Recently, it is observed that changes in the microbes present in the gut and the two-way interaction between microorganisms in the intestine and the brain could have an important function in the onset and advancement of these disorders.

11.2.2.1 Parkinson's Disease

In the context of Parkinson's disease (PD), there are observations suggesting that changes in the gut microorganisms could be involved in the onset and advancement of the condition. Numerous studies have noted discrepancies in the gut microbiota between individuals with PD and those without it. These alterations in the microorganisms present in the intestine can lead to the generation of metabolites, including SCFAs and LPSs, which have the potential to affect the structure of the gut barrier and initiate inflammation within the body. Inflammation and changes in gut permeability might contribute to the spread of pathological alpha-synuclein protein aggregates, a key characteristic of PD; this signal comes from the gut by the vagus nerve in the brain (Singh et al., 2022).

11.2.2.2 Alzheimer's Disease

In Alzheimer's disease, there is a connection to the accumulation of beta-amyloid plaques and tau tangles within the brain. Disturbances in the GBA might potentially function in the inflammation and neurodegeneration seen in Alzheimer's disease. Shifts in the makeup of the gut microbiota can result in the production of metabolites that impact the equilibrium between pro-inflammatory and anti-inflammatory compounds within the body. A compromised gut barrier can allow these metabolites, as well as inflammatory substances, to enter the bloodstream and potentially reach the brain, thereby promoting neuroinflammation and the accumulation of amyloid proteins(Liu et al., 2020).

11.2.2.3 Amyotrophic Lateral Sclerosis

ALS is marked by the deterioration of motor neurons. Although the exact cause of ALS remains unclear, researchers are keen to investigate the potential influence of disturbances in the GBA on its development. Changes in the microorganisms present in the gut and modifications in gut permeability have been noted in individuals with ALS. These changes might create metabolites and inflammatory substances that contribute to widespread inflammation and could potentially affect the central nervous system. These changes may produce metabolites and inflammatory agents that contribute to systemic inflammation and could potentially influence the central nervous system.

11.2.2.4 Huntington's Disease

Huntington's disease (HD) is identified by the buildup of abnormal mutant huntingtin protein in the brain. It is assumed that disruptions in the GBA play a role in the advancement of HD. The gut microbiota has the capacity to generate metabolites that impact the creation and clustering of mutant huntingtin protein. Additionally, inflammation in the gut can initiate a broader inflammatory reaction in the body, potentially exacerbating the neuroinflammation seen in HD (Love et al., 2022).

11.2.2.5 Multiple Sclerosis

Multiple sclerosis (MS) is an autoimmune ailment marked by the loss of myelin from nerve fibers in the central nervous system. There is interest in examining how disruptions in the GBA might function in the immune system dysfunction seen in MS. An imbalance in the gut microbiota, known as dysbiosis, can affect the equilibrium of immune cells. This imbalance can promote the development and exacerbation of MS (Parodi & Kerlero de Rosbo, 2021).

In all of these NDs, the mechanisms by which disruptions in gut–brain communication contribute to disease progression are complex and multifaceted. Inflammation, altered responses from the immune system, and the production of metabolites by microbes present in the intestine are fundamental elements linking the gut and the brain in these diseases. Moreover, the signals between the intestine and the brain are sent by the direct channel of the vagus nerve, potentially enabling disease-related factors to travel through this pathway. Comprehending these connections is essential for developing targeted therapies that could regulate the gut microbiota and reinstate proper gut–brain communication, potentially influencing the progression of NDs. However, it's important to acknowledge that this field of research is still emerging, and further investigations are required to completely understand the mechanisms at play and translate these discoveries into effective clinical interventions.

11.3 IMPACT OF DYSBIOSIS ON NEURONAL HEALTH AND DISEASE PROGRESSION

Dysbiosis, which signifies an irregularity in the gut microbiota, has risen as a significant element impacting not just gastrointestinal health but also multiple facets of neurological health. The GBA, a two-way communication system connecting the gut with the central nervous system, assumes a central role in facilitating these influences. Dysbiosis triggers a cascade of events with implications for neuronal health (Carding et al., 2015). Firstly, dysbiosis-induced inflammation and immune activation can have widespread effects (Levy et al., 2017). The gut houses a significant portion of the body's immune cells, and an imbalance in the microbiota can lead to an immune response that goes beyond the gut, contributing to systemic inflammation. This inflammation can influence the blood–brain barrier's integrity, potentially allowing harmful molecules to cross into the brain. Neuroinflammation, a prominent feature of numerous neurological disorders, is believed to be influenced, at least in part, by inflammation triggered by dysbiosis. Secondly, the gut microbiota's role in producing neuroactive compounds is of paramount importance. The generation of neurotransmitters such as serotonin can be altered by dysbiosis (Strandwitz, 2018). These compounds play essential roles in mood regulation, behavior, and cognitive function. Changes in their balance caused by dysbiosis have been linked to conditions such as depression, anxiety, and even neurodegenerative disorders. Furthermore, the gut microbiota's digestion of dietary fibers generates SCFAs, which have both local and systemic effects. SCFAs contribute to maintaining gut health and strengthening barrier function. Moreover, they can enter the bloodstream and impact the brain, influencing neuronal activity, inflammation, and even blood–brain barrier permeability. Dysbiosis

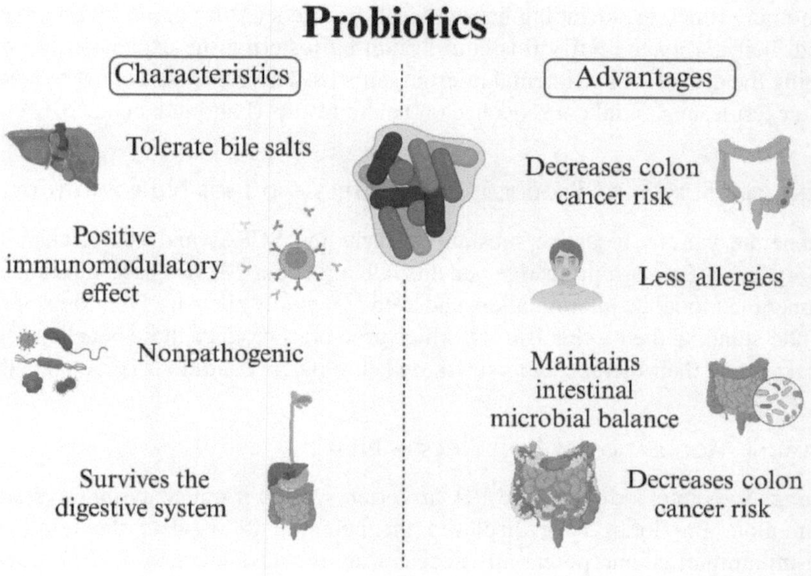

FIGURE 11.2 Characteristics and advantages of probiotics. The characteristics that are a must for the microbes to be called probiotics are tolerance to bile salts, nonpathogenic, survival of the digestive system's gastric juices, and positive immunomodulatory effect. The advantages the probiotics provide are a decrease in colon cancer risk, fewer allergies, and maintaining the microbial balance.

can disrupt this SCFA production, potentially altering their brain-related effects (Mirzaei et al., 2021). Neurodegenerative conditions such as PD and Alzheimer's disease have demonstrated connections with dysbiosis. Abnormal proteins associated with these diseases, including alpha-synuclein and beta-amyloid, could potentially migrate from the gut to the brain either through the vagus nerve or by way of inflammatory routes, contributing to the ongoing advancement of the diseases. Moreover, microorganisms present in the intestine's involvement in regulating the immune response and protein aggregation underscores its influence on the mechanisms of neurodegenerative disorders. Understanding the intricate links between dysbiosis and neuronal health offers avenues for potential interventions. Strategies such as dietary modifications, probiotics, and prebiotics are being explored to restore a balanced gut microbiota, aiming to diminish the detrimental outcomes of dysbiosis on neuronal function and disease progression. As research in this area advances, personalized approaches targeting the GBA hold promise for promoting neurological well-being and managing NDs (Figure 11.2).

11.3.1 Understanding Probiotics: Types and Mechanisms of Action

Probiotics refer to living microorganisms that, when provided in sufficient quantities, offer advantageous effects on the well-being of the host. They come in various strains, the most common being *Lactobacillus* and *Bifidobacterium* species (Prince et al., 2013). Understanding their mechanisms of action is essential to appreciate their therapeutic potential. Probiotics can engage with the host through various processes, such as modifying the gut microbiota, strengthening the intestinal barrier, and generating bioactive compounds that affect various physiological processes (Plaza-Diaz et al., 2019).

11.3.2 Restoring Gut Microbiota Balance with Probiotics

The equilibrium of the gut microbiota is a pivotal factor in preserving overall health. Dysbiosis, characterized by a disproportion in the composition of microbes present in the intestine, has been connected to many illnesses, including neurological disorders (Ahire et al., 2021). Probiotics have demonstrated their ability to rectify this equilibrium by fostering the expansion of good bacteria while impeding the growth of detrimental microorganisms. This reinstatement of balance in the gut microbes can exert a substantial consequence on health results (Fantinato et al., 2019).

11.3.3 Beneficial Substances Produced by Probiotics and Their Neuroprotective Effects

Probiotics generate various bioactive substances, including SCFAs and neurotransmitters, which have the ability to confer neuroprotective benefits (Chang et al., 2021). These substances can influence brain function, modulate inflammation, and even potentially alleviate symptoms of neurological disorders. Understanding the mechanisms by which probiotics produce these beneficial substances is crucial for harnessing their therapeutic potential in neurological conditions (Bu et al., 2022).

11.3.4 Immune Modulation by Probiotics in NDs

NDs, including Alzheimer's disease and PD, are often seen in immune system dysregulation and neuroinflammation. Probiotics have displayed the potential to regulate the immune response, diminishing inflammation, and potentially decelerating the advancement of these conditions (Ma et al., 2022).

11.3.5 Alleviating Oxidative Stress and Inflammation through Probiotics

Oxidative stress and inflammation are common factors in many health conditions, including NDs. Probiotics, through their anti-inflammatory properties and the production of antioxidants, have the potential to mitigate these processes (Petruzziello et al., 2023; Srivastav et al., 2019). Understanding how probiotics alleviate oxidative stress and inflammation provides insights into their therapeutic utility in many health disorders (Gangaraju et al., 2022).

11.4 PRECLINICAL AND CLINICAL EVIDENCE

11.4.1 Preclinical Studies on Probiotics and Neuroregeneration

Studies conducted in preclinical settings have indicated that probiotics may possess promising neurodegenerative properties. The application of probiotics has been demonstrated to improve glucose metabolism, reduce inflammation and oxidative stress, reduce the occurrence of neurodegeneration, and enhance both motor and non-motor functions in animal models of PD. Through the GBA, the gut microbiota plays a pivotal role in facilitating communication between the gut and the brain, thereby influencing the advancement of NDs (Tahmi et al., 2021). Furthermore, prebiotics, substances that encourage the proliferation of beneficial bacteria, have demonstrated the ability to enhance neurocognitive function and mitigate age-related neurodegeneration in animal models (Tahmi et al., 2021). Moreover, the imbalance in the microbiota–GBA and the existence of particular antibodies have been linked to the development of celiac disease and related neurological impairments (Durgante, 2019). In summary, preclinical investigations offer insights into the potential neurodegenerative impacts of probiotics and their relevance in the context of neurodegenerative disorders. Nevertheless, additional research is essential to validate these observations and translate them into practical clinical applications (Durgante, 2019).

11.4.2 Neurogenesis and Cognitive Function: Evidence from Experimental Models and Human Studies

Neurogenesis means the generation of fresh neurons from NSCs within the specialized neurogenic environment. It is essential for tissue regeneration, neural plasticity, and memory formation (Leta

TABLE 11.1
Some Preclinical Studies and Their Practical Applications

Insights	Practical Implications	References
Probiotics supplementation has shown the potential to improve cognitive function and reduce cognitive decline in preclinical and clinical studies.	Supplementing with probiotics could serve as a promising therapeutic strategy for addressing dementia and cognitive decline.	Liu et al. (2021)
An extensive examination of preclinical and clinical data indicates that probiotics show potential for generating anti-inflammatory and neurogenic effects in the context of Parkinson's disease.	Probiotics could potentially offer neurogenic and anti-inflammatory benefits for individuals with Parkinson's disease, potentially enhancing motor functions in this condition.	McAfoose and Baune (2009)
The paper explores the possible use of fecal microbiota transplantation in investigating neurodegenerative conditions, including dementia.	The gut microbiota might be implicated in neurodegenerative conditions, and microbiota-related therapies could represent a viable treatment avenue.	Yang et al. (2021)
The paper reviewed preclinical studies on prebiotics and age-related neurodegeneration, finding weak evidence of their efficacy in attenuating neurocognitive decline.	Prebiotic supplementation may improve neurocognitive function.	Takano (2018)
Probiotics and prebiotics hold promise for promoting neurodevelopment and potentially preventing and treating specific neurological disorders.	Bacteria can send signals to the brain, impacting various processes, and there is potential for neurological advantages associated with probiotics and prebiotics.	Macready et al. (2010)
The paper explores the potential benefits of using the probiotic *Lactobacillus fermentum* to enhance cognitive performance and bolster immune responses in an aged mouse model.	The probiotic *Lactobacillus fermentum* JDFM216 demonstrates an enhancement in cognitive behavior.	Macready et al. (2009)
This study investigates the outcomes of *Lactobacillus* and *Bifidobacterium* probiotics on cognitive ability and neurodegenerative factors in aged mice.	Supplementing with probiotics enhances physiological function and cognitive capabilities in older mice. These bacteria have the potential to serve as anti-aging agents.	Shabab et al. (2017)
The paper suggests that preclinical studies have shown effectiveness of probiotics on central nervous system function, including neuroregeneration.	Probiotics can improve psychiatric disorder-related behaviors.	Lyman et al. (2014)
The fundamental mechanisms of probiotics for their neuroprotective influence in neurological conditions affecting older adults encompass neural, hormonal, and immunological pathways.	Probiotics show promise as intervention therapy for neurological disorders.	Deshpande et al. (2006)
Probiotics and synbiotics have potential therapeutic effects on brain and nervous health, including neurodegenerative diseases like Alzheimer's.	Probiotics, prebiotics, and synbiotics may be effective in treating Alzheimer's disease. Microbiome modulation can improve cognitive function and metabolic activity.	Williams (2010)

(Continued)

TABLE 11.2 (*Continued*)
Clinical Trials Exploring the Effects of Probiotics on Neural Health

Probiotics	Clinical ID	Clinical Significance
The composition includes *Bifidobacterium animalis* subsp., fructo-oligosaccharides, and maltodextrin	NCT05173701	Assessing probiotics and the impact on the immune system of individuals with Parkinson's disease
Bifidobacterium species, *Lactobacillus plantarum*	NCT05145881	Examining the effectiveness of probiotic therapy in addressing Alzheimer's disease
Bifidobacterium triple viable capsules (BIFICO)	NCT04871464	The function and mechanism of probiotics in enhancing motor symptoms in Parkinson's disease
Lactobacillus plantarum PS128	NCT04722211	Assessing the clinical manifestations of Parkinson's disease following probiotic intervention
The liquid probiotic (Symprove)	NCT04140760	Assessing the potential enhancement of well-being in Parkinson's disease through a 12-week probiotic intervention
Proprietary probiotic	NCT03324399	Assessing the clinical results related to muscle strength, clinical global assessments, and spasticity in patients receiving an experimental probiotic
Bifidobacterium species, *L. plantarum*	NCT05568498	Examining the utilization of a multistrain oral probiotic as a therapeutic approach for managing depression in individuals diagnosed with Parkinson's disease
Streptococcus thermophilus, *Bifidobacterium* species, *L. plantarum*	NCT05521477	Exploring the impact of supplementing with probiotic SLAB51 on biomarkers associated with Alzheimer's disease
Multistrain probiotics capsules	NCT03377322	Examining the influence of probiotics on constipation in individuals with Parkinson's disease
Bifidobacterium	NCT03991195	Exploring the therapeutic potential of gut microbiota as a non-pharmacological way of addressing early Alzheimer's disease and understanding the potential neurological mechanisms involved
Lactobacillus reuteri, *Lactobacillus paracasei*, and *L. plantarum*	NCT04094129	Assessing the impact of Wismemo for Alzheimer's disease and dementia
L. casei	NCT04293159	Assessing the impact of probiotics on constipation among individuals diagnosed with Parkinson's disease
Lactobacillus acidophilus	NCT05576818	Examining the utilization of a synbiotic as a supplementary therapy in the management of Parkinson's disease

et al., 2021). Irregularities in neurogenesis are associated with a variety of conditions, such as neuropsychiatric disorders and NDs such as Alzheimer's disease. At the core of regulating neurogenesis is the neurogenic niche, which consists of glial and endothelial cells (Hang Mak et al., 2020; Sun et al., 2021). The cells within the niche react to external signals and uphold the internal necessities of the neurogenic process, thereby shaping the behavior of NSCs (Cerdó et al., 2017). Signaling through purinergic receptors, such as P2X7, P2Y1, A2A, A1, and P2Y13, is involved in both embryonic and adult neurogenesis (Park et al., 2020). The brain cavities and CSF also have a significant influence on neurogenesis, as CSF contains neurogenic signals that control neural precursor cell behavior (Ni et al., 2019). Understanding the regulation of neurogenesis by the neurogenic niche and CSF may provide insights into therapeutic strategies in neurological disorders.

Neurogenesis in model organisms has been extensively studied using various techniques (Wang et al., 2016). Research involving animal models, including mice and primates, has supplied proof of postnatal and adult neurogenesis taking place within the SVZ and SGZ (Sharma & Kaur, 2020). Immunohistochemistry studies on post-mortem human sections have also shown robust evidence for adult neurogenesis in the human brain stem cell niches (Arora et al., 2020). Organotypic cultures have served as dependable models for investigating the mechanisms of neurogenesis in both typical and diseased states (Ishimoto & Kato, 2021). However, it is important to consider species differences in adult neurogenesis, as different species may exhibit variations in where it occurs, how it works, and what it does. By taking a neuroethological approach and considering a larger, non-biomedical context, a comprehensive understanding of adult neurogenesis can be achieved.

Studies have offered indications that adult neurogenesis takes place within the key regions: the SGZ in the dentate gyrus and the SVZ (Morgun et al., 2019). However, recent findings have rekindled controversies regarding adult human SGZ neurogenesis (Li & Guo, 2021). Concrete proof of adult neurogenesis in humans has been challenging to obtain, but influential earlier studies and contemporary research have revealed that adult neurogenesis indeed transpires in the human dentate gyrus (Ribeiro et al., 2019). The presence of ongoing neurogenesis in the adult hippocampus, extending to the tenth decade of human life, has been documented. Additionally, deficits in this process have been noted in individuals with Alzheimer's disease (Gato et al., 2020). Studies employing immunohistochemistry on post-mortem human brain samples have presented proof of neurogenesis during both childhood and adulthood in the NSC niches of the human brain. Moreover, there are reports of adult neurogenesis taking place in the enteric nervous system. Within this context, glial cells and ICCs have been proposed as potential NSCs.

Cognitive function refers to the complex processes involved in thinking, learning, memory, and decision-making. It is influenced by various factors and can be measured using different methods. One approach is to use a cognitive function measurement device that acquires voice data, drawing data, and walking data to calculate evaluation values related to cognitive function. Another perspective highlights the dynamic interplay between multiple network interactions and systems within the brain, suggesting that cognitive function is the result of organization and interactions between various systems and subsystems (Pastorino et al., 2021). Metabolic syndrome has been observed to have lower cognitive function, particularly in cross-sectional studies, and certain components of metabolic syndrome, such as high blood pressure and hyperglycemia, are strong predictors of cognitive function (Pastorino et al., 2021). Cognitive functions, encompassing cognitive biases and executive functions, hold substantial sway over the potential for relapse in substance-related and addictive disorders. Transcranial current stimulation exhibits the potential to enhance these cognitive functions, offering promise in addiction treatment (Pastorino et al., 2021). Additionally, a cognitive function testing method involving image-based tests has been developed to assess cognitive function accurately (Pastorino et al., 2021).

Cognitive function studies using models have provided concrete evidence of human brain functioning. Models represent complex brain mechanisms using computational and mathematical equations, allowing for more accurate interpretation and analysis of cognitive functioning (Cavaliere et al., 2016). Physical performance tests have been used as simple means of predicting cognitive decline and developing predictive models for cognitive function. These tests have shown associations between better physical performance and slower cognitive decline over time (Cavaliere et al., 2016). Cytokines like IL-1β, IL-6, and TNF-α have been identified as participants in cognitive processes at the molecular level. This substantiates the concept of a cytokine model for understanding cognitive function (Nogueira et al., 2022). Research has demonstrated that diets high in fat can negatively affect the learning and memory abilities of rats. This suggests a potential connection between obesity and cognitive decline (Nogueira et al., 2022). Research employing PET has delved into the connections between monoamine neurotransmission and cognitive functions within psychiatric conditions. These studies provide valuable insights into not only the fundamental mechanisms at play but also potential avenues for therapeutic interventions in these disorders (Nogueira et al., 2022).

Emerging evidence from human studies suggests that certain dietary components, such as polyphenols, flavonoids, and micronutrients, may have a positive impact on cognitive function (Gault & Szele, 2021; Moreno-Jiménez et al., 2021). Epidemiological studies have shown a potential link between polyphenol intake and cognitive function (Kronenberg & Klempin, 2020). Clinical trials have also highlighted the capacity of certain polyphenols to positively impact distinct aspects of cognitive function (Kronenberg & Klempin, 2020). Nevertheless, there exists a notable absence of agreement in human research when it comes to determining the array of cognitive domains for assessment and the precise selection of tests to be utilized. In forthcoming research, it is imperative to carefully consider prior human studies and address pertinent matters such as the sensitivity of tasks, statistical robustness, and the potential for type I errors. By doing so, significant advancements can be made in comprehending the impacts of nutritional therapies on cognitive function.

11.4.3 Neuroinflammation and Neurotoxicity: Insights from Probiotic Interventions

The brain, the command center of the human body, is a dynamic and intricately organized structure. Like any other part of the body, it is not immune to threats or injuries. When the brain encounters these challenges, it mounts an immune response known as neuroinflammation (Kim et al., 2018). This process involves a complex interplay of immune cells, signaling molecules, and inflammatory pathways, all aimed at maintaining brain health and restoring equilibrium (Westfall et al., 2017). Within the intricate landscape of the brain's delicate neurons and intricate networks lies a hidden danger: neurotoxicity. This phenomenon refers to the process by which exposure to harmful substances or conditions leads to damage, dysfunction, or even death of neurons (Kesika et al., 2021). Neurotoxicity can arise from a variety of sources, both external and internal.

Neurological disorders, characterized by neuroinflammation and neurotoxicity, pose significant challenges to patients. As our understanding of the GBA deepens, emerging research suggests that the microbiota–gut–brain connection has a crucial function in influencing neuroinflammation and neurotoxicity (Kesika et al., 2021). Neuroinflammation represents a multifaceted immune reaction that takes place in the central nervous system, frequently initiated by factors like infections, injuries, or chronic ailments. Extended neuroinflammation has the potential to give rise to neurotoxicity, a phenomenon characterized by an excessive release of pro-inflammatory agents that can harm neurons and compromise overall brain performance. Neurotoxicity is linked to various neurological disorders.

Probiotics refer to living microorganisms that, when provided in sufficient quantities, provide advantages to the host's health (Suda & Matsuda, 2022). Probiotics, known for their potential to modulate gut microbiota, have gained attention as a novel approach to address these issues. Their potential to influence gut microbiota composition and function has led to investigations into their role in mitigating neuroinflammation and neurotoxicity (Suganya & Koo, 2020).

The immune system's intricate dance orchestrates both protection and potential harm to neurons. Probiotics enter the stage with precision immunomodulation, where they engage with immune cells and signaling pathways. By steering the immune response away from hyperactivity, these

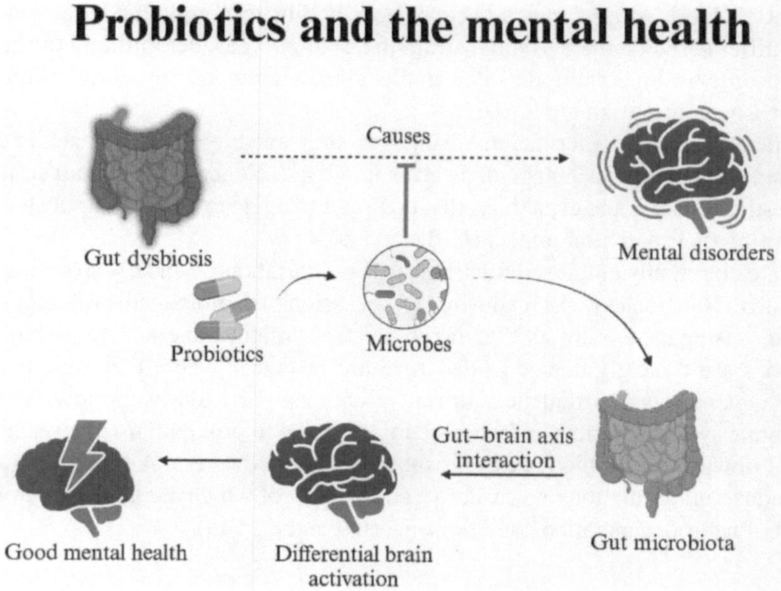

FIGURE 11.3 Probiotics and mental health. The gut dysbiosis causes various mental disorders. But the probiotics help to inhibit this gut dysbiosis, restoring the GBA that leads to good mental health.

microorganisms temper the flames of neuroinflammation. This calculated intervention holds the potential to quench the storm of cytokines that contribute to neurotoxicity. The gut, often referred to as the "second brain," houses a diverse community of microbes that profoundly influence health. Dysbiosis, the disruption of this delicate ecosystem, has been implicated in neurological disorders (Cepeda et al., 2017). Probiotics, akin to skilled gardeners, cultivate a flourishing microbial landscape (Suganya & Koo, 2020). By nurturing beneficial strains and curbing the overgrowth of harmful ones, they contribute to a balanced environment that indirectly shields against neuroinflammatory onslaughts.

Among the array of probiotic components, metabolites stand out as powerful messengers. SCFAs, generated as a result of probiotics fermenting dietary fibers, serve to expand their protective capabilities. SCFAs such as butyrate are renowned for their anti-inflammatory prowess (Cepeda et al., 2017). Their role in fostering an environment conducive to neuroprotection unveils a critical facet of probiotics' impact on neurotoxicity. Imagine the gut barrier as a fortified castle wall guarding against invading forces. Probiotics fortify this barrier, preventing the translocation of toxic molecules into the systemic circulation (Suda & Matsuda, 2022). This act of defense mitigates the systemic inflammation that can fan the flames of neuroinflammation. By reinforcing the gut's defenses, probiotics indirectly contribute to the preservation of neuronal health. The GBA orchestrates a symphony of neurotransmitters that influence mood and cognition. Probiotics play a harmonious role, contributing to the production of neurotransmitters like GABA and serotonin (Kesika et al., 2021). This harmonizing effect not only enhances emotional well-being but also impacts neuroinflammation. The modulation of neurotransmitter systems by probiotics creates a ripple effect, influencing the broader landscape of neurotoxicity.

11.5 CHALLENGES AND CONSIDERATIONS IN TRANSLATING PROBIOTIC THERAPIES

Although probiotics are widely acknowledged as harmless and can offer diverse health advantages, there are many hurdles associated with their utilization, which we will delve into below.

Varieties of probiotic strains can induce diverse bodily responses, and the suitable amount required may differ based on the particular strain in question. Thus, determining the best strain and dosage for a specific health condition can be challenging, leading to a broad spectrum of effectiveness in probiotic outcomes (Sun et al., 2021).

For probiotic bacteria to confer health advantages, they need to endure the acidic conditions of the stomach and successfully establish themselves in the gut. Nonetheless, not all strains can withstand this digestive journey, and even those that do might struggle to establish a substantial presence in the gut, limiting their potential impact (Hill et al., 2014).

Probiotics are commonly employed for relatively brief durations, typically spanning a few weeks to a few months. Nonetheless, the enduring repercussions of prolonged probiotic consumption remain unclear, raising the possibility that their advantages might wane with time (Hill et al., 2014). While probiotics are typically deemed safe, there are instances where they may lead to adverse reactions like bloating, gas, or diarrhea. In rare situations, particularly in individuals with compromised immune systems, serious infections can occur due to probiotic use. Nevertheless, despite these potential downsides, probiotics exhibit substantial effectiveness. A balanced gut microbiota is known to reduce inflammation and oxidative stress, both of which are critical factors associated with the onset of neurodegenerative conditions (Cortese et al., 2018).

11.5.1 Bioavailability and Formulation Challenges

As per the World Health Organization's definition, probiotics refer to living microorganisms given in adequate amounts to bestow health benefits upon the host. These advantageous bacteria have garnered substantial attention in the market, with their global market size surging from an estimated $3.3 billion in 2015 to $42.25 billion in 2017, and anticipated to reach $74.69 billion by 2025. Well-known strains such as *Lactobacillus*, *Bifidobacterium*, and *Saccharomyces* are frequently employed as probiotics. These organisms primarily inhabit the digestive tract and offer advantages such as producing substances that inhibit harmful bacteria, enhancing nutrient absorption, and deactivating toxin receptors. Immune response modulation is another crucial role of probiotics.

Incorporating probiotics into everyday foods enriches them with nutrients like fibers, vitamins, minerals, and antioxidants. Due to their proven safety and positive health effects, there is a significant demand for probiotics in functional foods and nutrition. This demand extends across various categories, including dairy, bakery, beverages, confectioneries, as well as fruits and vegetables. An ideal probiotic strain should thrive at its intended site, be side-effect-free, survive digestive conditions including bile acids, aid in lactose digestion, resist enteric pathogens, and offer various health effects like anti-colon cancer and antihypertensive impacts (Prakash et al., 2011).

The bioavailability of probiotics refers to their ability to survive digestion, reach the target site in the body, and exert their intended effects. Ensuring probiotics' bioavailability involves overcoming challenges such as surviving stomach acidity, interacting with other ingredients, and reaching the intended site in active form.

Various factors that impact probiotic bioavailability are formulation, strain selection, viability, delivery system, gut microenvironment, and patient factors.

Probiotics have even been explored for conditions like diabetes and obesity. Yet, a significant challenge lies in maintaining their viability and availability through stomach conditions and biological enzymes (Cortese et al., 2018). For meaningful health effects, a concentration of 108–109 CFUs per gram per day is generally deemed necessary. Achieving this viability may require innovative methods. Microencapsulation is a promising technique wherein probiotics are shielded with a protective layer, preventing direct contact with acids and enzymes that degrade them. This outer layer preserves the probiotics and their effectiveness, presenting a viable strategy to enhance probiotic efficiency (Mhatre & Gurav, 2020; Nagpal et al., 2012).

While there is promising data indicating the advantages of using probiotics in treating Alzheimer's disease, there are significant obstacles that must be addressed before probiotic treatment can be widely accepted in the medical field. At present, the United States Food and Drug Administration (US FDA) has granted approval to a restricted selection of probiotics that are deemed safe for inclusion in both food products and dietary supplements (Thursby & Juge, 2017). Nonetheless, the FDA has refrained from granting approval for the promotion of probiotics as risk reducers for diseases or as established treatments for pre-existing medical ailments. It's essential to recognize that while probiotics offer potential health benefits, there are associated hazards and ambiguities as well. Certain accounts have connected probiotic consumption with adverse outcomes such as sepsis, immune responses, and the transmission of genes that could contribute to antibiotic resistance (T et al., 2017).

These risks are particularly concerning for vulnerable populations such as the elderly, critically ill, and those with weakened immune systems, as probiotic use in these cases can lead to complications. Furthermore, the impact of probiotic supplementation can exhibit notable variations contingent upon the particular strains employed, potentially leading to unforeseen metabolic consequences. This lack of consensus in the field has led to uncertainty about the optimal formulation, dosage, and treatment schedule that can provide maximum benefits while minimizing potential side effects (Zmora et al., 2018).

Another limitation of using probiotics in Alzheimer's disease treatment is the unpredictable and temporary colonization of the gut lining. Different individuals may have varying levels of resistance to probiotic establishment in their gut microbiota, making it difficult to determine which specific probiotics within a multi-probiotic regimen are responsible for observed outcomes. Furthermore, there's a concern that excessive production of serotonin by gut microbiota could lead to serotonin syndrome in certain cases. This syndrome is linked to an abundance of serotonin receptors found both in the central nervous system and the peripheral areas, frequently stemming from the consumption of antidepressant medications that influence serotonin levels (Feeney, 2007).

11.5.2 Personalized Approaches for Probiotic Treatment

Creating probiotic strains tailored to individuals and employing precise, low-dose treatments for correcting the gut microbiome poses a significant challenge and opportunity in personalized nutrition and future medicine. Given the intricate nature of the microbiome, conducting clinical studies to identify those who respond best to specific strains and establishing personalized application protocols is complex. Understanding the mechanisms that govern interactions between bacteria and the host adds to the difficulty. Current evidence supports interventions that are highly personalized. With probiotic products' safety in mind, a broad group of potential consumers can benefit.

To achieve personalization, developing and using products derived from an individual's own microbial strains holds promise. Yet, it's crucial to strike a balance and avoid viewing the gut microbiota as a universal cure-all. A comprehensive and balanced approach (Precision, Predictive, Preventive, and Personalized Medicine) is necessary to minimize potential risks. Integrating these strategies will shape a realistic vision for the future, embracing the potential of probiotics while maintaining a cautious stance (Singh & Natraj, 2021).

11.5.3 Regulatory Aspects and Safety Considerations

The limited understanding of how probiotics function mechanistically poses a significant challenge in predicting the harmlessness of probiotic interventions. The multifaceted interaction between the gut's microbial community and various nutritional factors assumes a crucial role in the initiation and alteration of chronic degenerative conditions, encompassing immune and metabolic disorders. This dynamic interplay between the host and the gut's microbial environment represents a central factor influencing both general well-being and disease development (Gionchetti et al., 2007).

Whether probiotics produce protective or detrimental effects and stimulate or suppress the immune system in a host, depends on the complex interaction between signals sent by the microorganisms present in the intestine, the host's genetic constitution, and environmental influences. Numerous studies have indicated that particular probiotic bacteria can enhance the proliferation and activity of immune cells, evident in increased antibody and cytokine production. This augmentation improves the immune response's efficacy against pathogens. Conversely, some probiotics have exhibited the capacity to alleviate chronic inflammation and allergic reactions, conditions stemming from excessive immune responses. They accomplish this by reducing the activity of effector cells and encouraging tolerance mechanisms. As an example, in the treatment of inflammatory bowel diseases and the prevention of atopic dermatitis, a probiotic mixture known as VSL#3, consisting of eight bacterial strains, directly alleviates pro-inflammatory immune responses. This blend triggers the development of regulatory T cells carrying TGFβ, which act as protective agents when transferred to recipient mice. This suggests that specific probiotics may establish protective memory within the adaptive immune system (Di Giacinto et al., 2005; Kalliomäki et al., 2007).

Defining the precise relationships between the structure and function of probiotics within target populations becomes crucial to mitigate the risk of unintended adverse effects. Although probiotics generally exhibit a tendency to save the intestinal barrier, there might be instances where they don't restore the barrier's integrity, potentially even promoting translocation or causing infections themselves. Rare cases of sepsis arising from probiotic usage in patients with underlying conditions underscore this point. These instances underscore the need to comprehensively understand probiotic mechanisms concerning both the intestinal shield function and the host's immune function. This is compounded by the realization that outcomes are likely specific to each distinct probiotic strain or combination employed.

Individuals who may experience substantial advantages from probiotic therapy encompass those in critical medical conditions or those on the verge of entering such a state, such as individuals preparing for major abdominal surgery. During times of severe illness, it can be theorized that the gut plays a central role in the emergence of pathological conditions. Disruptions in the integrity of the gut barrier may be conjectured to initiate and sustain conditions such as sepsis, systemic inflammatory response syndrome, and multi-organ failure (Clark & Coopersmith, 2007). In such circumstances, the usually balanced interplay among the intestinal microbiota, epithelial cells, and the immune system experiences disruption.

In ill patients, the composition of the intestinal microbiota can undergo alterations due to several factors. These factors encompass the use of antibiotics of broad spectrum, variations in nutrient accessibility, fluctuations in gut movement, pH levels, and osmolarity, as well as the increased release of stress hormones like catecholamines (Alverdy et al., 2003). The impairment of the mucosal barrier creates an opening for opportunistic pathogens residing within the intestinal lumen to breach this barrier. This breach sets off a potent pro-inflammatory reaction, increasing the susceptibility to systemic inflammatory response syndrome.

Probiotic strains and combinations hold promise in reinstating this intricate three-part equilibrium. They can actively bolster colonization resistance by generating antimicrobial bacteriocins engaging in competitive growth (Liévin, 2000), and reducing the attachment and penetration of epithelial cells by pathogens (Resta-Lenert & Barrett, 2003; Sherman et al., 2005). Additionally, specific probiotics are known to have anti-apoptotic properties (Yan et al., 2007) and contribute to maintaining the structural integrity of the cytoskeleton and tight junctions (Petrof et al., 2004). Nevertheless, one of the most extensively researched and acknowledged functions of probiotics is their capacity to regulate the immune system. As an example, probiotics have shown the capacity to promote the release of anti-inflammatory cytokines, including IL-10 (Hart et al., 2004), regulate the functioning of human dendritic cells, and mitigate pro-inflammatory responses (Galdeano et al., 2007).

11.5.4 Future Directions and Research Priorities

Investigations regarding the application of probiotics for neuropathological conditions such as Alzheimer's disease and PD are currently underway, and a definitive assessment of their efficacy remains pending. Some studies suggest that probiotics might help by reducing inflammation, and oxidative stress, and enhancing gut microbiota, thereby possibly improving cognitive function. However, these findings are mostly derived from animal models, invertebrate studies, or small human trials. Further studies are necessary to establish their protection and potency. It's crucial to know that probiotics aren't a standalone cure for these conditions but could complement a holistic treatment plan including medications, lifestyle adjustments, and medical recommendations. While *Bifidobacterium* and *Lactobacillus* show potential, more substantial randomized trials are required to comprehensively grasp their benefits and limitations.

Probiotics have the potential to offer a robust strategy for addressing the disturbed gut equilibrium observed in PD. This approach may involve enhancing gut health, mitigating inflammation within the enteric nervous system, and reducing gut permeability. The initial clinical trial, which took place in 2011, showcased improvements in long-term constipation among individuals with PD who consumed fermented milk containing *Lactobacillus casei Shirota*. This improvement resulted in a reduction in abdominal discomfort and bloating (Gazerani, 2019).

A clinical trial showed that an ingestible tablet containing a probiotic formulation improved insulin resistance, sensitivity, and motor scores in patients with PD. Another study used a liquid probiotic formula called Symprove (K-1803), designed to maintain activity upon reaching the lower gut (Tamtaji et al., 2019).

In a *Caenorhabditis elegans* model, Bacillus subtilis probiotics hindered α-synuclein aggregation and cleared existing aggregates (Goya et al., 2020). An in vitro study found that certain *Lactobacillus* and *Bifidobacterium* probiotics reduced oxidative stress, inflammation, and harmful bacterial overgrowth in PD patients' blood cells (Goya et al., 2020).

Certain probiotic strains have the capability to restrain pathogens and generate tyrosine decarboxylase, an enzyme that converts levodopa into dopamine in the gut. This has the potential to address the reduced levels of levodopa observed in PD (van Kessel et al., 2019). Prolonged administration of six specific bacterial strains demonstrated neuroprotective effects and mitigated motor impairments in a genetic mouse model of PD (Hsieh et al., 2020; Nicola et al., 2016).

Probiotic combinations hold the promise of diminishing inflammation by encouraging the production of cytokines and alleviating oxidative stress by limiting the generation of reactive oxygen species (Nowak et al., 2019). Given that infections can accelerate PD progression, probiotics like VSL#3 controlled gene expression in the brain cortex, mitigating inflammation and enhancing neuronal function (Distrutti et al., 2013).

A recent discovery showed that the probiotic blend SLAB51 countered detrimental effects induced by 6-hydroxydopamine in PD models, displaying anti-inflammatory actions, restoring pro-survival pathways, safeguarding dopaminergic neurons, and improving behavior. These discoveries recommend that SLAB51 may have the ability to prevent or treat PD, highlighting how the adjustment of gut microbiota can impact pro-survival pathways that could potentially decelerate the advancement of PD.

Given the potential significance of probiotics in treating or preventing various illnesses, there's a call for focused research direction and guidance. The emphasis should be on addressing these medical gaps rather than commercial interests, leading to a more effective integration of probiotics into society. The foremost driver for research innovation and development should be meeting these unmet medical needs.

To accomplish this, research endeavors can be customized for three distinct population segments: infants, children, and adults/elderly. Within the infant category, there are three critical clinical areas that demand comprehensive research: (1) Addressing diarrhea, (2) tackling AAD, and (3) addressing NEC. For children, the focus should revolve around (1) addressing obesity, (2) managing AAD, and (3) handling diarrhea. In the context of adults, the priority areas should encompass (1) addressing AAD, (2) managing IBS, and (3) addressing Alzheimer's disease.

Considering the viewpoints of KOLs and patients/consumers, there is a notable requirement to bolster the clinical substantiation for probiotic products. The research also underscores the ongoing collaboration between KOLs and the industry in research and development (R&D). However, it appears that the perceived impact of KOLs on the research priorities of the industry remains somewhat limited. To ensure that the unaddressed needs of patients receive adequate attention, it is advisable for KOLs, who serve as advocates for patients, to assume a more substantial role in influencing the research agendas within the industry's R&D processes. This collaborative approach between experts and industry could result in more targeted and effective probiotic interventions that genuinely address medical needs.

Dementia is a widespread global issue, affecting around 24 million people (Reitz et al., 2011). Among various forms of dementia, Alzheimer's disease stands as the primary contributor, inflicting substantial societal, medical, and economic challenges. The absence of effective treatments has elevated Alzheimer's disease to a critical concern for many affluent nations, prompting focused attention on healthcare and social support. Although the investigation of the GBA and the modulation of gut health to mitigate or prevent neurophysiological disorders is in its early phases, an increasing body of evidence indicates that probiotics may present potential benefits in the management of Alzheimer's disease (Sindi et al., 2015).

As mentioned earlier, the human microbiome has the potential to impact a range of neurometabolic and neurochemical pathways, serving as a link between the gastrointestinal system and the central nervous system. A proposed mechanism behind the potential effectiveness of probiotics involves certain lactobacilli and bifidobacteria strains' capacity to generate GABA. Disruptions in the signaling of this neurotransmitter have been linked to Alzheimer's disease. Additionally, studies involving "germ-free" mice have indicated reduced levels of brain-derived neurotrophic factor, a phenomenon also witnessed in individuals with Alzheimer's disease.

The practical consequences of these discoveries still require further clarification. It is still unclear whether modifying the gut microbiota with probiotics can genuinely have a substantial function in preventing Alzheimer's disease or enhancing the quality of life for individuals living with this condition. However, KOLs in the field believe there is substantial potential to be gained from pursuing research in this domain (Bhattacharjee & Lukiw, 2013).

11.6 CONCLUSION

To combat the escalating public health concern of NDs, our journey has taken us through the intricate web of the GBA, exploring the profound association between microbiota and neurodegeneration. We have delved into the rationale behind harnessing the regenerative potential of probiotics, offering a glimmer of hope for those affected by these devastating conditions.

Through this chapter, we have traversed the landscape of gut–brain communication, uncovering the disruptive forces at play in NDs and the dire consequences of dysbiosis on neuronal health. We have illuminated the therapeutic potential of probiotics, shedding light on their various mechanisms of action, from restoring gut microbiota balance to producing beneficial substances that fortify the brain's defenses. We have seen how probiotics can act as immune modulators, soothing the fires of neuroinflammation and quenching the flames of oxidative stress.

The evidence presented in this chapter, both from preclinical studies and clinical trials (refer to Tables 11.1 and 11.2), offers promise for those seeking innovative approaches to neuroregeneration. We have witnessed the exciting potential of probiotics in promoting neurogenesis and preserving cognitive function, and we have gained insights into their ability to tame neuroinflammation and mitigate neurotoxicity.

Yet, in our pursuit of probiotic therapies, we cannot ignore the challenges that lie ahead. Bioavailability and formulation hurdles must be overcome, and personalized approaches must be tailored to individual needs. Regulatory considerations and safety concerns must guide the path forward as we navigate the complex terrain of probiotic treatments.

In conclusion, we summarize our core findings, underscoring the potential of probiotics as a therapeutic avenue for promoting neuronal health in NDs. The implications for clinical practice are profound, offering a glimmer of hope for patients and healthcare providers alike. The future beckons with exciting research priorities, calling upon the scientific community to unlock the full potential of probiotics in the pursuit of better neurological health.

In closing, the story of probiotics as a regenerative force in the realm of NDs is still unfolding. With each discovery, we inch closer to a brighter future where these microscopic warriors may hold the key to restoring and preserving the precious gift of neuronal health.

BIBLIOGRAPHY

Ahire, J. J., Jakkamsetty, C., Kashikar, M. S., Lakshmi, S. G., & Madempudi, R. S. (2021). In vitro evaluation of probiotic properties of Lactobacillus plantarum UBLP40 isolated from traditional indigenous fermented food. *Probiotics and Antimicrobial Proteins, 13*(5), 1413–1424. https://doi.org/10.1007/s12602-021-09775-7

Alverdy, J. C., Laughlin, R. S., & Wu, L. (2003). Influence of the critically ill state on host–pathogen interactions within the intestine: Gut-derived sepsis redefined. *Critical Care Medicine, 31*(2), 598–607. https://doi.org/10.1097/01.CCM.0000045576.55937.67

Arora, K., Green, M., & Prakash, S. (2020). The microbiome and Alzheimer's disease: Potential and limitations of prebiotic, synbiotic, and probiotic formulations. *Frontiers in Bioengineering and Biotechnology, 8*, 537847. https://doi.org/10.3389/fbioe.2020.537847

Bengmark, S. (2013). Gut microbiota, immune development and function. *Pharmacological Research, 69*(1), 87–113. https://doi.org/10.1016/j.phrs.2012.09.002

Bhattacharjee, S., & Lukiw, W. J. (2013). Alzheimer's disease and the microbiome. *Frontiers in Cellular Neuroscience, 7*, 153. https://doi.org/10.3389/fncel.2013.00153

Bu, Y., Liu, Y., Liu, Y., Wang, S., Liu, Q., Hao, H., & Yi, H. (2022). Screening and probiotic potential evaluation of bacteriocin-producing Lactiplantibacillus plantarum in vitro. *Foods, 11*(11), 1575. https://doi.org/10.3390/foods11111575

Carding, S., Verbeke, K., Vipond, D. T., Corfe, B. M., & Owen, L. J. (2015). Dysbiosis of the gut microbiota in disease. *Microbial Ecology in Health and Disease, 26*(0), 26191. https://doi.org/10.3402/mehd.v26.26191

Cavaliere, F., Benito-Muñoz, M., & Matute, C. (2016). Organotypic cultures as a model to study adult neurogenesis in CNS disorders. *Stem Cells International, 2016,* 3540568. https://doi.org/10.1155/2016/3540568

Cepeda, M. S., Katz, E. G., & Blacketer, C. (2017). Microbiome-gut-brain axis: Probiotics and their association with depression. *Journal of Neuropsychiatry and Clinical Neurosciences, 29*(1), 39–44. https://doi.org/10.1176/appi.neuropsych.15120410

Cerdó, T., Ruíz, A., Suárez, A., & Campoy, C. (2017). Probiotic, prebiotic, and brain development. *Nutrients, 9*(11), 1247. https://doi.org/10.3390/nu9111247

Chang, Y. H., Jeong, C. H., Cheng, W. N., Choi, Y., Shin, D. M., Lee, S., & Han, S. G. (2021). Quality characteristics of yogurts fermented with short-chain fatty acid-producing probiotics and their effects on mucin production and probiotic adhesion onto human colon epithelial cells. *Journal of Dairy Science, 104*(7), 7415–7425. https://doi.org/10.3168/jds.2020-19820

Clark, J. A., & Coopersmith, C. M. (2007). Intestinal crosstalk: A new paradigm for understanding the gut as the "motor" of critical illness. *Shock, 28*(4), 384–393. https://doi.org/10.1097/shk.0b013e31805569df

Cortese, Y. J., Wagner, V. E., Tierney, M., Devine, D., & Fogarty, A. (2018). Review of catheter-associated urinary tract infections and *in vitro* urinary tract models. *Journal of Healthcare Engineering, 2018,* 2986742. https://doi.org/10.1155/2018/2986742

Deshpande, A., Mina, E., Glabe, C., & Busciglio, J. (2006). Different conformations of amyloid β induce neurotoxicity by distinct mechanisms in human cortical neurons. *Journal of Neuroscience, 26*(22), 6011–6018. https://doi.org/10.1523/JNEUROSCI.1189-06.2006

Di Giacinto, C., Marinaro, M., Sanchez, M., Strober, W., & Boirivant, M. (2005). Probiotics ameliorate recurrent Th1-mediated murine colitis by inducing IL-10 and IL-10-dependent TGF-β-bearing regulatory cells. *Journal of Immunology, 174*(6), 3237–3246. https://doi.org/10.4049/jimmunol.174.6.3237

Dinan, T. G., & Cryan, J. F. (2012). Regulation of the stress response by the gut microbiota: Implications for psychoneuroendocrinology. *Psychoneuroendocrinology, 37*(9), 1369–1378. https://doi.org/10.1016/j.psyneuen.2012.03.007

Distrutti, E., Cipriani, S., Mencarelli, A., Renga, B., & Fiorucci, S. (2013). Probiotics VSL#3 protect against development of visceral pain in murine model of irritable bowel syndrome. *PLoS One, 8*(5), e63893. https://doi.org/10.1371/journal.pone.0063893

Durgante, H. (2019). A brief review of connectionist models in contrast with modelling cognition. *[International Journal]. Sleep Medicine and Disorders, 3*(1), 7–8. https://doi.org/10.15406/smdij.2019.03.00059

Fantinato, V., Camargo, H. R., & de Sousa, A. L. O. P. (2019). Probiotics study with Streptococcus salivarius and its ability to produce bacteriocins and adherence to KB cells. *Revista de Odontologia da UNESP, 48.* https://doi.org/10.1590/1807-2577.02919

Feeney, S. N. (2007). Serotonin syndrome. In *Pediatric clinical advisor* (pp. 516–517). Elsevier. https://doi.org/10.1016/B978-032303506-4.10295-0

Galdeano, C. M., de Moreno de LeBlanc, A., Vinderola, G., Bonet, M. E. B., & Perdigón, G. (2007). Proposed model: Mechanisms of immunomodulation induced by probiotic bacteria. *Clinical and Vaccine Immunology, 14*(5), 485–492. https://doi.org/10.1128/CVI.00406-06

Gangaraju, D., Raghu, A. V., & Siddalingaiya Gurudutt, P. (2022). Green synthesis of γ-aminobutyric acid using permeabilized probiotic *Enterococcus faecium* for biocatalytic application. *Nano Select, 3*(10), 1436–1447. https://doi.org/10.1002/nano.202200059

Gato, A., Alonso, M. I., Lamus, F., & Miyan, J. (2020). Neurogenesis: A process ontogenically linked to brain cavities and their content, CSF. *Seminars in Cell and Developmental Biology, 102,* 21–27. https://doi.org/10.1016/j.semcdb.2019.11.008

Gault, N., & Szele, F. G. (2021). Immunohistochemical evidence for adult human neurogenesis in health and disease. *Wires Mechanisms of Disease, 13*(6), e1526. https://doi.org/10.1002/wsbm.1526

Gazerani, P. (2019). Probiotics for Parkinson's disease. *International Journal of Molecular Sciences, 20*(17), 4121. https://doi.org/10.3390/ijms20174121

Gionchetti, P., Rizzello, F., Morselli, C., Poggioli, G., Tambasco, R., Calabrese, C., Brigidi, P., Vitali, B., Straforini, G., & Campieri, M. (2007). High-dose probiotics for the treatment of active pouchitis. *Diseases of the Colon and Rectum, 50*(12), 2075–2084. https://doi.org/10.1007/s10350-007-9068-4

Goya, M. E., Xue, F., Sampedro-Torres-Quevedo, C., Arnaouteli, S., Riquelme-Dominguez, L., Romanowski, A., Brydon, J., Ball, K. L., Stanley-Wall, N. R., & Doitsidou, M. (2020). Probiotic Bacillus subtilis protects against α-synuclein aggregation in C. elegans. *Cell Reports, 30*(2), 367–380.e7. https://doi.org/10.1016/j.celrep.2019.12.078

Gubert, C., Kong, G., Renoir, T., & Hannan, A. J. (2020). Exercise, diet and stress as modulators of gut microbiota: Implications for neurodegenerative diseases. *Neurobiology of Disease, 134,* 104621. https://doi.org/10.1016/j.nbd.2019.104621

Hang Mak, C. C., Hong Meng, H. Y., Yan Mak, J. W., Ko, O. H., Tao, Z., & Leung Chan, F. K. (2020). IDDF2020-ABS-0203 Investigating the evidence of prebiotic supplementation in the attenuation of age-related neurodegeneration in in vivo studies: A systematic review and meta-analysis with Bayesian inference. *Abstracts,* A64–A65. https://doi.org/10.1136/gutjnl-2020-IDDF.120

Hart, A. L., Lammers, K., Brigidi, P., Vitali, B., Rizzello, F., Gionchetti, P., Campieri, M., Kamm, M. A., Knight, S. C., & Stagg, A. J. (2004). Modulation of human dendritic cell phenotype and function by probiotic bacteria. *Gut, 53*(11), 1602–1609. https://doi.org/10.1136/gut.2003.037325

Hill, C., Guarner, F., Reid, G., Gibson, G. R., Merenstein, D. J., Pot, B., Morelli, L., Canani, R. B., Flint, H. J., Salminen, S., Calder, P. C., & Sanders, M. E. (2014). Expert consensus document. The international scientific association for probiotics and prebiotics consensus statement on the scope and appropriate use of the term probiotic. *Nature Reviews. Gastroenterology and Hepatology, 11*(8), 506–514. https://doi.org/10.1038/nrgastro.2014.66

Hsieh, T. H., Kuo, C. W., Hsieh, K. H., Shieh, M. J., Peng, C. W., Chen, Y. C., Chang, Y. L., Huang, Y. Z., Chen, C. C., Chang, P. K., Chen, K. Y., & Chen, H. Y. (2020). Probiotics alleviate the progressive deterioration of motor functions in a mouse model of Parkinson's disease. *Brain Sciences, 10*(4), 206. https://doi.org/10.3390/brainsci10040206

Ishimoto, T., & Kato, Y. (2021). *Regulation of neurogenesis by organic cation transporters: Potential therapeutic implications* (pp. 281–300). Springer. https://doi.org/10.1007/164_2021_445

Jandhyala, S. M., Talukdar, R., Subramanyam, C., Vuyyuru, H., Sasikala, M., & Nageshwar Reddy, D. (2015). Role of the normal gut microbiota. *World Journal of Gastroenterology, 21*(29), 8787–8803. https://doi.org/10.3748/wjg.v21.i29.8787

Kalliomäki, M., Salminen, S., Poussa, T., & Isolauri, E. (2007). Probiotics during the first 7 years of life: A cumulative risk reduction of eczema in a randomized, placebo-controlled trial. *Journal of Allergy and Clinical Immunology, 119*(4), 1019–1021. https://doi.org/10.1016/j.jaci.2006.12.608

Kamada, N., Chen, G. Y., Inohara, N., & Núñez, G. (2013). Control of pathogens and pathobionts by the gut microbiota. *Nature Immunology, 14*(7), 685–690. https://doi.org/10.1038/ni.2608

Kesika, P., Suganthy, N., Sivamaruthi, B. S., & Chaiyasut, C. (2021). Role of gut-brain axis, gut microbial composition, and probiotic intervention in Alzheimer's disease. *Life Sciences, 264*, 118627. https://doi.org/10.1016/j.lfs.2020.118627

Kim, N., Yun, M., Oh, Y. J., & Choi, H. J. (2018). Mind-altering with the gut: Modulation of the gut-brain axis with probiotics. *Journal of Microbiology, 56*(3), 172–182. https://doi.org/10.1007/s12275-018-8032-4

Kronenberg, G., & Klempin, F. (2020). Laying out the evidence for the persistence of neurogenesis in the adult human hippocampus. *European Archives of Psychiatry and Clinical Neuroscience, 270*(4), 497–498. https://doi.org/10.1007/s00406-019-01066-1

Leta, V., Ray Chaudhuri, K., Milner, O., Chung-Faye, G., Metta, V., Pariante, C. M., & Borsini, A. (2021). Neurogenic and anti-inflammatory effects of probiotics in Parkinson's disease: A systematic review of preclinical and clinical evidence. *Brain, Behavior, and Immunity, 98,* 59–73. https://doi.org/10.1016/j.bbi.2021.07.026

Levy, M., Kolodziejczyk, A. A., Thaiss, C. A., & Elinav, E. (2017). Dysbiosis and the immune system. *Nature Reviews Immunology, 17*(4), 219–232. https://doi.org/10.1038/nri.2017.7

Li, X. Y., He, C., Zhu, Y., & Lu, N. H. (2020). Role of gut microbiota on intestinal barrier function in acute pancreatitis. *World Journal of Gastroenterology, 26*(18), 2187–2193. https://doi.org/10.3748/wjg.v26.i18.2187

Li, Y., & Guo, W. (2021). Neural stem cell niche and adult neurogenesis. *The Neuroscientist: A Review Journal Bringing Neurobiology, Neurology and Psychiatry, 27*(3), 235–245. https://doi.org/10.1177/1073858420939034

Liévin, V., Peiffer, I., Hudault, S., Rochat, F., Brassart, D., Neeser, J. R., & Servin, A. L. (2000). Bifidobacterium strains from resident infant human gastrointestinal microflora exert antimicrobial activity. *Gut, 47*(5), 646–652. https://doi.org/10.1136/gut.47.5.646

Liu, S., Gao, J., Zhu, M., Liu, K., & Zhang, H. L. (2020). Gut microbiota and dysbiosis in Alzheimer's disease: Implications for pathogenesis and treatment. *Molecular Neurobiology, 57*(12), 5026–5043. https://doi.org/10.1007/s12035-020-02073-3

Liu, Y., Gu, N., Jiang, L., Cao, X., & Li, C. (2021). Predicting cognitive function based on physical performance: Findings from the China health and retirement longitudinal study. *Aging Clinical and Experimental Research, 33*(10), 2723–2735. https://doi.org/10.1007/s40520-021-01810-5

Love, C. J., Masson, B. A., Gubert, C., & Hannan, A. J. (2022). *The microbiota-gut-brain axis in Huntington's disease* (pp. 141–184). https://doi.org/10.1016/bs.irn.2022.06.005

Lyman, M., Lloyd, D. G., Ji, X., Vizcaychipi, M. P., & Ma, D. (2014). Neuroinflammation: The role and consequences. *Neuroscience Research, 79,* 1–12. https://doi.org/10.1016/j.neures.2013.10.004

Ma, X. Y., Son, Y. H., Yoo, J. W., Joo, M. K., & Kim, D. H. (2022). Citation: Tight junction protein expression-inducing probiotics alleviate TNBS-induced cognitive impairment with colitis in mice. *Nutrients, 14*(14), 2975. https://doi.org/10.3390/nu14142975

Macready, A. L., Butler, L. T., Kennedy, O. B., Ellis, J. A., Williams, C. M., & Spencer, J. P. E. (2010). Cognitive tests used in chronic adult human randomised controlled trial micronutrient and phytochemical intervention studies. *Nutrition Research Reviews, 23*(2), 200–229. https://doi.org/10.1017/S0954422410000119

Macready, A. L., Kennedy, O. B., Ellis, J. A., Williams, C. M., Spencer, J. P. E., & Butler, L. T. (2009). Flavonoids and cognitive function: A review of human randomized controlled trial studies and recommendations for future studies. *Genes and Nutrition, 4*(4), 227–242. https://doi.org/10.1007/s12263-009-0135-4

Martin, A. M., Sun, E. W., Rogers, G. B., & Keating, D. J. (2019). The influence of the gut microbiome on host metabolism through the regulation of gut hormone release. *Frontiers in Physiology, 10,* 428. https://doi.org/10.3389/fphys.2019.00428

McAfoose, J., & Baune, B. T. (2009). Evidence for a cytokine model of cognitive function. *Neuroscience and Biobehavioral Reviews, 33*(3), 355–366. https://doi.org/10.1016/j.neubiorev.2008.10.005

Mhatre, S., & Gurav, N. (2020). Enhancing bioavailability of probiotics using microencapsulation. *The Bombay Technologist, 67*(1). https://doi.org/10.36664/bt/2020/v67i1/151190

Mirzaei, R., Bouzari, B., Hosseini-Fard, S. R., Mazaheri, M., Ahmadyousefi, Y., Abdi, M., Jalalifar, S., Karimitabar, Z., Teimoori, A., Keyvani, H., Zamani, F., Yousefimashouf, R., & Karampoor, S. (2021). Role of microbiota-derived short-chain fatty acids in nervous system disorders. *Biomedicine and Pharmacotherapy, 139,* 111661. https://doi.org/10.1016/j.biopha.2021.111661

Moreno-Jiménez, E. P., Terreros-Roncal, J., Flor-García, M., Rábano, A., & Llorens-Martín, M. (2021). Evidences for adult hippocampal neurogenesis in humans. *Journal of Neuroscience, 41*(12), 2541–2553. https://doi.org/10.1523/JNEUROSCI.0675-20.2020

Morgun, A. V., Osipova, E. D., Boytsova, E. B., Shuvaev, A. N., Komleva, Y. K., Trufanova, L. V., Vais, E. F., & Salmina, A. B. (2019). Astroglia-mediated regulation of cell development in the model of neurogenic niche in vitro treated with Aβ1-42. *Biomeditsinskaya Khimiya, 65*(5), 366–373. https://doi.org/10.18097/pbmc20196505366

Nagpal, R., Kumar, A., Kumar, M., Behare, P. V., Jain, S., & Yadav, H. (2012). Probiotics, their health benefits and applications for developing healthier foods: A review. *FEMS Microbiology Letters, 334*(1), 1–15. https://doi.org/10.1111/j.1574-6968.2012.02593.x

Ni, Y., Yang, X., Zheng, L., Wang, Z., Wu, L., Jiang, J., Yang, T., Ma, L., & Fu, Z. (2019). *Lactobacillus* and *Bifidobacterium* improves physiological function and cognitive ability in aged mice by the regulation of gut microbiota. *Molecular Nutrition and Food Research, 63*(22), e1900603. https://doi.org/10.1002/mnfr.201900603

Nicola, S., Amoruso, A., Deidda, F., Pane, M., Allesina, S., Mogna, L., Del Piano, M., & Mogna, G. (2016). Searching for the perfect homeostasis. *Journal of Clinical Gastroenterology, 50*(suppl_2), S126–S130. https://doi.org/10.1097/MCG.0000000000000678

Nogueira, A. B., Hoshino, H. S. R., Ortega, N. C., dos Santos, B. G. S., & Teixeira, M. J. (2022). Adult human neurogenesis: Early studies clarify recent controversies and go further. *Metabolic Brain Disease, 37*(1), 153–172. https://doi.org/10.1007/s11011-021-00864-8

Nowak, A., Paliwoda, A., & Błasiak, J. (2019). Anti-proliferative, pro-apoptotic and anti-oxidative activity of *Lactobacillus* and *Bifidobacterium* strains: A review of mechanisms and therapeutic perspectives. *Critical Reviews in Food Science and Nutrition, 59*(21), 3456–3467. https://doi.org/10.1080/10408398.2018.1494539

Ojha, S., Patil, N., Jain, M., Kole, C., & Kaushik, P. (2023). Probiotics for neurodegenerative diseases: A systemic review. *Microorganisms, 11*(4), 1083. https://doi.org/10.3390/microorganisms11041083

O'Shea, E. F., Cotter, P. D., Stanton, C., Ross, R. P., & Hill, C. (2012). Production of bioactive substances by intestinal bacteria as a basis for explaining probiotic mechanisms: Bacteriocins and conjugated linoleic acid. *International Journal of Food Microbiology, 152*(3), 189–205. https://doi.org/10.1016/j.ijfoodmicro.2011.05.025

Park, M. R., Shin, M., Mun, D., Jeong, S. Y., Jeong, D. Y., Song, M., Ko, G., Unno, T., Kim, Y., & Oh, S. (2020). Probiotic Lactobacillus fermentum strain JDFM216 improves cognitive behavior and modulates immune response with gut microbiota. *Scientific Reports, 10*(1), 21701. https://doi.org/10.1038/s41598-020-77587-w

Parodi, B., & Kerlero de Rosbo, N. (2021). The gut-brain axis in multiple sclerosis. Is its dysfunction a pathological trigger or a consequence of the disease? *Frontiers in Immunology, 12*, 718220. https://doi.org/10.3389/fimmu.2021.718220

Pastorino, L., Grillo, F., Albertelli, M., Ghiorzo, P., & Bruno, W. (2021). Insights into mechanisms of tumorigenesis in neuroendocrine neoplasms. *International Journal of Molecular Sciences, 22*(19), 10328. https://doi.org/10.3390/ijms221910328

Petrof, E. O., Kojima, K., Ropeleski, M. J., Musch, M. W., Tao, Y., De Simone, C., & Chang, E. B. (2004). Probiotics inhibit nuclear factor-κB and induce heat shock proteins in colonic epithelial cells through proteasome inhibition. *Gastroenterology, 127*(5), 1474–1487. https://doi.org/10.1053/j.gastro.2004.09.001

Petruzziello, C., Saviano, A., & Ojetti, V. (2023). Probiotics, the immune response and acute appendicitis: A review. *Vaccines, 11*(7), 1170. https://doi.org/10.3390/vaccines11071170

Plaza-Diaz, J., Ruiz-Ojeda, F. J., Gil-Campos, M., & Gil, A. (2019). Mechanisms of action of probiotics. *Advances in Nutrition, 10*(suppl_1), S49–S66. https://doi.org/10.1093/advances/nmy063

Prakash, S., Tomaro-Duchesneau, C., Saha, S., & Cantor, A. (2011). The gut microbiota and human health with an emphasis on the use of microencapsulated bacterial cells. *Journal of Biomedicine and Biotechnology, 2011,* 981214. https://doi.org/10.1155/2011/981214

Prince, M., Bryce, R., Albanese, E., Wimo, A., Ribeiro, W., & Ferri, C. P. (2013). The global prevalence of dementia: A systematic review and metaanalysis. *Alzheimer's and Dementia, 9*(1), 63. https://doi.org/10.1016/j.jalz.2012.11.007

Reitz, C., Brayne, C., & Mayeux, R. (2011). Epidemiology of Alzheimer disease. *Nature Reviews. Neurology, 7*(3), 137–152. https://doi.org/10.1038/nrneurol.2011.2

Resta-Lenert, S., & Barrett, K. E. (2003). Live probiotics protect intestinal epithelial cells from the effects of infection with enteroinvasive Escherichia coli (EIEC). *Gut, 52*(7), 988–997. https://doi.org/10.1136/gut.52.7.988

Ribeiro, D. E., Glaser, T., Oliveira-Giacomelli, Á., & Ulrich, H. (2019). Purinergic receptors in neurogenic processes. *Brain Research Bulletin, 151,* 3–11. https://doi.org/10.1016/j.brainresbull.2018.12.013

Salzman, N. H. (2011). Microbiota–immune system interaction: An uneasy alliance. *Current Opinion in Microbiology, 14*(1), 99–105. https://doi.org/10.1016/j.mib.2010.09.018

Shabab, T., Khanabdali, R., Moghadamtousi, S. Z., Kadir, H. A., & Mohan, G. (2017). Neuroinflammation pathways: A general review. *International Journal of Neuroscience, 127*(7), 624–633. https://doi.org/10.1080/00207454.2016.1212854

Sharma, V., & Kaur, S. (2020). The effect of probiotic intervention in ameliorating the altered central nervous system functions in neurological disorders: A review. *Open Microbiology Journal, 14*(1), 18–29. https://doi.org/10.2174/1874285802014010018

Sherman, P. M., Johnson-Henry, K. C., Yeung, H. P., Ngo, P. S. C., Goulet, J., & Tompkins, T. A. (2005). Probiotics reduce enterohemorrhagic Escherichia coli O157:H7- and Enteropathogenic *E. coli* O127:H6-induced changes in polarized T84 epithelial cell monolayers by reducing bacterial adhesion and cytoskeletal rearrangements. *Infection and Immunity, 73*(8), 5183–5188. https://doi.org/10.1128/IAI.73.8.5183-5188.2005

Sindi, S., Mangialasche, F., & Kivipelto, M. (2015). Advances in the prevention of Alzheimer's disease. *F1000prime Reports, 7*, 50. https://doi.org/10.12703/P7-50

Singh, N., Singh, V., Rai, S. N., Mishra, V., Vamanu, E., & Singh, M. P. (2022). Deciphering the gut microbiome in neurodegenerative diseases and metagenomic approaches for characterization of gut microbes. *Biomedicine and Pharmacotherapy, 156,* 113958. https://doi.org/10.1016/j.biopha.2022.113958

Singh, T. P., & Natraj, B. H. (2021). Next-generation probiotics: A promising approach towards designing personalized medicine. *Critical Reviews in Microbiology, 47*(4), 479–498. https://doi.org/10.1080/1040841X.2021.1902940

Srivastav, S., Neupane, S., Bhurtel, S., Katila, N., Maharjan, S., Choi, H., Hong, J. T., & Choi, D. Y. (2019). Probiotics mixture increases butyrate, and subsequently rescues the nigral dopaminergic neurons from MPTP and rotenone-induced neurotoxicity. *Journal of Nutritional Biochemistry, 69,* 73–86. https://doi.org/10.1016/j.jnutbio.2019.03.021

Strandwitz, P. (2018). Neurotransmitter modulation by the gut microbiota. *Brain Research, 1693*(B), 128–133. https://doi.org/10.1016/j.brainres.2018.03.015

Suda, K., & Matsuda, K. (2022). How microbes affect depression: Underlying mechanisms via the gut–brain axis and the modulating role of probiotics. *International Journal of Molecular Sciences, 23*(3), 1172. https://doi.org/10.3390/ijms23031172

Suganya, K., & Koo, B. S. (2020). Gut–brain axis: Role of gut microbiota on neurological disorders and how probiotics/prebiotics beneficially modulate microbial and immune pathways to improve brain functions. *International Journal of Molecular Sciences, 21*(20), 7551. https://doi.org/10.3390/ijms21207551

Sun, P., Su, L., Zhu, H., Li, X., Guo, Y., Du, X., Zhang, L., & Qin, C. (2021). Gut microbiota regulation and their implication in the development of neurodegenerative disease. *Microorganisms, 9*(11), 2281. https://doi.org/10.3390/microorganisms9112281

Tahmi, M., Palta, P., & Luchsinger, J. A. (2021). Metabolic syndrome and cognitive function. *Current Cardiology Reports, 23*(12), 180. https://doi.org/10.1007/s11886-021-01615-y

Takano, H. (2018). Cognitive function and monoamine neurotransmission in schizophrenia: Evidence from positron emission tomography studies. *Frontiers in Psychiatry, 9*, 228. https://doi.org/10.3389/fpsyt.2018.00228

Tamtaji, O. R., Taghizadeh, M., Daneshvar Kakhaki, R., Kouchaki, E., Bahmani, F., Borzabadi, S., Oryan, S., Mafi, A., & Asemi, Z. (2019). Clinical and metabolic response to probiotic administration in people with Parkinson's disease: A randomized, double-blind, placebo-controlled trial. *Clinical Nutrition, 38*(3), 1031–1035. https://doi.org/10.1016/j.clnu.2018.05.018

Thursby, E., & Juge, N. (2017). Introduction to the human gut microbiota. *Biochemical Journal, 474*(11), 1823–1836. https://doi.org/10.1042/BCJ20160510

van Kessel, S. P., Frye, A. K., El-Gendy, A. O., Castejon, M., Keshavarzian, A., van Dijk, G., & El Aidy, S. (2019). Gut bacterial tyrosine decarboxylases restrict levels of levodopa in the treatment of Parkinson's disease. *Nature Communications, 10*(1), 310. https://doi.org/10.1038/s41467-019-08294-y

Wang, H., Lee, I. S., Braun, C., & Enck, P. (2016). Effect of probiotics on central nervous system functions in animals and humans: A systematic review. *Journal of Neurogastroenterology and Motility, 22*(4), 589–605. https://doi.org/10.5056/jnm16018

Westfall, S., Lomis, N., Kahouli, I., Dia, S. Y., Singh, S. P., & Prakash, S. (2017). Microbiome, probiotics and neurodegenerative diseases: Deciphering the gut brain axis. *Cellular and Molecular Life Sciences, 74*(20), 3769–3787. https://doi.org/10.1007/s00018-017-2550-9

Williams, N. T. (2010). Probiotics. *American Journal of Health-System Pharmacy, 67*(6), 449–458. https://doi.org/10.2146/ajhp090168

Yadav, M. K., Kumari, I., Singh, B., Sharma, K. K., & Tiwari, S. K. (2022). Probiotics, prebiotics and synbiotics: Safe options for next-generation therapeutics. *Applied Microbiology and Biotechnology, 106*(2), 505–521. https://doi.org/10.1007/s00253-021-11646-8

Yan, F., Cao, H., Cover, T. L., Whitehead, R., Washington, M. K., & Polk, D. B. (2007). Soluble proteins produced by probiotic bacteria regulate intestinal epithelial cell survival and growth. *Gastroenterology, 132*(2), 562–575. https://doi.org/10.1053/j.gastro.2006.11.022

Yang, W., Cui, K., Li, X., Zhao, J., Zeng, Z., Song, R., Qi, X., & Xu, W. (2021). Effect of polyphenols on cognitive function: Evidence from population-based studies and clinical trials. *Journal of Nutrition, Health and Aging, 25*(10), 1190–1204. https://doi.org/10.1007/s12603-021-1685-4

Zmora, N., Zilberman-Schapira, G., Suez, J., Mor, U., Dori-Bachash, M., Bashiardes, S., Kotler, E., Zur, M., Regev-Lehavi, D., Brik, R. B.-Z., Federici, S., Cohen, Y., Linevsky, R., Rothschild, D., Moor, A. E., Ben-Moshe, S., Harmelin, A., Itzkovitz, S., Maharshak, N., . . . Elinav, E. (2018). Personalized gut mucosal colonization resistance to empiric probiotics is associated with unique host and microbiome features. *Cell, 174*(6), 1388–1405.e21. https://doi.org/10.1016/j.cell.2018.08.041

12 Bio-Engineered Gut Microbiota for Drug Delivery

Novel Propitious Realm

Pawar Jayashree, Mulye Kalpita, Talker Judith, and Kotnis Ashwin

12.1 INTRODUCTION

The gastrointestinal (GI) tract of humans harbors a large number of strictly anaerobic microbes, with the presence of more than 50 bacterial phyla, dominated primarily by phyla Bacteroidetes and Firmicutes in varying proportions in each individual. The bacterial cells not only outnumber the host cells but also encode a substantially larger number of genes as compared to humans, which are able to carry out numerous functions that humans have limited ability for or are unable to perform (Bull & Plummer, 2014). Microbial colonization starts at birth and evolves over the course of a lifetime and is affected by endogenous and exogenous alterations. Over years of evolution, these microbes preferentially occupy different niches in the body and have found ways in which they can communicate with the host cells through the exchange of metabolites.

Since the past decade, the gut microbiota has surprised the medical research fraternity with the exemplary role the different members play in controlling numerous physiological processes. Specific bacterial populations within the gut microbiota have been identified that are directly influencing various cellular pathways and processes. An imbalance of gut microbiota has been seen contributing to numerous pathological conditions like immune disorders, inflammatory diseases, chronic infections, and behavioral disorders.

12.1.1 Influence of Diet on Gut Microbiota

Among many intrinsic and extrinsic factors that influence microbiota, dietary habits pose as the 'Lead hero'. Several studies have observed that dietary habits influence the gut microbiome under carefully monitored experimental conditions. Proteins, fats, and carbohydrates are three major constituents of any diet. However, the proportion, origin, and main supply resource ingredients fulfilling these dietary demands vary a lot, depending upon—geographic location, local culture, and obviously the availability of resources.

One crucial aspect that affects the human gut microbial diversity is the source of protein supplements as exemplified by an increased risk of IBD due to high total protein intake, particularly animal protein (Jantchou et al., 2010). Animal proteins have been reported to increase *Lactobacillus*, *Bacteroides*, *Alistipes*, *Bilophila*, *Clostridia*, *Roseburia*, and *Eubacterium rectale* in the gut. It has been shown that regular consumption of red meat augments the growth of some gut microbiota that elevate the levels of TMAO, a proatherogenic substance that increases the risk of cardiovascular disease (DeFilippis et al., 2015). Plant-derived proteins increase *Bifidobacterium* and *Lactobacillus* and decrease *Bacteroides* and *Clostridium perfringens*. It elevates levels of SCFAs, has a positive influence on the gut barrier, and has been linked with reduced inflammation and increased

DOI: 10.1201/9781003452249-12

regulatory T cells (Tregs), to maintain homeostasis and self-tolerance, which are positively influenced by plant-derived proteins.

Like protein, fat consumption also directs the prevalence of some species in microbiota. Several studies on the human population have observed that a diet that is high in fat content may increase both the overall anaerobic microbiota and Bacteroides. A diet that is low in fat content increases the amount of *Bifidobacterium* found in the feces, whereas a diet rich in saturated fat augments *Faecalibacterium prausnitzii*. Also, participants with a high-monounsaturated-fat diet showed a decreased load of total bacteria in the feces and low levels of plasma total and LDL cholesterol; however, the relative abundance of any bacterial species remained unchanged.

Carbohydrates are among the most well-studied macromolecules for their influence on gut microbial diversity. Carbohydrates are categorized into two groups: Digestible and non-digestible. Participants who were administered date fruits thus had high levels of carbohydrates, namely, sucrose, fructose, and glucose (which usually are the resultant products of enzymatic degradation of digestible carbohydrates), had relatively higher levels of bifidobacteria, and decreased levels of *Bacteroides*. Another study revealed that these bacterial changes were duplicated when lactose was added to the diet, which led to a decline in *Clostridium* species. One surprising finding with the addition of lactose was an increased fecal concentration of beneficial SCFAs (Francavilla et al., 2012) as lactose is usually considered an irritant of the GI tract (e.g., lactose intolerance) (Singh et al., 2017).

The most consistent and long-lasting influence on host immunity is diet. Altering the makeup of immune cells associated with the GI cavity can reduce inflammation, enhance antitumor immunity, and increase the therapeutic effects of cancer immunotherapy. The human microbiota, immune system, and metabolism all interact intricately. The gut-associated lymphoid tissue is a large and significant component of the immune system that regulates the immune responses at the local and systemic levels. Intraepithelial lymphocytes and IECs, which are immediately exposed to the contents of the lumen including metabolites produced by the gut microbes, are the first cells in the gut to develop innate immunity. IECs contain different types of cells such as the antimicrobial peptides releasing Paneth cells and goblet cells, which release mucus providing protective cover over the epithelial layer. There are a variety of immune cells, such as CD4+ and CD8+ T cells and B cells, innate lymphoid cells, and antigen-presenting cells in lamina propria (Gopalakrishnan et al., 2018).

Innate immunity is essential for recognizing and reacting to microbiota-derived products. Commensal microbiota inhabiting the gut lumen have profound effects systemically and on the local immune system, within the gut mucosa. Similarly, gut microbiota can change as a result of the immune system. IgA is secreted into the gut lumen by plasma cells in the lamina propria. Numerous antimicrobial peptides are secreted by Paneth cells, and their activity is increased in response to signals from nearby immune cells in response to the microbiota. Local DCs, which travel to the draining lymph nodes to activate naive T cells into effector T cells, Tregs, or Th17 cells, can be activated by bacterial metabolites or bacteria themselves. These cells can then migrate back to the gut mucosa or enter systemic circulation. Specific metabolites or bacterial byproducts can alter the DC in a fashion that allows them to skew toward a Treg versus Th17 phenotype. Tregs secrete IL-10, creating a local anti-inflammatory cytokine environment. Interleukin-17 produced by Th17 cells can increase Paneth cell production of antimicrobial peptides and can function in recruiting PMNs from the bloodstream. A small number of bacterial metabolites that enter the bloodstream directly have the potential to gradually change the systemic immune system. The recognition of microorganisms via PRRs ensures a perfect harmony between host and microbes. A vast family of extracellular and intracellular receptors known as PRRs are able to recognize particular MAMPs or microbe-associated molecular patterns. TLRs, CLRs, NOD-like receptors, and cytosolic sensors of DNA and RNA are examples of PRRs. Activation of PPRs leads to the induction of chemokines and cytokines necessary to orchestrate a protective immune response (Fukata & Arditi, 2013).

Studies on patients with hematologic malignancies who have undergone allogeneic stem cell transplant (allo-HSCT) revealed dysbiosis in the gut microbiome in response to cancer therapy. Dysbiosis and impaired systemic immunity were observed to be common in these patients. This can be due to treatment with immunomodulators, antibiotics, and radiation therapy that can impact the immune system and cause dysbiosis of the gut microbiota (Routy et al., 2017; Shono et al., 2016). A number of researchers have suggested a connection between dysbiosis and altered reactions, and also with therapeutic toxicity. Fecal sample analysis revealed a disruption of the gut microbiota's pre-HSCT state of balance, with reduced bacterial diversity and stability and a predominance of *Streptococcus*, *Enterococcus*, and other *Proteobacteria* (Holler et al., 2014; Taur et al., 2012), and reduction in *Faecalibacterium* and *Ruminococcus* that promote good health (Biagi et al., 2015). The high diversity of gut microbiome has been shown to impact the lives of long-term cancer survivors (Taur et al., 2014).

Apart from regulating the immune response, the gut microbiome manufactures a variety of metabolites from food components, host products, and other microbial metabolic intermediates. These metabolites have been demonstrated to have immunoprotective properties, for instance, bile acid derivatives, tryptophan metabolites, and SCFAs.

It has been noted that besides influencing local immunity, gut microbiota contributes to controlling systemic immune responses through various metabolites. The gut microbiota is also known to synthesize an array of biochemical metabolites that help a large number of metabolic processes that essentially sync with numerous events in the cell required for maintaining homeostasis. One such example is the fermentation of dietary fiber and intestinal mucus by the goblet cells that are in synergy with the prevalent gut microbiota. Supports the growth of unique microbes that produce SCFA and gases such as acetate, propionate, and butyrate.

12.1.1.1 Gut Microbiome Implicated in Human Diseases

Host genetics, immune responses, and diets affect the composition of gut microbiota. Individual members of gut microbiota, frequently in consortia having the metabolic and immune capacities, determine their role in host health and diseases.

12.1.2 Metabolic Diseases and Gut Microbes

The prevalence of metabolic illnesses has substantially increased worldwide. Metabolic illnesses include PCOS, obesity, cardiovascular diseases, non-alcoholic fatty liver disease (NAFLD), metabolic syndrome, T2DM, and atherosclerosis (Norman et al., 2007; Popkin et al., 2012; Younossi et al., 2016; Zheng et al., 2018; Virani et al., 2020). The gut microbiome is primarily implicated in metabolizing nutrients after diet consumption, the metabolism of xenobiotics and drugs, the preservation of the architecture and functionality of the GI tract, and the prevention of intestinal pathogenesis (Jandhyala et al., 2015).

Obesity is one of the common metabolic diseases attributed to complex gene–environment interactions. The global obesity epidemic, which is a result of lifestyle transitions, has also resulted in marked alterations in the composition of human gut microbiota. The upregulation of *Mollicutes* and downregulation of *Akkermansia*, *Faecalibacterium*, *Oscillobacter alisteripes*, and *Bacteroides thetaiotaomicron* have been observed.

It has been shown that the microbiome of obese people has a higher metabolic capacity to obtain energy from food. It is important to note that the microbiota influences the movement, use, and storage of collected energy. It is now widely accepted that the relative abundance of Bacteroidetes and Firmicutes, rather than the microbiome's overall composition, determines the phenotype of obesity.

The influence of gut microbiome has also been observed in another common disease of metabolism—NAFLD. NAFLD causes excessive lipid accumulation in the liver, which increases the synthesis and release of pro-inflammatory adipokines, thus causing insulin resistance and type 2 diabetes as a comorbidity (Reilly & Saltiel, 2017). Significant increase in the abundance of the phylum Bacteroidetes while reduction in Firmicutes has been observed in individuals with NAFLD (Wang et al., 2016). Intestinal dysbiosis has been observed in NAFLD and non-alcoholic steatohepatitis (NASH). The fecal microbiota of children with NAFLD showed decreased alpha diversity whereas those with NASH showed the lowest α-diversity. Other diseases such as PCOS showed notable alterations in the composition of gut microbiotas in a letrozole-induced mice model of PCOS, raising the possibility that dysbiosis of the gut microbiota and PCOS are related as reported by Kelley et al. (2016)

The inflammation caused by psychological stress has been shown to be regulated by the gut microbiome. Xu et al. (2020) in their study on mice models have discovered that the gut microbiota along with the IL-17/G-CSF pathway influenced the psychological stress on vaso-occlusion in sickle cell disease. The research has revealed an underappreciated mechanism by which stress controls inflammation by augmenting aged neutrophils through the synthesis of commensal SFB and G-CSF by Th17 cells.

In 1930, J.H. Stokes and D.M. Pillsbury first postulated the 'brain–gut–skin axis'. It was proposed that depressive and anxious mental states impact the GI tract functioning, alter the composition of the normal gut microbiota, increase the permeability of the intestine, and cause systemic inflammation. Increased gut epithelial permeability has been associated with systemic inflammation, which can impact the homeostasis of the skin by activating T cells, disturbing immunosuppressive cytokines, and affecting T regulatory cells that promote tolerance. Additionally, it has been proposed that changed concentrations of neurotransmitters produced by gut microbes can communicate with peripheral organs through as-yet-unidentified neural routes.

TABLE 12.1
List of Gut Microbiota Products and Their Impact on Health

Gut Microbiota Product	Influence on Health Outcome
Butyrate	Prevents gut microbial dysbiosis by maintaining oxygen balance in the gut and is required by epithelial cells that are active in β oxidation and utilize large amounts of oxygen
Acetate	Is a crucial and abundant metabolite required for the growth of other microbiota and the regulation of central appetite and lipid metabolism in peripheral tissues and lipogenesis; central appetite regulator
Propionate	Is a crucial metabolite transferred to the liver, for the regulation of gluconeogenesis and interaction with the fatty acid receptors in the gut that regulate the signaling pathways involved in food satiety
FBA	Decreases hepatic fat accumulation and insulin resistance
Trimethylamine	Oxidizes in the liver to trimethylamine-*N*-oxide
Indole propionic acid	Reduces the risk of type 2 diabetes
Tauroursodeoxycholic acid (TUDCA)	Increases the hepatic and muscle insulin sensitivity
Tauro beta muricholic acid	Decreases glucose intolerance
Glucourodeoxycholic acid (GUDCA)	Decreases hyperglycemia
Glycodeoxycholic acid (GDCA)	Decreases insulin resistance
HYA *N*-(1-carbamoyl-2-phenyl-ethyl) butyramide	Decreases obesity
Gut microbial enzymes	Contribute to bile acid metabolism
Ceramides	Induce cold-induced thermogenesis
Taurine, histamine, and spermine	Increase IL-18 levels
Indole 3 aldehyde	Increases IL-22 levels

TABLE 12.2
List of Microbes, Their Microbial Metabolites/Components with Targets, and Influence on Health Outcomes

Microbes	Microbial Component/ Metabolite/ Characteristic	Target/Function	Influence on Health Outcome
Intestinal microbiota	Flagellin	Binding TLR5 and NLRC4	Activate the immune machinery to fight pathogens; when administered intraperitoneally, flagellin confers resistance to rotavirus infection
Clostridium, Bifidobacterium, Ruminococcus, and Bacteroides	Adherence to epithelial cells	StimulatingT17 cells, T regulatory cells	Maintain homeostasis of the intestinal mucosa by inducing differentiation of Th17 and Treg cells
Gut microbiota	SCFA	Stimulating intestinal epithelial cells	Augment the synthesis of the antimicrobial peptides and mucus
		Stimulating colonic regulatory T cells	Play a role in the maturation and expansion of colonic regulatory T cells and reducing of local inflammatory responses to the gut microbes
		Stimulating intestinal cells and epithelial barrier	Induce proliferation and differentiation of epithelial cells
	Tryptophan metabolites (indoles)	Ligand for the aryl hydrocarbon receptor (AhR)	Are crucial for intestinal homeostasis and prevention of inflammatory bowel disease

According to a report by Yan et al. (2017) on the cutaneous microbiota, individuals with psoriasis tend to have higher relative abundances of *Streptococcus* and lower levels of *Propionibacterium* than controls. Psoriatic patients had a perturbed ratio of gut microbes *Firmicutes* and *Bacteroidetes* as compared to healthy individuals. Comparatively fewer actinobacteria were found in psoriasis patients than in healthy people.

The involvement of gut dysbiosis has been studied during the recent COVID-19 pandemic. The study by S. Ahlawat et al. (2020) concluded that the probable 'gut-lung axis' in COVID-19 involves the inhalation of SARS-CoV-2-laden-droplets exhaled from a SARS-CoV-2-infected person. The inhaled droplets result in the binding of the spike protein of SARS-CoV-2 to ACE2 for facilitating the entry inside the host cells. The overwhelmed immune system eventually releases pro-inflammatory cytokines that increase lung permeability, allowing the virus to travel through circulation and attach to ACE2 receptors which are abundantly located on colonic enterocytes. The binding of the virus to the enterocytes alters the permeability of the intestine, which causes the leaking of gut metabolites and related bacteria into the bloodstream. The microorganisms that are released and the byproducts they produce damage several organs, including the lungs. As a result, when individuals with COVID-19 disease present with diarrhea, a serious GI symptom, 'microbial dysbiosis' is suspected (Ahlawat et al., 2020).

12.2 APPLICATIONS OF ENGINEERED GUT MICROBES

12.2.1 Microbial Strains Used for Bioengineering: The Rising Stars of the Gutywood

Synthetic biology involves the engineering and synthesis of biological or biologically inspired complex systems that exhibit novel functions that do not exist naturally (Serrano, 2007). One significant application of synthetic biology is engineering microbiota for drug delivery. The strategy offers various advantages over the use of pre-, pro-, or synbiotics. For example, genetic engineering can instill novel functions that are not observed in the native/natural microbiota. Additional genetic elements like inducible promoters may allow better fine-tuning of gene expression and flexibility of the engineered bacteria in the host and environment.

Although genetic engineering tools have traditionally been using organisms like *E. coli*, *Lactobacillus*, and *Saccharomyces*, the focus has shifted to engineering the gut microbiota including *Bacillus* spp. and *Weissella* spp. after the developments in the field of human microbiome research (Ozdemir et al., 2018; Arnold et al., 2023). Being part of the gut environment, genetically engineered probiotic bacteria may survive better in the gut, portraying a 'colonization advantage'. They may thus continuously release the drug with the possibility of circumventing repeated dosing of the drug (Rutter et al., 2022; Arnold et al., 2023).

When compared to conventional drug delivery, employing gut microbes for drug delivery offers precise targeting and better control, along with the accomplishment of 'smart' drug delivery in complicated delivery environments of the body (Feng et al., 2023). Improved accessibility is another advantage, as the desired prebiotic/metabolite/drug is synthesized in situ (Chen et al., 2023). By engineering resident gut microbes, rather than conventional organisms, the intrinsic metabolic diversity of gut microbes can be harnessed without the requirement for complete rewiring of the metabolic pathways of a chassis organism.

Selecting appropriate microbial systems is important in the development of effective drug delivery systems. Commonly used strains and tools are described in the following box.

Bacteria: *E. coli* Nissle (1917) has been a preferred strain for probiotic engineering in many studies. It allows gene manipulation due to its highly researched genome, transcriptome, and metabolism pathways. It is non-invasive and non-uropathogenic, and it is quickly eliminated by general blood serum defense mechanisms. Interestingly, it possesses 'genomic islands'—gene clusters coding for microcin-producing genes, which suppress other enterobacteria. *E. coli* Nissle 1917 also bears a unique LPS located in the outer cell membrane, which plays a role in immunomodulation, especially, the anti-inflammatory properties of the strain with no immunotoxic effects. The strain is known to increase the synthesis of epithelial defensin and have a 'sealing effect' on the tight junctions of the enterocytes, which strengthens the epithelial barrier and eliminates 'leaky gut' symptoms. It stimulates the growth of the gut immune system in both animal models and newborn humans. Metabolic products of the strain have been shown to enhance the motility of the colon, which might be an added benefit for therapeutic application and utility in individuals with chronic constipation (Sonnenborn & Schulze, 2009).

Fungi: Fungi are eukaryotic organisms with gene expression mechanisms similar to humans, unlike bacteria. Better gene expression and post-translational modifications of the expressed protein/s and resistance to attack by bacteriophages are added advantages while using fungal systems (Durmusoglu et al., 2021; Bai et al., 2023). Although the quantity of fungi in the gut is much less compared with bacteria, they are approximately a hundred times more and have an important role in the ecosystem of the gut. Notably, most bacteria in the gut ecosystem are strict anaerobes, whereas many fungi, including *Saccharomyces species pluralis* (spp.), are facultative anaerobes compared to the gut bacteria, most of which are strict anaerobes. The fungi harbored in the gut offer numerous advantages for engineering applications. Fungi including *Penicillium camemberti* and *Aspergillus sojae* are part of our diets due to baking and brewing and are crucial components of a healthy gut microbiota.

Baker's yeast (*Saccharomyces cerevisiae*) has been traditionally utilized as a model organism in genetic and molecular biology studies due to its ease of culturing, non-pathogenic nature, and high growth rate. The availability of a wide array of mutants and genetic engineering tools is an added benefit while using this organism.

S. cerevisiae contains glucans as a major part of their cell wall, known to target the phagocytic cells. This property makes baker's yeast an excellent drug delivery carrier for molecules such as proteins, DNA, siRNA, and small drug molecules. Glucans and yeast cells have been widely used as carriers for targeted vaccine delivery for oral, topical mode.

Many of the present nano-therapies are available as intravenous injections which need more strict regulation and are less patient-friendly. The oral drug delivery route, in contrast, is better patient-compliant, economical, and safe with easy dosage regulation. The oral route of delivery available for yeast models, enabling rapid clearance of *S. cerevisiae* from the gut (Bai et al., 2023), makes it an ideal candidate for short and maneuverable biosensing applications and minimizing competition with other resident microbiota. It has been shown that subsequent to the administration of nanoparticle-loaded yeast capsules orally, they are transcytosed by M cells, followed by consecutive endocytosis by macrophages/monocytes, which further transport the particles to distant target sites of acute inflammation or tumor (Sabu et al., 2019).

The cytoplasmic contents of yeast cells are discarded by numerous physical treatments and chemical procedures to form the 'empty yeast microcapsule'. These especially have been proven to be an effective means to enclose positively and negatively charged (after treating them with polycations) particles. Multiple methods including standard mixing and spray drying are available to embed the pharmacological compounds in the yeast microcapsule. It should be noted that different methods are available for the immobilization of yeast cells, e.g., on a solid carrier surface using cross-linking agents, entrapment inside a porous polymer matrix, self-aggregation using a natural or artificial method, and mechanical containment within a solid barrier. All these add to the advantages of using this organism for drug delivery.

Saccharomyces boulardii is another probiotic yeast similar to *S. cerevisiae* that grows rapidly at 37°C, has efficient vectors available for introducing foreign genes, and is amenable to simple transformation protocols as well as CRISPR-mediated genome editing tools. Tools for the genetic modification of yeast have recently become available (Scott et al., 2021). The impact of various genetic elements including promoter region, terminator sequence, selection markers, and copy number control elements on the volume and variation of protein expression in this organism was investigated by Durmusoglu et al. in 2021. Furthermore, they have shown that *S. boulardii* colonization in germ-free mice can persist for over 30 days in spite of commensal bacteria competing for niche space. On the contrary, the duration of gut residence in both untreated and antibiotic-treated animals is only 12 days. The total content of β-carotene recovered in the feces of treated mice was 56-fold higher than the β-carotene present in the initial probiotic dose, demonstrating the success in engineering *S. boulardii* to synthesize small molecules like β-carotene in situ in the germ-free mouse gut. As a result, the research has created a 'synthetic toolkit' for gene manipulation in this.

Utilizing antibiotic-resistance genes as selectable markers in genetic engineering is well known. The introduction of such strains in the human body is a major issue of concern. Auxotrophic mutants of *S. boulardii* that can be used for selection of recombinants are available. Selection of auxotrophs is a safer and preferred strategy for this purpose as compared to selecting antibiotic resistant cells. This as an added advantage of using this organism for gut mycoflora engineering.

12.2.2 Techniques for Microbiota Engineering: The Tools of the Trade

12.2.2.1 The Yet Uncultured Microbiota: Black Box for Genetic Engineering?

Nearly 70% of the human gut microbes, including the majority of gut anaerobes, represent the 'novel' bacterial population, which has not yet been cultivated ex vivo. Although with 'culturomics' tools the number of pure microbial cultures obtained from the human gut has notably increased since 2012, there is a considerable number of human gut microbes yet to be isolated and cultured in vitro. Cultivation-independent strategies involving molecular methods have provided us the information about the vast diversity of gut microbiota, harnessing the immense repertoire of microbial functions, and need pure cultures for testing and modifying the candidate genes, proteins, or metabolic pathways. In spite of numerous novel approaches being undertaken for the cultivation of the gut microbiota, the cultivated members, so far, are quite less, especially the anaerobic members of the gut. Tremendous efforts are also being undertaken to bridge the cultivation-dependent and cultivation-independent strategies; for example, Yin et al. (2022) have used the recent 'single-cell droplet' approach to isolate the beneficial gut microbes. Newer and robust technologies, such as Raman spectroscopy, multicolor flow cytometry and cell sorter, and advanced microfluidic technologies, are also being used as powerful tools to study microbiome function at the single-cell level (Yuan et al., 2017) and for sorting cells (Huang et al., 2023). Figure 12.1 lists some of the highly promising approaches currently used for cultivating the 'yet uncultured' gut microbiota.

Mining the next generation of probiotic candidate microbes from the human gut, and further identifying suitable candidates for drug delivery, has indeed become a promising research hotspot. In view of these facts, one needs to first design methods to grow these 'yet uncultured' microbiota in the laboratory, to engineer them as chassis for drug delivery. Since not much is known about the

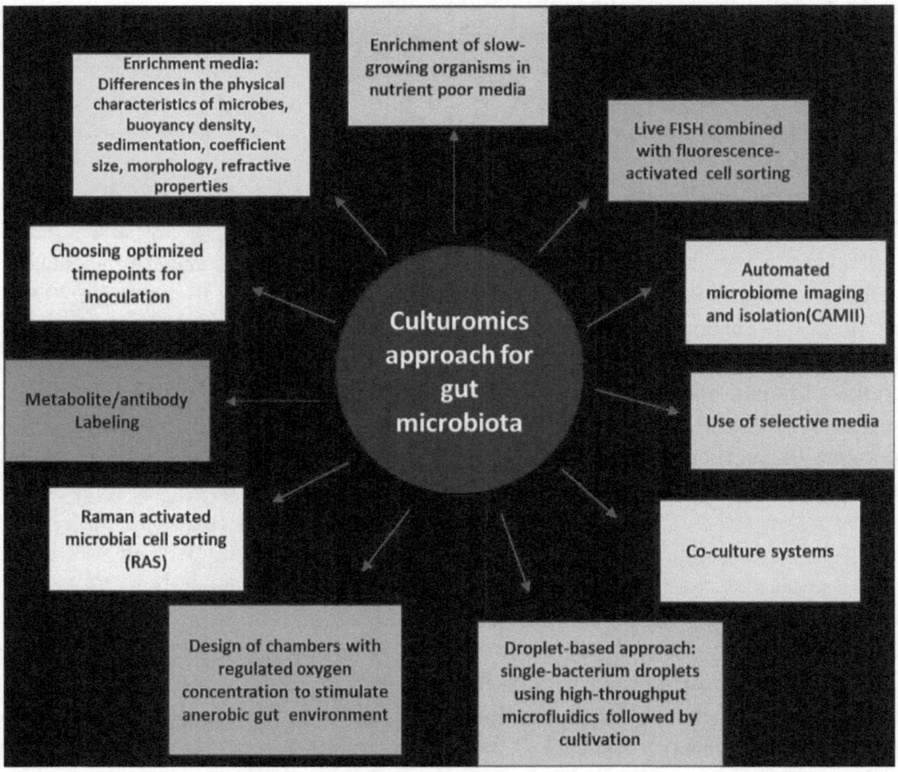

FIGURE 12.1 Novel methods for the cultivation of the 'yet uncultured' gut microbiota.

cultural, physiological, and genetic properties of these microbes, ambiguity exists regarding the exact protocols to be used for gene manipulation, which are still required to be developed for these 'novel microorganisms' (Arnold et al., 2022), while only a handful of bacterial commensals such as *Bacteroidetes* and model pathogens can be genetically manipulated at present.

12.2.2.2 Fecal Microbiota Transplant

Gut microbiome and microbial dysbiosis in humans play crucial roles in health and numerous diseases. Microorganisms in 'co-culture' or as 'consortia' are known to perform multiple vital functions as they coexist in populations, both densely crowded and sparse and diverse communities, resulting in growing efforts to utilize and coordinate this complex niche (Bittihn et al., 2018). Microbes in communities produce numerous metabolites, for communication during intra- or interspecies microbial interactions. Multiple factors including but not limited to physical interactions of the microbes through adhesion molecules, and special signaling biochemicals, could be responsible for such symbiotic/antagonistic interactions between microorganisms. Also, one organism individually or in a population can induce or inhibit the production of de novo products or biosynthetic pathways in other organisms or pathways many of which remain to be discovered as these are very intricate and difficult to grow in laboratory conditions (Zhang & Wang, 2016). Maximum utilization of such novel interactions microorganisms in a niche would be possible only by use of high-performance consortia, rather than isolated single organisms for particular applications.

Fecal microbiota transplantation (FMT) is a newly developed therapeutic approach that addresses dysbiosis of the gut microbiota by introducing healthy, pre-screened donor feces to a sick recipient in an attempt to mend the microbiota and treat the illness (Airola et al., 2023). FMT has shown promising results in the management of recurrent infection of *Clostridium difficile*, digestive system disorders including Crohn's disease, IBD, and ulcerative colitis. The objective of FMT is to re-establish gut homeostasis by re-introducing the community of organisms in the fecal material of healthy donors (Patwa et al., 2022).

Autologous FMT has been proposed by Ke et al. (2022) as a novel way to counteract the decrease of species in the human gut microbiome, which may increase vulnerability to numerous diseases. The hosts' stool samples would need to be taken and cryopreserved when they are younger and healthier for autologous FMT.

The most recent recommendations for practicing FMT as a treatment modality include a specific selection procedure for the donor based on a detailed clinical interview for diseases, biochemical and pathological analysis of blood and stool, and molecular testing of the stool sample on the day of each donation/administration of feces in the diseased patient recipient (Airola et al., 2023). In spite of these, FMT poses certain issues of serious concern. FMT involves the transfer of an undefined and inconsistent consortium of microbes that changes even in the same donor with changes in the diet of the donor, mode of administration, etc., questioning the precision and reproducibility of FMT.

FMT has been the subject of serious safety concerns, particularly in the case of immunocompromised patients. Additionally, substantial negative effects brought on by the transmission of enteropathogenic bacteria linked to FMT that are donor-derived and drug-resistant have been identified, resulting in significant morbidity and one reported death (Lamousé-Smith et al., 2021). All these incidents point toward a highly cautious use of FMT.

Megaprojects such as the iHMP, HMP, and MetaHit projects have provided enormous sequence information up to the species and strain-level alterations in the microbial community composition in healthy individuals and various disease cohorts using advanced computational methods and machine learning techniques. Advances in cultivating the yet uncultured microbiota have also taken leaps, which have enabled the development of both bacterial culture collections and stool banks (Lamousé-Smith et al., 2021).

A logical choice for the development of microbial drugs with potentially safer and more effective responses would be the use of synthetic microbial consortia of well-defined strains that have demonstrated measurable characteristics to treat disease and are able to multiply in the recipient upon administration to maintain the homeostasis (Lamousé-Smith et al., 2021; Tan et al., 2020).

In patients with liver disease, bacterial urease in the intestine results in hyperammonemia-associated encephalopathy and neurotoxicity due to the conversion of urea to ammonia and carbon dioxide in the patient's liver. Shen et al. (2015) have developed the ASF, a defined consortium of eight bacteria with minimal urease gene content and engineered murine gut microbiota to reduce urease activity. After receiving an inoculation of ASF, mice that had lost the majority of the gut microbiota underwent a long-lasting decrease in fecal urease activity and ammonia generation. In a mouse model of hepatic damage, ASF transplantation was found to be related to lower morbidity and death.

Tanoue et al. (2019) have used information from metagenomic datasets to constitute a consortium of 11 rare, low-abundance human-associated strains of bacteria from fecal specimens of healthy individuals whose inclusion criteria was the ability to generate interferon-γ-producing CD8 T cells in the intestine. The 11 bacteria chosen have been shown to act synergistically, participate in the induction, and do not cause inflammation. These 11 bacteria were able to colonize mice and augment host resistance against infection by *Listeria monocytogenes* and improve the therapeutic efficacy of immune checkpoint inhibitors in syngenic tumor models.

The use of synthetic, defined, gut microbial consortia thus seems to be a promising strategy as an alternative to FMT, which needs to be explored further as a treatment modality for different diseases.

12.2.2.3 Engineering the Gut Bacteria

Synthetic biology involves the deletion of bacterial genes responsible for pathogenicity, as well as the introduction of new gene circuits for introducing particular function/s to the chassis organism. Apart from utilizing these top-down approaches and bottom-up strategies, San León and Nogales (2022) have proposed a middle-out strategy combining these strategies to engineer novel synthetic microbial communities that harbor improved performance and have a broader scope of application.

Transformation, conjugation, and transduction are well-known methods for introducing foreign DNA into bacteria. Bacteria are known to vary in their ability to take up foreign DNA attributed to differences in cell envelope structure and composition, which impacts the cell wall permeability. Their capacity to maintain and tolerate exogenous DNA also varies and depends on multiple factors required including machinery for replication of plasmids, DNA recombination, and genome defense. The development of a 'universal genetic modification toolbox' has been largely hindered for gut microbiota because of these factors.

Transformation is probably the most widely exploited method for introducing the therapeutic gene into gut bacteria due to its simple setup. Bacteria may be naturally competent to take up the foreign DNA, or competency may be induced using certain buffers and physiological conditions. Foreign DNA may also be introduced by electroporation which is electric pulse-mediated cell membrane permeabilization. Transformation has been conducted in some gut microbes, *Bacteroidetes*, *Enterococcus*, and *Lactobacillus*. However, conjugation and transduction are other possible options that have been used comparatively less. Transduction is hindered in gut bacteria owing to the availability of known transducing bacteriophages. Knowledge about defined origins of replication is required while using conjugation, many times lacking in the case of gut bacteria. While conjugation is the method of choice for gut microbiota, another possibility is the use of ICEs, which integrate efficiently in the bacterial DNA and spread through the machinery of host replication and do not require selection for maintenance (Chen et al., 2023).

The genome defense systems in the form of RM system and CRISPR–CAS have an important role in the maintenance of the introduced DNA. The strategy of maintaining plasmids in *E. coli* strains to develop methylation patterns' for getting rid of the RM system is often followed for this purpose (Figure 12.2).

2.3. Genome engineering strategies: The therapeutic gene may be inserted into an appropriate plasmid vector. Despite being effective, plasmids may be less preferred due to instability, copy

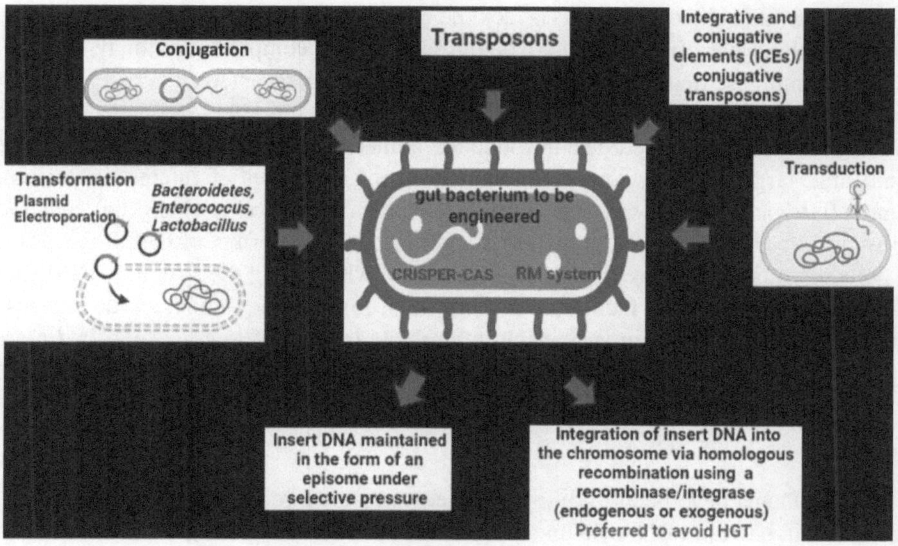

FIGURE 12.2 Methods to introduce the therapeutic gene into gut bacteria.

number variations, incompatible replication, requirement for constant pressure for selection, and concern about horizontal gene transfer. Systems that involve the integration of the foreign gene into bacterial chromosomes may solve many of these issues and hence are preferred. Genes can be deleted from or integrated into the bacterial chromosome using traditional double crossover homologous recombination methods. This method can even be used for poorly described bacteria, although the procedure is time-consuming and dependent on recombinogenic chassis organisms (Arnold et al., 2023).

Integrase-based systems can alternatively be used for the integration of the therapeutic gene. The *Bacteroides* mobilizable transposon integrase systems NBU1 and NBU2, which cause integration of foreign DNA within the host chromosome, are popular and utilized for engineering *Bacteroides*. Integration may also be mediated through the group II intron system, by using the Ll. LtrB group II intron from *Lactococcus lactis*. The 'ClosTron' technique, which is used to engineer numerous *Clostridium* species, relies on the intron-encoded protein LtrA to mediate self-insertion in a predetermined, target site in the host genome and which can be reprogrammed. 'Cre recombinase-lox P site'-based recombination is also being used for many host systems (Arnold et al., 2023).

12.2.3 The CRISPR–CAS System

The year 1987 witnessed a breakthrough invention of CRISPR (clustered regularly interspaced short palindromic repeats)-Cas system, which won the Nobel Prize in 2020 in the field of chemistry. CRISPR-CAS9 system was initially discovered as a bacterial adaptive immune mechanism that destroys previously encountered foreign DNA in the form of bacteriophages and plasmids, and it has now become a powerful gene modification tool in the form of 'genetic scissors' in various biological systems.

The Cas9-dependent type II-C system obtained from *Streptococcus pyogenes* was the first CRISPR–Cas system that was employed for gene engineering and is currently the most frequently utilized method. It comprises Cas9 nuclease (SpCas9) that acts along with an engineered sgRNA and guides SpCas9 to induce its activity after recognizing a target DNA sequence that is complementary to the sgRNA, which is adjacent to a PAM. DSBs are produced by activated SpCas9-sgRNA, and desirable insertions, deletions, and base substitutions are introduced by using the cellular DNA repair system. The majority of gut bacteria lack the necessary hardware to repair DSBs. As a result, exogenous recombinase is often required to be introduced. The components namely, sgRNA, nuclease, and the recombinase that are encoded on a plasmid are first transferred to the gut bacterium to be engineered for this purpose (Chen et al., 2023).

CRISPR-Cas9 has been used for introducing numerous genomic changes including insertions, small and large deletions, or single-point mutations in genes of interest in *Lactobacillus, Bacteroides, Enterococcus, Clostridium difficile* (as well as a few other clostridia), and *Klebsiella* to gain insight into the gene level, though off-targeting, the toxic effect of CRISPR-Cas9, and the induced double-strand breaks are the major issues faced while using the system. CRISPRi, a novel knockdown approach, has also facilitated a novel, high-throughput, genome-wide screens for the determination of gene function in various gut microbiota including *Bacillus subtilis, Enterobacter cloacae, E. coli*, and *Lactobacillus plantarum* (Chen et al., 2023).

12.2.4 Transposable Elements

Transposable elements have been traditionally used to insert foreign DNA sequences and disrupt genes of interest in bacterial DNA. To anticipate the function of different genetic elements in bacterial DNA, transposons have also been utilized in TIS techniques, which combine powerful genome-wide mutagenesis using transposons with high-throughput sequencing. To assign gene function and link phenotype to genotype, several variations of TIS have been used, including Tn-Seq, INSeq, TraDIS, HITS, and coupling of Tn-Seq with random DNA barcoding of each mutant (RB-TnSeq) (Cain et al., 2020; Chen et al., 2023).

To discover genetically tractable components, Rubin et al (2022) have recently devised a unique method called ET-seq, using non-targeted transposon insertions that were located and quantified after transferring to the microbial consortium. Post this, DART systems were used for precise DNA incorporation into cells of the organisms detected as 'tractable' by ET-seq. The technology has enabled 'organism-specific' as well as 'locus-specific' genetic manipulation in a community setting. It also allows for the incorporation of species- and site-specific alterations in a number of bacteria of the infant gut microbiota, as well as the measurement of gene fitness in a non-model bacterium and enrichment of the desired species. Importantly, the system does not require in vitro cultivation of the bacteria, a significant point, in view of the majority of gut bacteria remaining uncultivated so far.

Therapeutic gene expression in the chassis system also needs to be optimized to the required level. This has been obtained by the appropriate use of suitable systems in the form of promoters, transcription termination signals, codon usage, RBS engineering, and riboswitches (Arnold et al., 2023).

12.2.4.1 The Sense and Response Systems

Numerous studies have demonstrated the use of constitutive promoters to express therapeutic products from inserted foreign genes (Ho et al., 2018; Praveschotinunt et al., 2019; Rottinghaus et al., 2019), wherein the strength of the constitutive promoter is an important criterion to be considered (Ozdemir et al., 2018). Ozdemir et al. (2018) have tabulated various studies that have utilized constitutive therapeutic delivery systems. Once expressed to the required extent, the release of the therapeutically active form from the genetically engineered microbe into the milieu is another factor that merits attention. It can be attained either by cell lysis to liberate the therapeutic; or by secreting it out. Lysis is a less preferred method; as it requires a complex regulatory system to ensure lysis after sufficient protein has been produced or once a desired population density has been reached. Secretion mechanism is often used which makes use of ABC transporters in the bacterium, Sec systems, and the flagellar secretion apparatus (Ozdemir et al., 2018).

Although constitutively expressing the therapeutic gene is a quite straightforward strategy, it may lead to undesired expression in non-targeted tissues, exhibiting off-target effects with dangerous outcomes. By administrating an auxotrophic, invasive, and non-pathogenic *E. coli* to a mouse model through the oral route, Castagliuolo et al. (2005) successfully delivered a therapeutic gene to the colonic mucosa. As a consequence of mucosal barrier disruption during colitis, vector-specific mRNA transcripts could be recovered from the colon as well as from extra-colonic tissues. The problem was later solved by adopting an inflammation-induced promoter instead of the conventional constitutive promoter.

Such off-target effects of engineered bacteria might be more likely when administered intravenously. Systems that can detect environmental signals and respond in the form of regulated expression have been designed, which promote the production and targeting of therapeutic proteins to specific locations by accurate sensing of environmental stimuli, followed by feedback-regulated expression to prevent overproduction. Insulation of promoters and RBS to decrease the contextual effects of the neighboring DNA sequences, along with the development of customized transcriptional and translational elements, has helped derive robust systems with highly controllable and predictable expression (Ozdemir et al., 2018).

Sense and response systems in which the expression can be regulated in a desired manner offer many advantages as compared to the constitutive expression approach. Herein, the system can detect a stimulus in the form of detectable molecules or conditions in the host environment, or externally provided signals, to produce a designated response. High-level heterologous protein expression, for example, may burden the cellular system, leading to the accumulation of mutations. Biosensor systems with regulated expression, in contrast, provide better genetic stability of the engineered cell. Protein production in the body in a location-selective and disease-responsive manner can minimize the 'off-target effects' of the proteins, including toxicity and resistance due to accumulation. Biosensor systems also provide opportunities for biocontainment of the engineered microbe (Rottinghaus et al., 2019).

Biosensing is a highly promising approach in synthetic biology and tremendous work is going on to develop systems that sense a particular input to provide output in a finely regulated manner. 'Controllability over-engineered behaviors' and 'scalability of the engineered systems' are key aspects of these systems. The construction of finely tuneable switches that respond to different signals lies at the heart of sense and response systems. Many groups of scientists have been working on designing such elements that sense varied environmental signals in the form of particular temperature, light, chemical/biological compounds, etc., and exhibit anticipated response, for example, in vivo release of the therapeutic at the desired dose/location in the body/particular time.

Huang et al. (2016) have developed 'Swarmbot Technology': A combination of 'spatial arrangement to control the population dynamics' of a genetically engineered microbe with 'environment sensing'. *E. coli*, with added synthetic circuits encapsulated in permeable membranes can sense the local environment and respond consequently. The engineered microbe could thrive only when present at sufficiently high numbers in the milieu, cells escaping the capsule were killed as a result of reduced cell density. Thus, the system ensured the prevention of unintentional proliferation of the engineered bacteria, taking care of the safety concern.

To accurately control artificial circuits in animal tissues, Piraner et al. (2017) created 'temperature-inducible' bio-switches. TlpA, a *Salmonella typhimurium* transcriptional repressor, and TcI, a temperature-sensitive bacteriophage repressor, were able to trigger a thirtyfold induction of the reporter gene in response to a slight rise in temperature. They further produced mutant variants of these to fine-tune the activation threshold of each switch. The method was also paired with a gene encoding a bacterial toxin, creating a 'kill switch' that allowed altered bacteria to survive at the temperatures present in the digestive tract but caused them to perish upon expulsion. This created a biocontainment strategy for the engineered bacteria.

Naydich et al. (2019) have described gene expression platforms for varied human gut *Bacteroides*, which upon induction, can modulate the expression of genes up to 9,000-fold. By varying the inducer concentration, gene expression inside the gut could be regulated across three orders of magnitude and also completely repressed in vivo. Importantly, these panels have been shown to act even across diverse human gut *Bacteroides*.

TABLE 12.3
Studies Using Sense and Response Systems

Infection/Disease	Chassis Organism	Model System Tested	Input Signal	Engineered Gene	Output Signal	Result	References
Pseudomonas aeruginosa gut infections	Sense-kill genetic system in *E. coli* Nissle 1917	In vivo: *Caenorhabditis elegans*, mouse	*P. aeruginosa* release of N-acyl homoserine lactone (quorum-sensing system)	Anti-biofilm hydrolase, antimicrobial protein pyocin, *Pseudomonas*	Expression of cloned genes	Prophylactic and antimicrobial effects against *P. aeruginosa* infection	Hwang et al. (2017)
Antibiotic-resistant *Vibrio cholerae* in complex populations	Toxin-intein antimicrobial in donor strain *E. coli* β3914	In vivo: zebrafish and crustacean larvae	Master transcriptional activator ToxR	Conjugative plasmid carrying gyrase that inhibits CcdB toxin of *Vibrio fischeri*	Expression of cloned genes	Antibiotic-resistant *V. cholerae* receiving the plasmid were killed completely	López-Igual et al. (2020)
Crohn's disease	Pesudotactic *E. coli*	In vitro	Nitric oxide, a biomarker for Crohn's disease	Pore-forming protein Tol AIII+ granulocyte macrophage colony-stimulating factor (GM-CSF)	Expression of cloned genes	'Smart' probiotics for the treatment of Crohn's disease	McKay et al. (2018)
Inflammatory bowel disease (IBD)	*Saccharomyces cerevisiae*	Mouse	eATP generated in the inflamed gut during the course of the disease	Human P2Y2 purinergic receptor with ~1,000-fold increase in eATP sensitivity	Secretion of ATP-degrading enzyme apyrase, depleting the pro-inflammatory eATP and increasing the levels of immunosuppressive adenosine	Development of self-tunable anti-inflammatory probiotics	Scott et al. (2021)

Salmonella typhimurium infection	*Escherichia coli* Nissle	In vitro	Tetrathionate, a molecule generated in the inflamed gut during the course of *Salmonella* infection	Plasmid-producing microcin H47	Release of *S. typhimurium*-inhibiting microcin	Inhibition of *Salmonella* growth in the presence of tetrathionate	Palmer et al. (2018)
Candida albicans infection	*E. coli*	In vitro	Hydroxyphenylacetic acid (HPA) secreted by *Candida albicans*	HPA sensor coupled with the generation of cis-2-dodecenoic acid	Inhibition of expression of virulence gene and filamentation in *C. albicans*	Inhibition of hyphae formation and filamentation, virulence factor expression, and fungal-induced epithelial damage; protection of epithelial cells from fungal-mediated damage	Tscherner et al. (2019)
Vibrio cholerae infection	Wild-type *E. coli*	In vitro	Quorum-sensing molecule '*S*-3-hydroxytridecan-4-one' produced by *V. cholerae*	Expression of green fluorescent protein	Lysis protein 'Artilysin', an engineered fusion product of the outer membrane-targeting peptide and endolysin	Development of sense-and-kill probiotic	Jayaraman et al. (2017)
Infection by *Enterococcus faecalis* and multidrug-resistant *Enterococcus faecium*	*Lactococcus lactis*	In vitro	Enterococcal sex pheromone cCF10	cCF10-responsive conjugative plasmid and genes for bacteriocins: hiracin JM79, enterocin A, and enterocin P	Expression of bacteriocins	Detection of naturally produced cCF10 and bateriocins by *E. faecalis*	Borrero et al. (2015)

Designing accurately controllable and precisely expressing sense and response systems requires designing complex regulatory gene networks that process sensory information to control biological functions. Today, computational algorithms are being used to program such complex regulatory networks. Nielsen et al. (2016) have developed 'Cello', a hardware description language for programming living cells. It is based on Verilog for implementing the design of gene circuits that perform Boolean logic functions and applied principles of electronic design automation for enhancing the complexity of the circuit that is harnessed into the synthetic gene regulation. The user is required to specify the sensors, actuators, and 'user constraints file' specific to the organism, gate technology, and valid operating conditions. Cello then uses this input to design a specific DNA sequence encoding the desired circuit via a set of algorithms that parse the Verilog text, create the circuit diagram, assign gates, balance constraints to build the DNA, and simulate performance. Such circuits permit the integration of several stimuli for better control over therapeutic delivery. Transcriptional logic gates as well as translational logic circuits are being developed with ever-increasing complexity using such tools. The incorporation of modules that demonstrate different functionalities, such as memory, oscillation, counting, and orthogonal communication, can be increased (Ozdemir et al., 2018).

12.2.4.2 Microbial Cell Factories

Microbial cell factories use microbes that are engineered to harbor genes and circuits for metabolic pathways, or produce chemicals (proteins, metabolites) for the prevention and treatment of disease, as a 'production facility'. Using bacterial cells in the form of minicells, BGs or BMVs have unique advantages in drug delivery. Bacterial cells perform numerous biochemical reactions subsequent to drug delivery. These activities may be occurring naturally or may be engineered. Also, bacterial cells are self-sustainable and function based on their genetic material. Modification in the bacterial cell structure to adapt to the environment or modification of its genetic material makes them best suited as highly specific and sustainable delivery systems. Also, bacterial cells can interact with the surrounding milieu facilitating a precise response that could be otherwise challenging to mimic using the current system of drug delivery. Moreover, bacterial cells can inhabit the oral cavity, nasal cavity, and skin apart from the GI tract and thus can target a wide array of diseases (Shen et al., 2022). Representative studies using gut bacteria as cell factories for disease treatment have been briefed below.

Many studies have used gut microbiota for the treatment of the autosomal recessive genetic disorder phenylketonuria, in which an individual cannot metabolize phenylalanine due to mutation in the gene encoding PAH enzyme, resulting in neurotoxicity. If phenylketonuria is managed with treatment provided in the early stages of life, it is possible to mitigate severe neurological disorders. Diet modification (protein-restricted diets with amino acids supplemented with trace elements to prevent nutritional deficits) and the use of co-factors that increase the activity of phenylalanine-degrading enzymes, for example, sapoterin dihydrochloride, have been the traditional strategies for the treatment of PKU. These approaches, however, were insufficient to treat phenylketonuria.

In 2018, Isabella and her colleagues conducted genetic modifications on *Escherichia coli* Nissle 1917 (EcN), enabling it to express phenylalanine-metabolizing genes when exposed to low-oxygen conditions within the mammalian intestinal tract. The synthetic strain, 'SYNB1618' is plasmid- and antibiotic-resistance-free and can express relevant enzymes to decrease the levels of phenylalanine in the body. The probiotic not only showed promising results in animal models but is being evaluated in phase-2 clinical trials.

Durrer et al. (2017) cloned the gene coding for phenylalanine lyase from *Anabaena variabilis* (AvPAL) into *Lactobacillus reuteri* expressed under the control of *Lactobacillus* high production constitutive promoter. Experiments with animal models indicated reduced blood phenylalanine levels within three to four days of treatment with the engineered bacteria. The eventual loss of the engineered probiotic from the gut of treated animals, as well as the absence of any immune response to the engineered bacteria, indicated their safe use.

Although these studies open the possibility of utilizing a novel probiotic that is obtained by genetic engineering as a promising therapeutic modality for PKU, limited transmembrane transport of phenylalanine has been noticed limiting the optimal utility of the activity of the probiotic. To address this issue, Jiang et al. (2022) facilitated the expression of phenylalanine-metabolizing enzyme phenylalanine ammonia-lyase in two forms as 'intracellularly free' as well as 'cell surface-immobilized' enzyme in EcN. This led to the simultaneous degradation of phenylalanine, both intracellularly and extracellularly, thus addressing the challenge of phenylalanine transportation. Administration of the synthetic strain in mice decreased the levels of phenylalanine by 44.4% in the blood, independent of the protein consumption from the diet of the mice.

Many studies have focused on engineered gut microbiota for the treatment of obesity. In one such experiment, N-acyl phosphatidylethanolamines (NAPEs), the naturally occurring lipid satiety factors, were introduced into *E. coli* Nissle 1917. Mice who were fed a diet high in fat and administered genetically engineered bacteria in drinking water displayed less obesity, less food intake, insulin resistance, and hepatosteatosis than control mice. Furthermore, even after the synthetic probiotic was removed from the water source, the protective benefits continued for at least 4 weeks (Chen et al., 2014). Butyrate is known to be a key molecule in carbohydrate and fat metabolism, augmenting insulin secretion and reducing appetite, and playing a major role in the host gut-microbe metabolism axis. In another study, Wang et al. (2022) engineered *B. subtilis* to produce butyrate as a probiotic to prevent obesity. The altered strain was successful in lowering the rate of weight gain due to high-fat diets, improving insulin and glucose tolerance, modifying the composition of the gut microbiome, and altering the human metabolic pathways.

IBD is a chronic disorder that results in inflammation of the intestines and other parts of the digestive system. Although its specific cause is unknown, the ailment is thought to be an autoimmune condition where the body's immune system assaults healthy tissues in the digestive tract. Bloating, diarrhea, rectal bleeding, weight loss, anemia, abscesses, and fistulas are a few symptoms of IBD, with a higher probability of developing colon cancer. Although anti-inflammatory or immunosuppressive medications are presently used to treat IBD, Crohn's disease, and ulcerative colitis, they exhibit low efficacy and unfavorable outcomes.

The use of *L. lactis* which secretes anti-TNFα nanobody as well as other pro-inflammatory cytokine antibodies has been administered through the oral route and has been demonstrated to be a promising alternative for treating IBD without adverse effects. Apart from IL-10, LAB have also been used for the delivery of other anti-inflammatory cytokines like IL27 (Bron & Kleerebezem, 2018). Škrlec et al. (2018) have used engineered *L. lactis* as a vector to deliver BPC-157, a peptide with anti-inflammatory and antioxidant properties that does its function owing to display on the cell membrane and release by protease action or by secretion for treatment of IBD.

Contribution of engineered microbes has been analyzed in treatment of neuroinflammtory disorders. GLP-1 affects the central nervous system and has limited utility in the clinic due to its extremely short half-life. Chen et al. (2018) engineered two strains continuously expressing GLP-1 and intervention with these. These strains caused significant restoration of the spatial learning and memory deficit in mice, inhibited activation of glia and accumulation of Aβ, and downregulated levels of inflammatory mediators COX-2, TLR-4, TNF-a, and IL-1β. These observations indicate the safe and effective use of these genetically engineered microbes for neuroinflammation-related disorders such as AD.

Hyperuricemia is the second-largest metabolic disorder, resulting in increased levels of uric acid in serum, further leading to chronic kidney disease, cardiovascular disease, gout, and diabetes. Zhao et al. (2022) have developed a recombinant urate-degrading EcN containing a plasmid with a gene cassette encoding proteins required for metabolism of uric acid. The gene cassette in their study consisted of genes PucL and PucM from *B. subtilis*, known to catalyze a three-step uric acid degradation pathway. KatG gene from *E. coli* coding for enzyme catalase efficiently removed PucL-generated H_2O_2 back to O_2. The gene for bacterial hemoglobin Vhb from *Vitreoscilla* sp. was incorporated to degrade urate at low-oxygen levels. YgfU gene from *E. coli*, a proton gradient-dependent transporter for urate, was also added to the cassette, which increased urate uptake and compensated for the low affinity of the engineered enzyme toward urate. The recombinant strain effectively lowered the serum uric acid under normal oxygen and hypoxic (prevailing in animal intestine) conditions in mice, when administered in the gut or injected into the blood vessel.

The degradation of angiotensin II to angiotensin-(1-7) is catalyzed by the enzyme ACE2, resulting in decreased inflammation and oxidative stress that is augmented by angiotensin II. ACE2 thus plays a protective role in cardiovascular and metabolic diseases. Large-scale production of high-quality ACE2 is hindered due to sufficient target tissue bioavailability. This limitation has been overcome by Verma et al. (2019) by engineering *Lactobacillus paracasei* to utilize it as a live vector for oral delivery of human ACE2. *L. paracasei* efficiently expressed codon-optimized ACE2 as a fusion protein comprising of non-toxic subunit B of cholera toxin, which served as a carrier for transmucosal transport. Mice treated with the recombinant probiotic showed increased ACE2 activities in serum and tissues. Better tissue availability of ACE-2 also reduced diabetic complications in mice with diabetic retinopathy.

Probiotics have also been used for in situ production of vaccines. Gao et al. (2019) designed GM *Lactobacillus casei* (strain pPG-α/*L. casei* 393) constitutively expressing the α-toxin of *C. perfringens*. After oral administration of the probiotic vaccine to mice, the α-toxoid was reported to be constitutively expressed to provide significant immune protection by eliciting mucosal, humoral, and cellular immunity. Chamcha et al. (2015) also developed an oral probiotic vaccine against HIV using GM *Lactococcus lactis*, expressing the HIV-1 Gag-p24 fusion protein on the tip of the T3 pilus of *S. pyogenes*. Strong HIV-specific mucosal, humoral, and cellular immune responses in mice were reported indicating the prophylactic potential of the probiotic vaccine.

The probiotic bacteria thus hold a strong potential to serve as microbial cell factories for the in situ production of therapeutic proteins.

12.2.4.3 Bacteria as Chassis for Drug Delivery

In synthetic biology, the term 'chassis' denotes an organism that hosts and maintains the designed DNA construct(s) required for a specific function. The metabolic network of the selected chassis should express the engineered extraneous DNA/genetic component/s and support its function. It should ideally exhibit robust growth, uncomplicated regulation of gene expression, and no evolutionary process that could otherwise compromise the function of the exogenous gene circuits (Figure 12.3) (Mugwanda et al., 2023).

Various bacteria, viz. particular strains of *S. typhimurium*, *Listeria* spp., *Clostridium novyi*, and *E. coli*, by flagella and tactic responses, are well known to inherently target and colonize tumors, suppress cancerous growth and metastasis, and prolong survival after systemic infection in animal models of cancer (Duong et al., 2019; Feng et al., 2023). This unique ability to target and colonize tumors is a highly significant trait in cancer treatment, as the cell membranes of solid cancers are otherwise difficult to penetrate by functional proteins that can target critical cancer pathways (Zhou & Han, 2022). Conventional and modern treatment approaches face trouble due to the trafficking of the nanoparticles and proteins from early and late endosomes to lysosomes and their

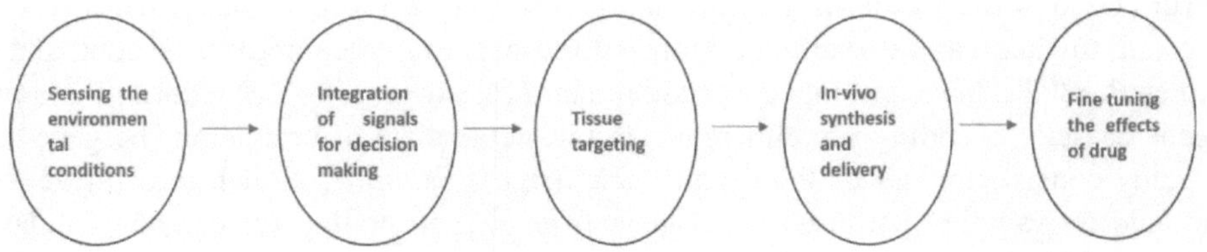

FIGURE 12.3 Steps involved in chassis development for drug delivery.

further degradation after cellular uptake. Bacterial systems mentioned earlier, importantly, are not limited by these mechanisms (Raman et al., 2021).

Strains of bacteria like *L. monocytogenes* or *Salmonella* spp. have been produced by attenuation or deletion of the virulence genes, which display reduced virulence and are used as 'chassis' for precise drug delivery to tumors. Owing to their affinity toward tumors, they might overcome the limitation of cellular penetration and thus optimize the therapeutic impact of the chemotherapeutic drugs while reducing the systemic toxicity to the individual undergoing therapy.

Genetic engineering has been applied to such 'chassis' organisms for multiple applications, obtaining attenuated strains without affecting their antitumor activity, introduction of particular nutrient-dependent mutations along with attenuation, as well as enhancement of tumor targeting. These tumor-targeting bacteria have served as chassis to deliver cytokines, cytotoxic compounds, immunomodulators, and enzymes that act upon and activate prodrugs, compounds that target tumor stroma and small interfering RNAs. Control over time, dose, and site for the release/in vivo production of the drug may also be achieved by using appropriate modules for the regulation of gene expression.

Various tumor-characteristic properties like hypoxia, acidosis, reduced glucose concentration due to the Warburg effect, and necrosis have been used for tumor targeting and regulation of gene expression, for example, the activation of hypoxia-inducible promoters by reduction of metabolites nitrate and fumarate in the hypoxic environment within tumor tissue, especially within the hypoxia rich regions within the tumor (Duong et al., 2019). The use of such tumor-targeting engineered 'smart bacteria' along with other cancer treatment strategies like chemotherapy, radiotherapy, and immunotherapy might prove to be a promising strategy for combating cancer. A few significant studies using bacteria as chassis for cancer treatment have been briefed next.

Ho et al. (2018) reprogrammed commensal EcN as a chassis for treating CRC, in view of its natural ability to prevent IBD and colonize the colon. The bacteria were engineered to bind specifically to the heparan sulfate proteoglycan on CRC cells and secrete myrosinase for the conversion of dietary glucosinolate to sulforaphane. The sulforaphane thus produced could inhibit growth and promote apoptosis in cancer cells. As a biocontainment strategy, the genetically engineered microorganisms were detached from the colorectal tissue upon clearance, and released in the feces. Cancer cell inhibition in vitro, smaller tumor size, and a seven-fold reduction in tumor occurrence in the murine CRC model were observed. Interestingly, the engineered probiotic could either be used as a supplement in the diet, along with a regular diet rich in cruciferous vegetables that are naturally rich in glucosinolate, which prevents CRC, or augment recovery post treatment in patients with CRCs.

Research by Raman et al. (2021) could be cited as an excellent example of using engineered tumor-targeting bacteria for cancer control. The authors have designed a non-pathogenic, therapeutic strain of 'ID *Salmonella*' to deliver proteins into solid cancers. The strain has been constituted by using genetic circuits to precisely regulate synthesis of protein drug, cellular invasiveness, and subsequent release of the protein drug. Instead of delivering synthesized drug/s, a novel strategy was utilized, wherein the organisms penetrated the tumor, divided at the site, and synthesized the drug in situ. This achieved multiple-fold higher drug concentrations at the target site. The released proteins were observed to be spread through the entire cytoplasm, remain bioactive, and interact with the specific cellular target molecules. The specially designed genetic circuit to autonomously promote protein release independent of external intervention led to protein drug delivery at the most appropriate time for each bacterium and ensured drug deposition only inside the cells and not in the extracellular milieu, avoiding toxic effects of the drug to normal cells and its release in healthy organs. Interestingly, after tumor invasion, when particular numbers of the strain were reached, lysis of the 'ID *Salmonella*' got triggered, thus making the strain self-limiting and safer than non-lysing Salmonellae. Notably, the use of the developed strain was reported to be safe, reduce tumor growth and metastasis, and increase survival in mouse models.

Wick et al. (2018) have developed an engineered strain of *Salmonella typhi*, VXM01, that was able to synthesize vascular endothelial growth factor-2, which is under clinical trials for the treatment of recurrent glioblastoma. The study explored the efficacy of the combination of *Salmonella typhi*, VXM01 with Avelumab (a checkpoint inhibitor), after administration of the standard treatment (Rutter et al., 2022).

Several studies on the effectiveness of engineered bacteria-based drug delivery systems that can improve the efficiency and accuracy of drug delivery in the treatment of cancer have shown encouraging results, many of which are being tested in clinical trials as well. However, according to clinical experimental data, the use of modified bacteria alone is not enough to treat tumors. Combining them with other therapies may yield better results (Feng et al., 2023).

Live bacteria have been used as chassis for drug delivery in the treatment of pathogenic infection, IBD, and metabolic diseases as well; these have been tabulated by Tan et al. (2020).

Naked nucleic acids like cDNAs and silencing RNAs used for therapeutic purposes are known to exhibit limited permeability through the cell membrane of cancer cells. 'Bactofection' is the use of live bacteria as vectors to deliver the DNA encoding therapeutic proteins in human cells. Bactofection has applications to administer either DNA encoding therapeutic proteins or tumor antigens. The bacteria used as vectors either are passively acquired by the immune cells or actively invade the cancer cells. *Salmonella* spp. and *L. monocytogenes* are used chassis for bactofection with applications in cancer treatment. Liang et al. (2018) constructed an attenuated mutant strain of *S. typhimurium* expressing anti-angiogenic agent 'endostatin' to inhibit tumor growth. Suppressed tumor growth, increased apoptosis, inhibition of angiogenesis within tumor tissues, and improved survival were noted in CT26 colon carcinoma and B16F10 melanoma mouse models.

12.2.4.4 Gut Bacteria in HM Poisoning

Environmental pollution by humans has led to increased concentrations of HMs like arsenic, cadmium, mercury, lead, aluminum, and chromium in water, air, and soil, building up their concentration in the food chain. This leads to their accumulation in plants and aquatic animals, which when consumed by humans leads to various adverse effects (Arun et al., 2021). HMs affect organs like the liver, kidneys, and lungs as well as various biochemical processes. When present in dangerous amounts, they have an effect on the nervous, circulatory, respiratory, and excretory systems of the organism. Neurons and muscles may deteriorate as a result of HM bioaccumulation, giving rise to symptoms that resemble those of Parkinson's and ADs, muscular dystrophy, and multiple sclerosis. Over time, DNA is destroyed by HM exposure, which eventually leads to cancer (Arun et al., 2021).

Human gut microbiota is known to be sensitive to high concentrations of HMs, which affects their growth, leading to dysbiosis. This in turn might be responsible for various diseases like IBD, cancers, atherosclerosis, obesity, liver diseases, kidney diseases, cardiac diseases, autism, epilepsy, and atopic dermatitis (Arun et al., 2021).

Several gut bacteria can inherently help in conditions of HM intoxication. The peptidoglycan and teichoic acids in bacterial cell walls can bind to the HM through ion-exchange interactions, nucleation reactions leading to precipitation, or complex formation via oxygen and nitrogen ligands. Organisms like *Pseudomonas* produce siderophores that can bind to iron as well as other HMs. Many different mechanisms such as decrease in pH, production of exopolysaccharides that bind the HM, alteration of physiological conditions, permeability of the gut, and production of enzymes for metabolism of HMs are employed by different gut bacteria to ameliorate the effects of HMs. Bacteria like *Lactobacillus species* can scavenge peroxide, superoxide, and hydroxyl free radicals, while *Bifidobacterium animalis* and *Lactobacillus rhamnosus* exhibit antioxidant activities, helping in dealing with oxidative stress (Monachese et al., 2012; Arun et al., 2021). In view of these inherent mechanisms, these gut bacteria seem to be a promising engineering chassis for designing next-generation probiotics with beneficial properties for heavy metal detoxification.

12.2.4.5 Gut Bacteria in Nanotechnology

Due to the nano-size and unique characteristics, nanomaterials have revolutionized the biomedical field by providing breakthrough applications in the form of mRNA vaccines using lipid nanoparticles for COVID-19, wearable smart sensors, devices, and wireless bandages that augment the healing of wounds. Thus, the technology holds huge promise in developing next-generation medical devices. Despite this promising scenario, nanomaterials possess certain pitfalls. Due to their nano-size, they are highly reactive, and readily interact with biomolecules when in contact with a physiological fluid. This in turn may lead to changes in their properties, leading to an unpredictable behavior and performance of the nano-system. Loss of active targeting, toxicity, changes in biodistribution, and changed pharmacological characteristics are a few serious consequences of this issue (Lateef et al., 2021).

Bacteria and fungi are known to play an important role in reactions such as oxidation, reduction, bio-absorption, and precipitation of metal ions even in the presence of high concentrations of dangerous metal ions, as previously described. They can not only create metal nanoparticles but also change metal into a non-toxic state. Gold, silver, silver-gold alloy, titanium oxide, selenium, tellurium, iron oxide, zinc oxide, and magnesium oxide nanoparticles have all been produced using probiotic bacteria species such as *Lactobacillus*, *Bacillus*, *Enterococcus*, and *Rhodobacter*. Nanoparticles synthesized by *Bifidobacterium* especially have been known to have antimicrobial, catalytic, anticoagulant, thrombolytic, cholesterol-reducing, antitumor, nano-preservative, larvicidal, antioxidant, and nutrient supplementing properties (Lateef et al., 2021). Gut bacteria, thus, have been used to synthesize nanomaterials.

Gold nanoparticles have been used in a novel application for tumor regression by the development of 'bacteria-mediated photothermal therapy'. *E. coli* MG1655 expressing antitumor molecules like TNF-α and cytolysin A in response to heat was decorated with photothermal gold nanoparticles. After the oral administration of engineered bacteria, NIR lasers were applied to kill the tumor cells. Upon irradiation, the gold nanoparticles absorbed and converted transdermal photons into local heat, which activated the expression of tumor-inhibiting molecules in the bacteria, leading to significant tumor killing as observed in mice models of breast cancer and colon cancer (Fan et al., 2018; Wang et al., 2021).

Apart from their use in nano-material synthesis, as well as sense and respond systems, gut bacteria themselves can also be used as alternative nano-carriers by virtue of inherent properties like self-propulsion and tactic responses. Bacteria have been used as nanomaterials in the form of BGs, minicells, and MVs. All of these represent bacteria-derived achromosomal particles, smaller than bacterial cells and having the size of nanoparticles (approximately 100 nm). They are widely employed as live, programmable drug delivery vehicles, better stable in physiological conditions as compared to chemically synthesized lipid particles. It is noteworthy that they do not possess the ability to replicate owing to lack of genomic DNA, but possess parts of the bacterial cell structure and function, an important consideration for safe and targeted drug delivery. They can also serve as carriers to deliver foreign antigens to antigen-presenting cells and augment the immune response, thus serving as potential vaccine candidates (Shen et al., 2022).

BGs are empty cell envelopes of bacterial cells that are formed by the bacteriophage φX174 lytic protein E in gram-negative bacteria, or using chemicals in gram-positive bacteria, 1–2 μm in size. Minicells, on the contrary, are nanosized bacterial cells, 100 to 400 nm, that are naturally produced during aberrant cell divisions (Shen et al., 2022). Minicells have been widely used for drug delivery in cancer treatment.

The miR-15/16 family has been reported to be highly downregulated with tumor suppressor function in MPM. miR-16 expression restoration was used as a novel approach for a therapeutic strategy for MPM by Reid et al. (2013), who administered miR-16 mimics packaged in minicells intravenously to xenograft-bearing nude mice resulting in the suppression of MPM tumors.

Whittle et al. (2015) have also synthesized exclusive minicells with bispecific proteins linked to the surface that target malignancies. Doxorubicin was encapsulated in these minicells in effective concentrations for chemotherapeutic application. Tumor regression was reported in mouse xenograft models of breast, lung, ovarian, and colon cancer with no evidence of toxicity. The ability of the system to pack a high concentration of up to one million drug molecules into a minicell was an added advantage.

Hancock et al. (2016) used intravesicle administration of VAX014 minicells as a post-operative adjuvant therapy for treating non-muscle invasive bladder cancer. VAX014 minicells represent recombinant *E. coli* bacterial minicells engineered to express invasin from *Yersinia pseudotuberculosis* to selectively target and deliver the bacterial protein toxin, PFO. VAX014 was observed to permeabilize target cell plasma membranes to simultaneously induce apoptosis and have a quick death rate for dissociated urothelial carcinoma cells. Single-dose in vivo pharmacology tests also indicated its ability to stop cancer growth, thus enhancing survival.

Until now, BCG was the only FDA-approved bacterium for non-muscle invasive bladder cancer. However, adverse cardiovascular complications have been reported due to systemic wrong dose administration of bacterial vectors. Bacteria-derived particles, due to their small size and inability to replicate and cause infection, in contrast, prove to be a safer alternative. Notably, minicells have been proven safe for systemic administration of drugs in three phase I clinical trials (Shen et al., 2022).

BMVs: BMVs represent bacteria-derived lipid-based spherical nanoparticles smaller than minicells, 20 to 400 nm in size. Most bacteria are naturally known to produce BMVs, which transport different cargo molecules to play a significant role in intercellular communication. Based on their origin, BMVs could be of different types, viz. OMVs, EOMVs, CMVs, and OIMVs (Shen et al., 2022).

Although BMVs are looked upon as alternative drug delivery vehicles, loading them with high concentrations of therapeutics through recombinant expression and contamination with bacterial endogenous impurities are major issues to be addressed (Shen et al., 2022).

12.2.4.6 Probiotic Micro-devices for Drug Delivery

For the efficacy of probiotic formulation, it is important to have viable probiotic bacteria at the point of consumption. There are reports that showed that probiotic bacteria have very short life spans in products they incorporate. Based on this observation, many have questioned the possibility of survival of these bacteria in the human gut. An approach that has recently become popular is microencapsulation, providing a physical barrier against adverse environmental conditions to these probiotic living cells increasing their chance of survival. Methods of microencapsulation of probiotic bacteria include spray drying, extrusion, emulsion, and phase separation.

Probiotic bacteria have been microencapsulated using kappa-carrageenan, gelatin, gellan gum, and starch, calcium alginate being the most widely used. Microencapsulation offers various advantages as compared to immobilization/entrapment procedures. The microcapsule provides a spherical, thin, robust, and semipermeable membranous wall to hold bacterial cells inside. Probiotic microorganisms can be subjected to small-scale laboratory processes using emulsion, extrusion, and/or coacervation after microencapsulation. It has, however, been difficult to produce enormous quantities of shelf-stable, viable probiotic bacterial cells required for industrial use for the creation of novel products (Kailasapathy, 2015).

Microencapsulated probiotics have been assessed in colon cancer therapeutics. A microencapsulated formulation of *L. acidophilus* was investigated for its possible antitumorigenic effects in Min (multiple intestinal neoplasia) mice with a germline Apc mutation, which naturally produces a number of pretumoric intestinal neoplasms (Prakash et al., 2011).

The efficacy of microencapsulated microbes has been evaluated for cardiovascular diseases as well. Bacterial cell-filled microcapsules were tested as a treatment strategy for decreasing cholesterol. Preliminary studies have implied that some lactobacilli possess a BSH enzyme that can significantly decrease cholesterol in vivo in cardiovascular disorders.

Numerous varieties of microcapsules are utilized for the targeted delivery of probiotic bacteria such as alginate–cellulose acetate phthalate, alginate–chitosan, alginate–chitosan–AcrylEze, alginate–chitosan alginate, alginate–chitosan Sureteric, alginate-coated gelatin, alginate–poly-l-lysine alginate, alginate–starch, gelatin–gum arabic–soluble starch, gelatin–toluene-2-4-diisocyanate, gellan–alginate, gellan–xanthan, genipin-crosslinked alginate–chitosan, pectin–casein, potato starch granules–amylose, and whey protein.

Extensive basic research followed by clinical trials is required to demonstrate the safety and efficacy of microencapsulated probiotic formulations. Nevertheless, probiotics are promising therapeutic formulations for the treatment and/or prevention of an array of human diseases.

12.2.4.7 GM Gut Microbiota under Clinical Trials

The microbiome-based therapeutic market has changed from 'emerging' to 'developing' as a result of clinical evidence and industrial partnerships, as proclaimed by GlobalData Pharmaceuticals. GlobalData also forecasts the market to be $1.554 billion in 2026. Oncology, dermatology, GI disease, and infectious disease are among the therapeutic areas of interest, which account for 33.3%, 24.0%, 16.0%, and 13.0% of the total products, respectively (https://www.clinicaltrialsarena.com/comment/microbiome-therapeutics-immuno-oncology-agents/). Genetically engineered microbes that have been created by addition, deletion, or alteration of the DNA of an organism, referred to as recombinant LBPs, are getting tested for their efficacy through multiple clinical trials.

Phase 1b, a multi-center, single-blinded, placebo-controlled trial was performed on locally advanced head and neck cancer participants who received induction with cisplatin, 5-fluorouracil, with or without docetaxel. AG013, an ActoBiotic, a mouth rinse consisting of GM *L. lactis* strain to secrete the mucosal protectant human trefoil factor 1, was tested for possible relief from oral mucositis. This convenient and cost-effective novel platform of drug delivery demonstrated AG013 to be safe and well tolerated. Preliminary data on efficacy suggested that AG013 may reduce chemotherapy-induced ulcerative oral mucositis (Limaye et al., 2013).

AG014 and AG 19 utilizing *Lactococcus lactis* chassis have been tested for GI inflammation in primary immunodeficiency and type 1 diabetes mellitus, respectively. Charbonneau et al. (2020) have enlisted engineered bacterial therapeutic ADXS-HOT, ADXS-HPV, and ADXS-PA based on *L. monocytogenes* chassis tested against non-small cell lung cancer, HPV-associated cancer, and metastatic prostate cancer, respectively.

The idea of using live bacteria to treat solid tumors was first stated more than a century ago. As a result of the hypoxic areas and aberrant blood vessel architecture, a necrotic core can be formed in solid tumors, which may favor obligate and facultative anaerobic bacteria. APS001F (*Bifidobacterium longum*), bacTRL-IL-12 (*B. longum*), and SYNB1891 (*E. coli* Nissle 1917) have been reported to be in clinical studies for treating solid cancers.

No recombinant LBPs have been approved for use in humans (Cs Charbonneau et al., 2020). The advancement in research would be influenced by the first proof of concept demonstration of an engineered bacterial therapeutic that impacts the disease and improves the survival and morbidity of the patients.

12.3 SAFETY, REGULATORY ISSUES, AND CHALLENGES

The traditional small- and large-molecule drug development requirements are not entirely applicable to LBPs, while the rules and regulations for their use are still being developed as these products are undergoing clinical trials. LBPs don't necessitate conventional drug toxicology studies, as they are considered natural inhabitants of the human body (Lamousé-Smith et al., 2021).

'Human Safety' has always been a prime concern while manipulating the gut microbial genome for drug delivery. Toxicity in humans due to using live bacteria has been shown to limit the dose and efficacy of the probiotic delivering the drug, leading even to the termination of clinical trials in some studies (Harimoto et al., 2022).

The possibility of transfer of the transgene from engineered bacteria to commensals of the gut is a vital issue to be tackled. GM *Bacteroides ovatus* with thymine less death was designed as a containment strategy by Wegmann et al. (2017). The strain was, however, observed to survive thymine starvation by exchange of genes with bacteria in the mammalian GI tract by horizontal gene transfer, resulting in transgene-carrying wild-type bacteria. This has caused concern regarding the instability of GM bacteria after entering the human system and their interaction with gut microbiota. The GeneGuard system by Wright et al. (2014) uses a noteworthy three-pronged approach that can prevent the escape of engineered plasmids into wild species by designing a mutually dependent strain and plasmid that are unable to survive without each other.

Integration of gene/s of interest into the bacterial genome rather than the use of plasmids is being advised to prevent horizontal gene transfer. This would not only lead to stable transformation but also reduce the risk of horizontal gene transfer. IS elements, phage integration systems, and homologous recombination-based systems are the possible tools for this purpose. Removal of the integrase gene while modifying the bacterial genome is also recommended for obtaining stable constructs (Zhou & Han, 2022; Plavec & Berlec, 2019).

'Biocontainment of the engineered strains' is another caution to be strictly followed. And whether the human body is capable of disseminating genetically engineered microorganisms into the surroundings through interspecies microbial exchange with other animals, such as pets, is yet another question. Bacteria with appropriate genetic modules may be designed, such that they survive only in the human body or specific tissues or organs of the human body, with limited or no viability outside these specific environments may be designed to tackle these concerns (Zhou & Han, 2022).

Although enormous sequence information data is available on the human microbiome, many members of the microbiota have not yet been cultivated in vitro. Also, standard protocols for exogenous DNA delivery, plasmid replication, and genomic integration into these organisms are limited. Gene-manipulation systems that work in diverse organisms might be helpful in this context. Computational biology also might help predict favorable and unfavorable modules/protocols for the selected chassis organism; for example, the 'RBS Calculator', a computational strategy that is based on the analysis of ribosome binding sites (RBS). It can be applied to predict translation rates of the proteins and design novel RBS that can regulate the rate of translation in a chassis organism. The development of similar tools would be crucial in engineering the 'yet uncultured' microbiota.

Whether the therapeutic gene is expressed using a simple constitutive or inducible promoter, or a complex sense and response system, it exerts metabolic stress on the host microorganism. The higher the stress, the more would be selective pressure to lose the system out of the cell or develop mutations that reduce its function. The issue might be addressed by limiting the production of the therapeutic until the host has grown enough and there is sufficient substrate in the environment. This strategy, however, may lead to changes in the dynamics of gene expression and might not be suitable for more complex systems (Ozdemir et al., 2018). An intricate balance between levels of expression of the therapeutic product and the long-term stability of the construct would be desired while designing these systems.

Although the sense and response systems have the advantage of precise delivery, compatibility issues might arise regarding ligand-receptor binding specificity, such as crosstalk between the components owing to common ancestry, DNA binding sequences that are unidentified or of unknown origin, etc.; and might be problematic during the actual clinical use.

Identifying the most suitable chassis is probably one of the most challenging tasks! An ideal drug delivery system aims at the delivery of the therapeutic agent to a particular site efficiently with the least toxicity. Precision targeting, drug solubility in the microenvironment, in vivo toxicity, and clearance of the drug after a certain period post-delivery are issues to be considered and worked upon while selecting the chassis organism and engineering the microorganisms (Sabu et al., 2019; Bai et al., 2023).

Survival of the introduced engineered bacteria within the anoxic environment of the gut is another challenge, where the introduced bacteria also need to outcompete the commensal flora already existing in the ecosystem (Bai et al., 2023). Modification of the bacterium to offer a competitive advantage over other microbiota members, such as the capacity to metabolize a particular carbon source that cannot be broken down by members of the endogenous community, has been a proposed strategy to ensure secure, reliable, and efficient engraftment. When fed with a special carbohydrate that was unavailable to the native microbiota, for instance, the porphyran utilization operon was incorporated into *B. thetaiotaomicron* to enable the engineered strain to occupy a metabolic niche and establish stably into a humanized mouse microbiome (Shepherd et al., 2018; Arnold et al., 2023). If native microbiota is engineered, the problem should be easier to solve because it may be innately well-adapted to the microenvironment and so overcome colonization resistance. This might, in turn, pave the way toward long-term stable engraftment without the necessity for regular dosing (Russel et al., 2022; Arnold et al., 2023).

Composition and functioning of the gut microbiota vary longitudinally (different regions from intestinal mucosa to lumen), as well as across latitudes (different parts of the digestive tract, from ileum to large intestine); making it a challenging task to determine 'how' and 'where' to deliver the engineered microbiota for most effective results.

Should one prefer a 'single strain', or 'keystone consortium of mutually supportive strains' for engineering and drug delivery is another key question that needs to be addressed. The gut environment is a complex ecosystem, with different microbes together being involved in overall functioning; community collaboration plays a significant function in forming the functional 'guilds'. Single strains might not survive in the competition or be as efficient.

The residence time of the engineered bacteria after introduction into the gut is another significant aspect to be given thought and, to a great extent, depends on the host chassis selected. Short residence time, for example, 48 hours, permits better reproducible and predictable pharmacological properties. However, repeated dosing might be required to reach the desired therapeutic effects (Rutter et al., 2022). Although strains with longer residence time in the gut may not require repeated dosing, they raise concerns regarding loss of function mutation and biocontainment; of both, the engineered organism as well as inserted genetic material.

The effect of the human genome on the delivered engineered flora would be another point to be investigated, as the final outcome would largely depend on this factor.

12.4 CONCLUSION

Research on the development and use of engineered human microbiota for therapeutic applications is growing at an enormous pace and attracting broad interest in view of their potential benefits. The dynamic host–microbe interactions being uncovered, integration of synthetic biology tools with computational biology and artificial intelligence, advances in cultivation and genetic engineering methods of gut microbiota, and huge omics data being decoded—all together are leading mankind to develop probiotics as advanced drug delivery systems for the treatment of challenging human diseases.

The use of synthetic microbial consortia for drug delivery, with each bacterium existing in the co-culture performing a unique role in the 'drug system' also might be foreseen as a promising treatment modality that needs to be thoroughly tested further.

Engineered gut bacteria, in isolation, as a naturally occurring consortium, or synthetically designed consortium might be used to treat HM toxicity in humans in the near future. AI and computational tools might be used to test the feasibility of existing pathways and/or design new synthetic pathways in gut bacteria for metal detoxification.

Though many engineered probiotic systems are under trial in the developed world, a lot of new gut microbes are yet to be explored for their potential from gut diversities prevailing in developing and underdeveloped countries that inhabit exclusive, native, conserved human communities.

As these regions of the globe have a rich, ancient cultural influence on the unique lifestyles of the population, it's worth exploring novel drug-delivering chassis for effective therapeutics for numerous diseases.

Ayurveda, the ancient Indian science of medicine, categorizes individuals into three prakritis—kapha, pitta, and vata. Although the core microbiome is similar in all individuals, prakriti-specific signature microbiota have been reported, for example, the prevalence of Paraprevotella and Christensenellaceae in vata individuals (Shalini et al., 2021). Engineered probiotics are thought to be the next generation of live biotherapeutics to target specific diseases (Huang et al., 2023). While we step forward toward personalized precision medicine and explore gut microbiota for drug delivery, the use of such prevalent microbiota for engineering purposes needs to be explored and may have a significant impact on the future of this field.

BIBLIOGRAPHY

Ahlawat, A., Wiedensohler, A., & Mishra, S. K. (2020). An overview on the role of relative humidity in airborne transmission of SARS-CoV-2 in indoor environments. *Aerosol and Air Quality Research, 20*(9), 1856–1861.

Airola, C., Severino, A., Porcari, S., Fusco, W., Mullish, B. H., Gasbarrini, A., Cammarota, G., Ponziani, F. R., & Ianiro, G. (2023). Future modulation of gut microbiota: From eubiotics to FMT, engineered bacteria, and phage therapy. *Antibiotics (Basel, Switzerland), 12*(5), 868. https://doi.org/10.3390/antibiotics12050868

Arnold, J., Glazier, J., & Mimee, M. (2023). Genetic engineering of resident bacteria in the gut microbiome. *Journal of Bacteriology, 205*(7), e00127-23. https://doi.org/10.1128/jb.00127-23

Arun, K. B., Madhavan, A., Sindhu, R., Emmanual, S., Binod, P., Pugazhendhi, A., . . . Pandey, A. (2021). Probiotics and gut microbiome– Prospects and challenges in remediating heavy metal toxicity. *Journal of Hazardous Materials, 420*, 126676.

Bai, X., Huang, Z., Duraj-Thatte, A. M., Ebert, M. P., Zhang, F., Burgermeister, E., Liu, X., Scott, B. M., Li, G., & Zuo, T. (2023). Engineering the gut microbiome. *Nature Reviews Bioengineering*, 1–15. https://doi.org/10.1038/s44222-023-00072-2

Biagi, E., Zama, D., Nastasi, C., Consolandi, C., Fiori, J., Rampelli, S., Turroni, S., Centanni, M., Severgnini, M., Peano, C., de Bellis, G., Basaglia, G., Gotti, R., Masetti, R., Pession, A., Brigidi, P., & Candela, M. (2015). Gut microbiota trajectory in pediatric patients undergoing hematopoietic SCT. *Bone Marrow Transplantation, 50*(7), 992–998. https://doi.org/10.1038/bmt.2015.16

Bittihn, P., Din, M. O., Tsimring, L. S., & Hasty, J. (2018). Rational engineering of synthetic microbial systems: From single cells to consortia. *Current Opinion in Microbiology, 45*, 92–99. https://doi.org/10.1016/j.mib.2018.02.009

Borrero, J., Chen, Y., Dunny, G. M., & Kaznessis, Y. N. (2015). Modified lactic acid bacteria detect and inhibit multiresistant enterococci. *ACS Synthetic Biology, 4*(3), 299–306. https://doi.org/10.1021/sb500090b

Bron, P. A., & Kleerebezem, M. (2018). Lactic acid bacteria for delivery of endogenous or engineered therapeutic molecules. *Frontiers in Microbiology, 9*, 1821. https://doi.org/10.3389/fmicb.2018.01821

Bull, M. J., & Plummer, N. T. (2014). Part 1: The human gut microbiome in health and disease. *Integrative Medicine (Encinitas, Calif.), 13*(6), 17–22.

Cain, A. K., Barquist, L., Goodman, A. L., Paulsen, I. T., Parkhill, J., & van Opijnen, T. (2020). A decade of advances in transposon-insertion sequencing. *Nature Reviews. Genetics, 21*(9), 526–540. https://doi.org/10.1038/s41576-020-0244-x

Castagliuolo, I., Beggiao, E., Brun, P., Barzon, L., Goussard, S., Manganelli, R., Grillot-Courvalin, C., & Palù, G. (2005). Erratum: Engineered E. coli delivers therapeutic genes to the colonic mucosa. *Gene Therapy, 12*(14), 1158. https://doi.org/10.1038/sj.gt.3302574

Charbonneau, M. R., Isabella, V. M., Li, N., & Kurtz, C. B. (2020). Developing a new class of engineered live bacterial therapeutics to treat human diseases. *Nature Communications, 11*(1), 1738. https://doi.org/10.1038/s41467-020-15508-1

Chamcha, V., Jones, A., Quigley, B. R., Scott, J. R., & Amara, R. R. (2015). Oral immunization with a recombinant Lactococcus lactis–expressing HIV-1 antigen on group A Streptococcus pilus induces strong mucosal immunity in the gut. *The Journal of Immunology, 195*(10), 5025–5034.

Chen, T., Tian, P., Huang, Z., Zhao, X., Wang, H., Xia, C., Wang, L., & Wei, H. (2018). Engineered commensal bacteria prevent systemic inflammation-induced memory impairment and amyloidogenesis via producing GLP-1. *Applied Microbiology and Biotechnology, 102*(17), 7565–7575. https://doi.org/10.1007/s00253-018-9155-6

Chen, Z., Guo, L., Zhang, Y., Walzem, R. L., Pendergast, J. S., Printz, R. L., Morris, L. C., Matafonova, E., Stien, X., Kang, L., Coulon, D., McGuinness, O. P., Niswender, K. D., & Davies, S. S. (2014). Incorporation of therapeutically modified bacteria into gut microbiota inhibits obesity. *Journal of Clinical Investigation, 124*(8), 3391–3406. https://doi.org/10.1172/JCI72517

Chen, Z., Jin, W., Hoover, A., Chao, Y., & Ma, Y. (2023). Decoding the microbiome: Advances in genetic manipulation for gut bacteria. *Trends in Microbiology*, *31*(11), 1143–1161. https://doi.org/10.1016/j.tim.2023.05.007

DeFilippis, F., Pellegrini, N., Vannini, L., Jefery, I. B., La Storia, A., . . . Laghi, L. (2015). High-level adherence to a Mediterranean diet beneficially impacts the gut microbiota and associated metabolome. *Gut*. http://gut.bmj.com/lookup/doi/10.1136/gutjnl-2015-309957

Duong, M. T. Q., Qin, Y., You, S. H., & Min, J. J. (2019). Bacteria-cancer interactions: Bacteria-based cancer therapy. *Experimental & Molecular Medicine, 51*(12), 1–15. https://doi.org/10.1038/s12276-019-0297-0

Durmusoglu, D., Al'Abri, I. S., Collins, S. P., Cheng, J., Eroglu, A., Beisel, C. L., & Crook, N. (2021). In situ biomanufacturing of small molecules in the mammalian gut by probiotic *Saccharomyces boulardii. ACS Synthetic Biology, 10*(5), 1039–1052. https://doi.org/10.1021/acssynbio.0c00562

Durrer, K. E., Allen, M. S., & Hunt von Herbing, I. (2017). Genetically engineered probiotic for the treatment of phenylketonuria (PKU); assessment of a novel treatment *in vitro* and in the PAHenu2 mouse model of PKU. *PLoS One, 12*(5), e0176286. https://doi.org/10.1371/journal.pone.0176286

Fan, J. X., Li, Z. H., Liu, X. H., Zheng, D. W., Chen, Y., & Zhang, X. Z. (2018). Bacteria-mediated tumor therapy utilizing photothermally-controlled TNF-α expression via oral administration. *Nano Letters, 18*(4), 2373–2380. https://doi.org/10.1021/acs.nanolett.7b05323

Feng, Z., Wang, Y., Xu, H., Guo, Y., Xia, W., Zhao, C., Zhao, X., & Wu, J. (2023). Recent advances in bacterial therapeutics based on sense and response. *Acta Pharmaceutica Sinica. B, 13*(3), 1014–1027. https://doi.org/10.1016/j.apsb.2022.09.015

Francavilla, R., Calasso, M., Calace, L., Siragusa, S., Ndagijimana, M., Vernocchi, P., Brunetti, L., Mancino, G., Tedeschi, G., Guerzoni, E., Indrio, F., Laghi, L., Miniello, V. L., Gobbetti, M., & De Angelis, M. (2012). Effect of lactose on gut microbiota and metabolome of infants with cow's milk allergy. *Pediatric Allergy and Immunology*, *23*(5), 420–427. https://doi.org/10.1111/j.1399-3038.2012.01286.x

Fukata, M., & Arditi, M. (2013). The role of pattern recognition receptors in intestinal inflammation. *Mucosal Immunology, 6*(3), 451–463. https://doi.org/10.1038/mi.2013.13

Gao, X., Ma, Y., Wang, Z., Bai, J., Jia, S., Feng, B., Jiang, Y., Cui, W., Tang, L., Li, Y., Wang, L., & Xu, Y. (2019). Oral immunization of mice with a probiotic *Lactobacillus casei* constitutively expressing the α-toxoid induces protective immunity against Clostridium perfringens α-toxin. *Virulence, 10*(1), 166–179. https://doi.org/10.1080/21505594.2019.1582975

Gopalakrishnan, V., Helmink, B. A., Spencer, C. N., Reuben, A., & Wargo, J. A. (2018). The influence of the gut microbiome on cancer, immunity, and cancer immunotherapy. *Cancer Cell, 33*(4), 570–580. https://doi.org/10.1016/j.ccell.2018.03.015

Hancock, B. M., McGuire, K. L., Tsuji, S., Reil, K., Hernandez, V., Giacalone, M. J., & Godbey, W. T. (2016). A single intravesical instillation of VAX014 inhibits orthotopic superficial bladder tumor implantation to increase survival. *Anticancer Research, 36*(12), 6243–6248. https://doi.org/10.21873/anticanres.11218

Harimoto, T., Hahn, J., Chen, Y. Y., Im, J., Zhang, J., Hou, N., Li, F., Coker, C., Gray, K., Harr, N., Chowdhury, S., Pu, K., Nimura, C., Arpaia, N., Leong, K. W., & Danino, T. (2022). A programmable encapsulation system improves delivery of therapeutic bacteria in mice. *Nature Biotechnology, 40*(8), 1259–1269. https://doi.org/10.1038/s41587-022-01244-y

Ho, C. L., Tan, H. Q., Chua, K. J., Kang, A., Lim, K. H., Ling, K. L., Yew, W. S., Lee, Y. S., Thiery, J. P., & Chang, M. W. (2018). Engineered commensal microbes for diet-mediated colorectal-cancer chemoprevention. *Nature Biomedical Engineering, 2*(1), 27–37. https://doi.org/10.1038/s41551-017-0181-y

Holler, E., Butzhammer, P., Schmid, K., Hundsrucker, C., Koestler, J., Peter, K., . . . Oefner, P. J. (2014). Metagenomic analysis of the stool microbiome in patients receiving allogeneic stem cell transplantation: loss of diversity is associated with use of systemic antibiotics and more pronounced in gastrointestinal graft-versus-host disease. *Biology of Blood and Marrow Transplantation*, *20*(5), 640–645.

Huang, H., Yin, H., & Zhang, X. (2023). Editorial: Engineering probiotics for multiple interventions on intestinal diseases. *Frontiers in Cellular and Infection Microbiology, 13,* 1138998. https://doi.org/10.3389/fcimb.2023.1138998

Huang, S., Lee, A. J., Tsoi, R., Wu, F., Zhang, Y., Leong, K. W., & You, L. (2016). Coupling spatial segregation with synthetic circuits to control bacterial survival. *Molecular Systems Biology, 12*(2), 859. https://doi.org/10.15252/msb.20156567

Hwang, I. Y., Koh, E., Wong, A., March, J. C., Bentley, W. E., Lee, Y. S., & Chang, M. W. (2017). Engineered probiotic Escherichia coli can eliminate and prevent *Pseudomonas aeruginosa* gut infection in animal models. *Nature Communications, 8*(1), 15028. https://doi.org/10.1038/ncomms15028

Isabella, V. M., Ha, B. N., Castillo, M. J., Lubkowicz, D. J., Rowe, S. E., Millet, Y. A., Anderson, C. L., Li, N., Fisher, A. B., West, K. A., Reeder, P. J., Momin, M. M., Bergeron, C. G., Guilmain, S. E., Miller, P. F., Kurtz, C. B., & Falb, D. (2018). Development of a synthetic live bacterial therapeutic for the human metabolic disease phenylketonuria. *Nature Biotechnology, 36*(9), 857–864. https://doi.org/10.1038/nbt.4222

Jandhyala, S. M., Talukdar, R., Subramanyam, C., Vuyyuru, H., Sasikala, M., & Nageshwar Reddy, D. (2015). Role of the normal gut microbiota. *World Journal of Gastroenterology, 21*(29), 8787–8803. https://doi.org/10.3748/wjg.v21.i29.8787

Jantchou, P., Morois, S., Clavel-Chapelon, F., Boutron-Ruault, M. C., & Carbonnel, F. (2010). Animal protein intake and risk of inflammatory bowel disease: The E3N prospective study. *American Journal of Gastroenterology*, *105*(10), 2195–2201. https://doi.org/10.1038/ajg.2010.192

Jayaraman, P., Holowko, M. B., Yeoh, J. W., Lim, S., & Poh, C. L. (2017). Repurposing a two-component system-based biosensor for the killing of Vibrio cholerae. *ACS Synthetic Biology, 6*(7), 1403–1415. https://doi.org/10.1021/acssynbio.7b00058

Jiang, Y., Sun, B., Qian, F., Dong, F., Xu, C., Zhong, W., Huang, R., Zhai, Q., Jiang, Y., & Yang, S. (2022). Expression of phenylalanine ammonia lyase as an intracellularly free and extracellularly cell surface-immobilized enzyme on a gut microbe as a live biotherapeutic for phenylketonuria. *Science China. Life Sciences, 66*(1), 127–136. https://doi.org/10.1007/s11427-021-2137-3

Kailasapathy, K. (2015). Biopolymers for administration and gastrointestinal delivery of functional food ingredients and probiotic bacteria. In *Functional polymers in food science: from technology to biology* (pp. 231–265).

Ke, S., Weiss, S. T., & Liu, Y. Y. (2022). Rejuvenating the human gut microbiome. *Trends in Molecular Medicine, 28*(8), 619–630. https://doi.org/10.1016/j.molmed.2022.05.005

Kelley, S. T., Skarra, D. V., Rivera, A. J., & Thackray, V. G. (2016). The gut microbiome is altered in a letrozole-induced mouse model of polycystic ovary syndrome. *PLoS One, 11*(1), e0146509. https://doi.org/10.1371/journal.pone.0146509

Lamousé-Smith, E., Kelly, D., & De Cremoux, I. (2021). Designing bugs as drugs: exploiting the gut microbiome. *American Journal of Physiology-Gastrointestinal and Liver Physiology*, *320*(3), G295–G303.

Lateef, A., Gueguim-Kana, E. B., Dasgupta, N., & Ranjan, S. (Eds.). (2021). *Microbial nanobiotechnology: Principles and applications*. Springer Nature.

Li, J., Zhao, F., Wang, Y., Chen, J., Tao, J., Tian, G., Wu, S., Liu, W., Cui, Q., Geng, B., Zhang, W., Weldon, R., Auguste, K., Yang, L., Liu, X., Chen, L., Yang, X., Zhu, B., & Cai, J. (2017). Gut microbiota dysbiosis contributes to the development of hypertension. *Microbiome, 5*(1), 14. https://doi.org/10.1186/s40168-016-0222-x

Liang, K., Liu, Q., Li, P., Han, Y., Bian, X., Tang, Y., & Kong, Q. (2018). Endostatin gene therapy delivered by attenuated Salmonella typhimurium in murine tumor models. *Cancer Gene Therapy, 25*(7–8), 167–183. https://doi.org/10.1038/s41417-018-0021-6

Limaye, S. A., Haddad, R. I., Cilli, F., Sonis, S. T., Colevas, A. D., Brennan, M. T., Hu, K. S., & Murphy, B. A. (2013). Phase 1b, multicenter, single blinded, placebo-controlled, sequential dose escalation study to assess the safety and tolerability of topically applied AG013 in subjects with locally advanced head and neck cancer receiving induction chemotherapy. *Cancer, 119*(24), 4268–4276. https://doi.org/10.1002/cncr.28365

López-Igual, R., Bernal-Bayard, J., Rodríguez-Patón, A., Ghigo, J. M., & Mazel, D. (2020). Engineered toxin–intein antimicrobials can selectively target and kill antibiotic-resistant bacteria in mixed populations. *Nature Biotechnology, 37*(7), 755–760. https://doi.org/10.1038/s41587-019-0105-3

McKay, R., Ghodasra, M., Schardt, J., Quan, D., Pottash, A. E., Shang, W., . . . & Bentley, W. E. (2018). A platform of genetically engineered bacteria as vehicles for localized delivery of therapeutics: Toward applications for Crohn's disease. *Bioengineering & Translational Medicine*, *3*(3), 209–221.

Monachese, M., Burton, J. P., & Reid, G. (2012). Bioremediation and tolerance of humans to heavy metals through microbial processes: A potential role for probiotics? *Applied and Environmental Microbiology, 78*(18), 6397–6404. https://doi.org/10.1128/AEM.01665-12

Mugwanda, K., Hamese, S., Van Zyl, W. F., Prinsloo, E., Du Plessis, M., Dicks, L. M. T., & Thimiri Govinda Raj, D. B. (2023). Recent advances in genetic tools for engineering probiotic lactic acid bacteria. *Bioscience Reports, 43*(1). https://doi.org/10.1042/BSR20211299

Naydich, A. D., Nangle, S. N., Bues, J. J., Trivedi, D., Nissar, N., Inniss, M. C., Niederhuber, M. J., Way, J. C., Silver, P. A., & Riglar, D. T. (2019). Synthetic gene circuits enable systems-level biosensor trigger discovery at the host–microbe interface. *M-Systems, 4*(4), 10–1128. https://doi.org/10.1128/mSystems.00125-19

Nielsen, A. A., Der, B. S., Shin, J., Vaidyanathan, P., Paralanov, V., Strychalski, E. A., Ross, D., Densmore, D., & Voigt, C. A. (2016). Genetic circuit design automation. *Science (New York, NY), 352*(6281), aac7341. https://doi.org/10.1126/science.aac7341

Norman, R. J., Dewailly, D., Legro, R. S., & Hickey, T. E. (2007). Polycystic ovary syndrome. *Lancet (London, England), 370*(9588), 685–697. https://doi.org/10.1016/S0140-6736(07)61345-2

Ozdemir, T., Fedorec, A. J. H., Danino, T., & Barnes, C. P. (2018). Synthetic biology and engineered live biotherapeutics: Toward increasing system complexity. *Cell Systems, 7*(1), 5–16. https://doi.org/10.1016/j.cels.2018.06.008

Palmer, J. D., Piattelli, E., McCormick, B. A., Silby, M. W., Brigham, C. J., & Bucci, V. (2018). Engineered probiotic for the inhibition of *Salmonella* via tetrathionate-induced production of microcin H47. *ACS Infectious Diseases, 4*(1), 39–45. https://doi.org/10.1021/acsinfecdis.7b00114

Patwa, S. A., Ward, C., & Kelly, C. R. (2022). FMT: What's Next? A narrative review of fecal microbiota transplantation in *Clostridium difficile* infection and inflammatory bowel disease. *Rhode Island Medical Journal, 105*(9), 20–24.

Piraner, D. I., Abedi, M. H., Moser, B. A., Lee-Gosselin, A., & Shapiro, M. G. (2017). Tunable thermal bioswitches for *in vivo* control of microbial therapeutics. *Nature Chemical Biology, 13*(1), 75–80. https://doi.org/10.1038/nchembio.2233

Plavec, T. V., & Berlec, A. (2019). Surface anchoring on *Lactococcus lactis* by covalent isopeptide bond. *Acta Chimica Slovenica, 66*(1), 18–27. https://doi.org/10.17344/acsi.2018.4422

Popkin, B. M., Adair, L. S., & Ng, S. W. (2012). Global nutrition transition and the pandemic of obesity in developing countries. *Nutrition Reviews, 70*(1), 3–21. https://doi.org/10.1111/j.1753-4887.2011.00456.x

Prakash, S., Tomaro-Duchesneau, C., Saha, S., & Cantor, A. (2011). The gut microbiota and human health with an emphasis on the use of microencapsulated bacterial cells. *Journal of Biomedicine and Biotechnology*, *2011*.

Praveschotinunt, P., Duraj-Thatte, A. M., Gelfat, I., Bahl, F., Chou, D. B., & Joshi, N. S. (2019). Engineered E. coli Nissle 1917 for the delivery of matrix-tethered therapeutic domains to the gut. *Nature Communications, 10*(1), 5580. https://doi.org/10.1038/s41467-019-13336-6

Raman, V., Van Dessel, N., Hall, C. L., Wetherby, V. E., Whitney, S. A., Kolewe, E. L., Bloom, S. M. K., Sharma, A., Hardy, J. A., Bollen, M., Van Eynde, A., & Forbes, N. S. (2021). Intracellular delivery of protein drugs with an autonomously lysing bacterial system reduces tumor growth and metastases. *Nature Communications, 12*(1), 6116. https://doi.org/10.1038/s41467-021-26367-9

Reid, G., Pel, M. E., Kirschner, M. B., Cheng, Y. Y., Mugridge, N., Weiss, J., Williams, M., Wright, C., Edelman, J. J., Vallely, M. P., McCaughan, B. C., Klebe, S., Brahmbhatt, H., MacDiarmid, J. A., & van Zandwijk, N. (2013). Restoring expression of miR-16: A novel approach to therapy for malignant pleural mesothelioma. *Annals of Oncology, 24*(12), 3128–3135. https://doi.org/10.1093/annonc/mdt412

Reilly, S. M., & Saltiel, A. R. (2017). Adapting to obesity with adipose tissue inflammation. *Nature Reviews. Endocrinology*, *13*(11), 633–643. https://doi.org/10.1038/nrendo.2017.90

Rottinghaus, A. G., Amrofell, M. B., & Moon, T. S. (2019). Biosensing in smart engineered probiotics. *Biotechnology Journal, 15*(10), e1900319. https://doi.org/10.1002/biot.201900319

Routy, B., Letendre, C., Enot, D., Chénard-Poirier, M., Mehraj, V., Séguin, N. C., Guenda, K., Gagnon, K., Woerther, P. L., Ghez, D., & Lachance, S. (2017). The influence of gut-decontamination prophylactic antibiotics on acute graft-versus-host disease and survival following allogeneic hematopoietic stem cell transplantation. *Oncoimmunology, 6*(1), e1258506. https://doi.org/10.1080/2162402X.2016.1258506

Rubin, B. E., Diamond, S., Cress, B. F., Crits-Christoph, A., Lou, Y. C., Borges, A. L., Shivram, H., He, C., Xu, M., Zhou, Z., Smith, S. J., Rovinsky, R., Smock, D. C. J., Tang, K., Owens, T. K., Krishnappa, N., Sachdeva, R., Barrangou, R., Deutschbauer, A. M., . . . Doudna, J. A. (2022). Species- and site-specific genome editing in complex bacterial communities. *Nature Microbiology, 7*(1), 34–47. https://doi.org/10.1038/s41564-021-01014-7

Russell, B. J., Brown, S. D., Siguenza, N., Mai, I., Saran, A. R., Lingaraju, A., . . . & Zarrinpar, A. (2022). Intestinal transgene delivery with native E. coli chassis allows persistent physiological changes. *Cell, 185*(17), 3263–3277.

Rutter, J. W., Dekker, L., Owen, K. A., & Barnes, C. P. (2022). Microbiome engineering: Engineered live biotherapeutic products for treating human disease. *Frontiers in Bioengineering and Biotechnology, 10,* 1000873. https://doi.org/10.3389/fbioe.2022.1000873

Sabu, C., Mufeedha, P., & Pramod, K. (2019). Yeast-inspired drug delivery: Biotechnology meets bioengineering and synthetic biology. *Expert Opinion on Drug Delivery, 16*(1), 27–41. https://doi.org/10.1080/17425247.2019.1551874

San León, D., & Nogales, J. (2022). Toward merging bottom–up and top–down model-based designing of synthetic microbial communities. *Current Opinion in Microbiology, 69,* 102169. https://doi.org/10.1016/j.mib.2022.102169

Scott, B. M., Gutiérrez-Vázquez, C., Sanmarco, L. M., da Silva Pereira, J. A., Li, Z., Plasencia, A., Hewson, P., Cox, L. M., O'Brien, M., Chen, S. K., Moraes-Vieira, P. M., Chang, B. S. W., Peisajovich, S. G., & Quintana, F. J. (2021). Self-tunable engineered yeast probiotics for the treatment of inflammatory bowel disease. *Nature Medicine, 27*(7), 1212–1222. https://doi.org/10.1038/s41591-021-01390-x

Serrano, L. (2007). Synthetic biology: Promises and challenges. *Molecular Systems Biology, 3,* 158. https://doi.org/10.1038/msb4100202

Shalini, T. V., Jnana, A., Sriranjini, S. J., Tanwar, A. S., Brand, A., Murali, T. S., Satyamoorthy, K., & Gangadharan, G. G. (2021). Exploring the signature gut and oral microbiome in individuals of specific Ayurveda prakriti. *Journal of Biosciences, 46*(3), 54. https://doi.org/10.1007/s12038-021-00182-2

Shen, H., Aggarwal, N., Wun, K. S., Lee, Y. S., Hwang, I. Y., & Chang, M. W. (2022). Engineered microbial systems for advanced drug delivery. *Advanced Drug Delivery Reviews, 187,* 114364. https://doi.org/10.1016/j.addr.2022.114364

Shen, T. C. D., Albenberg, L., Bittinger, K., Chehoud, C., Chen, Y. Y., Judge, C. A., Chau, L., Ni, J., Sheng, M., Lin, A., Wilkins, B. J., Buza, E. L., Lewis, J. D., Daikhin, Y., Nissim, I., Yudkoff, M., Bushman, F. D., & Wu, G. D. (2015). Engineering the gut microbiota to treat hyperammonemia. *The Journal of Clinical Investigation, 125*(7), 2841–2850. https://doi.org/10.1172/JCI79214

Shepherd, E. S., Deloache, W. C., Pruss, K. M., Whitaker, W. R., & Sonnenburg, J. L. (2018). An exclusive metabolic niche enables strain engraftment in the gut microbiota. *Nature, 557*(7705), 434–438. https://doi.org/10.1038/s41586-018-0092-4

Shono, Y., Docampo, M. D., Peled, J. U., Perobelli, S. M., Velardi, E., Tsai, J. J., Slingerland, A. E., Smith, O. M., Young, L. F., Gupta, J., Lieberman, S. R., Jay, H. V., Ahr, K. F., Porosnicu Rodriguez, K. A., Xu, K., Calarfiore, M., Poeck, H., Caballero, S., Devlin, S. M., . . . Jenq, R. R. (2016). Increased GVHD-related mortality with broad-spectrum antibiotic use after allogeneic hematopoietic stem cell transplantation in human patients and mice. *Science Translational Medicine, 8*(339), 339ra71. https://doi.org/10.1126/scitranslmed.aaf2311

Singh, R. K., Chang, H. W., Yan, D. I., Lee, K. M., Ucmak, D., Wong, K., Abrouk, M., Farahnik, B., Nakamura, M., Zhu, T. H., Bhutani, T., & Liao, W. (2017). Influence of diet on the gut microbiome and implications for human health. *Journal of Translational Medicine, 15*(1), 1–17. https://doi.org/10.1186/s12967-017-1175-y

Škrlec, K., Ručman, R., Jarc, E., Sikirić, P., Švajger, U., Petan, T., Perišić Nanut, M., Štrukelj, B., & Berlec, A. (2018). Engineering recombinant *Lactococcus lactis* as a delivery vehicle for BPC-157 peptide with antioxidant activities. *Applied Microbiology and Biotechnology, 102*(23), 10103–10117. https://doi.org/10.1007/s00253-018-9333-6

Sonnenborn, U., & Schulze, J. (2009). The nonpathogenic Escherichia coli strain Nissle 1917-features of a versatile probiotic. *Microbial Ecology in Health and Disease, 21*(3–4), 122–158. https://doi.org/10.3109/08910600903444267

Stokes, J. H., & Pillsbury, D. M. (1930). The effect on the skin of emotional and nervous states: III. Theoretical and practical consideration of a gastro-intestinal mechanism. *JAMA Dermatology, 22,* 962–993.

Tan, Y., Shen, J., Si, T., Ho, C. L., Li, Y., & Dai, L. (2020). Engineered live biotherapeutics: Progress and challenges. *Biotechnology Journal, 15*(10), e2000155. https://doi.org/10.1002/biot.202000155

Tanoue, T., Morita, S., Plichta, D. R., Skelly, A. N., Suda, W., Sugiura, Y., Narushima, S., Vlamakis, H., Motoo, I., Sugita, K., Shiota, A., Takeshita, K., Yasuma-Mitobe, K., Riethmacher, D., Kaisho, T., Norman, J. M., Mucida, D., Suematsu, M., Yaguchi, T., . . . Honda, K. (2019). A defined commensal consortium elicits CD8 T cells and anti-cancer immunity. *Nature, 565*(7741), 600–605. https://doi.org/10.1038/s41586-019-0878-z

Taur, Y., Jenq, R. R., Perales, M. A., Littmann, E. R., Morjaria, S., Ling, L., Gobourne, A., Viale, A., Dahi, P. B., Ponce, D. M., Barker, J. N., Giralt, S., van den Brink, M., & Pamer, E. G. (2014). The effects of intestinal tract bacterial diversity on mortality following allogeneic hematopoietic stem cell transplantation *Blood, The Journal of the American Society of Hematology, 124*(7), 1174–1182. https://doi.org/10.1182/blood-2014-02-554725

Taur, Y., Xavier, J. B., LiPuma, L., Ubeda, C., Goldberg, J., Gobourne, A., Lee, Y. J., Dubin, K. A., Socci, N. D., Viale, A., Perales, M. A., Jenq, R. R., van den Brink, M. R., & Pamer, E. G. (2012). Intestinal domination and the risk of bacteremia in patients undergoing allogeneic hematopoietic stem cell transplantation. *Clinical Infectious Diseases: An Official Publication of the Infectious Diseases Society of America, 55*(7), 905–914. https://doi.org/10.1093/cid/cis580

Tscherner, M., Giessen, T. W., Markey, L., Kumamoto, C. A., & Silver, P. A. (2019). A synthetic system that senses *Candida albicans* and inhibits virulence factors. *ACS Synthetic Biology, 8*(2), 434–444. https://doi.org/10.1021/acssynbio.8b00457

Verma, A., Xu, K., Du, T., Zhu, P., Liang, Z., Liao, S., Zhang, J., Raizada, M. K., Grant, M. B., & Li, Q. (2019). Expression of human ACE2 in Lactobacillus and beneficial effects in diabetic retinopathy in mice. *Molecular Therapy. Methods and Clinical Development, 14,* 161–170. https://doi.org/10.1016/j.omtm.2019.06.007

Virani, S. S., Alonso, A., Benjamin, E. J., Bittencourt, M. S., Callaway, C. W., Carson, A. P., Chamberlain, A. M., Chang, A. R., Cheng, S., Delling, F. N., Djousse, L., Elkind, M. S. V., Ferguson, J. F., Fornage, M., Khan, S. S., Kissela, B. M., Knutson, K. L., Kwan, T. W., Lackland, D. T., Lewis, T. T., . . . American Heart Association Council on Epidemiology and Prevention Statistics Committee and Stroke Statistics Subcommittee. (2020). Heart disease and stroke statistics-2020 update: A report from the American heart association. *Circulation, 141*(9), e139–e596. https://doi.org/10.1161/CIR.0000000000000757

Wang, B., Jiang, X., Cao, M., Ge, J., Bao, Q., Tang, L., Chen, Y., & Li, L. (2016). Altered fecal microbiota correlates with liver biochemistry in nonobese patients with non-alcoholic fatty liver disease. *Scientific Reports*, *6,* 32002. https://doi.org/10.1038/srep32002

Wang, L., Cheng, X., Bai, L., Gao, M., Kang, G., Cao, X., & Huang, H. (2022). Positive interventional effect of engineered butyrate-producing bacteria on metabolic disorders and intestinal flora disruption in obese mice. *Microbiology Spectrum, 10*(2), e0114721. https://doi.org/10.1128/spectrum.01147-21

Wang, L., Qin, W., Xu, W., Huang, F., Xie, X., Wang, F., Ma, L., & Zhang, C. (2021). Bacteria-mediated tumor therapy via photothermally-programmed cytolysin A expression. *Small, 17*(40), e2102932. https://doi.org/10.1002/smll.202102932

Wegmann, U., Carvalho, A. L., Stocks, M., & Carding, S. R. (2017). Use of genetically modified bacteria for drug delivery in humans: Revisiting the safety aspect. *Scientific Reports, 7*(1), 2294. https://doi.org/10.1038/s41598-017-02591-6

Whittle, J. R., Lickliter, J. D., Gan, H. K., Scott, A. M., Simes, J., Solomon, B. J., MacDiarmid, J. A., Brahmbhatt, H., & Rosenthal, M. A. (2015). First in human nanotechnology doxorubicin delivery system to target epidermal growth factor receptors in recurrent glioblastoma. *Journal of Clinical Neuroscience, 22*(12), 1889–1894. https://doi.org/10.1016/j.jocn.2015.06.005

Wick, W., Osswald, M., Wick, A., & Winkler, F. (2018). Treatment of glioblastoma in adults. *Therapeutic Advances in Neurological Disorders, 11*. https://doi.org/10.1177/1756286418790452

Wright, O., Delmans, M., Stan, G. B., & Ellis, T. (2014). GeneGuard: A modular plasmid system designed for biosafety. *ACS Synthetic Biology*, *4*(3), 307–316. https://doi.org/10.1021/sb500234s

Xu, C., Lee, S. K., Zhang, D., & Frenette, P. S. (2020). The gut microbiome regulates psychological-stress-induced inflammation. *Immunity, 53*(2), 417–428.e4. https://doi.org/10.1016/j.immuni.2020.06.025

Yan, D., Issa, N., Afifi, L., Jeon, C., Chang, H. W., & Liao, W. (2017). The role of the skin and gut microbiome in psoriatic disease. *Current Dermatology Reports, 6*(2), 94–103. https://doi.org/10.1007/s13671-017-0178-5

Yin, J., Chen, X., Li, X., Kang, G., Wang, P., Song, Y., Ijaz, U. Z., Yin, H., & Huang, H. (2022). A droplet-based microfluidic approach to isolating functional bacteria from gut microbiota. *Frontiers in Cellular and Infection Microbiology, 12,* 920986. https://doi.org/10.3389/fcimb.2022.920986

Younossi, Z. M., Koenig, A. B., Abdelatif, D., Fazel, Y., Henry, L., & Wymer, M. (2016). Global epidemiology of nonalcoholic fatty liver disease—meta-analytic assessment of prevalence, incidence, and outcomes. *Hepatology*, *64*(1), 73–84.

Yuan, G. C., Cai, L., Elowitz, M., Enver, T., Fan, G., Guo, G., Irizarry, R., Kharchenko, P., Kim, J., Orkin, S., Quackenbush, J., Saadatpour, A., Schroeder, T., Shivdasani, R., & Tirosh, I. (2017). Challenges and emerging directions in single-cell analysis. *Genome Biology, 18*(1), 84. https://doi.org/10.1186/s13059-017-1218-y

Zhang, H., & Wang, X. (2016). Modular co-culture engineering, a new approach for metabolic engineering. *Metabolic Engineering, 37,* 114–121. https://doi.org/10.1016/j.ymben.2016.05.007

Zhao, R., Li, Z., Sun, Y., Ge, W., Wang, M., Liu, H., Xun, L., & Xia, Y. (2022). Engineered *Escherichia coli* Nissle 1917 with urate oxidase and an oxygen-recycling system for hyperuricemia treatment. *Gut Microbes, 14*(1), 2070391. https://doi.org/10.1080/19490976.2022.2070391

Zheng, Y., Ley, S. H., & Hu, F. B. (2018). Global aetiology and epidemiology of type 2 diabetes mellitus and its complications. *Nature Reviews. Endocrinology, 14*(2), 88–98. https://doi.org/10.1038/nrendo.2017.151

Zhou, Y., & Han, Y. (2022). Engineered bacteria as drug delivery vehicles: Principles and prospects. *Engineering Microbiology, 2*(3), 100034. https://doi.org/10.1016/j.engmic.2022.100034

13 Application of Probiotics in Food Industry

A Promising Scope for Improving Food Quality

Rafael Audino Zambelli and Luciana Gama de Mendonça

13.1 INTRODUCTION

Consumer perceptions have changed dramatically over the past decade. Concern is increasingly common with health and longevity. In this way, the use of functional, fortified, and nutraceutical foods has gained the interest of part of the population, mainly with a focus on disease prevention (Ferreira et al., 2020; Chen & Hu, 2020). The increase in consumer interest is evidenced by the growing number of probiotic products on the market and the number of companies that have started to research and develop products containing probiotics in their formulations.

Probiotic goods are subject to varying regulations depending on the country. However, several countries still do not have specific laws for the commercialization of this type of product. In the European Union, for example, functional statements regarding health benefits for products classified as probiotics require endorsement from the EFSA. This authority has released a roster of microbial cultures that do not need to undergo a safety assessment; however, this does not imply that the product is exempt from inspection and examination of claims (Kolaček et al., 2017; Domínguez-Díaz et al., 2020).

The exploration of probiotics and their possible uses has garnered considerable interest across multiple domains, such as medicine, nutrition, and the food sector (Angelin & Kavitha, 2020). Investigations into the advantageous effects of microorganisms within the human body have roots in the 19th century. The inaugural documented observation was made by Doderlein in 1892. Subsequently, Metchnikoff delved into the functional characteristics of bacteria sourced from fermented milk (Anukam & Reid, 2007; Santacroce et al., 2021).

Probiotics are categorized as living microorganisms that, when consumed in suitable amounts, can bestow beneficial health effects upon individuals, and they have been linked to various favorable health outcomes, such as better intestinal health, alleviation of digestive discomfort, mitigation of intestinal inflammation, reinforcement of the immune system, and support for cardiovascular well-being (Oniszczuk et al., 2021). Among the main functions of probiotics, maintenance and balance of the gut microbiota and a decrease in the incidence of chronic non-communicable diseases can be mentioned, as well as reducing the appearance of allergies (Lim & Kim, 2017; Gu et al., 2023). It offers a means to modulate and improve the composition and activity of the gut microbiota. When ingested in sufficient quantities, probiotics can elicit advantageous impacts on human health (Sánchez et al., 2017).

After adults consume probiotics, the microorganisms initiate the colonization process in the gastrointestinal tract (Plaza-Diaz et al., 2019). Maintaining a healthy microflora of the gastrointestinal tract produces a number of benefits in the human body, such as eliminating bacteriocins and fighting pathogenic microflora, which reduces the number of diseases that affect the digestive system, destroys components that are not broken down by enzymes, and can promote the synthesis

 DOI: 10.1201/9781003452249-13

of micronutrients such as amino acids and vitamins, in addition to improving the absorption of microelements in the intestinal walls (Yao et al., 2020).

Some countries already have their own regulations for the characterization of probiotics as functional food, in particular, Italy, Brazil, and Canada can be mentioned. These countries have established a minimum amount necessary to obtain the benefits which must be confirmed through scientific studies in humans or animals, and companies must ensure that the amount of microorganisms must be maintained until the end of the product's shelf life (Xavier-Santos et al., 2020).

13.2 DEFINITION AND CLASSIFICATION OF PROBIOTICS

Initially, probiotics were comprised of a solitary type of microorganism, predominantly from the *Saccharomyces* or *Lactobacillus* groups. As scientific exploration advanced, multiple experiments were undertaken and subsequently synthesized in meta-analyses, unearthing the advantages linked to these probiotics. Notably, they demonstrated efficacy in alleviating infectious diarrhea and post-antibiotic diarrhea, while also effectively tackling colitis associated with *Clostridium difficile* infections. These revelations underscored the effectiveness of probiotics in managing gastrointestinal concerns and promoting gut well-being (Goldenberg et al., 2017).

As outlined by the ISAPP, probiotics are living microorganisms that offer beneficial effects when administered in appropriate proportions and can provide some benefit to the host, such as improving gastrointestinal health through improved immune and digestive function and mucosal protection (Khalesi et al., 2019). This definition provides health professionals, researchers, industry, legislators, and consumers with more assertive guidelines for the definitions and forms of use of probiotics (Ma et al., 2023).

For probiotic microorganisms to genuinely contribute to health improvements, they need to withstand the challenging conditions of the human stomach and gastrointestinal tract. Hence, a valid probiotic assertion should encompass attributes such as resilience against gastric acid, resistance to bile salts, successful passage through the upper gastrointestinal tract, as well as the capability to establish colonies and proliferate within the intestine (Wan et al., 2018).

The beneficial effects of probiotic bacteria become noticeable when a significant number of viable bacteria, amounting to at least 10^7 colony-forming units per milliliter of the product, remain viable throughout the entirety of the product's shelf life (Baruah et al., 2022).

Figure 13.1 illustrates the primary reasons for incorporating probiotics in clinical scenarios.

13.2.1 Types of Probiotic Microorganisms

Most of the probiotic microorganisms belong to the intestinal microbiota. They are mainly the gram-positive LAB: *Lactobacillus*, *Carnobacterium*, *Leuconostoc*, *Enterococcus*, *Pedicoccus*, *Streptococcus*, *Lactococcus*, *Tetragenococcus*, *Saccharomyces*, *Bacillus*, and *Escherichia coli*. It is important to note that bacteria have different properties and effects on the body and not every strain is considered probiotic (Jach et al., 2013; Fijan, 2014).

Lactobacillus are the most used and studied group of bacteria with the objective of being probiotics. They are found in the human intestine and are present in fermented foods such as yogurt and cheese. Different strains of *Lactobacillus* may offer some health benefits, such as aiding in the digestion of lactose, improving gut health, controlling some types of cancers, and reducing blood cholesterol (Das et al., 2022). Because of their long history of safe use, several strains of *Lactobacillus* are classified as GRAS foods.

This class of microorganisms belongs to LAB, presents characteristics of gram-positive bacillus, is non-sporulated, and has negative catalase and oxidase (Coudeyras et al., 2008).

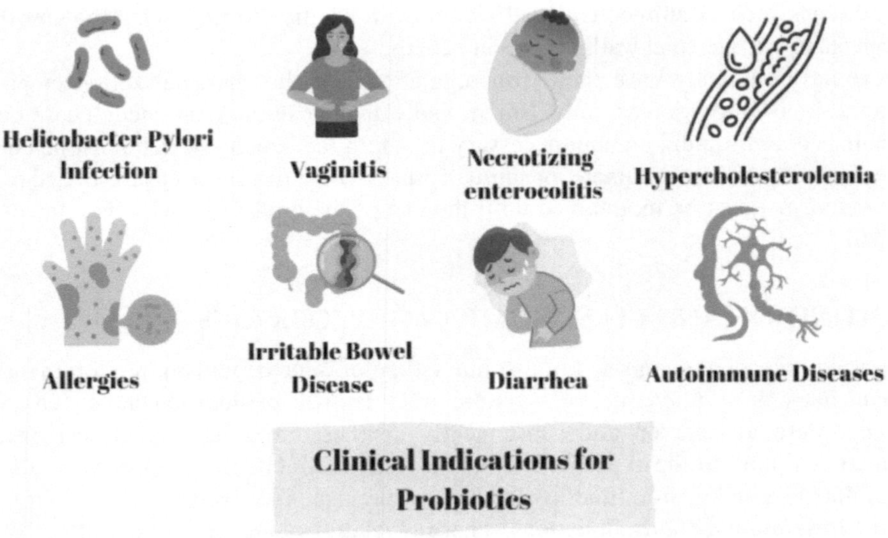

FIGURE 13.1 Clinical indications for probiotics use.

TABLE 13.1
Most Used Probiotic Microorganisms

Probiotic Genera	References
Lactobacillus	Rasaei et al. (2023) and Islam et al. (2023).
Bifidobacterium	Soares et al. (2019) and Di Gioia et al. (2014).
Enterococcus	Barbosa et al. (2014) and Abedini et al. (2023).
Lactococcus	Lei et al. (2022) and Baig et al. (2022).
Bacillus	Rasaei et al. (2023) and Zhao et al. (2023).
Pediococcus	Lee et al. (2014) and Vieira et al. (2020).
Streptococcus	Fei et al. (2023) and Li et al. (2022)
Escherichia	Wu et al. (2023)

These microorganisms engage in the metabolic breakdown of carbohydrates, leading to the production of acid. *Lactobacillus* species are broadly categorized into three groups based on their metabolic pathways. One subset comprises obligate homofermentative species, which exclusively ferment carbohydrates to generate lactic acid as the primary byproduct. Notable examples within this category include LA and *Lactobacillus salivarius.* Conversely, the facultative homofermentative group ferments carbohydrates to yield a combination of ethanol, lactic acid, carbon dioxide, and acetic acid as end products. *Lactobacillus casei* and *Lactobacillus plantarum* fall into this group. Lastly, the obligate heterofermentative group carries out carbohydrate fermentation, resulting in the production of lactic acid, ethanol, carbon dioxide, and acetic acid. *Lactobacillus reuteri* and *Lactobacillus fermentum* exemplify this particular metabolic category (De Angelis & Gobbetti, 2016).

These microorganisms have the capability to establish themselves in various regions of the human body, notably in the oral cavity, female genital tract, and gastrointestinal tract. The interaction with humans is characterized as mutualistic, wherein *Lactobacillus* species offer support to the host in breaking down dietary substances, while the host provides habitat and nourishment for the microorganisms' sustenance and proliferation (Heeney et al., 2018).

In this way, they produce lactic acid and regulate intestinal pH levels, providing a hostile environment for pathogenic bacteria (Panwar et al., 2021). Some strains of *Lactobacillus* have been shown to modulate the immune system, helping to strengthen the body's defenses against infections and pathogens (Mazziotta et al., 2023) and can be beneficial in managing diarrhea, including cases related to antibiotic use. They help restore the balance of gut bacteria disrupted by antibiotics (Kopacz & Phadtare, 2022).

A specific strain of *E. coli* known as *E. coli* Nissle 1917 has been researched extensively for its probiotic properties, especially in supporting gut health and treating certain gastrointestinal conditions. This non-pathogenic gram-negative strain is employed to address various gastrointestinal issues, including diarrhea and uncomplicated diverticular disease (Behrouzi et al., 2020). The antimicrobial properties of this microorganism include the immediate effect and stimulation of the creation of a defense system by the cells of the intestinal epithelium, in addition to increasing the positive effects in type 2 diabetes (Wehkamp et al., 2004).

It's important to emphasize that probiotics are generally distinguished by their genus, species, and specific strain nomenclature. This distinction is significant as diverse strains within a single species can yield differing health outcomes. Moreover, the potential health advantages associated with probiotics are often contingent on the specific strain, underscoring the importance of selecting the appropriate probiotic strain tailored to a particular health issue (Parker et al., 2018).

13.3 IMPACT OF PROBIOTICS ON GUT HEALTH

The ingestion of fermented foods has been linked to numerous health advantages, attributed to the presence of bioactive elements generated during the fermentation process, as well as the live probiotics they contain, being considered effective in the fight against chronic non-communicable diseases, IBS, anorexia, diabetes, and cardiovascular diseases (Patel et al., 2023). Probiotics and prebiotics have diverse mechanisms of action that can positively influence human health. These mechanisms encompass the inhibition of detrimental bacterial growth, reinforcement of barrier function, immune system modulation, and augmentation of metabolic processes (Guarner et al., 2012).

The intestinal tract is a multifaceted and ever-changing milieu that has developed distinct immunocellular attributes over time, primarily as a result of constant interaction with a diverse array of pathogens and antigens; thus, several classes of immune cells in the intestine play important roles in regulating host immunity and neutralizing possible infections (Sharifi-Rad et al., 2020; Zhou et al., 2020).

The microbiota present in the gut consists of a sensitive ecosystem of beneficial, neutral, and potentially pathogenic microorganisms. Some factors associated with human life such as a nutrient-poor diet, use of antibiotics, stress, and infections can unbalance the balance of the gut microbiota, which leads to an excessive growth of harmful bacteria. The composition of the intestinal microbiota can vary according to age, lifestyle, dietary habits, gender, and ethnicity. This variation is considered normal from a physiological point of view; however, it can lead to intestinal and extraintestinal disorders (Rinninella et al., 2019). In addition, probiotics can improve immunity, maintain the epithelial barrier, modulate the immune system, and inhibit the adhesion of pathogens to the intestinal surface (Wang et al., 2021).

Figure 13.2 presents the main beneficial actions of probiotics along the gastrointestinal tract.

The probiotic's mechanism of action to maintain intestinal health lies in the competition for the substrate necessary for the fermentation process with pathogenic microorganisms. In this way, probiotics prevent the adhesion of pathogenic bacteria to host cells, in addition to releasing metabolites with a protective effect in the intestine (Hemaiswarya et al., 2013; Plaza-Diaz et al., 2019).

The intestinal barrier functions as a protective shield, safeguarding the organism from the external environment and upholding the integrity of the epithelial lining. This intricate defense system encompasses the mucosal layer, immunoglobulin A (IgA), antimicrobial proteins, and the adhesive complex of epithelial junctions. When this barrier becomes compromised, whether through any

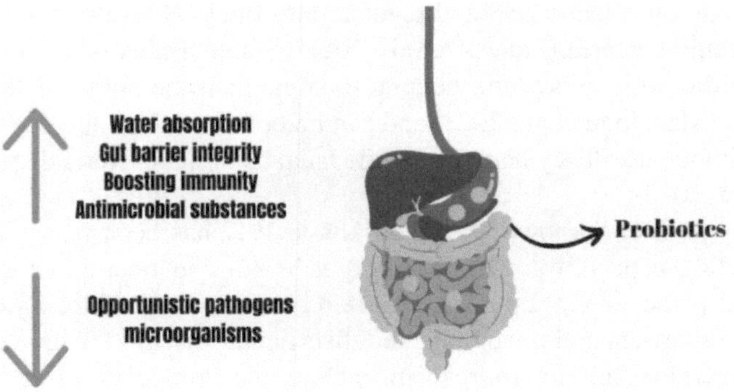

FIGURE 13.2 Action of probiotics in the gastrointestinal tract.

means, it allows bacteria and dietary antigens to penetrate the submucosal layer, inciting inflammatory reactions that give rise to various intestinal disorders (Sartor et al., 2006). The immunoglobulin A (IgA) antibody holds a pivotal position within the adaptive immune system, notably within mucosal regions. These antibodies are primarily manufactured by plasma cells situated in the intestinal lamina propria, shaping dimers united by a connecting chain. The process of transporting dimeric IgA across IECs and releasing it into the intestinal lumen is facilitated by its interaction with the polymeric immunoglobulin receptor (Xiong & Hu, 2015).

The intestinal epithelial tissue exhibits several physical adaptations to promote separation from the connective tissue of the host and the external environment. This structural barricade comprises a stratum of epithelial cells, their intercellular connections, and the mucous layer enveloping the epithelial surface (Artis & Grencis, 2008).

Probiotics can play a significant role in intestinal mucosa adhesion, which refers to the ability of beneficial microorganisms to adhere to the lining of the intestinal mucosa. This adhesion is essential for probiotics to exert their health benefits effectively. When probiotics adhere to the intestinal mucosa, they can interact more closely with the gut epithelial cells and modulate various physiological processes (Monteagudo-Mera et al., 2019). The attachment of probiotic bacteria to the intestinal mucosa is crucial for their establishment, as well as for modulating the immune system and resisting pathogens. This adherence process is intertwined with probiotic advantages and impacts, serving as a fundamental factor in the assessment and choice of novel probiotic strains (Popowska et al., 2017). This competitive exclusion can prevent harmful microbes from attaching to the intestinal mucosa and reduce their potential to cause infections or diseases (Tegegne & Kebede, 2022).

The adhesion of these microorganisms enables them to engage with the gut-associated lymphoid tissue. Through these interactions with immune cells, probiotics play a constructive role in shaping the immune response and mitigating inflammation within the intestinal environment (Mazziotta et al., 2023).

13.3.1 Role of Gut Microbiota in Digestive Health

Intestinal microorganisms constitute a vital component of the intestinal barrier, contributing significantly to the preservation of its normal functioning. These microorganisms are plentiful within the host's intestines, establishing a symbiotic relationship through colonization (Gou et al., 2022).

Probiotics possess the capacity to shape the makeup of gut microbiota by fostering an equilibrium and restraining the growth of potentially detrimental bacteria within the gastrointestinal tract. Research indicates that probiotic varieties such as LA and *L. casei* can enhance the presence of advantageous LAB, while concurrently diminishing the prevalence of fecal coliforms and anaerobic bacteria in the intestinal environment (Galdeno et al., 2016).

The gastrointestinal mucosa holds immense significance as one of the primary defense sites within the human body. It presents an interface where foreign antigens, microbes, parasites, and potential pathogens can closely engage with the host's immune system. Structurally, it forms a semi-permeable barrier that facilitates nutrient absorption and immune surveillance by curbing the entry of harmful antigens and microbes. The gastrointestinal mucosal barrier is constructed from four essential components. First, the commensal microbiota plays a pivotal role. Second, the mucus layer contains molecules that secrete IgA and peptides endowed with antimicrobial properties. The third element is the monolayer of IECs. Lastly, the lymphoid tissue encompasses diverse populations of immune cells, situated within compartments distributed throughout the length of the gastrointestinal tract (Vancamelbeke & Vermeire, 2017).

The gut microbiota holds a crucial function in upholding general health and overall well-being. Restoring and maintaining gut microbial balance is one of the key roles of probiotics. When this microbial balance is disrupted, it can lead to various health issues (Thursby & Juge, 2017). The cooperation between probiotics fosters the proliferation of beneficial bacteria and hinders the progression of harmful bacteria. This interaction arises through several mechanisms:

13.4 COMPETITIVE EXCLUSION

Several strategies have been developed to reduce the population of pathogenic and undesirable bacteria in the gastrointestinal tract from food sources. However, many of them depend on the natural competition of bacteria to eliminate pathogens that affect food safety and consumer health. Therefore, probiotics have been developed and classified as competitive exclusion cultures in the pathogen reduction strategy (Callaway et al., 2008).

Competitive exclusion refers to the capability of specific probiotic microorganisms to outcompete harmful or pathogenic bacteria in the gastrointestinal tract through competitive interactions. When probiotics are introduced into the gut, they compete with undesirable microorganisms for nutrients, adhesion sites on the gut lining, and other essential resources. This competition can help prevent harmful bacteria from establishing and thriving in the gut, thereby promoting a healthier gut microbial balance (Binda et al., 2020).

Probiotic bacteria can consume nutrients and occupy niches in the gut, reducing the availability of resources for harmful bacteria, which helps limit their growth. Certain strains of probiotics synthesize antimicrobial compounds, including bacteriocins, organic acids, and hydrogen peroxide, that possess the ability to impede the proliferation of pathogens (Sudheer et al., 2022). Nonetheless, the efficacy of distinct probiotic strains can differ, necessitating further research to enhance comprehension of their modes of operation and potential uses. (McFarland et al., 2018).

13.5 PRODUCTION OF ANTIMICROBIAL SUBSTANCES

Probiotic bacteria have gained recognition for their capacity to generate antimicrobial compounds, a pivotal factor contributing to their aptitude in bolstering gastrointestinal well-being and counteracting detrimental pathogens. These antimicrobial agents assume a crucial role in curbing the growth and actions of harmful bacteria and other microorganisms within the gut (Amara & Shibl, 2015). Among the notable antimicrobial substances synthesized by probiotics are bacteriocins, hydrogen peroxide, SCFAs, and organic acids.

Bacteriocins are small proteinaceous compounds with antimicrobial properties that are produced by certain probiotic bacteria. These compounds can selectively target and kill specific pathogenic bacteria, while sparing beneficial bacteria. Bacteriocins contribute to the preservation of a harmonious gut microbiota by diminishing the presence of detrimental organisms (Darbandi et al., 2022).

Probiotic microorganisms have the capability to generate organic acids, including acetic acid, lactic acid, and propionic acid, through the fermentation of carbohydrates. These organic acids establish an acidic milieu within the gut, creating an inhospitable setting for the proliferation of numerous pathogenic bacteria. Additionally, organic acids can help improve the gut barrier function and reduce the risk of harmful bacteria crossing into the bloodstream (Wang et al., 2021). In the small intestine, microorganisms with probiotic action have the ability to ferment non-digestible carbohydrates, such as inulin, galactose, oligosaccharides containing xylose from various plant sources, and fructo-oligosaccharides to meet energy needs (Hutkins et al., 2016).

Some probiotic strains, particularly certain *Lactobacillus* species, produce hydrogen peroxide as a byproduct of their metabolic processes. Hydrogen peroxide possesses antimicrobial attributes and aids in regulating the expansion of detrimental bacteria within the gut (Dempsey & Corr, 2022).

Specific strains of advantageous bacteria, such as *Bifidobacterium* and select *Lactobacillus* species, engage in dietary fiber fermentation, yielding SCFAs like butyrate, acetate, and propionate. SCFAs confer an array of health advantages, including fortifying the integrity of the gut lining, augmenting immune function, modulating inflammation, and cultivating a gut environment conducive to the proliferation of beneficial bacteria while impeding the growth of detrimental ones (Silva et al., 2020).

It can also exert its antimicrobial effects simply by outcompeting harmful bacteria for available nutrients in the gut. By consuming the available resources, probiotics limit the growth and survival of pathogenic bacteria that depend on the same nutrients. The production of antimicrobial substances by probiotics is one of the mechanisms through which these beneficial microorganisms contribute to a balanced gut microbiota and support overall gut health. However, the effects of probiotics can be strain-specific (Fijan, 2023).

13.6 MODULATION OF GUT pH

The presence and actions of probiotics can induce modifications in the acidity of the intestinal milieu. The pH balance within the gastrointestinal tract assumes a pivotal role in molding the constitution and functions of the gut microbiota, influencing both the proliferation of beneficial bacteria and the viability of detrimental counterparts. The pH can be changed by some controls such as organic food production, use of specific nutrients, fermentation intensity, interaction with host cells, and buffering capacity (Zheng et al., 2020).

The adjustment of gut pH through the influence of probiotics contributes to fostering a more favorable gut milieu. This modulation encourages the proliferation of beneficial bacteria while restraining the growth of detrimental ones. A balanced gut microbiota with an appropriate pH level is associated with improved digestion, enhanced nutrient absorption, strengthened gut barrier function, and a reduced risk of gastrointestinal disorders (Peng et al., 2020).

Several bacteria considered probiotics produce organic acids during the fermentation of carbohydrates. These acids promote the reduction of the pH of the intestine, making it more acidic. Consequently, a mildly acidic setting typically fosters the proliferation of advantageous bacteria, while hampering the development of numerous pathogenic counterparts that thrive in less acidic conditions (You et al., 2022).

Probiotic bacteria compete with other microorganisms, including harmful ones, for available nutrients in the gut. By utilizing these nutrients, probiotics can limit the growth of potentially harmful bacteria that may contribute to a less desirable gut pH (Liao & Nyachoti, 2017).

Probiotics are involved in the fermentation process in the gut. As they ferment dietary fibers and other substrates, they produce various metabolites, including SCFAs. SCFAs have a direct impact on gut pH. These SCFAs help maintain an optimal pH for the growth of beneficial bacteria while discouraging the proliferation of harmful ones (Kumar et al., 2022).

It can interact with the cells lining the intestinal wall. These interactions can stimulate the secretion of certain substances that regulate pH levels in the gut and help maintain a balanced gut environment (Carabotti et al., 2015).

Some probiotic strains possess the ability to resist changes in pH, acting as buffers in the gut environment. This buffer capacity can help stabilize the pH and prevent significant fluctuations, which is beneficial for the gut microbiota (Sylvain et al., 2016).

13.7 IMMUNOMODULATION

Probiotics can exert immunomodulatory effects, meaning they can influence and regulate the immune system's activity. These effects can be beneficial in maintaining immune homeostasis, enhancing immune responses against pathogens, and potentially managing immune-related disorders (Raheem et al., 2021).

The immune-regulating capabilities of probiotics have prompted research into their potential as supplementary agents for addressing a range of immune-associated conditions, encompassing allergies, inflammatory bowel disorders, and respiratory infections. Moreover, probiotics could potentially contribute to enhancing immune activity within susceptible groups, like the elderly and individuals undergoing medical treatments that compromise the immune system (Cristofori et al., 2021).

In this case, the immunomodulatory properties of probiotics are the result of some mechanisms: regulation of immune cell activity, cytokine production, enhanced barrier function, regulation of toll-like receptors, anti-inflammatory effects, and promotes the induction of regulatory T cells (Galdeno et al., 2019).

Probiotics have the capacity to engage with immune cells situated in the gut-associated lymphoid tissue, encompassing structures like Peyer's patches and lymph nodes embedded in the intestinal wall. Through interactions with immune components such as T cells, B cells, and antigen-presenting cells, probiotics are capable of contributing to the equilibrium between pro-inflammatory and anti-inflammatory reactions. The gut serves as a primary locus for the interplay between probiotics and the immune system, primarily due to the substantial presence of immune cells within the gut-associated lymphoid tissue (Yousefi et al., 2018).

In addition, these microorganisms can influence the process of cytokine secretion, which are signaling molecules that mediate immune responses. Certain probiotics stimulate the synthesis of anti-inflammatory cytokines, such as IL-10, while concurrently dampening the expression of pro-inflammatory cytokines such as TNF-α and IL-6 (Azad et al., 2018).

Probiotics hold the capacity to enhance the performance of the intestinal barrier by promoting the production of tight junction proteins and mucus. This reinforcement aids in upholding gut integrity and diminishing inflammation. Furthermore, probiotics can engage with TLRs present in immune cells. By engaging these receptors, probiotics can influence immune responses, including the activation of specific immune pathways (Gou et al., 2022).

Regulatory T cells (Tregs) constitute a distinct and crucial subset of T cells with a pivotal responsibility in preserving immune tolerance and curbing excessive immune reactions. These cells are integral for regulating the immune system and averting autoimmune responses. Studies have demonstrated that probiotics possess the capability to stimulate and advance the maturation of regulatory T cells, thereby contributing to their immunomodulatory influence (Rocamora-Reverte et al., 2021).

The triggering of regulatory T cells through probiotics is a promising area of research in the field of immunology. It suggests that probiotics can potentially be used as therapeutic agents to help modulate immune responses and manage immune-related disorders, such as autoimmune diseases and allergies (Bubnov et al., 2015).

13.8 RESTORATION AFTER DISRUPTION

Probiotics have been studied for their potential to aid in the restoration of gut health after disruptions, such as those caused by antibiotics, infections, or dietary changes. When the natural balance of gut microbiota is disturbed, it can lead to dysbiosis and various gastrointestinal issues. Recent discoveries concerning the structure and operational aspects of the microbiome have underscored the considerable impact that diet can exert on the makeup of the gut microbiota. This, in a cyclical manner, subsequently influences the well-being of both humans and animals. Disruptions in the delicate balance between microbes and their hosts can lead to various disease conditions, including chronic inflammation, autoimmune disorders, and neurological issues (Hemarajata & Versalovic, 2013). In addition to their direct influence on shaping the gut microbiota composition, probiotics might have an impact on the broader metabolic functioning of intestinal microbiomes (McNulty et al., 2011).

One of the mechanisms is the replenishment of beneficial bacteria as a way of recomposing the gastrointestinal flora. Probiotics contain live beneficial bacteria that can help replenish the gut with strains that are temporarily reduced or altered during disruptions. By introducing these beneficial microbes, probiotics can support the restoration of a balanced gut microbiota. In this case, specific strains of beneficial bacteria obtained from the consumption of probiotic foods are introduced into the gastrointestinal tract and restart the colonization process, helping to replenish populations of beneficial microorganisms that may have been reduced or disrupted (Huang et al., 2022).

13.9 FERMENTATION OF DIETARY FIBERS

Dietary fiber constitutes a prominent non-digestible constituent within diets, synergistically interconnecting with various physiological elements within the digestive tract. This collaboration extends to configuring the digesta, which holds significance in terms of satiety and the regulation of food consumption. Furthermore, dietary fiber partakes in the modulation of digestive processes, facilitating improved management of lipid and glucose levels circulating in the bloodstream. Additionally, it serves as a substrate for the microbial fermentation processes facilitated by probiotics, contributing to the mitigation of colon cancer risk and aiding in bowel regularity. These fibers, characterized by their distinct chemical structure and molecular weight, yield elevated digestive viscosity, ultimately leading to a diminished glycemic response (Mudgil & Barak, 2013; Williams et al., 2017; Nascimento et al., 2019).

The fermentation of dietary fibers by probiotics constitutes a pivotal metabolic activity that unfolds within the gastrointestinal tract. Specific strains of probiotic bacteria, like certain varieties of *Lactobacillus* and *Bifidobacterium*, harness dietary fibers as an energy source and engage in fermentation processes to enzymatically deconstruct these intricate carbohydrates into more elementary compounds. Throughout this fermentation, probiotics generate a range of metabolites, among them SCFAs, as exemplified by (Shah et al., 2020).

The fermentation of dietary fibers by probiotics yields advantages not only for the probiotic bacteria but also for the host's gastrointestinal well-being. The resulting SCFAs serve as an energy resource for the cells that line the intestinal barrier, contributing to enhanced nutrient uptake. Furthermore, this process aids in upholding a harmonious gut microbiota by fostering the proliferation of beneficial bacteria. The fermentation of dietary fibers by probiotics encompasses a cascade of metabolic activities executed by these advantageous microorganisms within the gastrointestinal tract (Markowiak-Kopeć & Śliżewska, 2020).

Initially, probiotic bacteria release specific enzymes to carry out the process of decomposition of complex dietary fibers into smaller, digestible components by the bacteria, in order to help access the nutrients present in dietary fibers (Saarinen et al., 2012).

Once the fibers are broken down, probiotics use oligosaccharides and other fermentable carbohydrates as an energy source. Among the final products of fermentation are the SCFAs, which will be used as a source of energy for the cells that line the intestinal wall, promoting the maintenance of the health of the enterocytes. In addition, they play an important role in regulating the intestine, maintaining a slightly acidic pH, favoring the growth of beneficial bacteria, and inhibiting the growth of pathogens (Simpson & Campbell, 2015).

SCFAs have the ability to interact with the immune system by influencing immune responses and promoting balanced immune function by reducing gut inflammation. In general, each of the SCFAs produced during dietary fiber fermentation has unique and specific roles in promoting health. Collectively, they play a fundamental role in supporting gut well-being. For instance, since all SCFAs are weak acids, they contribute to lowering the colonic pH. This decrease in pH is beneficial as it can inhibit the growth of harmful pathogenic bacteria like Enterobacteriaceae, which are sensitive to low pH levels (den Besten et al., 2013).

13.10 CROSS-FEEDING

Cross-feeding stands as a notable occurrence observed within probiotic bacteria and other constituents of the gut microbiota. This phenomenon delineates the cooperative metabolic interactions transpiring amid diverse microorganisms within the gut environment. Probiotic microorganisms engage in the fermentation process to yield specific metabolites, which subsequently function as substrates or nourishment for other advantageous microbes present in the gut (Cheng et al., 2020). Microbial cross-feeding manifests as a sequential procedure where microorganisms establish interactions by utilizing molecules generated during the metabolic activities of one microbe (designated as the provider or producer). These molecules subsequently undergo further metabolic transformation by another microorganism (termed the receiver or beneficiary) (Smith et al., 2019).

The notion that cross-feeding influences microbiome composition has been substantiated through both theoretical deliberations and practical investigations. This understanding has emerged through the utilization of a systems biology approach to microbial communities, which is referred to as microbial systems ecology. This approach entails scrutinizing comprehensive omics data in an integrated manner (Montaigne et al., 2021).

Bifidobacteria emerge as early inhabitants of the mammalian gut, capitalizing on their capacity to degrade intricate carbohydrates to facilitate colonization. Their prominence within the initial gut microbiota can be attributed, in part, to their aptitude for tapping into glycans within the gut environment via mutually beneficial cross-feeding or resource-sharing interactions. This phenomenon underscores a sort of "social conduct" exhibited among diverse bifidobacterial strains, wherein they collaborate to exploit and harness available resources. The intricate interplays and genetic strategies orchestrated by bifidobacteria offer insights into their adeptness in adapting to the gut milieu and their pivotal role as indispensable components of the gut microbiota. Deeper investigations in this domain are imperative for a comprehensive grasp of the mechanisms underpinning these intriguing behaviors and their potential implications for gut health (Turroni et al., 2017).

Boger et al. (2018) explored the co-cultivation of *L. salivarius* and *Lactobacillus paracasei* in the presence of inulin, leading to encouraging outcomes in terms of the second strain's beneficial interactions with the first. This synergy was facilitated by the presence of an extracellular exo-inulinase. The phenomenon of cross-feeding was contingent upon the specific carbohydrate type and its corresponding chain length.

Probiotics can bring about various modifications in the gut microbiota, causing a more balanced and diverse microbial ecosystem. Microbiome modulation can occur through two primary mechanisms: first, directly via the influence of dietary constituents on the metabolic functions and composition of the microbiome; and second, indirectly by shaping the gut's physiological aspects to induce alterations in the environment within the intestinal lumen, subsequently affecting the microbiome. In both cases, dietary choices play a crucial role in shaping the gut microbiome and its functions, which can have significant implications for overall health and well-being (Basu & Donaldson, 2003).

The gut microbiota population is perpetually in flux and tailored to each individual, molded by an array of elements like dietary patterns, interactions with ingested probiotics, prevailing intestinal circumstances, and other host-specific factors. This ever-evolving essence of the microbiota signifies their potential to incorporate novel strains "transiently" into the ecosystem. These variations amplify the diversity and intricacy of the gut's microbial assembly, a pivotal factor in nurturing gut health and overall holistic wellness (Zhang et al., 2016).

Different probiotic strains have unique effects on the gut microbiota. Some strains may have a more significant impact on specific bacterial groups, while others might influence the overall diversity of the microbiome. It's important to consider the strain specificity of probiotics when choosing appropriate supplements or foods.

13.11 APPLICATION OF PROBIOTICS IN FOOD SAFETY AND PRESERVATION

Probiotics have been explored for their potential applications in food safety and preservation due to their beneficial effects on gut health and antimicrobial properties.

Food safety is jeopardized by various factors, including chemical, biological, and physical hazards. Among these, biological hazards, particularly bacteria, play a significant role in causing food spoilage and foodborne illnesses. In recent years, a novel approach has emerged, utilizing probiotics and postbiotics, to address this issue. Probiotics and postbiotics are known for their potent antimicrobial properties, offering a promising method to control the growth of pathogenic microorganisms and prevent food contamination. This innovative approach has the potential to enhance food safety and minimize the risks associated with foodborne diseases (Rad et al., 2021).

Generally, the probiotics offered on the market are linked to beverages and dairy products, however, they are unsuitable for individuals who have casein allergies, lactose intolerant, or who are adherents of the vegan diet (Vasudha & Mishra, 2013). In this context, other fermented products have been the target of the application of probiotic cultures such as kombucha (Filho et al., 2023).

One of the mechanisms that LAB use to collaborate with food safety is the massive production of lactic acid through carbohydrate fermentation. This process is defined as food acidification (Bintsis et al., 2018). The production of lactic acid by these microorganisms allows the appearance of acidic conditions in fermented foods, making the environment hostile to pathogenic and spoilage microorganisms. Therefore, reduced pH values improve the hygienic-sanitary properties of foods and prolong their shelf life (Papadimitriou et al., 2016).

The utilization of probiotics as biocontrol agents within the realm of aquaculture is witnessing an upward trajectory, driven by the escalating demand for ecologically conscious and sustainable approaches in aquaculture endeavors. Probiotics present numerous merits as supplements, encompassing the augmentation of the nutritional quality of aquaculture yields, the curbing of detrimental pathogen expansion, and the enhancement of the immune defense mechanisms in aquatic organisms. Consequently, the integration of probiotics into aquaculture practices holds the potential to foster more healthful and sustainable production techniques, concurrently championing ecological harmony (Soliman et al., 2019).

The beneficial microorganisms extracted from the intestinal tract of healthy shrimp exhibited notable efficacy in impeding the growth of Vibrio pathogens, as evidenced by substantial inhibition zones. The *Vibrio* pathogens in question, including *Vibrio alginolyticus*, *Vibrio parahaemolyticus*, *Vibrio harveyi*, and *Vibrio cholera* were isolated and cultivated on TCBS media. Employing the well-diffusion technique, three distinct strains, specifically *L. paracasei*, *Lactobacillus rhamnosus*, and *Pediococcus acidilactici*, consistently manifested consistent probiotic activity against the targeted pathogens (Rajyalakshmi et al., 2021).

In the context of biological control, probiotic yeasts or products containing yeast cell walls have been utilized to combat mycotoxins. Various yeast strains have shown effectiveness in transforming toxins into non-toxic or less-toxic substances, and some can also inhibit the growth of filamentous fungi. Incorporating yeasts into different technological processes can directly hinder the synthesis of toxins by specific fungi. Additionally, certain yeast species have the capability to accumulate mycotoxins from agricultural products, effectively detoxifying them in the process. This approach shows promise as a natural and eco-friendly method to address mycotoxin contamination in various settings (Pfliegler et al., 2015).

Based on the recent research findings, both probiotic bacteria and yeast strains demonstrated effective inhibition of toxigenic fungi growth. These probiotics showed a significant decrease in mycotoxin production. Notably, *L. plantarum* displayed the most substantial reduction, with a 64.51% decrease in AFS production by *A. flavus* and an 87.21% decrease in OTA production by *P. nordicum*. The potential of probiotics as a valuable strategy for controlling mycotoxin production and reducing the impact of toxigenic fungi in various applications (Ab El-Fadeel et al., 2022).

Biological approaches encompass the utilization of naturally derived compounds from plants, animals, and microorganisms, capable of impeding the proliferation of pathogenic microorganisms within food. Among the antimicrobial methodologies are the incorporation of probiotics, bacteriophages, and their corresponding metabolites (Seal et al., 2018; Agripoulou et al., 2020). These antimicrobial agents encompass natural or synthetic substances or metabolites, adept at restraining or eradicating the growth of pathogenic microorganisms, all without recourse to antibiotics, as elucidated by Lewis (2013).

Strains of *Lactobacillus* were subject to scrutiny regarding their capacity to generate antimicrobial compounds exhibiting effectiveness against *E. coli, Shigella sonnei*, and *Salmonella typhimurium*. These strains demonstrated potent antimicrobial attributes against *S. sonnei*, particularly under conditions of increased acidity. Furthermore, the production of the observed antimicrobial agents was contingent upon the organic acids synthesis, most notably lactic acid, as indicated in the study conducted by Zhang et al. (2011).

13.11.1 Nutritional Enhancement Through Probiotics

The concept of nutritional enhancement utilizing probiotics entails harnessing advantageous microorganisms to elevate the nutritional quality and facilitate the health advantages of food items (Amara & Shibl, 2015).

The process of fermentation enables the removal of antinutrients from food, potentially resulting in the production of bioactive substances like vitamins, enzymes, minerals, and peptides (Kumari et al., 2022). In this context, probiotics assume a pivotal role in preserving the harmonious bacterial equilibrium within the intestine, thereby fostering diversity and balance (Wang et al., 2021).

13.11.2 Probiotics as Vitamin Producers

Probiotics, notably specific bacterial strains, possess a remarkable capability to generate vitamins within the human body. These vitamins play a pivotal role in various physiological processes, underpinning overall well-being (LeBlanc et al., 2017). The synthesis of vitamins by probiotic bacteria within the intestinal milieu offers a natural and advantageous avenue for enriching human vitamin levels. Certain strains of probiotic bacteria, particularly those belonging to *Lactobacillus* and *Bifidobacterium*, exhibit the proficiency to produce an array of vitamins, including B vitamins and vitamin K2 (menaquinone) (Barkhidarian et al., 2021; Molina et al., 2012).

By producing these vitamins within the gut, probiotics contribute to the overall nutrient balance and can potentially supplement the dietary intake of these essential vitamins. This is particularly significant in cases where dietary sources of vitamins may be limited or not well absorbed by the body (Pham et al., 2021).

The synthesis of vitamins by probiotics constitutes an integral facet of the complex symbiotic interaction between these advantageous bacteria and the human host. As probiotics establish residence within the gastrointestinal tract and engage with dietary components, they actively contribute to the host's comprehensive nutritional well-being and provide bolstering assistance to a diverse array of physiological functions (Hou et al., 2022).

Retinoids, commonly known as vitamin A, assume pivotal roles in a multitude of cellular functions distributed across the body. Within the gastrointestinal tract, their significance becomes particularly pronounced in processes such as mucin synthesis, cellular proliferation, and cellular differentiation. These aspects hold a critical importance in preserving the standard barrier functionality of the intestines. In instances where the intestinal mucosal function experiences disruption, it has the potential to induce changes in the permeability of the intestinal epithelium and hinder the generation of biochemical substances that engage with gut microorganisms. Consequently, the status of vitamin A within the body can wield influence over the gut microbiome through its impact on the integrity of the intestinal mucosal barrier. This intricate correlation underscores the interconnectedness of nutrition, gut health, and the microbial ensemble residing within the intestinal realm (Huda et al., 2019; Pham et al., 2021).

Li et al. (2017) investigated extracellular strains of *Lactobacillus* regarding the production of vitamin B12 and its characteristics of tolerance and environmental stresses, bile salts, and gastric acid. *L. plantarum* strains showed high extracellular production of B12 under environmental stress and showed good viability to gastric acid and bile salts. In another study, Li et al. (2017) identified five strains of Enterococcus strains isolated from infant feces that were identified as B12 producers, among them, *Enterococcus faecium*, which produced the highest amount (~ 500 μg/L).

13.11.3 Enhancement of Mineral Bioavailability by Probiotics

Bacteria exert substantial influence over the bioavailability and bioaccessibility of minerals, a phenomenon that can be further heightened through processes like cereal fermentation and crop germination. Probiotics, in particular, have demonstrated the capacity to exert a positive impact on the accessibility of minerals such as iron, calcium, selenium, and zinc by engaging with the gut microbiome and its metabolic functions. The existing body of scientific knowledge underscores the advantageous implications of bacteria in elevating mineral bioaccessibility and bioavailability, thereby rendering support to both the human gut microbiome and overall well-being. These discoveries underscore the significance of contemplating probiotics and bacterial fermentation techniques as prospective avenues to amplify mineral assimilation and utilization, ultimately contributing to enhanced nutritional outcomes and holistic wellness (Bielik & Kolisek, 2021).

Probiotic bacteria, especially LAB, produce organic acids throughout the fermentation. These organic acids help to lower the pH in the gut, creating an acidic environment that aids in the solubilization of minerals, particularly calcium, iron, and magnesium. Solubilized minerals are more readily absorbed by the body (Lau et al., 2021). Some probiotics have the ability to form complexes with minerals through the chelation process, which involves the binding of minerals with organic molecules, favoring their stability and bioavailability to be absorbed by the human body (Dinu et al., 2022). When probiotics encounter mineral ions in the gut, the chelating agents produced by the bacteria form stable complexes with the minerals. These complexes prevent the minerals from precipitating or binding to other compounds that might hinder their absorption (Tsafrakidou et al., 2020).

In this way, solubilized minerals are more available for absorption by the lining of the intestine and can be used more efficiently by the body, since, by forming stable chelates, probiotics collaborate to shield minerals from reacting with other substances, which can prevent their absorption. This results in improved bioavailability, with more chelated minerals being absorbed. In turn, this improved bioavailability can positively affect many physiological processes in the body, for example, increased calcium absorption supports bone health, while improved iron absorption helps prevent anemia (Scholz-Ahrens et al., 2007; Skrypnik & Suliburska, 2017).

Among the chelating agents produced by probiotics, organic acids stand out, especially lactic, citric, acetic, and malic acids. These acids have several carboxyl groups in their structures, which can form strong bonds with metal ions, promoting chelation. Many traditional fermented foods, such as yogurt, kefir, sauerkraut, and kimchi, are rich in probiotics and can contribute to mineral chelation. The fermentation process leads to the production of chelating agents, increasing the nutritional quality of these foods (Ke et al., 2018; Soemarie et al., 2021).

The probiotic chelation efficacy can fluctuate among individuals owing to variations in gut microbiota makeup, genetic influences, and dietary patterns. As a consequence, the advantages derived from chelation could exhibit more notable outcomes in certain individuals compared to others (Chen et al., 2022).

13.12 PROBIOTICS IN THE FUNCTIONAL FOODS

Functional foods constitute a distinct class of edibles, encompassing both unprocessed and processed variants, which constitute a vital component of everyday dietary practices. Beyond merely providing vital nutritional components, these foods harbor the potential to confer beneficial effects on the well-being of the individual consumer. Their utilization can play a role in mitigating the likelihood of specific illnesses by augmenting the immune system's prowess in thwarting and combating infections attributed to pathogens. Furthermore, functional foods might also lend a hand in the management or alleviation of conditions that engender functional disruptions within the host's physiological framework (Granato et al., 2020).

Functional foods enriched with probiotics assume a pivotal function in fostering equilibrium within the host's gastrointestinal microbiota. A wealth of extensive investigations has substantiated the compelling merits associated with probiotics, encompassing an array of advantageous outcomes. These encompass the thwarting of diverse intestinal disorders, fortification against specific cancer forms, stimulation of immune responsiveness, mitigation of symptomatic manifestations linked to IBS, curtailment of cholesterol levels, and engagement in other pivotal physiological mechanisms (Saulnier et al., 2009; Zommiti et al., 2020).

Certain constituents and compounds present in food possess the potential to exert adverse influences on the development and viability of probiotics. Among these, a notable category is that of polyphenolic compounds, commonly prevalent in plant-derived food items. Renowned for their antioxidant attributes, polyphenols are frequently associated with diverse health advantages. However, investigations have unveiled inhibitory ramifications of polyphenolic compounds on LAB, a subgroup of beneficial probiotics. The presence of polyphenols within the gut milieu might impede the expansion and function of these probiotic microorganisms, potentially diminishing their efficacy in fostering gut well-being. This underscores the critical significance of recognizing the interplay between probiotics and specific nutritional constituents during the formulation of probiotic-enriched foods or supplements (Rodríguez et al., 2009; Palanivelu et al., 2022).

Chosen strains of LAB with well-established probiotic attributes exhibit a range of health advantages, notably their capacity to foster equilibrium within the intestinal microbiota through the suppression of detrimental pathogenic proliferation. Extensive scrutiny of these strains has underscored their favorable impact on gut well-being (Dicks & Botes, 2010).

Thanks to their advantageous attributes, specific probiotic LAB strains find application as starter cultures in the creation of functional foods, which are foods that offer supplementary health advantages beyond fundamental nutrition. Probiotic-containing foods, such as yogurt, kefir, and fermented vegetables, are examples of functional foods that utilize probiotic LAB as starter cultures. These probiotic-containing foods are not only delicious but also promote gut health and overall well-being (Damián et al., 2022).

During the formulation of a functional fermented beetroot beverage, the utilization of two distinct probiotic strains was integrated. These strains encompassed the ABT-5 probiotic formulation, encompassing *Streptococcus thermophilus,* BB-12, and LA-5, alongside the singular presence of LA-5.

The fermentation process played a crucial role in bringing about several positive attributes in the final product. As a result of the fermentation process, the beverage's antioxidant capacity experienced enhancement. Probiotic fermentation can release bioactive compounds that contribute to antioxidant properties, enhancing the potential health benefits of the beverage. The zinc content of the beverage was also increased through fermentation. Probiotic bacteria have the ability to release bound zinc from food matrices, making it more bioavailable for absorption in the digestive system. The fermentation process improved the organoleptic properties of the beverage, including taste, flavor, and consistency. During fermentation, lactate is formed as a byproduct, which can enhance the taste and tanginess of the beverage, making it more palatable (Abdo et al., 2020).

Strains of *Lactobacillus* species have shown promise in exerting beneficial effects on individuals with diet-induced obesity. These probiotics have the potential to reduce body fat percentage, particularly by reducing the size of white adipose tissue cells. Given the significant potential of dietary-based approaches in effectively managing type 2 diabetes, researchers are actively exploring methods to safely and efficiently modify human gut microflora. To advance our understanding in this field, future research endeavors should prioritize investigating the immunomodulatory, complex hormonal, and metabolic mechanisms underlying the interaction between gut microbiota and the host across various tissues. By gaining insights into these intricate processes, we can unlock new avenues for improving human health and addressing conditions related to obesity and metabolic disorders. For meaningful clinical applications, it is essential that treatments be thoroughly evaluated through well-designed trials that focus on patient-oriented endpoints (Larsen et al., 2010; Begum et al., 2017).

13.13 CONCLUSION

The incorporation of probiotics into food products represents a promising and versatile approach to enhancing food quality and promoting consumer health. Probiotics, as live microorganisms, exert numerous beneficial effects when consumed in adequate amounts. Their ability to promote a balanced gut microbiota stands out as a primary benefit, leading to improved digestive health, enhanced nutrient absorption, and strengthened immune function.

Probiotics have a vital role in ensuring food safety and preservation, showcased by their antimicrobial attributes capable of restraining the proliferation of detrimental bacteria and pathogens. Moreover, their ability to heighten the bioavailability of specific nutrients also contributes to the nutritional worth of food items.

The probiotics application in the food industry is diverse, with potential incorporation into various food items such as fermented foods, beverages, dairy products, baked goods, and snacks. However, successful integration necessitates careful consideration of various factors, including regulatory requirements, labeling guidelines, and consumer acceptance.

As research and technological advancements continue, the future is promising for the expanded incorporation of probiotics into food products, offering consumers a broader range of functional and health-promoting choices. Probiotics represent a significant step toward a healthier and more diversified food landscape, benefiting both the food industry and consumers alike.

BIBLIOGRAPHY

Abdo, E., El-Sohaimy, S., Shaltout, O., Abdalla, A., Zeitoun, A. (2020). Nutritional evaluation of beetroots (*Beta vulgaris* L.) and its potential application in a functional beverage. *Plants, 9*(12), 1752–1761. https://doi.org/10.3390/plants9121752

Abedini, R., Zaghari, G., Jabbari, L., Salekdeh, G. H., & Hashemi, M. (2023). A potential probiotic *Enterococcus faecium* isolated from camel rumen, fatty acids biotransformation, antilisteria activity and safety assessment. *International Dairy Journal, 145,* 706–714. https://doi.org/10.1016/j.idairyj.2023.105706

Ab EL-Fadeel, R. H., Ahmed Shalaby, S. O., Arafa Mohamed, M. M., & Khater, K. (2022). Biological control of some types of mycotoxins by probiotic bacteria and yeast strains. *Egyptian Journal of Dairy Science, 21,* 67–75. https://doi.org/10.21608/ejds.2022.171199.1008

Agriopoulou, S., Stamatelopoulou, E., Sachadyn-Król, M., & Varzakas, T. (2020). Lactic acid bacteria as antibacterial agents to extend the shelf life of fresh and minimally processed fruits and vegetables: Quality and safety aspects. *Microorganisms, 8*(6), 88–96. https://doi.org/10.3390/microorganisms 8060952

Amara, A. A., & Shibl, A. (2015). Role of probiotics in health improvement, infection control and disease treatment and management. *Saudi Pharmaceutical Journal, 23*(2), 107–114. https://doi.org/10.1016/j.jsps.2013.07.001

Angelin, J., & Kavitha, M. (2020). Exopolysaccharides from probiotic bacteria and their health potential. *International Journal of Biological Macromolecules, 162*(2), 853–865. https://doi.org/10.1016/j.ijbiomac.2020.06.190

Anukam, K. C., & Reid, G. (2007). Probiotics: 100 years (1907–2007) after Elie Metchnikoff's observation. *Communicating Current Research and Educational Topics and Trends in Applied Microbiology, 1*, 466–474.

Artis, D., & Grencis, R. K. (2008). The intestinal epithelium: Sensors to effectors in nematode infection. *Mucosal Immunology, 1*(4), 252–264. https://doi.org/10.1038/mi.2008.21

Azad, A. K., Sarker, M., & Wan, D. (2018). Immunomodulatory effects of probiotics on cytokine profiles. *BioMed Research International, 29,* 806–813.

Baig, M. A., Turner, M. S., Liu, S. Q., Shah, N. N., & Ayyash, M. M. (2022). Heat, cold, acid, and bile salt induced differential proteomic responses of a novel potential probiotic *Lactococcus garvieae* C47 isolated from camel milk. *Food Chemistry, 397,* 774–782. https://doi.org/10.1016/j.foodchem.2022.133774

Barbosa, J., Borges, S., & Teixeira, P. (2014). Selection of potential probiotic *Enterococcus faecium* isolated from Portuguese fermented food. *International Journal of Food Microbiology, 191,* 144–148. https://doi.org/10.1016/j.ijfoodmicro.2014.09.009

Barkhidarian, B., Roldos, L., Iskandar, M. M., Saedisomeolia, A., & Kubow, S. (2021). Probiotic supplementation and micronutrient status in healthy subjects: A systematic review of clinical trials. *Nutrients, 13*(9), 3001–3010. https://doi.org/10.3390/nu13093001

Baruah, R., Ray, M., & Halami, P. M. (2022). Preventive and therapeutic aspects of fermented foods. *Journal of Applied Microbiology, 132*(5), 3476–3489. https://doi.org/10.1111/jam.15444

Basu, T. K., & Donaldson, D. (2003). Intestinal absorption in health and disease: Micronutrients. *Best Practice and Research. Clinical Gastroenterology, 17*(6), 957–979. https://doi.org/10.1016/s1521-6918(03)00084-2

Begum, P., Madhavi, G., Rajagopal, S., Viswanath, B., Razak, M., & Venkataratnamma, V. (2017). Probiotics as functional foods potential effects on human health and its impact on neurological diseases. *International Journal of Nutrition, Pharmacology, Neurological Diseases, 7*(2), 23–33. https://doi.org/10.4103/ijnpnd.ijnpnd_90_16

Behrouzi, A., Mazaheri, H., Falsafi, S., Tavassol, Z. H., Moshiri, A., & Siadat, S. D. (2020). Intestinal effect of the probiotic Escherichia coli strain Nissle 1917 and its OMV. *Journal of Diabetes and Metabolic Disorders, 19*(1), 597–604. https://doi.org/10.1007/s40200-020-00511-6

Bielik, V., & Kolisek, M. (2021). Bioaccessibility and bioavailability of minerals in relation to a healthy gut microbiome. *International Journal of Molecular Sciences, 22*(13), 6803–6812. https://doi.org/10.3390/ijms22136803

Binda, S., Hill, C., Johansen, E., Obis, D., Pot, B., Sanders, M. E., Tremblay, A., & Ouwehand, A. C. (2020). Criteria to qualify microorganisms as "probiotic" in foods and dietary supplements. *Frontiers in Microbiology, 11,* 88–101. https://doi.org/10.3389/fmicb.2020.01662

Bintsis, T. (2018). Lactic acid bacteria as starter cultures: An update in their metabolism and genetics. *AIMS Microbiology, 4*(4), 665–684. https://doi.org/10.3934/microbiol.2018.4.665

Boger, M. C. L., Lammerts van Bueren, A. L., & Dijkhuizen, L. (2018). Cross-feeding among probiotic bacterial strains on prebiotic inulin involves the extracellular exo-inulinase of *Lactobacillus paracasei* Strain W20. *Applied and Environmental Microbiology, 84*(21), 820–831. https://doi.org/10.1128/AEM.01539-18

Bubnov, R. V., Spivak, M. Y., Lazarenko, L. M., Bomba, A., & Boyko, N. V. (2015). Probiotics and immunity: Provisional role for personalized diets and disease prevention. *EPMA Journal, 6*(1), 14–22. https://doi.org/10.1186/s13167-015-0036-0

Callaway, T. R., Edrington, T. S., Anderson, R. C., Harvey, R. B., Genovese, K. J., Kennedy, C. N., Venn, D. W., & Nisbet, D. J. (2008). Probiotics, prebiotics and competitive exclusion for prophylaxis against bacterial disease. *Animal Health Research Reviews, 9*(2), 217–225. https://doi.org/10.1017/S1466252308001540

Carabotti, M., Scirocco, A., Maselli, M. A., & Severi, C. (2015). The gut-brain axis: Interactions between enteric microbiota, central and enteric nervous systems. *Annals of Gastroenterology, 28*(2), 203–209.

Chen, J., & Hu, L. (2020). Nanoscale delivery system for nutraceuticals: Preparation, application, characterization, safety, and future trends. *Food Engineering Reviews, 12*(3), 14–31.

Chen, R., Tu, H., & Chen, T. (2022). Potential application of living microorganisms in the detoxification of heavy metals. *Foods, 11*(13), 1905–1917. https://doi.org/10.3390/foods11131905

Cheng, C. C., Duar, R. M., Lin, X., Perez-Munoz, M. E., Tollenaar, S., Oh, J. H., Pijkeren, J. P., Li, F., Sinderen, D. V., Ganzle, M. G., & Walter, J. (2020). Ecological importance of cross-feeding of the intermediate metabolite 1,2-propanediol between bacterial gut symbionts. *Applied and Environmental Microbiology, 86*(11), 190–220. https://doi.org/0.1128/AEM.00190-20

Coudeyras, S., Marchandin, H., Fajon, C., & Forestier, C. (2008). Taxonomic and strain-specific identification of the probiotic strain *Lactobacillus rhamnosus* 35 within the *Lactobacillus casei* group. *Applied and Environmental Microbiology, 74*(9), 2679–2689. https://doi.org/10.1128/AEM.02286-07

Cristofori, F., Dargenio, V. N., Dargenio, C., Miniello, V. L., Barone, M., & Francavilla, R. (2021). Anti-inflammatory and immunomodulatory effects of probiotics in gut inflammation: A door to the body. *Frontiers in Immunology, 12,* 578–589. https://doi.org/10.3389/fimmu.2021.578386

Damián, M. R., Cortes-Perez, N. G., Quintana, E. T., Ortiz-Moreno, A., Garfias Noguez, C., Cruceño-Casarrubias, C. E., Sánchez Pardo, M. E., & Bermúdez-Humarán, L. G. (2022). Functional foods, nutraceuticals and probiotics: A focus on human health. *Microorganisms, 10*(5), 1065–1079. https://doi.org/10.3390/microorganisms10051065

Darbandi, A., Asadi, A., Ari, M. M., Ohadi, E., Talebi, M., Zadeh, M. H., Emamie, A. D., Ghanavati, R., & Kakan, M. (2022). Bacteriocins: Properties and potential use as antimicrobials. *Journal of Clinical Laboratory Analysis, 36*(1), 240–252. https://doi.org/10.1002/jcla.24093

Das, T. K., Pradhan, S., Chakrabarti, S., Mondal, K. C., & Ghosh, K. (2022). Current status of probiotic and related health benefits. *Applied Food Research, 2*(2), 185–210. https://doi.org/10.1016/j.afres.2022.100185

De Angelis, M., & Gobbetti, M. (2016). *Lactobacillus* SPP: General characteristics. In *Reference module in food science* (p. 120). Elsevier.

Dempsey, E., & Corr, S. C. (2022). *Lactobacillus* spp. For gastrointestinal Health: Current and Future Perspectives. *Frontiers in Immunology, 13,* 840–852. https://doi.org/10.3389/fimmu.2022.840245

den Besten, G., van Eunen, K., Groen, A. K., Venema, K., Reijngoud, D. J., & Bakker, B. M. (2013). The role of short-chain fatty acids in the interplay between diet, gut microbiota, and host energy metabolism. *Journal of Lipid Research, 54*(9), 2325–2340. https://doi.org/10.1194/jlr.R036012

Dicks, L. M. T., & Botes, M. (2010). Probiotic lactic acid bacteria in the gastro-intestinal tract: Health benefits, safety and mode of action. *Beneficial Microbes, 1*(1), 11–29. https://doi.org/10.3920/BM2009.0012

Di Gioia, D., Strahsburger, E., Lopez de Lacey, A. M. L., Bregola, V., Marotti, I., Aloisio, I., Biavati, B., & Dinelli, G. (2014). Flavonoid bioconversion in *Bifidobacterium pseudocatenulatum* B7003: A potential probiotic strain for functional food development. *Journal of Functional Foods, 7,* 671–679. https://doi.org/10.1016/j.jff.2013.12.018

Dinu, L. D., Avram, I., Pelinescu, D. R., & Vamanu, E. (2022). Mineral-enriched postbiotics: A new perspective for microbial therapy to prevent and treat gut dysbiosis. *Biomedicines, 10*(10), 2392–2401. https://doi.org/10.3390/biomedicines10102392

Domínguez Díaz, L., Fernández-Ruiz, V., & Cámara, M. (2020). The frontier between nutrition and pharma: The international regulatory framework of functional foods, food supplements and nutraceuticals. *Critical Reviews in Food Science and Nutrition, 60*(10), 1738–1746. https://doi.org/10.1080/10408398.2019.1592107

Fei, Z., Xie, D., Wang, M., Zhang, Y., Zhang, H., Du, Q., & Jin, P. (2023). Enhanced biotransformation of bioactive components and volatile compounds of bamboo (*Phyllostachys glauca McClure*) leaf juice fermented by probiotic *Streptococcus thermophiles. LWT—Food Science and Technology, 173,* 114–119. https://doi.org/10.1016/j.lwt.2022.114363

Ferreira, C. M., de Lima, S. B., Zambelli, R. A., & Afonso, M. R. A. (2020). Efeito da farinha mista de subprodutos vegetais em pães tipo forma. *Brazilian Journal of Development, 6*(2), 8710–8724. https://doi.org/10.34117/bjdv6n2-254

Fijan, S. (2014). Microorganisms with claimed probiotic properties: An overview of recent literature. *International Journal of Environmental Research and Public Health, 11*(5), 4745–4767. https://doi.org/10.3390/ijerph110504745

Fijan, S. (2023). Probiotics and their antimicrobial effect. *Microorganisms, 11*(2), 528–540. https://doi.org/10.3390/microorganisms11020528

Filho, A. A. L. A., Sousa, P. H. M., Vieira, I. G. P., Fernandas, V. B., Cunha, F. E. T., Magalhães, F. E. A., & da Silva, L. M. R. (2023). Kombucha and kefir fermentation dynamics on cashew nut beverage (*Anacardium occidentale* L.). *International Journal of Gastronomy and Food Science, 33,* 88–110.

Galdeano, C. M., Cazorla, S. I., Lemme Dumit, J. M., Vélez, E., & Perdigón, G. (2019). Beneficial effects of probiotic consumption on the immune system. *Annals of Nutrition and Metabolism, 74*(2), 115–124. https://doi.org/10.1159/000496426

Galdeno, C. M., Nuñez, I. N., & Perdigón, G. (2016). Malnutrition: Role of the diet on the microbiota and in the functioning of the gut immune system. *SM Journal of Public Health and Epidemiology, 2,* 1023–1029.

Goldenberg, J. Z., Yap, C., Lytvyn, L., Lo, C. K., Beardsley, J., & Mertz, D. (2017). Probiotics for the prevention of *Clostridium difficile*-associated diarrhea in adults and children. *Cochrane Database of Systematic Reviews, 12,* 88–112.

Gou, H. Z., Zhang, Y. L., Ren, L. F., Li, Z. J., & Zhang, L. (2022). How do intestinal probiotics restore the intestinal barrier? *Frontiers in Microbiology, 13,* 929–939. https://doi.org/10.3389/fmicb.2022.929346

Granato, D., Barba, F. J., Ovacevic, D. B., Lorenzo, J. M., Cruz, A. G., & Putnik, P. (2020). Functional foods: Product development, technological trends, efficacy testing, and safety. *Annual Review of Food Science and Technology*, *11*, 93–118.

Gu, S., Yang, D., Liu, C., & Xue, W. (2023). The role of probiotics in prevention and treatment of food allergy. *Food Science and Human Wellness, 12*(3), 681–690. https://doi.org/10.1016/j.fshw.2022.09.001

Guarner, F., Khan, A. G., Garisch, J., Eliakim, R., Gangl, A., Thomson, A., Krabshuis, J., Lemair, T., Kaufmann, P., De Paula, J. A., Fedorak, R., Shanahan, F., Sanders, M. E., Szajewska, H., Ramakrishna, B. S., Karakan, T., & Kim, N. (2012). World gastroenterology organisation global guidelines: Probiotics and prebiotics October 2011. *Journal of Clinical Gastroenterology, 46*(6), 468–481. https://doi.org/10.1097/MCG.0b013e3182549092

Heeney, D. D., Gareau, M. G., & Marco, M. L. (2018). Intestinal Lactobacillus in health and disease, a driver or just along for the ride? *Current Opinion in Biotechnology, 49,* 140–147. https://doi.org/10.1016/j.copbio.2017.08.004

Hemaiswarya, S., Rajal, R., Ravikumari, R., & Carvalho, I. S. (2013). Mechanism of action of probiotics. *Brazilian Archives of Biology and Technology, 56*(1), 12–20.

Hemarajata, P., & Versalovic, J. (2013). Effects of probiotics on gut microbiota: Mechanisms of intestinal immunomodulation and neuromodulation. *Therapeutic Advances in Gastroenterology, 6*(1), 39–51. https://doi.org/10.1177/1756283X12459294

Hou, K., Wu, Z. X., Chen, X. Y., Wang, J. Q., Zhang, D., Xiao, C., Zhu, D., Koya, J. B., Wei, L., Li, J., & Chen, Z. S. (2022). Microbiota in health and diseases. *Signal Transduction and Targeted Therapy, 7*(1), 135–142. https://doi.org/10.1038/s41392-022-00974-4

Huang, Y., Lin, X., Yu, S., Chen, R., & Chen, W. (2022). Intestinal engineered probiotics as living therapeutics: Chassis selection, colonization enhancement, gene circuit design, and biocontainment. *ACS Synthetic Biology, 11*(10), 3134–3153. https://doi.org/10.1021/acssynbio.2c00314

Huda, M. N., Ahmad, S. M., Kalanetra, K. M., Taft, D. H., Alam, M. J., Khanam, A., Raqib, R., Underwood, M. A., Mills, D. A., & Stephensen, C. B. (2019). Neonatal vitamin A supplementation and vitamin A status are associated with gut microbiome composition in Bangladeshi infants in early infancy and at 2 years of age. *Journal of Nutrition, 149*(6), 1075–1088. https://doi.org/10.1093/jn/nxz034

Hutkins, R. W., Krumbeck, J. A., Bindels, L. B., Cani, P. D., Fahey, G., Goh, Y. J., Hamaker, B., Martens, E. C., Mills, D. A., Rastal, R. A., Vaughan, E., & Sanders, M. E. (2016). Prebiotics: Why definitions matter. *Current Opinion in Biotechnology, 37,* 1–7. https://doi.org/10.1016/j.copbio.2015.09.001

Islam, S., Biwas, S., Jabin, T., Moniruzzaman, M., Biswas, J., Uddin, S. Akthar-E-Ekram, M., Elgorban, A.M., Ghodake, G., Syed, A., Saleh, A., & Zaman, S. (2023). Probiotic potential of Lactobacillus plantarum DMR14 for preserving and extending shelf life of fruits and fruit juice. *Helyion*, *9*(6), 173–184.

Jach, M., Los, R., Maj, M., & Malm, A. (2013). Probiotics—technological and manufacturing aspects. *Postępy Mikrobiologii, 52,* 161–170.

Ke, W., Ding, W., Xu, D., Shah, M. N., Zhang, P., & Guo, X. (2018). Influences of addition of malic acid or citric acid, Lactobacillus plantarum and their mixtures on fermentation quality, proteolysis and fatty acid composition of ensiled alfalfa. *Archives of Animal Nutrition, 72*(6), 492–502. https://doi.org/10.1080/1745039X.2018.1510156

Khalesi, S., Bellissimo, N., Vandelanotte, C., Williams, S., Stanley, D., & Irwin, C. (2019). A review of probiotic supplementation in healthy adults: Helpful or hype? *European Journal of Clinical Nutrition, 73*(1), 24–37. https://doi.org/10.1038/s41430-018-0135-9

Kolaček, S., Hojsak, I., Berni Canani, R., Guarino, A., Indrio, F., Orel, R., Pot, B., Shamir, R., Szajewska, H., Vandenplas, Y., van Goudoever, J. V., & Weizman, Z. (2017). Commercial probiotic products: A call for improved quality control. A position paper by the ESPGHAN working group for probiotics and prebiotics. *Journal of Pediatric Gastroenterology and Nutrition, 61*(1), 117–124. https://doi.org/10.1097/MPG.0000000000001603

Kopacz, K., & Phadtare, S. (2022). Probiotics for the prevention of antibiotic-associated diarrhea. *Healthcare, 10*(8), 1450–1465. https://doi.org/10.3390/healthcare10081450

Kumar, D., Lal, M. K., Dutt, S., Raigond, P., Changan, S. S., Tiwari, R. K., Chourasia, K. N., Mangal, V., & Singh, B. (2022). Functional fermented probiotics, prebiotics, and synbiotics from non-dairy products: A perspective from nutraceutical. *Molecular Nutrition and Research, 66*(14), 81–93. https://doi.org/10.1002/mnfr.202101059

Kumari, R., Sanjukta, S., Sahoo, D., & Rai, A. K. (2022). Functional peptides in Asian protein rich fermented foods: Production and health benefits. *Systems Microbiology and Biomanufacturing, 2*(1), 1–13. https://doi.org/10.1007/s43393-021-00040-0

Larsen, N., Vogensen, F. K., van den Berg, F. W. J., Nielsen, D. S., Andreasen, A. S., Pedersen, B. K., Al-Soud, W. A., Sørensen, S. J., Hansen, L. H., & Jakobsen, M. (2010). Gut microbiota in human adults with Type 2 diabetes differs from non-diabetic adults. *PLoS One, 5*(2), 985–997. https://doi.org/10.1371/journal.pone.0009085

Lau, S. W., Chong, A. Q., Chin, N. L., Talib, R. A., & Basha, R. K. (2021). Sourdough microbiome comparison and benefits. *Microorganisms, 9*(7), 1355–1362. https://doi.org/10.3390/microorganisms9071355

LeBlanc, J. G., Chain, F., Martín, R., Bermúdez-Humarán, L. G., Courau, S., & Langella, P. (2017). Beneficial effects on host energy metabolism of short-chain fatty acids and vitamins produced by commensal and probiotic bacteria. *Microbial Cell Factories, 16*(1), 79–88. https://doi.org/10.1186/s12934-017-0691-z

Lee, K. W., Park, J. Y., Sa, H. D., Jeong, J. H., Jin, D. E., Heo, H. J., & Kim, J. H. (2014). Probiotic properties of *Pediococcus* strains isolated from jeotgals, salted and fermented Korean sea-food. *Anaerobe, 28,* 199–206. https://doi.org/10.1016/j.anaerobe.2014.06.013

Lei, W., Hao, L., You, S., Yao, H., Liu, C., & Zhou, H. (2022). Partial purification and application of a bacteriocin produced by probiotic *Lactococcus lactis* C15 isolated from raw milk. *LWT—Food Science and Technology, 169,* 917–922. https://doi.org/10.1016/j.lwt.2022.113917

Lewis, K. (2013). Platforms for antibiotic discovery. *Nature Reviews. Drug Discovery, 12*(5), 371–387. https://doi.org/10.1038/nrd3975

Li, P., Gu, Q., Wang, Y., Yu, Y., Yang, L., & Chen, J. V. (2017). Novel vitamin B12-producing Enterococcus spp. And preliminary in vitro evaluation of probiotic potentials. *Applied Microbiology and Biotechnology, 101*(15), 6155–6164. https://doi.org/10.1007/s00253-017-8373-7

Li, P., Gu, Q., Yang, L., Yu, Y., & Wang, Y. (2017). Characterization of extracellular vitamin B12 producing *Lactobacillus plantarum* strains and assessment of the probiotic potentials. *Food Chemistry, 234,* 494–501. https://doi.org/10.1016/j.foodchem.2017.05.037

Li, X., Fields, F. R., Ho, M., Marshall-Hudson, A., Gross, R., Casser, M. E., & Naito, M. (2022). Safety assessment of *Streptococcus salivarius* DB-B5 as a probiotic candidate for oral health. *Food and Chemical Toxicology, 153,* 277–284.

Liao, S. F., & Nyachoti, M. (2017). Using probiotics to improve swine gut health and nutrient utilization. *Animal Nutrition, 3*(4), 331–343. https://doi.org/10.1016/j.aninu.2017.06.007

Lim, S. M., & Kim, D. H. (2017). Bifidobacterium adolescentis IM38 ameliorates high-fat diet-induced colitis in mice by inhibiting NF-κB activation and lipopolysaccharide production by gut microbiota. *Nutrition Research, 41*(1), 86–96. https://doi.org/10.1016/j.nutres.2017.04.003

Ma, T., Shen, X., Shi, X., Sakandar, H. A., Quan, K., Li, Y., Jin, H., Kwok, L. Y., Zhang, H., & Sun, Z. (2023). Targeting gut microbiota and metabolism as the major probiotic mechanism: An evidence-based review. *Trends in Food Science and Technology, 138,* 178–198. https://doi.org/10.1016/j.tifs.2023.06.013

Markowiak-Kopeć, P., & Śliżewska, K. (2020). The effect of probiotics on the production of short-chain fatty acids by human intestinal microbiome. *Nutrients, 12*(4), 1107–1118. https://doi.org/10.3390/nu12041107

Mazziotta, C., Tognon, M., Martini, F., Torreggiani, E., & Rotondo, J. C. (2023). Probiotics mechanism of action on immune cells and beneficial effects on human health. *Cells, 12*(1), 184–195. https://doi.org/10.3390/cells12010184

McFarland, L. V., Evans, C. T., & Goldstein, E. J. C. (2018). Strain-specificity and disease-specificity of probiotic efficacy: A systematic review and meta-analysis. *Frontiers in Medicine, 5,* 124–132. https://doi.org/10.3389/fmed.2018.00124

McNulty, N., Yatsunenko, T., Hsiao, A., Faith, J., Muegge, B., & Goodman, A. (2011). The impact of a consortium of fermented milk strains on the gut microbiome of gnotobiotic mice and monozygotic twins. *Science Translational Medicine, 3,* 106–112.

Molina, V., Médici, M., Font de Valdez, G. F., & Taranto, M. P. (2012). Soybean-based functional food with vitamin B12-producing lactic acid bacteria. *Journal of Functional Foods, 4*(4), 831–836. https://doi.org/10.1016/j.jff.2012.05.011

Montaigne, V., Vannier, N., Vanderkoornhuyse, P., & Hacquard, S. (2021). Microbial systems ecology to understand cross-feeding in microbiomes. *Frontiers in Microbiology, 12,* 780–791.

Monteagudo-Mera, A., Rastall, R. A., Gibson, G. R., Charalampopoulos, D., & Chatzifragkou, A. (2019). Adhesion mechanisms mediated by probiotics and prebiotics and their potential impact on human health. *Applied Microbiology and Biotechnology, 103*(16), 6463–6472. https://doi.org/10.1007/s00253-019-09978-7

Mudgil, D., & Barak, S. (2013). Composition, properties and health benefits of indigestible carbohydrate polymers as dietary fiber: A review. *International Journal of Biological Macromolecules, 61,* 1–6. https://doi.org/10.1016/j.ijbiomac.2013.06.044

Nascimento, N. P., de Oliveira, M. M. C., Nascimento, C. P., da Costa, J. M. C., Zambelli, R. A., & da Silva, E. M. C. (2019). Biscoito salgado adicionado de surimi e tomate em pó: Aceitabilidade na alimentação escolar. *Revista Brasileira de Ciências Agrárias, 14*(2), 5635–5641.

Oniszczuk, A., Oniszczuk, T., Gancarz, M., & Szymańska, J. (2021). Role of gut microbiota, prebiotics and prebiotics in cardiovascular diseases. *Molecules, 26*(4), 1172–1179. https://doi.org/10.3390/molecules26041172

Palanivelu, J., Thanigaivel, S., Vickram, S., Dey, N., Mihaylova, D., & Desseva, I. (2022). Probiotics in functional foods: Survival assessment and approaches for improved viability. *Applied Sciences, 12*(1), 455–466. https://doi.org/10.3390/app12010455

Panwar, H., Rokana, N., Aparna, S. V., Kaur, J., Singh, A., Singh, J., Singh, K. S., Chaudhary, V., & Puniya, A. K. (2021). Gastrointestinal stress as innate defence against microbial attack. *Journal of Applied Microbiology, 130*(4), 1035–1061. https://doi.org/10.1111/jam.14836

Papadimitriou, K., Alegría, Á., Bron, P. A., De Angelis, M., Gobbetti, M., Kleerebezem, M., Lemos, J. A., Linares, D. M., Ross, P., Stanton, C., Turroni, F., van Sinderen, D., Varmanen, P., Ventura, M., Zuñiga, M., Tsakalidou, E., & Kok, J. (2016). Stress physiology of lactic acid bacteria. *Microbiology and Molecular Biology Reviews, 80*(3), 837–890. https://doi.org/10.1128/MMBR.00076-15

Parker, E. A., Roy, T., D'Adamo, C. R., & Wieland, L. S. (2018). Probiotics and gastrointestinal conditions: An overview of evidence from the Cochrane Collaboration. *Nutrition, 45,* 125–134. https://doi.org/10.1016/j.nut.2017.06.024

Patel, P., Butani, K., Kumar, A., Singh, S., & Prajapati, B. G. (2023). Effects of fermented food consumption on non-communicable diseases. *Foods, 12*(4), 687–695. https://doi.org/10.3390/foods12040687

Peng, M., Tabashsum, Z., Anderson, M., Truong, A., Houser, A. K., Padilla, J., Akmel, A., Bhatti, J., Rahaman, S. O., & Biswas, D. (2020). Effectiveness of probiotics, prebiotics, and prebiotic-like components in common functional foods. *Comprehensive Reviews in Food Science and Food Safety, 19*(4), 1908–1933. https://doi.org/10.1111/1541-4337.12565

Pfliegler, W. P., Pusztahelyi, T., & Pócsi, I. (2015). Mycotoxins—Prevention and decontamination by yeasts. *Journal of Basic Microbiology, 55*(7), 805–818. https://doi.org/10.1002/jobm.201400833

Pham, V. T., Dold, S., Rehman, A., Bird, J. K., & Steinert, R. E. (2021). Vitamins, the gut microbiome and gastrointestinal health in humans. *Nutrition Research, 95,* 35–53. https://doi.org/10.1016/j.nutres.2021.09.001

Plaza-Diaz, J., Ruiz-Ojeda, F. J., Gil-Campos, M., & Gil, A. (2019). Mechanism of action of probiotics. *Advances in Nutrition, 10*(1), 49–56. https://doi.org/10.1093/advances/nmy063

Popowska, M., Krawczyk-Balska, A., Ostrowski, R., & Desvaux, M. (2017). INLL from Listeria monocytogenes is involved in biofilm formation and adhesion to mucin. *Frontiers in Microbiology, 8,* 660–672. https://doi.org/10.3389/fmicb.2017.00660

Rad, A. H., Aghebati-Maleki, L., Kafil, H. S., Gilani, N., Abbasi, A., & Khani, N. (2021). Postbiotics, as dynamic biomolecules, and their promising role in promoting food safety. *Biointerface Research in Applied Chemistry, 11*(6), 14529–14544. https://doi.org/10.33263/BRIAC116.1452914544

Raheem, A., Liang, L., Zhang, G., & Cui, S. (2021). Modulatory effects of probiotics during pathogenic infections with emphasis on immune regulation. *Frontiers in Immunology, 12,* 616713. https://doi.org/10.3389/fimmu.2021.616713

Rajyalakshmi, K., Babu, M. K., Shabana, S., & Satya, A. K. (2021). Identification and screening of probiotics as a biocontrol agent against pathogenic vibriosis in shrimp aquaculture. *Annals of the Romanian Society for Cell Biology, 25*(6), 12292–12305.

Rasaei, D., Hosseinian, S. A., Asasi, K., Shekarforoush, S. S., & Khodakaram-Tafti, A. (2023). The beneficial effects of spraying of probiotic Bacillus and Lactobacillus bacteria on broiler chickens experimentally infected with avian influenza virus H9N2. *Poultry Science, 102*(7), 102669. https://doi.org/10.1016/j.psj.2023.102669

Rinninella, E., Raoul, P., Cintoni, M., Franceschi, F., Miggiano, G. A. D., Gasbarrini, A., & Mele, M. C. (2019). What is the healthy gut microbiota composition? A changing ecosystem across age, environment, diet, and diseases. *Microorganisms, 7*(1), 14–22. https://doi.org/10.3390/microorganisms7010014

Rocamora-Reverte, L., Melzer, F. L., Wurzner, R., & Weinberger, B. (2021). The complex role of regulatory T cells in immunity and aging. *Frontiers in Immunology, 11,* 90–101.

Rodríguez, H., Curiel, J. A., Landete, J. M., de las Rivas, B., López de Felipe, F. L., Gómez-Cordovés, C., Mancheño, J. M., & Muñoz, R. (2009). Food phenolics and lactic acid bacteria. *International Journal of Food Microbiology, 132*(2–3), 79–90. https://doi.org/10.1016/j.ijfoodmicro.2009.03.025

Saarinen, M. T., Lahtinen, S. J., Sørensen, J. F., Tiihonen, K., Ouwehand, A. C., Rautonen, N., & Morgan, A. (2012). Treatment of bran containing bread by baking enzymes; effect on the growth of probiotic bacteria on soluble dietary fiber extract *in vitro. Bioscience, Biotechnology, and Biochemistry, 76*(6), 1135–1139. https://doi.org/10.1271/bbb.110977

Sánchez, B., Delgado, S., Blanco-Míguez, A., Lourenço, A., Gueimonde, M., & Margolles, A. (2017). Probiotics, gut microbiota, and their influence on host health and disease. *Molecular Nutrition and Food Research, 61*(1), 85–99. https://doi.org/10.1002/mnfr.201600240

Santacroce, L., Inchingolo, F., Topi, S., Del Prete, R., Di Cosola, M., Charitos, I. A., & Montagnani, M. (2021). Potential beneficial role of probiotics on the outcome of COVID-19 patients: An evolving perspective. *Diabetes and Metabolic Syndrome. Clinical Research Review, 15*(3), 295–301. https://doi.org/10.1016/j.dsx.2020.12.040

Sartor, R. B. (2006). Mechanisms of disease: Pathogenesis of Crohn's disease and ulcerative colitis. *Nature Clinical Practice. Gastroenterology and Hepatology, 3*(7), 390–407. https://doi.org/10.1038/ncpgasthep0528

Saulnier, D. M., Spinler, J. K., Gibson, G. R., & Versalovic, J. (2009). Mechanisms of probiosis and prebiosis: Considerations for enhanced functional foods. *Current Opinion in Biotechnology, 20*(2), 135–141. https://doi.org/10.1016/j.copbio.2009.01.002

Scholz-Ahrens, K. E., Ade, P., Marten, B., Weber, P., Timm, W., Açil, Y., Glüer, C. C., & Schrezenmeir, J. (2007). Prebiotics, probiotics, and Synbiotics affect mineral absorption, bone mineral content, and bone structure. *Journal of Nutrition, 137*(3), 838–846. https://doi.org/10.1093/jn/137.3.838S

Seal, B. S., Drider, D., Oakley, B. B., Brüssow, H., Bikard, D., Rich, J. O., Miller, S., Devillard, E., Kwan, J., Bertin, G., Reeves, S., Swift, S. M., Raicek, M., & Gay, C. G. (2018). Microbial-derived products as potential new antimicrobials. *Veterinary Research, 49*(1), 66–72. https://doi.org/10.1186/s13567-018-0563-5

Shah, B. R., Li, B., Al Sabbah, H. A., Xu, W., & Mráz, J. (2020). Effects of prebiotic dietary fibers and probiotics on human health: With special focus on recent advancement in their encapsulated formulations. *Trends in Food Science and Technology, 102,* 178–192. https://doi.org/10.1016/j.tifs.2020.06.010

Sharifi-Rad, J., Rodrigues, C. F., Stojanović-Radić, Z., Dimitrijević, M., Aleksić, A., Neffe-Skocińska, K., Zielińska, D., Kołożyn-Krajewska, D., Salehi, B., Milton Prabu, S. M., Schutz, F., Docea, A. O., Martins, N., & Calina, D. (2020). Probiotics: Versatile bioactive components in promoting human health. *Medicina, 56*(9), 433–442. https://doi.org/10.3390/medicina56090433

Silva, Y. P., Bernardi, A., & Frozza, R. L. (2020). The role of short-chain fatty acids from gut microbiota in gut-brain communication. *Frontiers in Endocrinology, 11,* 25. https://doi.org/10.3389/fendo.2020.00025

Simpson, H. L., & Campbell, B. J. (2015). Review article: Dietary fibre–microbiota interactions. *Alimentary Pharmacology and Therapeutics, 42*(2), 158–179. https://doi.org/10.1111/apt.13248

Skrypnik, K., & Suliburska, J. (2017). Association between the gut microbiota and mineral metabolism. *Journal of the Science of Food and Agriculture, 98*(7), 2449–2460. https://doi.org/10.1002/jsfa.8724

Smith, N. W., Shorten, P. R., Altermann, E., Roy, N. C., & McNabb, W. C. (2019). The classification and evolution of bacterial cross-feeding. *Frontiers in Ecology and Evolution, 7,* 153–162. https://doi.org/10.3389/fevo.2019.00153

Soares, M. B., Martinez, R. C. R., Pereira, E. P. R., Balthazar, C. F., Cruz, A. G., Ranadheera, C. S., & Sant'Ana, A. S. (2019). The resistance of *Bacillus, Bifidobacterium,* and *Lactobacillus* strains with claimed probiotic properties in different food matrices exposed to simulated gastrointestinal tract conditions. *Food Research International, 125,* 542–550. https://doi.org/10.1016/j.foodres.2019.108542

Soemarie, Y. B., Milanda, T., & Barliana, M. I. (2021). Fermented Foods as probiotics: A review. *Journal of Advanced Pharmaceutical Technology and Research, 12*(4), 335–339. https://doi.org/10.4103/japtr.japtr_116_21

Soliman, W. S., Shaapan, R. M., Mohamed, L. A., & Gayed, S. S. R. (2019). Recent biocontrol measures for fish bacterial diseases, in particular to probiotics, bio-encapsulated vaccines, and phage therapy. *Open Veterinary Journal, 9*(3), 190–195. https://doi.org/10.4314/ovj.v9i3.2

Sudheer, S., Gangwar, P., Usmani, Z., Sharma, M., Sharma, V. K., Sana, S. S., Almeida, F., Dubey, N. K., Singh, D. P., Dilbaghi, N., Khayat, K., H. R. K., Gupta, V. K., Singh, B. N., Khayatkashani, M., & Nabavi, S. M. (2023). Shaping the gut microbiota by bioactive phytochemicals: An emerging approach for the prevention and treatment of human diseases. *Biochimie, 193,* 38–63. https://doi.org/10.1016/j.biochi.2021.10.010

Sylvain, F. E., Cheaib, B., Llewellyn, M., Correia, T. G., Fagundes, D. B., Val, A. L., & Derome, N. (2016). pH drop impacts differentially skin and gut microbiota of the Amazonian fish tambaqui (*Colossoma macropomum*). *Scientific Reports, 6,* 320–331.

Tegegne, B. A., & Kebede, B. (2022). Probiotics, their prophylactic and therapeutic applications in human health development: A review of the literature. *Heliyon, 8*(6), e09725. https://doi.org/10.1016/j.heliyon.2022.e09725

Thursby, E., & Juge, N. (2017). Introduction to the human gut microbiota. *Biochemical Journal, 474*(11), 1823–1836. https://doi.org/10.1042/BCJ20160510

Tsafrakidou, P., Michaelidou, A. M., & G Biliaderis, C. G. (2020). Fermented cereal-based products: Nutritional aspects, possible impact on gut microbiota and health implications. *Foods, 9*(6), 734–742. https://doi.org/10.3390/foods9060734

Turroni, F., Milani, C., Duranti, S., Mahony, J., Sinderen, D. V., & Ventura, M. (2017). Glycan utilization and cross-feeding activities by *bifidobacteria. Trends in Microbiology, 26*(4), 18–29.

Vancamelbeke, M., & Vermeire, S. (2017). The intestinal barrier: A fundamental role in health and disease. *Expert Review of Gastroenterology and Hepatology, 11*(9), 821–834. https://doi.org/10.1080/17474124.2017.1343143

Vasudha, S., & Mishra, H. N. (2013). Non-dairy probiotic beverages. *International Food Research Journal,* 7–15.

Vieira, K. C. O., Ferreira, C. S., Bueno, E. B. T., De Moraes, Y. A., Toleto, A. C. C. G., Nagasaki, W. R., Pereira, V. C., & Winkelstroter, L. K. (2020). Development and viability of probiotic orange juice supplemented by *Pediococcus acidilactici* CE 51. *LWT—Food Science and Technology, 130,* 637–642.

Wan, M. L., Forsythe, S. J., & El-Nezami, H. (2018). Probiotics interaction with foodborne pathogens: A potential alternative to antibiotics and future challenges. *Critical Reviews in Food Science and Nutrition, 72,* 1–14.

Wang, X., Zhang, P., & Zhang, X. (2021). Probiotics regulate gut microbiota: An effective method to improve immunity. *Molecules, 26*(19), 6076–6088. https://doi.org/10.3390/molecules26196076

Wang, Y., Wu, J., Lv, M., Shao, Z., Hungwe, M., Wang, J., Bai, X., Xie, J., Wang, Y., & Geng, W. (2021). Metabolism characteristics of lactic acid bacteria and the expanding applications in food industry. *Frontiers in Bioengineering and Biotechnology, 9,* 285–299. https://doi.org/10.3389/fbioe.2021.612285

Wehkamp, J., Harder, J., Wehkamp, K., Wehkamp-von Meissner, B. W., Schlee, M., Enders, C., Sonnenborn, U., Nuding, S., Bengmark, S., Fellermann, K., Schröder, J. M., & Stange, E. F. (2004). NF-κB- and AP-1-mediated induction of human beta Defensin-2 in intestinal epithelial cells by *Escherichia coli* Nissle 1917: A novel effect of a probiotic Bacterium. *Infection and Immunity, 72*(10), 88–101. https://doi.org/10.1128/IAI.72.10.5750-5758.2004

Williams, B. A., Grant, L. J., Gidley, M. J., & Mikkelsen, D. (2017). Gut fermentation of dietary fibres: Physicochemistry of plant cell walls and implications for health. *International Journal of Molecular Sciences, 18*(10), 2203–2212. https://doi.org/10.3390/ijms18102203

Wu, S., Zhang, Q., Cong, G., Xiao, Y., Shen, Y., Zhang, S., Zhao, W., & Shi, S. (2023). Probiotic *Escherichia coli* Nissle 1917 protect chicks from damage caused by *Salmonella enterica serovar enteritidis* colonization. *Animal Nutrition, 14,* 831–839. https://doi.org/10.1016/j.aninu.2023.06.001

Xavier-Santos, D., Bedani, R., Lima, E. D., & Saad, S. M. I. (2020). Impact of probiotics and prebiotics targeting metabolic syndrome. *Journal of Functional Foods, 64*(1), 103–112. https://doi.org/10.1016/j.jff.2019.103666

Xiong, N., & Hu, S. (2015). Regulation of intestinal IgA responses. *Cellular and Molecular Life Sciences, 72*(14), 2645–2655. https://doi.org/10.1007/s00018-015-1892-4

Yao, M., Xie, J., Du, H., McClements, D. J., Xiao, H., & Li, L. (2020). Progress in microencapsulation of probiotics: A review. *Comprehensive Reviews in Food Science and Food Safety, 19*(2), 857–874. https://doi.org/10.1111/1541-4337.12532

You, S., Ma, Y., Yan, B., Pei, W., Wu, Q., Ding, C., & Huang, C. (2022). The promotion mechanism of prebiotics for probiotics: A review. *Frontiers in Nutrition, 9,* 1000517. https://doi.org/10.3389/fnut.2022.1000517

Yousefi, B., Eslami, M., Ghasemian, A., Kokhaei, P., Salek Farrokhi, A. S., & Darabi, N. (2018). Probiotics importance and their immunomodulatory properties. *Journal of Cellular Physiology, 234*(6), 8008–8018. https://doi.org/10.1002/jcp.27559

Zhang, C., Derrien, M., Levenez, F., Brazeilles, R., Ballal, S. A., Kim, J., Degivry, M. C., Quéré, G., Garault, P., van Hylckama Vlieg, J. E., Garrett, W. S., Doré, J., & Veiga, P. (2016). Ecological robustness of the gut microbiota in response to ingestion of transient food-borne microbes. *ISME Journal, 10*(9), 2235–2245. https://doi.org/10.1038/ismej.2016.13

Zhang, Y., Zhang, L., Du, M. Yo, H. Guo, C. Tuo, Y. Han, X. Li, J. Zhang, L., & Yang L. (2011). Antimicrobial activity against Shigella sonnei and probiotic properties of wild lactobacilli from fermented food. *Microbiological Research, 167*(1), 27–31. https://doi.org/10.1016/j.micres.2011.02.006

Zhao, N., Yu, T., & Yan, F. (2023). Probiotic role and application of thermophilic Bacillus as novel food materials. *Trends in Food Science and Technology, 138,* 1–15. https://doi.org/10.1016/j.tifs.2023.05.020

Zheng, D., Liwinski, T., & Elinav, E. (2020). Interaction between microbiota and immunity in health and disease. *Cell Research, 30*(6), 492–506. https://doi.org/10.1038/s41422-020-0332-7

Zhou, B., Yuan, Y., Zhang, S., Guo, C., Li, X., Li, G., Xiong, W., & Zeng, Z. (2020). Intestinal flora and disease mutually shape the regional immune system in the intestinal tract. *Frontiers in Immunology, 11,* 575. https://doi.org/10.3389/fimmu.2020.00575

Zommiti, M., Feuilloley, M. G. J., & Connil, N. (2020). Update of probiotics in human world: A nonstop source of benefactions till the end of time. *Microorganisms, 8*(12), 1907–1917. https://doi.org/10.3390/microorganisms8121907

14 Evolutionary Trends in Probiotics

Scope and State of the Art

Sadma Parveen and Rizwan Ahamad

14.1 INTRODUCTION

Probiotics are living microorganisms that are consumed with the aim of changing the gut flora in a way that has positive health effects. Today's probiotic supplements come in a diversity of formulations and contain a wide range of bacterial and fungal species. Microbials were initially used inadvertently years ago when a tribe discovered the health benefits of consuming fermented foods. These early fermented foods are the immediate ancestors of contemporary probiotic-containing foods and goods (Hunter, 2008). Yogurt and fermented milk have been consumed by humans throughout history in a variety of ways, according to both myth and fact.

The metabolic process known as fermentation is how an organism turns a carbohydrate, usually sugar or starch, across an acid or alcohol. These metabolic by-products prevent the rotting of fermented foods by lowering pH and a variety of other effects. The term "fermentation" originates from the Latin word fermentum, denoting the process of boiling. The term was bestowed to it upon the observation that mixtures of crushed grapes, when kept in large containers, produced effervescence like boiling. Although the precise origins of human use of the fermentation process remain uncertain, it is widely recognized as a time-honored technique for preserving food. Dehydration is often acknowledged as the only conventional technique for preserving food. The technology of fermentation is believed to have originated in the Indus Valley Civilization, based on compelling evidence. Several artifacts suggest that fermentation was perhaps used in ancient times in Egypt and the Middle East (McGovern, 2009). The first records of fermentation may be traced back to 6000 B.C. in the Fertile Crescent, namely in southern Mesopotamia, along the Tigris and Euphrates rivers (Kiple & Ornelas, 2000). The consumption of Laban Rayeb and Laban Khad, two types of fermented milk from ancient Egypt, dates back to as early as 7000 B.C. (Kosikowski, 1977).

Although chance most likely recreates a significant act in the development of fermentation, the method gained popularity not merely because it kept food but because it offered a diversity of flavors, it might have helped digestion and/or had other discerned positive ramifications. Oral communication served as the primary means of transmission for the next generations. Depending on the raw materials, the environment, and regional taste preferences, humans were enjoying an extensive range of fermented foods and beverages by the Middle Ages (Table 14.1).

14.1.1 Evolution of Probiotics Throughout the Years

Figure 14.1 illustrates the historical development of probiotics across time.

14.1.2 Fermented Milk

Between 5000 and 8000 B.C., man began raising domestic animals in Asia and/or North East Africa. Written in India before 2000 B.C., the Vedic hymns reveal that Hindus have used fermented milk products from ancient times (Wilson, 1900). The Egyptians, Greeks, and Romans, among

DOI: 10.1201/9781003452249-14

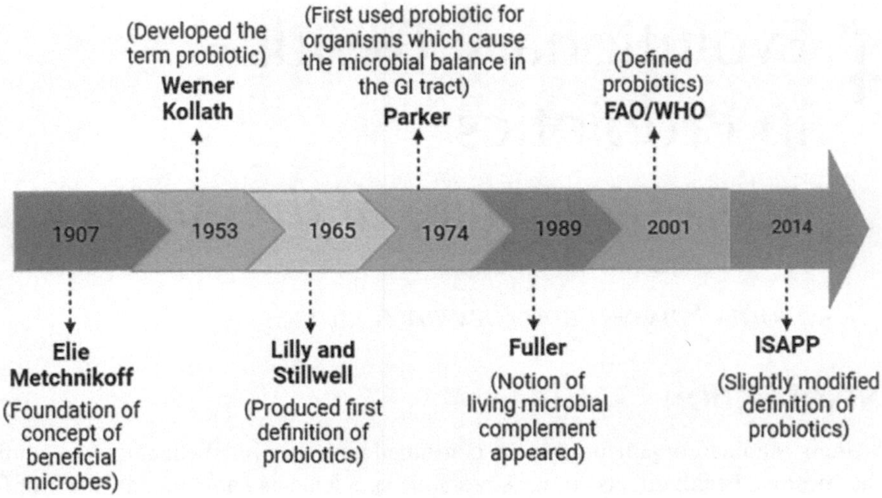

FIGURE 14.1 The evolution of probiotics over the years.

TABLE 14.1
Various Types of Fermented Food Used in Different Civilizations

S. No.	Frequently Employed Fermented Food Products
1	Bread
2	Soy sauce
3	Vegetables
4	Sausage
5	Beer and wine
6	Chocolate
7	Milk and cheese

many others, left many records between 2000 and 3000 B.C. that show milk, cheese, and butter were often consumed (Breasted, n. d.). For instance, Sumerians traveled through vast desert swaths carrying milk in sheep stomach-made sacks. The milk was fermented into curd by the enzymes in the stomach wall, improving the flavor and shelf life. According to Genesis 18, 1–8, which is from the 13th century B.C. version of the Bible, "Abraham made an offering to God, showed in an oak wood, fermented milk." For their taste and health advantages, fermented milk products were used routinely at this time in practically every society. Different names have been used to refer to these comparable compounds because of geographic remoteness and cultural variations (Table 14.2). Hippocrates, the Greek physician credited with coining the phrase "All disease begins in the gut," regarded fermented milk as a couple, a food item and a remedy besides the ability to treat intestinal diseases. According to the Roman historian Plinius, it was asserted that fermented milk products could potentially serve as a remedy for gastroenteritis (Suvarna & Boby, 2005).

14.1.3 Fermented Vegetables

Food fermentation of some kind has been created by almost all civilizations. Throughout history, the inhabitants of China, Japan, and Korea have predominantly utilized agitation as a key method for pickling various vegetables, including turnips, cabbage, cucumbers, eggplant, onions, squash, and carrots. Over 6,000 years have passed since cabbage was first fermented, according to records in China. When the Great Wall of China was being built (about 300 B.C.), Chinese laborers were frequently given fermented vegetables to help with their health and well-being (Yokotsuka & Sasaki, 1985). Sauerkraut, a lacto-fermented cabbage product, is mentioned in several Roman sources that also describe its "delicious taste" and therapeutic benefits. During his extensive travels, the Emperor Tiberius the Roman emperor, was known to regularly carry sauerkraut as part of his provisions. During their extensive voyages, Captain James Cook and the others consumed sauerkraut as a preventive measure against scurvy, a disease, approximately two millennia after the aforementioned events (Saloheimo, 2005).

14.1.4 Bread

Hieroglyphics from ancient Egypt offer the first descriptions of bread-making. The Egyptians learned that if the dough was not handled for a few hours before baking, the finished bread would be lighter and airier. Instead of fermentation, they attributed this event to a heavenly mechanism (Kiple & Ornelas, 2000). This custom extended to other nations as the Egyptians expanded their kingdom and seized additional areas. It is known that the Romans utilized wine-derived yeasts to bake bread from matured dough. Like yeast, leaven was a soft, fermented dough-like substance that was frequently mentioned in the Bible.

14.1.5 Beer and Wine

The nomadic lifestyle of hunter-gatherer tribes gave way to the more stable lifestyle of farmers between 9000 and 7000 B.C. The initial domestic cereal crops, according to many historians, are what led to the invention of beer and winemaking. The oldest indications of the production and consumption of beer date back to China, more than 7,000 years ago. Four thousand years ago, yeast was utilized in Egypt to make beer and as a leavening agent, according to the archaeological record (McGovern, 2009). It is known that the Greeks and Romans utilized starter organisms for inoculating fresh fruit juice for fermentation centuries later (Kiple & Ornelas, 2000).

14.2 MECHANISMS OF ACTION

How probiotics function is an often-asked question. There is no one solution because there are several strains and product compositions. There is a belief that all the drug's mechanisms of action

TABLE 14.2
Several Names of Fermented Milk Throughout Different Regions of the Globe

S. No.	Fermented Dairy Product	Country
1	Zabadi	Egypt
2	Dahi	India
3	Taettermjolk	Scandinavia
4	Kumiss	Mangolia
5	Cieddu	Italy
6	Kefir	Balkan
7	Koumiss	Russia
8	Doogh	Iran

are well known; therefore, probiotics should function similarly. Warfarin, a medication prescribed to reduce the risk of cardiac events, functions by inhibiting the synthesis of specific clotting factors dependent on vitamin K. This interference results in a reduction of the body's ability to produce blood clots, ultimately mitigating the likelihood of pathological clot formation. Such knowledge was gained through research on both humans and animals, and it may have been simpler to demonstrate because of the way of action. However, not all medications must have this characteristic. Data on the use of the well-researched drug aspirin to prevent cardiovascular disease, whose mechanisms are thought to be known, are inconclusive (*Aspirin Therapy in Primary Cardiovascular Disease Prevention: A Position Paper of the European* Society *of Cardiology Working Group on Thrombosis | Journal of the American College of Cardiology*, n.d.).

There are genetic and functional differences between bacterial strains such as *Lactobacillus reuteri* SD2112 and *L. reuteri* RC-14 (Cadieux et al., 2008), the former microorganism is believed to generate reuterin, which is considered essential for eradicating pathogens within the GIT (Langa et al., 2014). On the other hand, the latter microorganism produces bio-surfactants that hinder the adherence of uropathogens (*Interference in Initial Adhesion of Uropathogenic Bacteria and Yeasts to Silicone Rubber by A Lactobacillus Acidophilus Biosurfactant | Microbiology Society*, n.d.). This highlights even more that, when explaining mechanisms of action, one must refrain from using the broad word "probiotics," although attempting to identify the strains. Having stated that there are widespread advantages associated with probiotics that have a common mechanism for improving the environment in the gut and promoting both a healthy digestive system and immune structure (Hill et al., 2014). This culmination was supported by effective meta-analyses and anti-infectious diarrhea, diarrhea brought on by antibiotics, transit through the intestines, IBD, and other circumstances. This does not imply that specific mechanisms have been established or that they are the same for all conditions. The lack of recombinant strains makes it difficult to carry out such efforts in people, although a rat study convincingly demonstrated that *Listeria monocytogenes* was inhibited by a bacteriocin generated by *Ligilactobacilus salivarius* UCC118 (Corr et al., 2007).

Atopic dermatitis patients were treated for 12 weeks with *L. salivarius* LS01 and *Bifidobacterium breve* BR03, which reduced gut microbial migration and stimulated an immune result as evidenced by amelioration of Th17/Treg and Th1/Th2 ratios (Iemoli et al., 2012), according to a study. Even though strain knock-outs weren't considered, this did propose mechanistic pathways. Additional human research backs up the idea that better barrier function prevents illness (*Pro- and Synbiotics to Control Inflammation and Infection in . . . : Journal of Trauma and Acute Care Surgery*, n.d., Giamarellos-Bourboulis et al., 2009).

It is challenging to assess and draw broad generalizations about how probiotics manipulate and regulate the immune system. Based on the host and maybe the delivery route, the same strain may increase antibacterial activity, the Th1 response (Reid & Kirjaivanen, 2005); (Irvine et al., 2010), along with anti-inflammatory, Th2 response (Bisanz et al., 2014; Yang et al., 2014) or regulatory action (Lorea Baroja et al., 2007). Probiotic strains like *Lactobacillus rhamnosus* GG might communicate with the host through a variety of methods, and the host can react in a variety of ways as well, as an excellent review succinctly demonstrates (Segers & Lebeer, 2014). It may be argued that the strain can evaluate the niche it is settled in and respond appropriately. This implies that it may reduce inflammation while also inducing Th1 responses, two seemingly incompatible strategies. The fact that LGG shortens the length of diarrhea (Aggarwal et al., 2014) but does not relieve constipation (Gan et al., 2014) demonstrates specificity.

The capacity of some probiotic strains to exert effects away from the site of treatment is a fascinating feature. This could happen if the organisms are transferred, from a nursing woman's intestines to her mammary glands (Arroyo et al., 2010) Or it could be brought on by the creation of molecules that are absorbed across the gut or that directly or indirectly affect host chemicals (Barbonetti et al., 2013). Examples of the latter are compounds that promote cardiac remodeling after cardiac ligation by raising the adiponectin leptin ratio (Gan et al., 2014) and compounds found in colostrum that may reduce the possibility of gestational diabetes mellitus (Luoto et al., 2010). Another example is lowering blood cholesterol, which can be accomplished through the assimilation of cholesterol, the creation of substances that hinder 3-hydroxy-3-methylglutaryl coenzyme A, deconjugation caused by bile salt hydrolase activity, and reduction in intestine levels of DCA (Guo et al., 2012; Tomaro-Duchesneau et al., 2014). Probiotic strains' capacity to lessen the critical and length of respiratory tract infection is an example of a distant site impact that is probably mediated by an increase in immune mediators (Zhao et al., 2022).

The fact that in proportion organisms, comparable to the quantities in the niche into which they are getting inside, can impart advantages is a remarkable and recurrent result in probiotic studies. This is valid for the densely populated digestive tract when only a small amount (10^9–10^{10} per mL) of probiotics is administered. The healthy vagina, when examined under a microscope, has relatively few lactobacilli, indicating that the sheer number of them is not the main concern. Competition trials have demonstrated that modest amounts of lactobacilli on surfaces can compete and displace greater amounts of pathogens (Reid, 2006; Reid & Tieszer, 1993). A possible method of displacement (Velraeds et al., 1996) could be the creation of biosurfactant molecules, but there are undoubtedly other options (Reid et al., 2011).

The compounds that probiotics make, like neurochemicals (Lyte, 2011) or what they invigorate the host to produce, seem to arrive in the brain preferably via the vagus nerve system, especially in the case of remote places like the brain where the probiotics themselves does not travel (Forsythe et al., 2014). This could be the most fascinating molecular area of probiotic study since it must deal with the organ that regulates a lot of what people do. It appears possible that drastically altering the gut microbiota via transplanting or injection of probiotic strains expressing components could not only affect daily habitat and memory (Messaoudi et al., 2011) but also what we eat and when we eat it, as well as how quickly or slowly pathological changes take place(*EBSCO host | 108831983 | Bacteria Need "Sleep" Too?: Microbiome Circadian Rhythmicity, Metabolic Disease, and Beyond.*, n.d.).

14.2.1 Probiotics Function in Human Health: Biological Mechanisms

Through their biological actions in the body, probiotics have a few positive effects on health. According to the "Human Microbiome Project," there are around ten times as many different bacteria living in the human body's tissues as there are human cells (Juturu & Wu, 2018). These bacteria also contain helpful microorganisms that are essential to maintaining human health. Probiotic bacteria generate postbiotic-like enzymes, SCFAs, and lactic acid and emit antimicrobial ligands that eradicate harmful bacterial strains; however, the precise mechanism of action is not entirely understood. They are referred described as "natural preservatives" because of their bacteriocins (Juturu & Wu, 2018). Probiotics have been associated with the modulation of nutrient availability, inhibition of infectious bacterial attachment in the colonic lumen, and enhancement of mucus production as a means to compete with pathogens. The production of mucus enhances the integrity of the intestinal epithelial cells barrier, thereby promoting immune system activation (Monteagudo-Mera et al., 2019).

Probiotics enhance the absorption of minerals and vitamins within the human body and mitigate the presence of pollutants through the utilization of supplementary enzymatic mechanisms, such as bile salt hydrolase (Skrypnik et al., 2019). Certain probiotics possess the ability to produce and release metabolites with antioxidant and anticarcinogenic properties, thereby contributing to the treatment of various diseases. After receiving antibiotics, the gut flora can be replenished with the use of endogenous probiotic supplements. Probiotics can be used before, during, or after antibiotic therapy to prevent antibiotic-related diarrhea. Additionally, it has been discovered by researchers that some pathways linked to probiotics transmission of nerve impulses throughout the nervous system's core may encourage possible healing effects on neuropsychiatric illnesses and ailments brought on by stress (Spencer & Hu, 2020).

Probiotics improve digestive health, but they also affect brain function, aid in the treatment of IBS, lower blood levels of low-density lipoprotein, protect women from yeast- and bacteria-based urinary tract infections, mitigate the occurrence of pancreatitis and enhance pancreatic well-being, improve respiratory tract health, restrict tumorigenesis, control immune responses, and support metabolic homeostasis (Lavelle & Sokol, 2020). Additionally, probiotics help treat metabolic conditions like non-alcoholic fatty liver disease, diabetes, cardiovascular illnesses, oral *Candida* infections, cancer, and periodontitis, among others (Nyvad & Takahashi, 2020). The choice of suitable probiotic strains and genera is crucial for various applications since different strains have varied health benefits (Aceti et al., 2018).

The relevance of probiotics in human healthiness, or the physiologic effects of probiotics, can be defined in terms of their metabolic activities, which are the basis for the biological impacts of probiotics. These outcomes are characterized as follows.

14.2.2 Modulation

Probiotics affect neural networks that either stimulate or decrease the control of processes, resulting in metabolic modulations (Sanders et al., 2018). Intestinal epithelial cells' barrier activities can be modified by probiotics' capacity to attach to the intestinal wall for immigration and to interact with natural immune reactions, which enhances the host's health. These modulatory mechanisms improve immunity (immunomodulation) by assisting in antagonism against pathogens (Suez et al., 2019). They also increase antioxidant potential, enhance nervous reflexes, improve intestinal transit, vascular endothelial cell supervision, regulation of blood pressure, modulation of cholesterol levels, and the preservation of a dynamic equilibrium between healthy and damaged cells (Ma et al., 2019).

14.2.3 Synthesis

The manufacturing of bioactive metabolites is a crucial function performed by probiotics as part of their mode of action. As an illustration, the cytokine secretion by BNL1059, CRL1528, LDR0723, and RGS1746 strains of *L. salivarius* is mediated by specific strain mechanisms, while the production of vitamins such as vitamin B2 and vitamin K2 by *Bacillus subtilis* and vitamin B12 by *Bacillus megaterium* occurs through species-specific mechanisms. Additionally, the synthesis of SCFAs is achieved via a non-specific mechanism (Tungland, 2018).

14.2.4 Absorption

Probiotics can improve the metabolism and bioavailability of micronutrients. Significant amounts of iron are absorbed in the form of Fe^{2+}; nevertheless, in the intestinal mucosa, iron interacts with apoferritin to change Fe^{2+} into Fe^{3+} (ferritin). Probiotics in the gut microbiota can aid in the conversion of Fe^{3+} to Fe^{2+}, which increases iron absorption in the duodenum. According to Hoppe et al. (Hoppe et al., 2015), consumption of lactic acid bacteria enhances the relative bioavailability of iron and the rate at which it is absorbed through extracellular enzymes. Similar findings were made by Dubey et al. (Dubey & Patel, 2018), who discovered that probiotics have a significant impact on calcium uptake and colonic fermentation-mediated calcium absorption. Probiotics play a role in the production and absorption of vitamin D; according to a different study by Costanzo et al. (2018), these illustrations clarify how probiotics work to increase the body's ability to absorb vitamins and minerals.

14.2.5 Prophylaxis

Probiotics' prophylactic mechanism aids in illness prevention and lowers the probability of contracting infections, viral infections, type 1 allergies, and cancer. According to Monteagudo-Mera et al.(2019), probiotic prophylaxis is used to prevent bacterial vaginosis. Significantly, numerous interventional research studies are being carried out to determine the efficacy of probiotic sanitation. To investigate the effectiveness of a synbiotic supplement against neonatal sepsis, Panigrahi et al. (2017) escorted randomized clinical trials that had been submitted under NIH clinicaltrials.gov. Significant reductions were seen between culture-positive and culture-negative cases of sepsis, as reported. Current clinical studies are examining the impact of probiotic interventions on the modification of the microbiome and the avoidance of serious infections, namely pneumonia, in patients with multiple traumas. Additionally, these trials are examining the impact of the probiotic oral mixture Labinic in inhibiting sepsis infection through the establishment of the ESBL triggered by Enterobacteriaceae.

14.3 PROBIOTIC ENCAPSULATION: NEED AND IMPORTANT FACTORS

The alimentary canal presents plenty of stress conditions to probiotics that are consumed orally. For instance, the pH levels in the body's digestive system can vary. The pH of the mouth is roughly 6–7, that of the stomach is 1–3, and that of the small and large intestines is between 6 and 7 (Cieplak et al., 2018). Maintaining the survival of probiotic bacteria reaching the large intestine is difficult due to the lower pH control in the gut and higher bile salt concentration in the small intestine.

Therefore, proper probiotic protection is essential throughout the creation of any useful probiotic food item. The viability of probiotics is influenced by various factors beyond those inherent to the body. These elements encompass the rectifying temperature, pH level of the encapsulating or matrix substance, oxygen concentration within the product, the existence of rival bacteria, and the harmful effects of metabolites. When storing items, it is important to consider both the ambient temperature and the moisture content of the environment. Additionally, the survival and revival of dried probiotics are correlated with their rehydration and solubility properties (Broeckx et al., 2016).

Various methods have been created to increase the ability of probiotics to withstand external stress, consequently boosting the colonization of the gut microbiota by alterations to the food matrix and the application of process engineering techniques. Regarding technological performance and probiotic stability, food matrix composition and selection are crucial factors (Sun et al., 2020).

Probiotics can be protected, their stability can be improved, and they can benefit from focused distribution when they are encapsulated as powder formulations. It's crucial to establish microbial stability, efficacy, functionality, safety, and targeting ability throughout the encapsulation procedure to optimize a probiotics encapsulation methodology (*Nutrients | Free Full-Text | Probiotics in Food Systems: Significance and Emerging Strategies Towards Improved Viability and Delivery of Enhanced Beneficial Value*, n.d.). In accordance with the FAO/WHO recommendation, Figure 14.2 explains the several screening sections that are involved. An encapsulation strategy should take the following factors into account to maintain the distinctive qualities of probiotics.

1. **Probiotics' Stability**: assurance of enhanced vitality retention of the encapsulated probiotic bacterium.
2. **Probiotics' Performance**: After encapsulation, serviceable properties such as adherence to mucus, aggregation, resistance to bile salts, stomach acids, and digestive enzymes, as well as antibacterial action against possible pathogens, should all be kept.
3. **Safety with Efficacy**: The probiotic variant needs to be effective, non-toxicogenic, safe, and free of sludge. It should also maintain its therapeutic potency after being encapsulated.
4. Capability of targeting the colon to promote gut flora has positive health impacts, as well as increased tolerance to environmental stress.

Probiotics have been encapsulated using a variety of methods (Figure 14.3). The primary objective of all these strategies is to safeguard the viability and stability of probiotics. The distinct conceptual

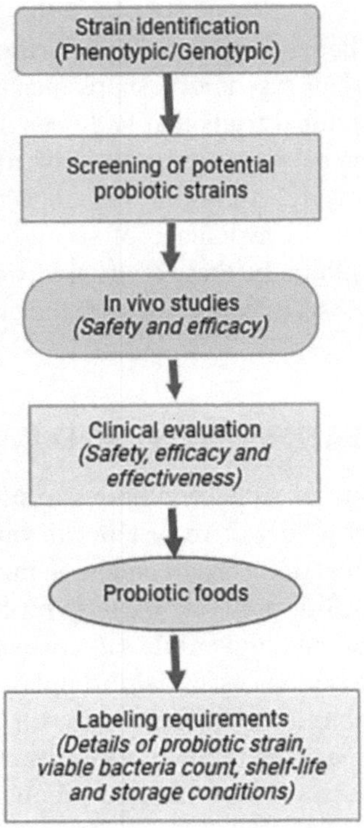

FIGURE 14.2 The evaluation process of probiotics, as outlined in the recommendations established by the Food and Agriculture Organization (FAO) and the World Health Organization (WHO), encompasses many stages that include screening sections dedicated to assessing both the operational and the security aspects of these microorganisms.

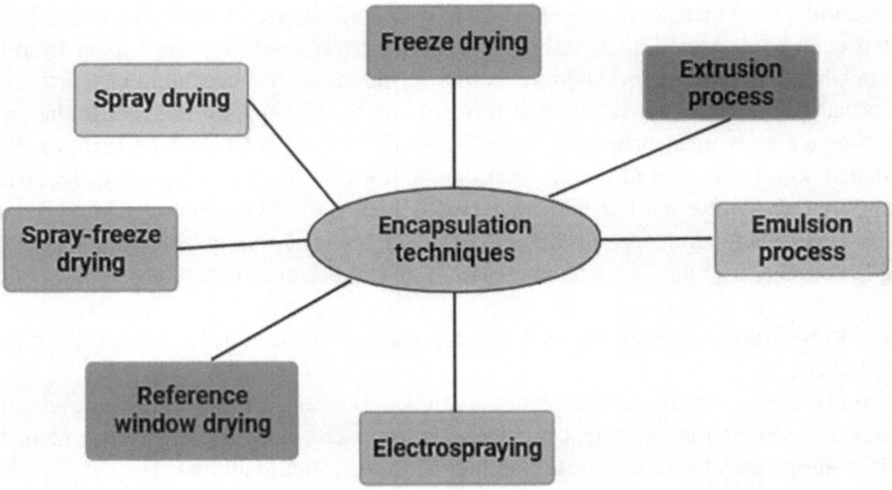

FIGURE 14.3 Various techniques used for the encapsulation of probiotics.

framework of each approach directly influences the overall quality of the end output. Processing conditions are thought to be the main determinants of the probiotics' capacity to maintain their quality and viability after being encapsulated. Additionally, numerous materials for walls have been examined for their potential use as coatings or protective agents in the encasing of probiotics. These substances are derived from food fibers, proteins, polysaccharides, and synthetic polymers. The decision is typically made based on a substance's usability, film-forming capacity, solubility, stability, digestion, and releasing qualities. The necessary qualities can also be achieved through the utilization of a variety of wall materials or the incorporation of emulsifiers.

However, many well-established probiotic encapsulation strategies have taken only probiotics' ability to survive into account and not their qualities or effectiveness. Probiotics' surface characteristics and functionality may be affected after encapsulation or drying. Probiotic properties including aggregation, antagonistic activity, intestinal mucus adhesion capacity, and bile salt hydrolase activity may be impacted by this. Future research must therefore investigate the functional properties of encapsulated probiotics along with their ability to survive, for a better understanding of the health advantages of probiotics.

14.4 THE MARKETING OF PROBIOTICS

In 1906, the French organization "Le Fermente" introduced a fermented milk beverage (Lactobacilline) that consisted of *Lactobacillus delbruekii* and *Streptococcus thermophilus*; Isaac Carasso launched merchandising yogurt making in Spain in 1919 in a similar fashion. The presence and viability of living organisms within these products, as well as their ability to withstand passage through the upper GIT, remain uncertain. As a result, fermented milk known as Yakult is frequently cited as the first probiotic to be sold commercially (Roy, 2005).

Early in the 20th century, probiotic-infused fermented milk was promoted as a treatment for intestinal illnesses. Focus has gradually switched to the ability of the mentioned bacteria to survive in the gastrointestinal system and the conveyor food to benefit the host. Due to the strains of World War II, the Great Depression, and the disclosure and widespread use of numerous antibiotics, interest in probiotics rapidly waned from the late 1930s onward. However, there have been several global trends from the 1980s to the present, including a rise in antimicrobial resistance, the dearth of medicine research and development pertaining to infectious diseases, the exorbitant prices associated with newly developed antibiotics, and the disparities in the attainability and employment of conventional infection averting measures. As a result, captivation in probiotics has once more surged because it is commonly believed that using them might help prevent and possibly treat a range of infections without the need for antibiotics. After the DSHEA was passed in 1994, sales of goods labeled as probiotics experienced a sharp increase. Due to this regulation, these substances could be sold as dietary supplements without having to pass the strict tests required to be approved as prescription medications. Since then, probiotic product marketing and sales in the US have increased dramatically. Probiotic food, supplements, and ingredient sales were valued at $14.9 billion globally in 2007 and are anticipated to rise to $19.6 billion by 2013. It is equivalent to a 4.3% compound annual growth rate (Hati et al., 2015).

14.5 PROBIOTICS CURRENT STANDING IN AN ARRAY OF DISEASES

Probiotics appear to hold promise for either decreasing the duration of infections or preventing them. The safety and effectiveness of probiotics in treating a variety of disorders are now being investigated in several laboratory research and clinical trials. Theorizing the immunomodulatory effects discovered in laboratory research with the output in living soul trials is one of the main hurdles we have today in the field of probiotics. The differences between research conducted in laboratories and clinical trials are via a variety of factors, together with genetics and microbial diversity. The function of probiotics has changed because of meta-analysis of clinical trials that used different strains.

14.5.1 Antibiotic-Associated Diarrhea

Research has shown that the administration of antibiotics can alter the composition of the intestinal microbiota inside the host, resulting in a reduction in amylolytic task, increased proteolytic activity, and decreased synthesis of SCFAs. To prevent or lessen the AAD, several probiotic organisms are being investigated in numerous clinical trials involving both children and adults. A meta-analysis was conducted to examine the efficacy of *S. boulardii* in avoiding AAD in randomized clinical trials. The results indicated that *S. boulardii* demonstrated significant protective effects against AAD, particularly when a greater number of strain-specific studies were included in the analysis (McFarland, 2010). A total of 10.2 individuals were mandated to cease a single occurrence of AAD. LGG has demonstrated its superiority over sugar pills or no therapies in decreasing antibiotic-associated diarrhea among pediatric and adult populations, as evidenced by multiple randomized control trials (Wenus et al., 2008).

14.5.2 *C. difficile* Infection

The use of probiotics in the averting, diagnosis, and management of CDI and perennial CDI has been researched. *S. boulardii*, a probiotic yeast, has been demonstrated in in-vitro experiments to digest *C. difficile* toxins A and B and enhance the levels of anti-toxin secretory IgA. According to studies, LGG increases mucin expression and reduces bacterial adhesion (Naaber et al., 1998). Several randomized controlled studies have been conducted using CDI or *C. difficile* neurotoxin procurement as the major or auxiliary endpoint (Hickson et al., 2007). Except for one experiment, none of them have demonstrated analytically significant reduction in CDI or *C. difficile* toxin uptake. In a random controlled trial conducted on individuals with persistent CDI, it was observed that the administration of high-dose vancomycin (2 grams/d) in combination with the probiotic *S. boulardii* resulted in an analytically significant decrease in the recurrence rate, as juxtaposed with the use of a lower dose of vancomycin or a medication called metronidazole with *Lactobacillus*.

14.5.3 Necrotizing Enterocolitis

The presence of NEC in premature infants is associated with an increased risk when their mothers receive broad-spectrum antibiotics during pregnancy or when the infants themselves receive antibiotics shortly after birth. This increased risk is attributed to changes in the composition of the intestinal microbiota, highlighting the significance of bacterial colonization patterns in the development of NEC. When *Bifidobacterium* species and *Lactobacillus acidophilus* are administered as a prophylactic treatment in neonates with birth weights below 1,500 grams, there is a lower relative risk of NEC and death, according to several meta-analyses. The administration of probiotics increased the risk of sepsis among newborns with birth weights under 750 grams (Lin et al., 2008).

14.5.4 Inflammatory Bowel Disease

In patients with UC, *Lactobacillus paracasei* showed immunomodulatory benefits by lowering pro-inflammatory cytokines in the vital fluid. In UC people, VSL#3 upregulates IL-12p40 production while downregulating IL-10 production by the lamina propria. However, none of the clinical trials (Marteau et al., 2006) were able to show any appreciable reduction in IBD symptoms compared to placebo. To prove that probiotics are superior to placebo or anti-inflammatory drugs like steroids, we need a variety of sizable research studies and meta-analyses. Probiotics do not now play a part in the induction or maintenance phases of remission for inflammatory bowel disorders.

14.5.5 Irritable Bowel Syndrome

IBS is a major universal digestive disease in both developed and underdeveloped countries, and treating it costs a lot of money. In the absence of an underlying organic condition, IBS is identified by the diagnostic scale of chronic, recurrent bouts of stomach pain or displeasure with disturbed bowel manner. Additionally, bloating sensations with or beyond obvious stomach distension, elevated anxiety, and a few extraintestinal symptoms are frequently seen. Even while a slew of research on both humans and animals points to altered gut flora in IBS patients, it is still unclear whether this is the result of the condition or its root cause (Rhee et al., 2009). The occurrence of IBS is more frequent after gastroenteritis. Potential factors contributing to IBS include abnormal lactulose breath tests caused by an overgrowth of bacteria in the small intestine, inflammation of the intestines, and changes in the makeup of the intestinal microbiota (*Abnormal Breath Testing in IBS: A Meta-Analysis | SpringerLink*, n.d.). The only probiotic to significantly reduce IBS symptoms is *Bifidobacterium infantis* 35624, according to a systematic analysis of numerous randomized controlled studies (Brenner et al., 2009).

14.5.6 Acute Pancreatitis

The prevalence of infectious complications in cases with acute necrotizing pancreatitis is notably high, with death rates reaching up to 80%. These complications are considered the most prevalent and severe adverse outcomes associated with this condition. It has been established that bacterial translocation has a significant role in the development of infectious complications in individuals with acute chronic necrotizing pancreatitis. Probiotics with or without prebiotics have been proven in several randomized controlled trials (Wan et al., 2021) to lessen the infectious consequences in individuals with acute severe pancreatitis. In a multicenter, double-blind, placebo-controlled clinical research by Besselink et al. (PROPATRIA trial) (*[Probiotic Prophylaxis in Patients with Predicted Severe Acute Pancreatitis: A Randomised, Double-Blind, Placebo-Controlled Trial].—Abstract—Europe PMC*, n.d.), the study included the random assignment of 296 individuals diagnosed with AP to different treatment groups either a placebo or enteral probiotic therapy for 28 days (a preparation containing multiple species of probiotics). Infectious complexity rates among the probiotic cohort and the placebo counterparts (30% vs. 28%) were not different, according to this study. Bowel ischemia occurred in nine individuals (eight of whom passed away) in the probiotics group but not in the placebo group.

Surprisingly, individuals who received probiotic treatment had a mortality rate that was much greater than patients who received a placebo (16% vs. 6%). The design and execution of this study have drawn criticism, including improper blinding, inadequate divulging of serious adverse events, an elevation in sample number following the research was initiated, the replacement of the population from "severe pancreatitis" with "predicted severe pancreatitis," and improper implementation of the intentional treatment investigation (*Dutch Probiotics Study Is Criticised for Its "Design, Approval, and Conduct" | The BMJ*, n.d.). Additionally, the people in the Besselink group meet with more pressure and a greater variety of probiotic organisms. Prophylactic antibiotics have not been shown to have a substantial positive impact on those suffering from necrotizing AP in randomized controlled studies or meta-analyses.

14.5.7 Ventilator-Associated Pneumonia

In the US, VAP is the most common illness picked up in hospitals. In addition to extending the time spent on automatic ventilation, the duration of residence in the ICU, and the possibility of lung activity recovery, it also raises mortality risk by a factor of 2–10 (Safdar et al., 2005). Although the pathophysiology of VAP is complicated, it often entails biofilm formation, microaspiration of contaminated secretions, and invasion of the aero-intestinal tract with pathogenic bacteria. The use of probiotics in preventing ICU mortality, VAP and hospital death as major or auxiliary endpoints has been investigated in a plethora of randomized control trials. The rate of VAP, the term of stay in the ICU, and *Pseudomonas aeruginosa* colonization of the respiratory tract all significantly decreased in a meta-analysis of 12 randomized controlled trials (Kollef, 2004), but there was insignificant improvement in-hospital mortality, ICU mortality, or hospital duration of stay.

14.5.8 Obesity and Insulin Resistance

The microbiota's makeup differs not just from individual to individual but also throughout every segment of the digestive system. The makeup of the gut microbiota is significantly influenced by genotype, as shown in research involving monozygotic twins. Bacteroidetes and Firmicutes make up over 90% of the entire microbiota, making them the most prevalent phylum (Candela et al., 2010). Although the species makeup of the gut microbiota varies greatly, healthy people often have similar functional gene profiles (microbiomes). Diet likely has a significant impact on how the gut microbiota is made up. *Prevotella* enterotype was linked to low levels of protein and fat intake and high levels of carbohydrates, whereas the presence of bacteroides enterotype has been associated with increased consumption of trans fats and proteins in the diet (Jumpertz et al., 2011).

The study observed a correlation between alterations in the bacterial makeup of the gut microbiota and fluctuations in the caloric intake of the diet throughout a span of three days. In overweight adolescents who achieved weight loss by a combination of a low-calorie diet and regular exercise, a significant reduction in fecal Enterobacteriaceae and sulfate-reducing bacteria was seen. Interestingly, Roux-en-Y gastric bypass operation has been linked to a rise in harmful gut bacteria and a decline in helpful species. There exists a divergence of opinions on the specific bacterial patterns that are associated with resistance to insulin and obesity. Obesity is characterized by low-grade, chronic inflammation accompanied by metabolic disturbances. Metabolic endotoxemia refers to the condition characterized by an observed increase in the levels of overall microbes, gram-negative bacteria, and bacteria such as *E. coli* DNA in the ileal mucosa, pus, and mesenteric adipose tissue (*Intestinal Mucosal Adherence and Translocation of Commensal Bacteria at the Early Onset of Type 2 Diabetes: Molecular Mechanisms and Probiotic Treatment | EMBO Molecular Medicine*, n.d.). This condition, also known as metabolic bacteremia, has been demonstrated to induce an augmented permeability of the gut and elevated levels of lipopolysaccharide in the bloodstream, indicating the presence of low-grade endotoxinemia. Lipopolysaccharide is a significant constituent of the outer membrane of gram-negative bacteria. The interaction between metabolic endotoxemia and starting insulin levels, insulin aversion, and triglyceride and cholesterol levels is seen to be favorable in individuals with type 2 diabetes. The role of pattern-recognition receptor TLR5, which is a component of the innate immune system, has been shown to influence the underlying microbial makeup and the emergence of insulin resistance. In this paper, hyperplasia, obesity, and insulin resistance were all seen in TLR5–/– animals. Insulin resistance was present in even thin TLR5–/– mice. Obesity has not been averted by food restriction, although insulin aversion has. Hyperphagia, obesity, and insulin resistance were produced when the gut microbiota from TLR5–/– mice was transplanted into wild-type mice with no germs. Treatment with antibiotics reduced insulin resistance, obesity, and hyperphagia in TLR5–/– mice (Vijay-Kumar et al., 2010, p. 5). This implies a strong connection between insulin resistance, innate immunity, and gut microbiota.

In research on school-aged children, the number of *Bifidiobacterium* spp. The fecal data from newborns were greater in kids who retained their usual weight at age 7 than in children who were gaining weight. According to this study, overweight is preceded by an abnormal gut microbial makeup. Additionally, *Bifidiobacterium* spp. is more prevalent in normal weight compared to overweight women and in pregnant women who gained less weight. It has been demonstrated that the abundance of inulin-type fructans with prebiotic characteristics leads to an increase in *Bifidiobacterium* spp. (Gibson & Roberfroid, 1995). The effect became apparent during a couple of days and vanished a week after the treatment was stopped (Luoto et al., 2010). Ingesting a daily quantity of 200 grams of boiled milk containing LG2055 for a period of 12 weeks was shown to significantly reduce body weight, waist circumference, and abdominal visceral and subcutaneous fat area in a double-blind, randomized, placebo-controlled trial.

The handling of obesity and insulin resistance may involve nutritional and pharmaceutical interventions aimed at the gut flora. A wide range of scientific disciplines, including gastroenterology, immunology, endocrinology, and microbiology, are involved in this fascinating and diverse area of research.

14.6 EXPANDING APPLICATIONS OF PROBIOTICS

Probiotics were first described by Fuller in 1989 as "a live microbial feed additive that benefits the host animals by enhancing their intestinal microbial balance" (Fuller, 1989). In 2001, the Joint Expert Consultation of the Food and Agricultural Organizations of the United Nations and the WHO put up a standardized definition, which was refined to read as follows: "a live bacteria that, when ingested in adequate amounts, confer a health benefit on the host." The majority of these criteria were entirely kept in the 2014 consensus statements from the International Scientific Association for Probiotics and Prebiotics (Colin et al., 2014).

Probiotics' primary positive impacts on the body include the suppression of potential gastrointestinal infections, strengthening of the epithelial barrier, and modification of immunity. The primary mechanism behind the host's defense against pathogenic microbes in the intestine is probiotic strains' contention with bacteria for essential spots on the mucosa. SCFAs-like acetic acid and organic acids like lactic acid that probiotic bacteria release are thought to have a substantial bactericidal effect on infections. Probiotics must be in a "living" form to defend their hosts from pathogens, as is stressed in the description of probiotics, as dead probiotic strains are unable to precisely connect to the mucosa or produce organic acids.

It has long been believed that probiotics should be used only in the gut because the original concept of probiotics placed a strong emphasis on their positive effects on enhancing intestinal microbial ecology. The number of bacteria in the gut can exceed 10^{12}/gram of feces (Simon & Gorbach, 1984), indicating an elevated level of colonization. In contrast, the stomach's bacterial bulk, where probiotic strains might be effective, is quite modest. When tested using culture techniques, the amount of native bacteria in a healthy stomach's gastric juice is at most 10^3/mL. The heightened acidity in the stomach caused by the generation of gastric acid leads to a discernible depletion in the population of gastric bacteria residing in the stomach. Consequently, this acidity also diminishes or stops the beneficial impacts exerted by probiotic strains quickly post their introduction into the stomach. Due to these circumstances, the usage of probiotics in the GIT or the small intestine at the proximal end has been deemed impracticable.

For probiotic strains to elicit therapeutic benefits inside the GIT, it is essential that they establish proximity to the mucosa (Suez et al., 2019). This may be achieved via two mechanisms: either by demonstrating a preference for the surface mucus coating or by clinging to the epithelial cell divisions. The observed results include contact-dependent immunomodulation, the synthesis of organic acids at concentrations that are efficacious, and the competitive reduction of adherence of pathogenic bacteria to the mucosa.

It is challenging for probiotic bacteria to get near the gastric mucosa because peristaltic motions tend to be more regular and active in the stomach than in the intestine. Additionally, because of this, using stomach probiotics is challenging. Another angle is that the introduction of foreign microorganisms can readily alter the tiny size of the stomach's resident microbiota. Because it is much smaller than the gut microbiota, these transient microorganisms (such as food additives or unintentional pollutants) have a significantly bigger impact on the bacteria residing in the upper GIT.

The same issue arises when probiotics are administered to the upper GIT, so they are not interfered with by significant quantities of the gut's diverse and resilient microbiota. If the potential strains exhibit resistance to high acidity and can reach the gastric mucosa, it may be more advantageous to provide probiotics by injection into the upper gastrointestinal system rather than applying them directly to the gut. Because powerful gastric acid kills many ingested germs, the stomach is an unbearable place for most microbes. Gastric fluid has a pH of 1–2, indicating high acidity, during the morning period of fasting. *Lactobacilli* and *bifidobacteria* possess exceptional resistance to acidity in its totality. Both bacterial groups have the ability to endure and thrive in an acidic environment characterized by a pH range of 3–4 (Marteau et al., 1997). It is important to note, however, that this level of acidity is not as extreme as the peak stomach acidity, which typically falls within the pH range of 1–2. To identify a probiotic strain that is well-suited for the stomach and can withstand a pH of about 2, it is necessary to conduct a screening process including potential probiotic strains.

Upon examination via culture methods, it has been shown that the genus *Lactobacillus* is among the uppermost bacterial groups present in the gastric region. Hence, the most optimal *Lactobacillus* strains are likely to be those employed as digestive probiotics. Furthermore, it was shown that adult mice reared in a SPF environment did not exhibit any presence of *H. pylori* infection in their stomachs (Kabir et al., 1997). In contrast, mice that were reared in a sterile environment exhibited heightened susceptibility to infection upon receiving an oral administration of *H. pylori.* The findings of this animal study indicate that mice with a substantial amount of native lactobacilli in their stomach, above 108 CFU/gram tissue, exhibited protection against *H. pylori* infection. *Lactobacillus gasseri* OLL2716 (LG21) is an exemplary probiotic strain that has the potential for gastric applications (Sakamoto et al., 2001). Among a selection of around 2,000 strains of lactobacilli, this particular strain was selected. Both the ability to tolerate acidity and the capability to adhere to the gut mucosa were variables considered throughout the selection process. Throughout the stationary growth phase, LG21 has been seen to survive in culture broth at a pH of 2.5, which is comparable to the acidity level found in GF. To mitigate the effects of acid stress, LG21 employs many defensive strategies, including the activation of cationic ATP-binding circuit exporter genes and the suppression of genes accomplished with transcriptional and protein coalescence. The acid response to stress is often crucial for lactobacilli due to their consistent production of significant quantities of organic acids during metabolic activity in their environment. In the absence of this protective mechanism, the presence of an acidic environment impedes the growth of lactobacilli and may potentially lead to their extinction.

Endoscopy clearly showed probiotic colonization of mucosa in a few studies. It was demonstrated that LG21 strains ingested by a yogurt beverage could reach the mucosal layer of the human stomach using biopsy samples acquired by upper GI endoscopy (Fujimura et al., 2006). This fine topical investigation was made possible via non-contact pressure catapulting and laser-assisted microdissection.

14.7 FUTURE PROSPECTS AND POSSIBILITIES OF PROBIOTICS

Genetically engineered probiotic organisms have the capacity to significantly transform and expand the scope of probiotic functionality by the targeted delivery of anti-inflammatory chemicals or other biologically significant substances to the inflamed mucosa. The concept in question has been shown by Steidler et al. (2000) via the use of *Lactococcus lactis*, a strain that has been genetically engineered to produce interleukin-10, while still meeting the necessary standards for food-grade use. The therapeutic effectiveness of intragastrically administered conventional steroids was shown to be comparable to that of the experimental treatment in two animal models of IBD. Although many people seem to have doubts about the appropriateness of genetically modified food-grade organisms, and a number of safety issues still need to be resolved, this strategy has clear benefits. These include administration to the location of mucosal inflammation that is organ-specific, convenient, and economical. The use of cell surface proteins for the purpose of attaching therapeutically significant compounds and afterward displaying them on the surface of bacteria is an alternative approach via which probiotic organisms convey biotherapeutic substances to the mucosal lining of the GIT. Therefore, the modification of surface proteins via the creation of hybrid proteins eliminates the need for genetically modified organisms in food, therefore addressing the concerns associated with genetically modified food that are prevalent among a significant portion of the population (Leenhouts et al., 1999).

14.8 CONCLUSION

The role of probiotics has been gradually developing over the past two to three decades and is currently being explored in a variety of gastrointestinal and non-gastrointestinal illnesses. To get dependable results across a range of medical conditions, it is necessary to conduct substantial, randomized trials that use a placebo control group and focus on a single strain of therapy. These studies should also adhere to defined protocols for dosage, formulation, and duration of treatment. It is now challenging to suggest a specific probiotic for a given ailment because the preparation and dosage may not be readily available on the market. One of the key areas of biomedical research is the collaboration of the gut microbiota and its host to engage in reciprocal control. More study is needed to determine their relation to human disorders. The therapeutic efficacy of probiotics in inflammatory illnesses is anticipated to be limited, but nonetheless considerable, in the absence of genetic alteration or surface protein modification. However, with carefully thought out, monitored research studies assessing efficacy in properly classified patients, the field of probiotics can advance over the next ten years. This needs to be supported by a clearer understanding of the mechanisms behind probiotic action, as is made possible by decoding the proteomes and genomes of distinct probiotic strains. In conclusion, because microorganisms make up a significant physical portion of the GIT and other places, it is crucial that specialists recognize their existence and think about the potential roles they may play in health and disease. Rapid diagnostic techniques will soon be accessible to inform on the microbiome's contents, and while instructions will be provided with the results, having some background in this sector could make life much simpler for those who understand the results. The novelty of the microbiome is that its makeup and functionality will likely be correlated with health, unlike conventional clinical microbiology which has associated one pathogen alongside a disease. The use of probiotics as therapeutic agents or preventive measures for maintaining health will necessitate extensive documentation of the strains, product composition, and how they act. This encompassing review elucidates the value of probiotics in preserving human well-being, as well as the need to encapsulate probiotics to get the intended outputs. The comprehension of the complex route and diverse stress conditions inside the oral gastrointestinal system of the human body provides insight into the need for encapsulation. Probiotics have demonstrated potential for protection and target delivery by encapsulation. Encapsulation techniques significantly impact probiotics, some of which have only been studied in-depth in the laboratory thus far.

BIBLIOGRAPHY

Abnormal breath testing in IBS: A meta-analysis | SpringerLink. (n.d.). Retrieved September 28, 2023, from https://link.springer.com/article/10.1007/s10620-010-1276-4

Aceti, A., Beghetti, I., Maggio, L., Martini, S., Faldella, G., & Corvaglia, L. (2018). Filling the gaps: Current research directions for a rational use of probiotics in preterm infants. *Nutrients, 10*(10), article 10. https://doi.org/10.3390/nu10101472

Aggarwal, S., Upadhyay, A., Shah, D., Teotia, N., Agarwal, A., & Jaiswal, V. (2014). Lactobacillus GG for treatment of acute childhood diarrhoea: An open labelled, randomized controlled trial. *The Indian Journal of Medical Research, 139*(3), 379–385.

Amar, J., Chabo, C., Waget, A., Klopp, P., Vachoux, C., Bermúdez-Humarán, L. G., Smirnova, N., Bergé, M., Sulpice, T., Lahtinen, S., Ouwehand, A., Langella, P., Rautonen, N., Sansonetti, P. J., . . . Burcelin, R. (2011). Intestinal mucosal adherence and translocation of commensal bacteria at the early onset of type 2 diabetes: Molecular mechanisms and probiotic treatment. *EMBO Molecular Medicine, 3*(9), 559–572. https://doi.org/10.1002/emmm.201100159

Arroyo, R., Martín, V., Maldonado, A., Jiménez, E., Fernández, L., & Rodríguez, J. M. (2010). Treatment of infectious mastitis during lactation: Antibiotics versus oral administration of lactobacilli isolated from breast milk. *Clinical Infectious Diseases, 50*(12), 1551–1558. https://doi.org/10.1086/652763

Aspirin therapy in primary cardiovascular disease prevention: A position paper of the European Society of Cardiology working group on thrombosis | *Journal of the American College of Cardiology*. (n.d.). Retrieved September 27, 2023 https://www.jacc.org/doi/abs/10.1016/j.jacc.2014.03.049

Barbonetti, A., Vassallo, M. R. C., Cinque, B., Filipponi, S., Mastromarino, P., Cifone, M. G., Francavilla, S., & Francavilla, F. (2013). Soluble products of Escherichia coli induce mitochondrial dysfunction-related sperm membrane lipid peroxidation which is prevented by lactobacilli. *PLoS One, 8*(12), e83136. https://doi.org/10.1371/journal.pone.0083136

Bisanz, J. E., Seney, S., McMillan, A., Vongsa, R., Koenig, D., Wong, L., Dvoracek, B., Gloor, G. B., Sumarah, M., Ford, B., Herman, D., Burton, J. P., & Reid, G. (2014). A systems biology approach investigating the effect of probiotics on the vaginal microbiome and host responses in a double blind, placebo-controlled clinical trial of post-menopausal women. *PLoS One, 9*(8), e104511. https://doi.org/10.1371/journal.pone.0104511

Breasted, J. H. (n.d.). *Ancient records of Egypt*. Retrieved September 28, 2023, from https://cir.nii.ac.jp/crid/1130000796231474688

Brenner, D. M., Moeller, M. J., Chey, W. D., & Schoenfeld, P. S. (2009). The utility of probiotics in the treatment of irritable bowel syndrome: A systematic review. *Official Journal of the American College of Gastroenterology: ACG, 104*(4), 1033.

Broeckx, G., Vandenheuvel, D., Claes, I. J. J., Lebeer, S., & Kiekens, F. (2016). Drying techniques of probiotic bacteria as an important step towards the development of novel pharmabiotics. *International Journal of Pharmaceutics, 505*(1–2), 303–318. https://doi.org/10.1016/j.ijpharm.2016.04.002

Cadieux, P., Wind, A., Sommer, P., Schaefer, L., Crowley, K., Britton, R. A., & Reid, G. (2008). Evaluation of reuterin production in urogenital probiotic Lactobacillus reuteri RC-14. *Applied and Environmental Microbiology, 74*(15), 4645–4649. https://doi.org/10.1128/AEM.00139-08

Candela, M., Maccaferri, S., Turroni, S., Carnevali, P., & Brigidi, P. (2010). Functional intestinal microbiome, new frontiers in prebiotic design. *International Journal of Food Microbiology, 140*(2–3), 93–101. https://doi.org/10.1016/j.ijfoodmicro.2010.04.017

Cieplak, T., Soffer, N., Sulakvelidze, A., & Nielsen, D. S. (2018). A bacteriophage cocktail targeting Escherichia coli reduces E.coli in simulated gut conditions, while preserving a non-targeted representative commensal normal microbiota. *Gut Microbes, 9*(5), 391–399. https://doi.org/10.1080/19490976.2018.1447291

Corr, S. C., Li, Y., Riedel, C. U., O'Toole, P. W., Hill, C., & Gahan, C. G. M. (2007). Bacteriocin production as a mechanism for the anti-infective activity of Lactobacillus salivarius UCC118. *Proceedings of the National Academy of Sciences of the United States of America, 104*(18), 7617–7621. https://doi.org/10.1073/pnas.0700440104

Costanzo, M., Cesi, V., Palone, F., Pierdomenico, M., Colantoni, E., Leter, B., Vitali, R., Negroni, A., Cucchiara, S., & Stronati, L. (2018). Krill oil, vitamin D and Lactobacillus reuteri cooperate to reduce gut inflammation. *Beneficial Microbes, 9*(3), 389–399. https://doi.org/10.3920/BM2017.0078

Dubey, M. R., & Patel, V. P. (2018). Probiotics: A promising tool for calcium absorption. *The Open Nutrition Journal, 12*(1), 59–69. https://doi.org/10.2174/1874288201812010059

Dutch probiotics study is Criticised for its "design, approval, and conduct". (n.d.). *The BMJ*. Retrieved September 28, 2023, from https://www.bmj.com/content/340/bmj.c77.full

EBSCO host | 108831983 | bacteria need "sleep" too? Microbiome circadian rhythmicity *Metabolic disease, and beyond*. (n.d.). Retrieved September 28, 2023, from https://web.p.ebscohost.com/abstract?direct=true&profile=ehost&scope=site&authtype=crawler&jrnl=08332207&AN=108831983&h=ekaQJVu%2bBkMJax85Y2OoP4k%2bLm06gk11u7bzaVjbBp212kcqstcnxI6Te2arpOOdVdaDATih37%2fqBS9ObJnmHQ%3d%3d&crl=c&resultNs=AdminWebAuth&resultLocal=ErrCrlNotAuth&crlhashurl=login.aspx%3fdirect%3dtrue%26profile%3dehost%26scope%3dsite%26authtype%3dcrawler%26jrnl%3d08332207%26AN%3d108831983

Forsythe, P., Bienenstock, J., & Kunze, W. A. (2014). Vagal pathways for microbiome-brain-gut axis communication. In M. Lyte & J. F. Cryan (Eds.), *Microbial endocrinology: The microbiota-gut-brain axis in health and disease* (pp. 115–133). Springer. https://doi.org/10.1007/978-1-4939-0897-4_5

Fujimura, S., Kato, S., Oda, M., Miyahara, M., Ito, Y., Kimura, K., Kawamura, T., Ohnuma, M., Tateno, H., & Watanabe, A. (2006). Detection of Lactobacillus gasseri OLL2716 strain administered with yogurt drink in gastric mucus layer in humans. *Letters in Applied Microbiology, 43*(5), 578–581. https://doi.org/10.1111/j.1472-765X.2006.02017.x

Fuller, R. (1989). Probiotic in man and animals. *Journal of Applied Bacteriology, 66*(5), 131–139.

Gan, X. T., Ettinger, G., Huang, C. X., Burton, J. P., Haist, J. V., Rajapurohitam, V., Sidaway, J. E., Martin, G., Gloor, G. B., Swann, J. R., Reid, G., & Karmazyn, M. (2014). Probiotic administration attenuates myocardial hypertrophy and heart failure after myocardial infarction in the rat. *Circulation Heart Failure, 7*(3), 491–499. https://doi.org/10.1161/CIRCHEARTFAILURE.113.000978

Giamarellos-Bourboulis, E. J., Bengmark, S., Kanellakopoulou, K., & Kotzampassi, K. (2009). Pro-and synbiotics to control inflammation and infection in patients with multiple injuries. *Journal of Trauma and Acute Care Surgery*, *67*(4), 815–821. https://doi.org/10.1097/TA.0b013e31819d979e

Gibson, G. R., & Roberfroid, M. B. (1995). Dietary modulation of the human colonic microbiota: Introducing the concept of prebiotics. *Journal of Nutrition, 125*(6), 1401–1412. https://doi.org/10.1093/jn/125.6.1401

Guo, C. F., Zhang, L. W., Han, X., Yi, H. X., Li, J. Y., Tuo, Y. F., Zhang, Y. C., Du, M., Shan, Y. J., & Yang, L. (2012). Screening for cholesterol-lowering probiotic based on deoxycholic acid removal pathway and studying its functional mechanisms in vitro. *Anaerobe, 18*(5), 516–522. https://doi.org/10.1016/j.anaerobe.2012.08.003

Hati, S., Mandal, S., & Prajapati, J. B. (2015). Methods for improving survival of probiotics against harsh environments. *International Journal of Fermented Foods*, *4*(1and 2), 1–13. http://dx.doi.org/10.5958/2321-712X.2015.00001.0

Hickson, M., D'Souza, A. L., Muthu, N., Rogers, T. R., Want, S., Rajkumar, C., & Bulpitt, C. J. (2007). Use of probiotic Lactobacillus preparation to prevent diarrhoea associated with antibiotics: Randomised double blind placebo controlled trial. *BMJ, 335*(7610), 80. https://doi.org/10.1136/bmj.39231.599815.55

Hill, C., Guarner, F., Reid, G., Gibson, G. R., Merenstein, D. J., Pot, B., Morelli, L., Canani, R. B., Flint, H. J., Salminen, S., Calder, P. C., & Sanders, M. E. (2014). The international scientific association for probiotics and prebiotics consensus statement on the scope and appropriate use of the term probiotic. *Nature Reviews Gastroenterology and Hepatology, 11*(8), 506–514. https://doi.org/10.1038/nrgastro.2014.66

Hoppe, M., Önning, G., Berggren, A., & Hulthén, L. (2015). Probiotic strain Lactobacillus plantarum 299v increases iron absorption from an iron-supplemented fruit drink: A double-isotope cross-over single-blind study in women of reproductive age. *British Journal of Nutrition, 114*(8), 1195–1202. https://doi.org/10.1017/S000711451500241X

Hunter, B. T. (2008). *Probiotic foods for good health: Yogurt, sauerkraut, and other beneficial fermented foods*. Basic Health Publications, Inc.

Iemoli, E., Trabattoni, D., Parisotto, S., Borgonovo, L., Toscano, M., Rizzardini, G., Clerici, M., Ricci, E., Fusi, A., De Vecchi, E., Piconi, S., & Drago, L. (2012). Probiotics reduce gut microbial translocation and improve adult atopic dermatitis. *Journal of Clinical Gastroenterology, 46*, S33–S44 https://doi.org/10.1097/MCG.0b013e31826a8468

Interference in initial adhesion of uropathogenic bacteria and yeasts to silicone rubber by A Lactobacillus acidophilus biosurfactant | Microbiology Society. (n.d.). Retrieved September 28, 2023 https://www.microbiologyresearch.org/content/journal/jmm/10.1099/00222615-47-12-1081

Irvine, S. L., Hummelen R., Hekmat, S., W. N. Looman, Habbema, J. D. F., & Reid, G Irvine, S. L., Hummelen, R., Hekmat, S., Looman, C. W., Habbema, J. D., & Reid, G. (2010). Probiotic yogurt consumption is associated with an increase of CD4 count among people living with HIV/AIDS. *Journal of Clinical Gastroenterology, 44*(9), e201–e205 https://doi.org/10.1097/MCG.0b013e3181d8fba8

Jumpertz, R., Le, D. S., Turnbaugh, P. J., Trinidad, C., Bogardus, C., Gordon, J. I., & Krakoff, J. (2011). Energy-balance studies reveal associations between gut microbes, caloric load, and nutrient absorption in humans. *The American Journal of Clinical Nutrition, 94*(1), 58–65. https://doi.org/10.3945/ajcn.110.010132

Juturu, V., & Wu, J. C. (2018). Microbial production of bacteriocins: Latest research development and applications. *Biotechnology Advances, 36*(8), 2187–2200. https://doi.org/10.1016/j.biotechadv.2018.10.007

Kabir, A. M., Aiba, Y., Takagi, A., Kamiya, S., Miwa, T., & Koga, Y. (1997). Prevention of Helicobacter pylori infection by lactobacilli in a gnotobiotic murine model. *Gut, 41*(1), 49–55. https://doi.org/10.1136/gut.41.1.49

Kiple, K. F., & Ornelas, K. C. (2000). *The Cambridge world history of food*. Cambridge University Press.

Kollef, M. H. (2004). Prevention of hospital-associated pneumonia and ventilator-associated pneumonia. *Critical Care Medicine, 32*(6), 1396–1405. https://doi.org/10.1097/01.CCM.0000128569.09113.FB

Kosikowski, F. V. (1977). *Cheese and fermented milk foods* (2nd ed.). https://www.cabdirect.org/cabdirect/abstract/19770434950

Langa, S., Martín-Cabrejas, I., Montiel, R., Landete, J. M., Medina, M., & Arqués, J. L. (2014). Short communication: Combined antimicrobial activity of reuterin and diacetyl against foodborne pathogens. *Journal of Dairy Science, 97*(10), 6116–6121. https://doi.org/10.3168/jds.2014-8306

Lavelle, A., & Sokol, H. (2020). Gut microbiota-derived metabolites as key actors in inflammatory bowel disease. *Nature Reviews Gastroenterology & Hepatology, 17*(4), article 4. https://doi.org/10.1038/s41575-019-0258-z

Leenhouts, K., Buist, G., & Kok, J. (1999). Anchoring of proteins to lactic acid bacteria. *Antonie van Leeuwenhoek, 76*(1–4), 367–376. https://doi.org/10.1023/A:1002095802571

Lin, H. C., Hsu, C. H., Chen, H. L., Chung, M. Y., Hsu, J. F., Lien, R., Tsao, L. Y., Chen, C. H., & Su, B. H. (2008). Oral probiotics prevent necrotizing enterocolitis in very low birth weight preterm infants: A multicenter, randomized, controlled trial. *Pediatrics, 122*(4), 693–700. https://doi.org/10.1542/peds.2007-3007

Lorea Baroja, M., Kirjavainen, P. V., Hekmat, S., & Reid, G. (2007). Anti-inflammatory effects of probiotic yogurt in inflammatory bowel disease patients. *Clinical and Experimental Immunology, 149*(3), 470–479. https://doi.org/10.1111/j.1365-2249.2007.03434.x

Luoto, R., Kalliomäki, M., Laitinen, K., & Isolauri, E. (2010). The impact of perinatal probiotic intervention on the development of overweight and obesity: Follow-up study from birth to 10 years. *International Journal of Obesity, 34*(10), article 10. https://doi.org/10.1038/ijo.2010.50

Lyte, M. (2011). Probiotics function mechanistically as delivery vehicles for neuroactive compounds: Microbial endocrinology in the design and use of probiotics. *Bioessays, 33*(8), 574–581. https://doi.org/10.1002/bies.201100024

Ma, C., Zhang, S., Lu, J., Zhang, C., Pang, X., & Lv, J. (2019). Screening for cholesterol-lowering probiotics from lactic acid bacteria isolated from corn silage based on three hypothesized pathways. *International Journal of Molecular Sciences, 20*(9), article 9. https://doi.org/10.3390/ijms20092073

Marteau, P., Lémann, M., Seksik, P., Laharie, D., Colombel, J. F., Bouhnik, Y., Cadiot, G., Soulé, J. C., Bourreille, A., Metman, E., Lerebours, E., Carbonnel, F., Dupas, J. L., Veyrac, M., Coffin, B., Moreau, J., Abitbol, V., Blum-Sperisen, S., & Mary, J. Y. (2006). Ineffectiveness of Lactobacillus johnsonii LA1 for prophylaxis of postoperative recurrence in Crohn's disease: A randomised, double blind, placebo controlled GETAID trial. *Gut, 55*(6), 842–847. https://doi.org/10.1136/gut.2005.076604

Marteau, P., Minekus, M., Havenaar, R., & Huis In't Veld, J. H. J. (1997). Survival of lactic acid bacteria in a dynamic model of the stomach and small intestine: Validation and the effects of bile. *Journal of Dairy Science, 80*(6), 1031–1037. https://doi.org/10.3168/jds.S0022-0302(97)76027-2

McFarland, L. V. (2010). Systematic review and meta-analysis of Saccharomyces boulardii in adult patients. *World Journal of Gastroenterology : WJG, 16*(18), 2202–2222. https://doi.org/10.3748/wjg.v16.i18.2202

McGovern, P. E. (2009). *Uncorking the past: The quest for wine, beer, and other alcoholic beverages*. University of California Press.

Messaoudi, M., Violle, N., Bisson, J. F., Desor, D., Javelot, H., & Rougeot, C. (2011). Beneficial psychological effects of a probiotic formulation (Lactobacillus helveticus R0052 and Bifidobacterium longum R0175) in healthy human volunteers. *Gut Microbes, 2*(4), 256–261. https://doi.org/10.4161/gmic.2.4.16108

Monteagudo-Mera, A., Rastall, R. A., Gibson, G. R., Charalampopoulos, D., & Chatzifragkou, A. (2019). Adhesion mechanisms mediated by probiotics and prebiotics and their potential impact on human health. *Applied Microbiology and Biotechnology, 103*(16), 6463–6472. https://doi.org/10.1007/s00253-019-09978-7

Naaber, P., Mikelsaar, R. H., Salminen, S., & Mikelsaar, M. (1998). Bacterial translocation, intestinal microflora and morphological changes of intestinal mucosa in experimental models of Clostridium difficile infection. *Journal of Medical Microbiology, 47*(7), 591–598. https://doi.org/10.1099/00222615-47-7-591

Nutrients | Free full-text | Probiotics in food systems: Significance and emerging strategies towards improved viability and delivery of enhanced beneficial value. (n.d.). Retrieved September 28, 2023, from https://www.mdpi.com/2072-6643/11/7/1591

Nyvad, B., & Takahashi, N. (2020). Integrated hypothesis of dental caries and periodontal diseases. *Journal of Oral Microbiology, 12*(1), 1710953. https://doi.org/10.1080/20002297.2019.1710953

Panigrahi, P., Parida, S., Nanda, N. C., Satpathy, R., Pradhan, L., Chandel, D. S., Baccaglini, L., Mohapatra, A., Mohapatra, S. S., Misra, P. R., Chaudhry, R., Chen, H. H., Johnson, J. A., Morris, J. G., Paneth, N., & Gewolb, I. H. (2017). A randomized synbiotic trial to prevent sepsis among infants in rural India. *Nature, 548*(7668), article 7668. https://doi.org/10.1038/nature23480

Probiotic prophylaxis in patients with predicted severe acute pancreatitis: A randomised, double-blind, placebo-controlled trial. (n.d.). *Abstract—Europe PMC*. Retrieved September 28, 2023, from https://europepmc.org/article/med/18438065

Reid, G. (2006). Exclusion of uropathogen adhesion to polymer surfaces by Lactobacillus acidophilus. *Canadian Journal of Infectious Diseases and Medical Microbiology, 17*(5), 291–295. https://doi.org/10.1155/2006/934626

Reid, G., & Kirjaivanen, P. (2005, November). Expression of antimicrobial defense factors in vaginal mucosa following exposure to Lactobacillus rhamnosus GR-1. *Canadian Family Physician, 51* 1477–1479.

Reid, G., & Tieszer, C. (1993). Preferential adhesion of urethral bacteria from a mixed population to a urinary catheter. *Cells and Materials, 3*(2). https://digitalcommons.usu.edu/cellsandmaterials/vol3/iss2/9

Reid, G., Younes, J. A., Van der Mei, H. C., Gloor, G. B., Knight, R., & Busscher, H. J. (2011). Microbiota restoration: Natural and supplemented recovery of human microbial communities. *Nature Reviews in Microbiology, 9*(1), article 1. https://doi.org/10.1038/nrmicro2473

Rhee, S. H., Pothoulakis, C., & Mayer, E. A. (2009). Principles and clinical implications of the brain–gut–enteric microbiota axis. *Nature Reviews. Gastroenterology and Hepatology, 6*(5), article 5. https://doi.org/10.1038/nrgastro.2009.35

Roy, D. (2005). Technological aspects related to the use of bifidobacteria in dairy products. *Le Lait, 85*(1–2), 39–56. https://doi.org/10.1051/lait:2004026

Safdar, N., Dezfulian, C., Collard, H. R., & Saint, S. (2005). Clinical and economic consequences of ventilator-associated pneumonia: A systematic review. *Critical Care Medicine, 33*(10), 2184–2193. https://doi.org/10.1097/01.CCM.0000181731.53912.D9

Sakamoto, I., Igarashi, M., Kimura, K., Takagi, A., Miwa, T., & Koga, Y. (2001). Suppressive effect of Lactobacillus gasseri OLL 2716 (LG21) on Helicobacter pylori infection in humans. *Journal of Antimicrobial Chemotherapy, 47*(5), 709–710. https://doi.org/10.1093/jac/47.5.709

Saloheimo, P. (2005). Captain Cook used sauerkraut to prevent scurvy. *Duodecim; lääketieteellinen aikakauskirja, 121*(9), 1014–1015.

Sanders, M. E., Merenstein, D., Merrifield, C. A., & Hutkins, R. (2018). Probiotics for human use. *Nutrition Bulletin, 43*(3), 212–225. https://doi.org/10.1111/nbu.12334

Segers, M. E., & Lebeer, S. (2014). Towards a better understanding of Lactobacillus rhamnosus GG—host interactions. *Microbial Cell Factories, 13*(1), S7. https://doi.org/10.1186/1475-2859-13-S1-S7

Simon, G. L., & Gorbach, S. L. (1984). Intestinal flora in health and disease. *Gastroenterology, 86*(1), 174–193.

Skrypnik, K., Bogdański, P., Schmidt, M., & Suliburska, J. (2019). The effect of multispecies probiotic supplementation on iron status in rats. *Biological Trace Element Research, 192*(2), 234–243. https://doi.org/10.1007/s12011-019-1658-1

Spencer, N. J., & Hu, H. (2020). Enteric nervous system: Sensory transduction, neural circuits and gastrointestinal motility. *Nature Reviews Gastroenterology and Hepatology, 17*(6), article 6. https://doi.org/10.1038/s41575-020-0271-2

Steidler, L., Hans, W., Schotte, L., Neirynck, S., Obermeier, F., Falk, W., Fiers, W., & Remaut, E. (2000). Treatment of murine colitis by Lactococcus lactis secreting interleukin-10. *Science, 289*(5483), 1352–1355. https://doi.org/10.1126/science.289.5483.1352

Suez, J., Zmora, N., Segal, E., & Elinav, E. (2019). The pros, cons, and many unknowns of probiotics. *Nature Medicine, 25*(5), article 5. https://doi.org/10.1038/s41591-019-0439-x

Sun, X., Acquah, C., Aluko, R. E., & Udenigwe, C. C. (2020). Considering food matrix and gastrointestinal effects in enhancing bioactive peptide absorption and bioavailability. *Journal of Functional Foods, 64,* 103680. https://doi.org/10.1016/j.jff.2019.103680

Suvarna, V. C., & Boby, V. U. (2005). Probiotics in human health: A current assessment. *Current Science, 88*(11), 1744–1748.

Tomaro-Duchesneau, C., Jones, M. L., Shah, D., Jain, P., Saha, S., & Prakash, S. (2014). Cholesterol assimilation by *Lactobacillus* probiotic bacteria: An *in vitro* investigation. *BioMed Research International, 2014,* e380316. https://doi.org/10.1155/2014/380316

Tungland, B. (2018). Short-chain fatty acid production and functional aspects on host metabolism. In *Human microbiota in health and disease: From pathogenesis to therapy* (pp. 37–106). Academic Press, Elsevier Inc.

Velraeds, M. M., van der Mei, H. C., Reid, G., & Busscher, H. J. (1996). Inhibition of initial adhesion of uropathogenic Enterococcus faecalis by biosurfactants from Lactobacillus isolates. *Applied and Environmental Microbiology, 62*(6), 1958–1963. https://doi.org/10.1128/aem.62.6.1958-1963.1996

Vijay-Kumar, M., Aitken, J. D., Carvalho, F. A., Cullender, T. C., Mwangi, S., Srinivasan, S., Sitaraman, S. V., Knight, R., Ley, R. E., & Gewirtz, A. T. (2010). Metabolic syndrome and altered gut microbiota in mice lacking toll-like receptor 5. *Science, 328*(5975), 228–231. https://doi.org/10.1126/science.1179721

Wan, Y.-D., Zhu, R.-X., Bian, Z.-Z., & Sun, T.-W. (2021). Effect of probiotics on length of hospitalization in mild acute pancreatitis: A randomized, double-blind, placebo-controlled trial. *World Journal of Gastroenterology*, *27*(2), 224–232. https://doi.org/10.3748/wjg.v27.i2.224

Wenus, C., Goll, R., Loken, E. B., Biong, A. S., Halvorsen, D. S., & Florholmen, J. (2008). Prevention of antibiotic-associated diarrhoea by a fermented probiotic milk drink. *European Journal of Clinical Nutrition, 62*(2), article 2. https://doi.org/10.1038/sj.ejcn.1602718

Wilson, E. (1900). *Sacred books of the east: Comprising the Vedic hymns, Zend-avesta, Dhammapada, Upanishads, the Koran and the life of Buddha*. Colonial Press.

Yang, S., Li, W., Challis, J. R. G., Reid, G., Kim, S. O., & Bocking, A. D. (2014). Probiotic Lactobacillus rhamnosus GR-1 supernatant prevents lipopolysaccharide-induced preterm birth and reduces inflammation in pregnant CD-1 mice. *American Journal of Obstetrics and Gynecology, 211*(1), 44.e1–44.e12. https://doi.org/10.1016/j.ajog.2014.01.029

Yokotsuka, T. (1985). Fermented protein foods in the Orient, with emphasis on shoy and miso in Japan. In*Microbiologyoffermentedfoods*(pp.197–247).Springer.https://doi.org/10.1007/978-1-4613-0309-1_12

Zhao, Y., Dong, B. R., & Hao, Q. (2022). Probiotics for preventing acute upper respiratory tract infections. *Cochrane Database of Systematic Reviews, 8*. https://doi.org/10.1002/14651858.CD006895.pub4

15 Probiotics
Conclusion and Future Perspective

Dhananjay Sharma, Gowhar Rashid, and Luxita Sharma

15.1 INTRODUCTION

Exaggerated research in recent years has more attention as it confirms the beneficial importance of the microbial population of the gastrointestinal (GI) tract. The thoughts of probiotics probably date back to 1908, when Bulgarian peasants increased their lives by the inclusion of fermented milk products in their diets, as suggested by Elie Metchnikoff (a Noble Prize winner) (*The Prolongation of Life : Optimistic Studies/by Élie Metchnikoff ; English Translation Edited by P. Chalmers Mitchell. | Wellcome Collection*, n.d.). He advocated that life longevity was due to the high intake of fermented milk products, and also considered a substitute of gut microbes by yogurt bacteria (Holzapfel & Schillinger, 2002). The term "probiotic" was first termed in 1954 by Vergin in his document "Anti-und Probiotika," where he compared the disadvantageous effect of antibiotics with other antimicrobial components to the gut microflora (Markowiak & Ślizewska, 2017), whereas, in 1965, Lilly and Stillwell explained that microorganisms are responsible for the growth of other microbes (Lilly & Stillwell, 1965). More precisely, in 1992, Fuller explained probiotics as a live microbial feed complement that constructively improves the healthy microbial content in animal intestines (McFarland, 2015).

Modern probiotics started at the beginning of 19's (1907) with the pioneering studies of Russian scientist Elie Metchnikoff, working at Pasteur Institute in Paris. Louis Pasteur pointed out that microbes are accountable for the fermentation process, whereas Metchnikoff carried out the probable effect of these microorganisms on human health. He also claimed that the toxins released from bacterial decomposition in the large intestine and their circulation in the body cause aging. The modification of microbial flora in the intestine depends on the food that makes them adopt, measure, and replace the harmful microbes with beneficial microbes. So, the said sentences describe well the concept of "probiotics" (Gasbarrini et al., 2016).

We have discussed the historical concept and how probiotics developed. Now we will discuss the possible health benefits and future prospects of probiotics. The repetitive use of antibiotics, irradiation, and immunosuppressive therapies may cause an alteration in the GI microflora composition. Therefore, the introduction of beneficial bacterial species in the GI tract could be beneficial to re-establish microbial harmony and prevent the disease (Vanderhoof & Young, 1998); these probiotics have recently received increasing attention not only in a varied range of biomedical applications such as tissue repair and tissue regeneration and also as an antimicrobial agent and in several disease treatments. This chapter will basically focus on the recent development and future perspective of probiotics.

15.1.1 Brief Overview of Probiotics

The term "probiotic" is made up of two words "pro" (Latin) and "bios" (Greek), meaning "for life" (Reid et al., 2003). True probiotics are basically safe, of human origin, and vector free; they probably provide resistance against pathogenicity, antibiotics, or toxicity factors (Plaza-Diaz et al., 2019).

Fuller defined probiotics as "a live microbial feed supplement which beneficially affects the host animal by improving its intestinal microbial balance" (McFarland, 2015).

DOI: 10.1201/9781003452249-15

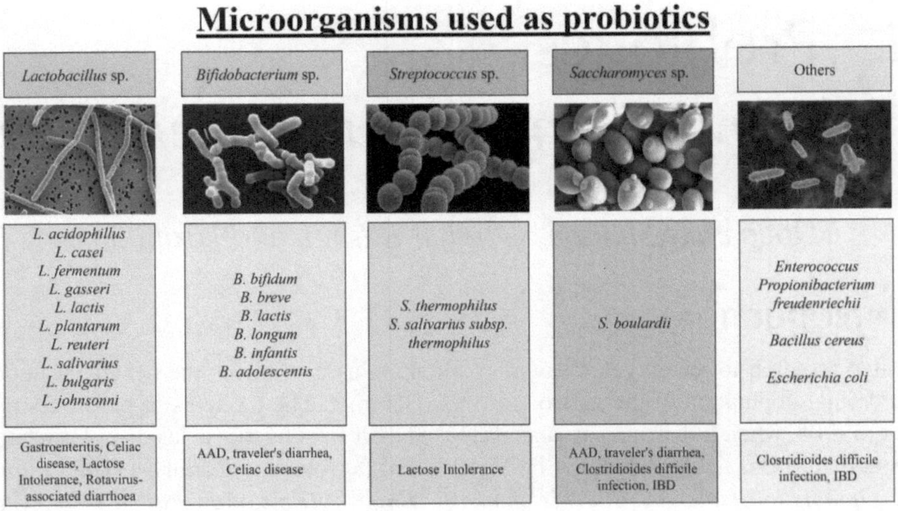

FIGURE 15.1 Some probiotic microorganisms and their effectiveness in diseases.

The expert panel of the FAO and WHO, 2001, explains probiotics as "live microorganisms which when administered in adequate amounts confer a health benefit on the host," whereas the definition is reiterated by replacing "which" with "that" in the said definition (Hill et al., 2014).

Stavropoulou and Bezirtzoglou (2020) state that probiotic flora are non-pathogenic living microbes, which when given in an adequate amount (10^6 viable CFU/g) would be helpful to the host by improving microbial balance in the gut and also partaking in various metabolism (Stavropoulou & Bezirtzoglou, 2020). Figure 15.1 illustrates some probiotic microorganisms and their effectiveness in diseases.

15.1.2 Importance of Studying Probiotics

More than 100 bacterial species naturally and predominantly constitute intestinal microbiota. The probiotic bacteria are those who are expected to exhibit possible health benefits to the host by means of modulation of intestinal microbiota and are included in this category. The species belonging to the genera *Lactobacillus* (such as *Lactobacillus plantarum*, *Lactobacillus casei*, and *Lactobacillus acidophilus*) and *Bifidobacterium* (*Bifidobacterium bifidum*, *Bifidobacterium longum*, and *Bifidobacterium lactis*) have been reported as a beneficial probiotic strain (Kailasapathy & Chin, 2000; Shi et al., 2016).

There are several criteria used to select a beneficial probiotic bacterial strain based on safety issues. Aforementioned two genera of bacteria are considered safe and for long-term use. All species of *Bacillus* are not considered safe, but a few species of *Bacillus* such as *Bacillus licheniformis* is reported as safe and can be used as probiotics, additionally the species belongs to *Bacillus*; i.e., *Bacillus cereus* is linked with health issues and may cause food-borne diseases (Leuschner & Robinson, 2010; Shi et al., 2016).

The microorganism meets the criteria for GRAS and can be used in probiotic preparation. The probiotics should be resistant to gastric enzymes such as pancreatic juices, bile, and hydrochloric acids. Along with this the probiotics should be immune system stimulators and anti-carcinogenic, have good intestinal permeability, and produce lactic acids. The main properties that probiotics should have are to survive in any medium whether acidic (stomach) or alkaline (duodenum). The microorganisms used in the probiotic preparation include both single and mixed cultures of live microorganisms. The lactic acid bacteria that are present in food include fermented milk, sausage, wine, fruit juices, and cheese (Gupta & Garg, 2009). An adequate dose of 5 billion CFU/day of the probiotic has been recommended for good health benefits, for at least five days (Grölund & Lehtonen, n.d.).

15.2 MECHANISM OF ACTION

15.2.1 Colonization and Normalization of Perturbed Intestinal Microbial Communities

Microbiome play an important role related to digestion and metabolism of food, development, and in immune system. So, early colonization of a child's GI tract is likely to be a determining factor in later life (Yang et al., 2016). The assemblage of GI microbiota begins before childbirth and continues to childhood. There are several factors that affect the colonization of intestinal microbiota such as genetic constituents, methods of childbirth, antibiotics used, types of feeding, and mental and physical health of the mother (Hesla et al., 2014).

The colonization may be affected by the bacterial isolates of umbilical cord blood, meconium, and placenta. The bacteria existing in the vagina and mother milk are important for the colonization of gut microbiota. These bacteria blow out from the GI tract to extra digestive sites via DCs, because these bacteria can easily penetrate the epithelium and take out the bacteria from the intestinal lumen (Plaza-Diaz et al., 2019).

The crucial process in the colonization is the adhesion of microbes to the host surface. Pili is a polymeric hair-like structure protruding from the bacterial surface, which helps to bind the bacteria with the host surface. These adhesion processes identify various types of host molecules such as transmembrane proteins (cadherin or integrins) and extracellular matrixes (such as fibronectin, collagen, elastin, or laminin) (Ribet & Cossart, 2015). The process of bacterial colonization starts just after or administration of probiotic strains. Most of the studies evaluated and assessed that the proper administration of microbial strain increases microbial colonization (Plaza-Diaz et al., 2019). The administration of such strains (*Lactobacillus gasseri* $CECT_{5714}$ and *Lactobacillus coryniformis* $CECT_{5711}$) in adults shows the increased production of short-chain fatty acids (SCFAs), fecal moisture, stool volume, and defecation (Olivares et al., 2006).

15.2.2 Competitive Exclusion of Pathogens and Bacteriocin Production

"Competitive exclusion" is the term that describes the condition where one species of bacteria will compete with the other species more vigorously to adopt the receptor site in the intestinal tract (Bermudez-Brito et al., 2012). The known mechanism behind the competitive exclusion of pathogens includes the reduction of luminal pH; production of bacteriocin, organic acids, hydrogen peroxide, and amines; and competition for nutritional sources. These bacteriocins are known to be secreted by lactobacilli and bifidobacteria, a kind of antimicrobial peptide that is composed of 30–60 amino acids and cationic in nature. They also provide "colonization resistance," preventing the entry of enteric pathogens. They act on the bacterial cytoplasmic membrane by targeting vesicles to disrupt the proton-motive force (Bermudez-Brito et al., 2012; Umu et al., 2017). Some of the species (*L. acidophilus* and *L. plantarum*) produce these compounds that inhibit the growth of *Clostridium difficile*, *Helicobacter*, rotavirus, *Escherichia coli*, and *Shigella* species in some GI difficulties and fight against uropathogens (Kumar et al., 2016; Mokoena, 2017).

The in vitro on human mucosal material (Hirano et al., 2003; Tuomola et al., 1999) and chicken and pig mucosal material in vivo studies (Genovese et al., 2000; Hirn et al., 1992) have demonstrated the probiotic bacteria as a competitive exclusion to the pathogens. One study shows that *Lactobacillus rhamnosus* has a strong adhering capacity that inhibits the incorporation of enterohemorrhagic *E. coli* in the human intestine (Hirano et al., 2003).

15.2.3 Enzymatic Activities and Production of Volatile Fatty Acids

In the gut lumen, the probiotics enzyme activity plays a significant role in the biological effect. More than 20 different types of enzymatic activities are exhibited by bifidobacteria and lactobacilli, among which beta-galactosidase activity is the most archetypal (Plaza-Diaz et al., 2019). In the intestine, the glucuronidated metabolites are hydrolyzed by intestinal bacteria into a toxic form that may cause intestinal damage. The low activity of beta-glucuronidase in the fecal material increases the carcinogens in the colonic lumen (D. H. Kim & Jin, 2001), whereas the supplementation of *B. longum* may alter the intestinal microbiota and may reduce the beta-glucuronidase activity that inhibits aberrant crypt formation in colon carcinogenesis (Kulkarni & Reddy, 1994).

A randomized control trial shows that the administration of *L. gasseri* $CECT_{5714}$ and *L. coryniformis* $CECT_{5711}$ increases the butyrate content in the feces compared to the control (received yogurt) (Olivares et al., 2006). The probiotic experimental group showed higher production of acetic acid and propionic acid after two weeks of treatment, whereas the production of butyric acid was still much higher in the treated group than the control, at the end of the washout period (Macfarlane & Macfarlane, 2003).

15.2.4 Cell Adhesion and Mucin Production

There are some specific rudiments that need to be addressed when we are indicating any microbial strain as a probiotic. Among these, adhesion is one of them, because it helps in mucosal colonization and further interaction between administered probiotics and the host. It also helps in the modulation of pathogen antagonism and immune system activation. Mucin (a complex glycoprotein mixture, a main component of the mucous) is secreted by the intestinal epithelial cells to evade the adhesion of pathogenic bacteria. *Lactobacillus* secretes some protein that promotes such kind of adhesion, which facilitates the attachment to the mucosal layer (Plaza-Diaz et al., 2019). Probiotics such as *L. plantarum* induce MUC2 and MUC3 mucin, which inhibits the adherence of enteropathogenic *E. coli* and enhances the mucosal layer and glycocalyx lying over the intestinal epithelium of microbial binding site by *Lactobacillus* spp. That provides the defense against pathogenic bacterial invasion (Bermudez-Brito et al., 2012). The probiotics help to maintain the epithelial barriers and increase the epithelial cell activation in response to bacterial invasion. The mechanism of the action of the probiotics is elaborately illustrated in Figure 15.2.

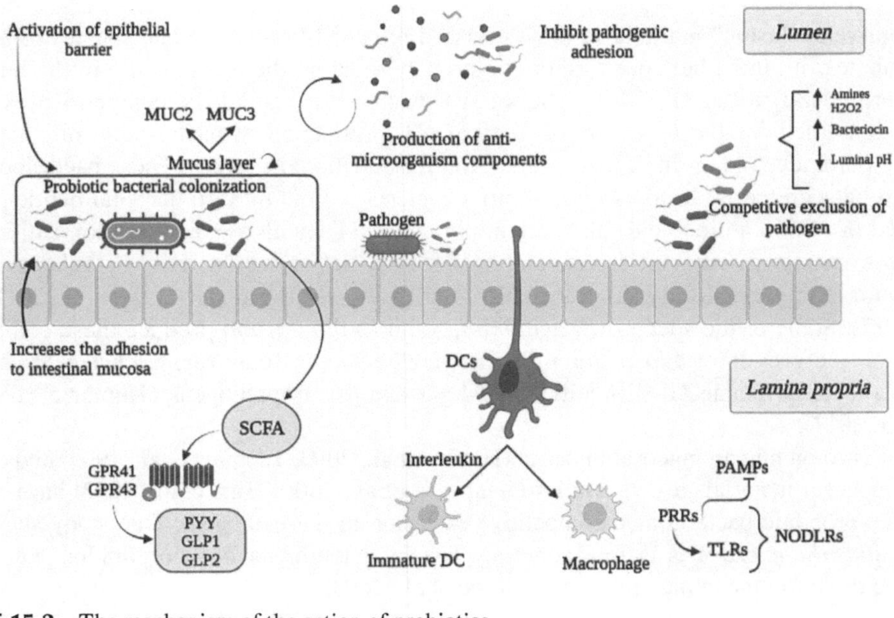

FIGURE 15.2 The mechanism of the action of probiotics.

15.2.5 Modulation of the Immune System

Several studies have demonstrated that probiotic bacteria modulate the immune system by producing molecules with an anti-inflammatory and immunomodulatory function that stimulates the immune cells. Probiotic bacteria's interaction with epithelial cells and DCs along with macrophages and lymphocytes produces immunomodulatory effects (D'Amelio & Sassi, 2017). The mechanism behind the action of the probiotics is the regulation of the immune response of the host cells. As we know the immune system works in two ways: innate and adaptive ways. The adaptive immune response is antigen-specific and depends upon B and T lymphocytes, whereas the innate immune system responds to the common structure (PAMPs). PRRs bind to PAMPs, which provide the first response to the entered pathogen. PRRs encompass the nucleotide-binding oligomerization domain, lectins, and adhesion molecules (Gómez-Llorente et al., 2010). Consequently, PRRs encompass the TLRs. TLRs are transmembrane proteins that are articulated on numerous immune and non-immune cells such as natural killer cells, DCs, macrophages, epithelial cells, fibroblast cells, and B-cells. The PRRs and TLRs both include NODLRs, which protect the cytoplasmic spaces (Claes et al., 2015). PRRs have also been designated as an important factor for formylated peptide, C-type lectin, intracellular IL-1 converting enzyme protease-activating, and retinoic acid inducible-like helicases. The probiotics help to maintain the host immune at equilibrium by modulating the immune responses by developing T-helper cells and T-regulatory cells (Hevia et al., 2015; Yousefi et al., 2015).

15.3 USES AND OTHER BENEFITS OF PROBIOTICS

15.3.1 Antibiotic-Associated Diarrhea

Antibiotics are the most common drug prescribed to children; even more than 50% of all children have received one course in at least 18 years. The most common antibiotics known to us are amoxicillin, azithromycin, clavulanate, and amoxicillin. Over or unused doses may cause AAD, which affects ≈11% of all children and ≈18% of children aged less than 2 years (Mantegazza et al., 2018).

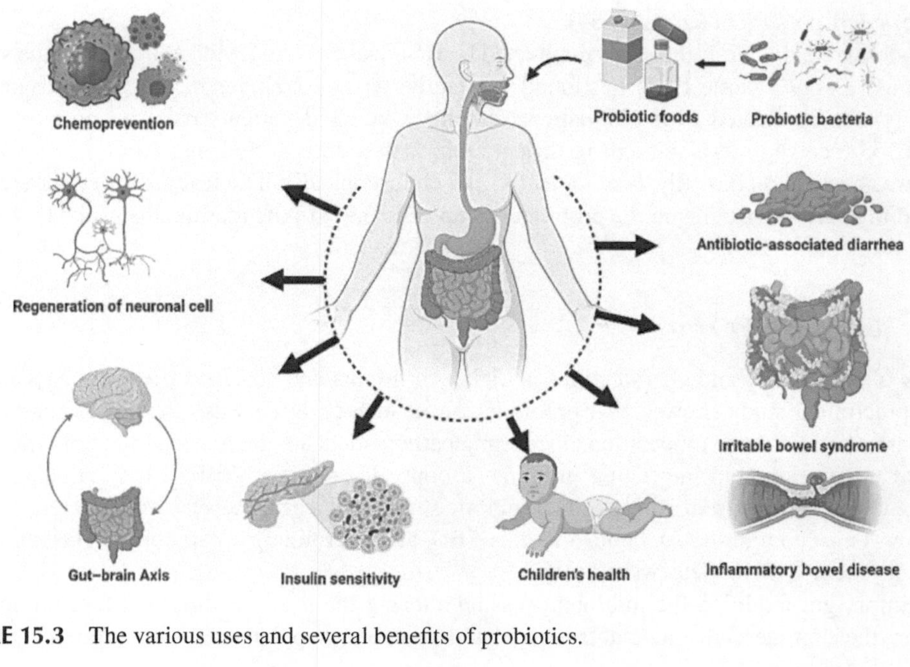

FIGURE 15.3 The various uses and several benefits of probiotics.

Various studies show that the use or supplementation of probiotics reduces the risk and frequency of AAD. A meta-analysis examined seven randomized control trials with a sample size of 881 and concluded that the probiotic use was effective in the treatment of AAD (RR = 0.396; CI 95%, 0.27–0.57) (Cremonini et al., 2002).

Lactobacillus GG, *Saccharomyces boulardii*, and *Enterococcus faecium* (SF68 strain) are mostly recommended for the prevention of AAD. *C. difficile colitis* is generally used for gastroenteritis treatment by oral rehydration therapy. When someone is suffering from both AAD and traveler's diarrhea, then *Saccharomyces cerevisiae* variant boulardii CNCM I_{1079} is generally recommended for effective treatment. For the effective treatment of travellers' diarrhea, the recommended bacterial strains are *Lactobacillus* $rosell_{52}$, *L.* $rosell_{11}$, and *Bifidobacterium* $rosell_{175}$ (Stavropoulou & Bezirtzoglou, 2020). The several uses and benefits of probiotics inclusion in the diet are illustrated in Figure 15.3.

15.3.2 Irritable Bowel Syndrome

Abdominal pain and IBS, jointly called functional bowel disorder, are the most common conditions reported by gastroenterologists. It affects ≈10% of all school-aged children, similarly to adults. The report of IBS identified in China in children is about 13%, in the USA 10%, and 6% in Sri Lanka (Sandhu & Paul, 2014). The probiotic use in IBS is not fully established. Some studies show that it is effective in lowering the related symptoms of IBS, whereas some lack the evidence. A meta-analysis included 20 trials (randomized, controlled, and blinded) based on 1,404 patients supplemented with probiotics. The result shows that probiotics were effective in improving the global IBS symptoms (RR = 0.78, CI 95%, 0.62–096) compared with placebo. It was found to reduce IBS-associated pains but was not effective in additional symptoms such as diarrhea, bloating, and flatulence (McFarland & Dublin, 2008).

15.3.3 Inflammatory Bowel Disease

IBD is collectively a disease that includes ulcerative colitis, Crohn's disease, and pouchitis. The main cause of IBD is unknown, but the disharmony of intestinal microflora may be one of the main reasons for IBD. The probiotic supplementation may exert a positive effect by incorporating the intestinal microflora (Schultz et al., 2003).

A randomized, double-blind study conducted by Rembacken et al. (1999) showed that the supplementation of *E. coli* (Nissle 1917) was found as effective as mesalazine in ulcerative colitis patients. The study was conducted over 327 patients among which 162 patients received probiotic drug/day and 165 received mesalazine drug thrice a day with a dose of 500 mg. After 12 months, the patient was evaluated clinically, histologically, and endoscopically. The result showed that relapses occurred in 36.4% of patients in the probiotic group and 33.9% in the mesalazine group ($p = 0.003$) (Rembacken et al., 1999).

15.3.4 Children's Health

The risk of respiratory and GI infections is higher in infants and children attending daycare centers. A preclinical study showed that probiotic use in such children was effective in maintaining the perturbed microbiota composition, decreasing pathogenic load, decreasing infection, increasing intestinal maturation, and improving immune response (Szajewska, 2016). Many clinical studies showed that the administration of specific probiotic strains reduces the severity of different pathologies such as nosocomial, AAD, colic, allergies, IBD, and necrotizing enterocolitis (Hashemi et al., 2016; Hojsak et al., 2018; Szajewska, 2016).

The infant gut modified the microbial session altering the breastfeeding and formula feeding. However, the commercially available formulated probiotic supplements with probiotic bacteria show the little-known ability to have a prolonged impact on the child's gut microbial configuration, effectiveness, and functionality (Bazanella et al., 2017).

15.3.5 Gut–Brain Axis and Mental Health

For the past few decades, probiotics have attracted much attention and interest in the treatment and prevention of neurological diseases. Recent several studies showed the possible role of probiotics in the pathogenesis of the brain disorder and neurological problems (Ghaisas et al., 2016; Umbrello & Esposito, 2016; Wang & Kasper, 2014). It is considered that there is a reciprocal link between the CNS, gut, and microbiota, so that is why it is called the "microbiota–gut–brain axis." It is nothing but a model representing the association between the brain and intestinal microflora (Ghaisas et al., 2016; Wang & Kasper, 2014).

The disharmony of intestinal and vaginal microflora may interfere with physical and psychological health and may cause stress. Under that situation, it is found that the putrefactive bacteria (*Clostridium* spp.) are in higher numbers. Studies show that the inclusion of *L. rhamnosus* regulates the transcript of GABA receptors and consequently emotional behavior. The alteration in intestinal microbiota also affects the GABA, which transmits the signal to the brain via enteric nerves (Konstandi et al., 2009; Tsiotsias et al., 2009). A cohort study conducted on children suffering from ASD when treated with *L. acidophilus* Rosell-11 for two months found improvement in antisocial behavior, concentration problems, and communication (Kałuzna-Czaplińska & Błaszczyk, 2012).

15.3.6 Insulin Sensitivity and Improvement

The gut microbiome plays an important role in diabetes management. Several studies in animal models showed that the intake of probiotics (*Lactobacillus* and *Bifidobacterium* spp.) helps to prevent or reduce the severity of diabetes (type II). The lactic acid bacteria display antioxidant activity, as the diabetic patients have a systematic inflammation with a high level of proinflammatory cytokines (TNF-α, IL-6, IKKb, and JNK), which employ a negative impact on insulin. So the treatment with lactic acid bacteria helps to modulate this inflammatory status (Bordalo Tonucci et al., 2017; Stavropoulou & Bezirtzoglou, 2020). A study shows that the supplementation of *Akkermansia muciniphila* for three months lowered the plasma lipopolysaccharide and improved insulin sensitivity (Depommier et al., 2019).

The bacteria help in the production of SCFA, which helps in binding to specific GPRs, such as GPR-41 and GPR-43, leading to an increase in the secretion of polypeptide YY and GLP 1 & 2 (GLP1 & GLP2), which are involved in the regulation of insulin sensitivity (Rastelli et al., 2019). (Polypeptide YY also known as peptide tyrosine (PYY) residue, is a 36-amino acid peptide synthesized and released from specialized enteroendocrine cells encoded by the *PYY* gene). The process of mechanism is illustrated in Figure 15.2.

15.3.7 Chemoprevention in Cancer

Among all types of cancer, GI cancers are the most prevalent, accounting for 20% of all cancers, and, among them, 9% causes death worldwide. The microbial disharmony is linked with GI cancer. As shown by some investigators, probiotics hold pro-apoptotic and anti-proliferative properties against GI cancer (Liong, 2008; Rafter, 2004). Another study shows that fermented milk with *L. casei*, *B. longum*, and *L. acidophilus* showed a potential effect on tumor cell apoptosis (Lee et al., 2019).

Additionally, in the cellular line, the bacterial strain of *B. adolescentis* SPM0212 effectively inhibits the propagation of three human colonic cancer cells (HT-29, Caco-2, and SW 480) (Y. Kim et al., 2008). A similar study showed that the *L. paracasei* IMPC2.1 and *L. rhamnosus* GG strain exhibited a proliferative and pro-apoptotic effect against colonic and gastric cancer (Orlando et al., 2012). Moreover, *B. polyfermenticus* showed anticancer activities in human colon cancer cells (Ma et al., 2010).

15.3.8 Regeneration of Neuronal Cell

The etiologies for the neurodegenerative disease are still unclear, but there would be lifestyle and genetic factors involved in it. The alteration in the gut microbiota may disturb the gut–brain axis. This alteration may bring human disorders comprising metabolic, cancer, autoimmune, and neurodegenerative disorders (Castelli et al., 2021). The microbiota reserve maintains the intestinal microbiota balance that improves the epithelial tight junction that reduces gut permeability. In the case of cellular damage multiple immune and inflammatory factors are produced that activate inflammatory cytokines that damage the CNS (both spinal nerve and vagus nerve) (Stavropoulou & Bezirtzoglou, 2020).

Probiotics have been found positive effects on the progression of autoimmune myasthenia gravis (Chae et al., 2012), motor behavior, and autoimmune encephalomyelitis (Kwon et al., 2013). Furthermore, the probiotics seem to have a positive impact on cognition and neuroprotective properties. *Clostridium butyricum* attenuates cerebral ischemia injury and *Bifidobacterium* cognitive function (Savignac et al., 2015; Sun et al., 2016).

15.4 THE EVOLUTIONARY TREND IN PROBIOTICS

Probiotics have established intensifying attention in the current years in the healthcare, scientific, and public arenas. The probiotics are currently well established for the consumers and the research community too. The consumption of probiotics with food or supplementation includes a wide range of beneficial effects such as improving gut microbiota harmony; inhibiting the growth of pathogenic bacteria; improving immunity; preventing IBD, AAD, and metabolic diseases; maintaining serum cholesterol; improving mental health; and reducing hypertension (Soomro et al., 2001).

The public perception of microorganisms increased the publicity around the microbiome research. At the mark of these advances, public consciousness and acceptance of probiotics continue to enlarge. The industrial growth for probiotics increased ≈7% annually over the next eight years (Cunningham et al., 2021).

Traditionally, *Lactobacillus*, *Bifidobacterium*, and other lactic acid-producing bacteria isolated from fermented dairy products have been used as probiotics but with the advancement of technologies and discovery approaches able to produce new potential probiotic strains. The advancement of inexpensive complete genome sequencing and influential cultivation methods has permitted a new range of microorganisms and isolation. This process leads to next-generation probiotics development for the human microbiome with advanced health benefits (O'Toole et al., 2017). Several bacteria such as *Faecalibacterium prausnitzii*, *A. muciniphila*, *Eubacterium* spp., *Roseburia intestinalis*, and *Bacteroides* spp. have been isolated from the human intestine due to their great health benefits (Brodmann et al., 2017; O'Toole et al., 2017). A promising probiotic, namely, *A. muciniphila*, was isolated in 2004 and has been tested on animal models and shown to avert the development of obesity; with bacterial pasteurization, the efficacy and stability of the species increases and is also effective in other metabolic diseases (Depommier et al., 2019). This species was previously in the marketplace with multispecies synbiotic preparation containing *Clostridium beijerinckii*, *Anaerobutyricum hallii*, *C. butyricum*, inulin, and *B. longum* subsp. *infantis* showed a beneficial impact on type 2 diabetes treatment (Perraudeau et al., 2020).

15.5 SAFETY AND SIDE EFFECTS OF PROBIOTICS

Mostly probiotics are considered safe for humans isolated from fermented foods. But, still, supervision should be taken while supplementing the probiotics to the immunocompromised or severely ill patients.

The US FDA and GRAS have been applied to specific probiotic organism use (*Generally Recognized as Safe (GRAS) | FDA*, n.d.). A literature search including 622 studies shows that the six genera of *Saccharomyces*, *Enterococcus*, *Lactobacillus*, *Bifidobacterium*, *Bacillus*, and *Streptococcus* were reported to be safe and no evidence of increased risk (Hempel et al., 2011).

According to a report by WHO and FAO, 2002, states that probiotics are responsible for four types of side effects (Doron & Snydman, 2015):

- Systemic infection
- Deleterious metabolic activities
- Excessive immune stimulation in susceptible one
- Gene transfer

Common health disorders associated with the unsafe intake of probiotics (*Lactobacillus*) noted are sepsis, liver abscess, and endocarditis; furthermore, *S. boulardii* is reported with fungemia (Snydman, 2008). The common side effects of probiotics are rash, nausea, flatulency, constipation, infection, and hiccups (Islam, 2016).

15.6 GUIDANCE FOR PHYSICIANS REGARDING PROBIOTICS

As we know probiotics are nothing but a live microorganism. There might be a possibility to infect the host, so that's why different probiotics have different safety profiles. As a probiotic, the issues of safety become more prominent when it's an *Enterococcus* spp.

A safety guideline for the use of the probiotic is recommended by FAO and WHO that the strains should have a qualified minimum with a series of tests like toxin production, infectivity in an immune-compromised animal model, toxin production, human side effects, antibiotic-resistance pattern, metabolic activities, and adverse outcome in consumers.

There are some guidelines that a probiotic and its product should meet:

- The microbes must be alive and in adequate numbers during administration.
- Strain must be genetically identified by latest terminology used for classifying the microbes (such as number, letter, or names).
- To designate a strain as a probiotic, it must have passed clinical studies (using humans, livestock, companion animals, etc.).
- One strain that may be beneficial for one condition might not be for another application.
- It should be classified as a strain for the use of humans as a probiotic with standardized testing.
- A proper probiotic strain (such as lactobacilli and bifidobacteria), daily dosage, regulated intake (such as 1–4 times/day), time of dose intake (before, during, or after the meal), and method of provision (capsule, powder, or tablet form) should be prescribed.

15.7 FUTURE DIRECTIONS

Since the term "probiotics" was defined, the research investigation of modulation and administration of microbiome to human health has been advancing at a rapid rate. For effective use and to increase the activity, the bacterial products are incorporated in the food in various ways such as fermented products and microencapsulate and as an inactivator for the better stability of food products. This activity increases the diversity of metabolites that demonstrate the beneficial health benefits to humans. Nevertheless, many studies (in vivo and in vitro) have been conducted on the animal model, which cannot totally ensure similar benefits to humans, so a deep and essential investigation is needed.

The in vivo molecular elucidation will help to classify a true probiotic and also to pick the most appropriate ones for the handling of a specific disease. So this is important to understand that how probiotics operate has catalyzed underlying host–microbe interaction. Not only is the mechanism of the action of the probiotic needed but also novel strategies should be developed for the better action and treatment of the diseases.

On the other hand, many studies are present that claim the foods incorporated by the probiotic show various health benefits such as gut microbiota regulation, reduced GI stress, and antidiabetic, anti-cancerous, antiobesity, psychobiotic, and antiviral activities. Along with these results, many clinical studies have related to the mechanism of the probiotic action. Therefore, in the future, more clinical experiment is required to adhere to these issues and reply to all the answers without any questions and also strongly bind the losing ends between the mechanism of action and beneficial health benefits. So, therefore, it would be a significant opportunity for the food industry and research in food science, medicine, and nutrition.

15.7.1 Biomedical Application of Probiotics

Bacterial therapy is a smart platform that delivers and produces healing agents. A monotherapy or combination therapy provides innovation for the treatment of a range of diseases. The integration of synthetic biological technology helps to secrete the chemotaxis and biomolecules to outperform the conventional diagnostic and therapeutic, therefore, need the facilitation in clinical application. The oral administration of bacteria compared to injection-administered bacteria shows more improvement in patients' compliance and reduces the systemic risk of infection. Moreover, the orally administered microbes lead to substantial loss of viability due to the highly acidic and bile salt content environment of the stomach and intestine. Therefore, a need for an appropriate biomaterial in probiotic microencapsulation arises to minimize and control cell death during GI passage (Li et al., 2020; Zhu et al., 2021).

Biosurfactants have been increasingly used for industrial and environmental applications, but now it has also been used in the medicinal field, but the studies are limited. The probiotic biosurfactant holds anti-adhesive, antibiofilm, antimicrobial, and antitumor potential (Fariq & Saeed, 2016). Figure 15.4 illustrates the different applications and future perspectives of probiotics in different fields.

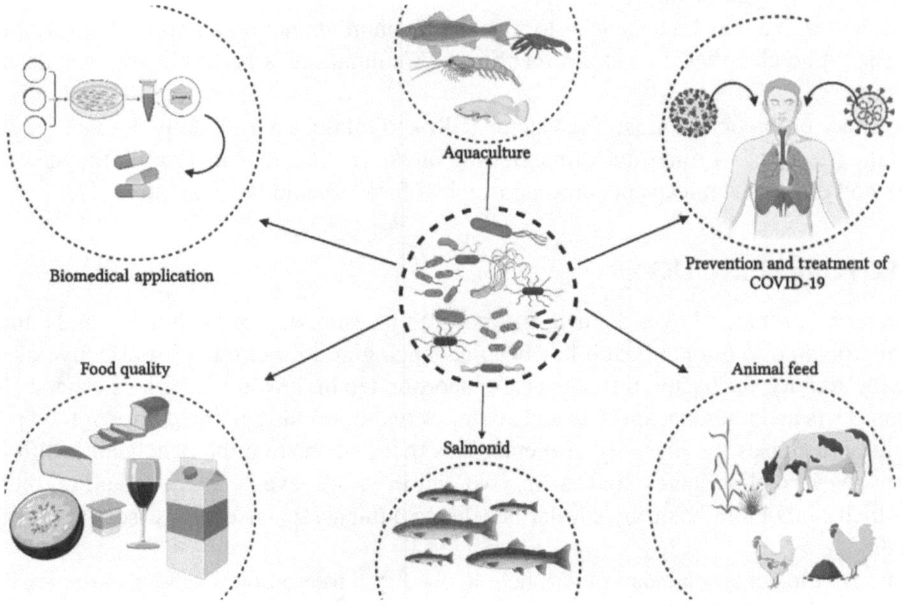

FIGURE 15.4 Application of probiotics in different fields and future perspectives.

15.7.2 Improving Food Quality with Probiotics

Thousands of years ago, the most famous Greek philosopher and father of medicine, Hippocrates said, "Let food be thy medicine, and let medicine be thy food"; the same concept is emerging with food but with the advanced term "functional foods." A functional food or superfood is a food that contains nutrients along with a health-prominent component. So a food can become functional by adding or incorporating it with probiotics (Soccol et al., n.d.).

The main aim of adding probiotics is to produce novel products with high nutritional value, food fermentation, improved sensory characteristics, and safety aspects. A number of studies concluded that fermented foods are associated with microbial communities because their components are linked with health benefits. Several studies concluded that the probiotic strain is incorporated in fermented milk, yogurt, cheese, dairy desserts, ice cream, and others. Nowadays, with the advancement of technologies and market demands, people are also moving toward non-dairy beverages as an alternative to milk products (due to lactose intolerance and other milk protein allergy issues). Some of the probiotics used in dairy, non-dairy, and beverages are mentioned in Table 15.1.

TABLE 15.1
Probiotics Used in Dairy, Non-dairy, and Beverages to Increase the Food Quality and Nutritional Values

Type of Product	Probiotic Microorganism	References
Yakult milk	*Lactobacillus casei* Shirota	Di Cerbo and Palmieri (2019)
Yo-plus Yogurt	*Bifidobacterium animalis* subsp. *lactis*, *Streptococcus thermophilus*, and *Actobacillus bulgaricus*	
Activa yogurt	*Bifidobacterium animalis* DN-173010 and *Bifidus regularis* in addition to *Streptococcus thermophilus* and *Lactobacillus bulgaricus*	
Gefilus juice	*Lacticaseibacillus Rhamnosus* GG	
Kefir drinks	*L. acidophilus*, *L. casei* subsp. *pseudoplantarum*, *Lactobacillus brevis*, *Candida pseudotropicalis*, *Lacticaseibacillus casei*, *L. casei* subsp. *rhamnosus*, *L. paracasei* subsp. *paracasei*, *Lactobacillus delbrueckii* subsp. *lactis*, *Fragilis/marxianus*, *S.* subsp. *Torulopsis holmii*, *L. kefiranofaciens* subsp. *Kefirgranum* subsp. *Nov*, *L. lactis*, *Lactiplantibacillus plantarum*, *L. lactis var. diacetylactis*, *L. lactis* subsp. *cremoris*, *Lactobacillus lactis*, *Enterococcus*, *Leuconostoc mesenteriodes*, *Cystopteris tenuis*, *Kluyveromyces marxianus* var. *marxianus*, *Lactobacillus bulgaricus*, *Kluyveromyces Lactobacillus lactis*, *Saccharomyces carlsbergensis*, *Saccharomyces unisporus*, *Debaryomyces hansenii*, *Zygosaccharomyces rouxii*	
Ice cream	*Lactobacillus reuteri*, *L. plantarum* 299v, *Lactobacillus rhamnosus* LGG,	Soccol et al. (n.d.)
Condensed yogurt (Kashk)	*L. acidophilus* La5, and *Bifidobacterium animalis* subsp. *lactis* BB-12	Razmpoosh et al. (2020)
Soy isoflavone beverage	*L. casei* (Shirota)	Toi et al. (2013)
Cashew yogurt	*L. rhamnosus* ATCC 53103, *L. plantarum* ATCC 14917, and *L. casei* ATCC 393	Shori et al. (2022)
Kimchi	*L. plantarum* PMO08	J. Kim et al. (2019)
Fruit juice beverages	*L. rhamnosus* GG, *L. casei* shirota, *L. plantarum*, and *L. acidophilus*	Sireswar et al. (2017)

15.7.3 Probiotics in Aquaculture

The utilization of probiotics in the aquaculture sector is progressive; several studies have been performed, and many studies are in the queue. Some studies show that the probiotic addition to water on a routine basis increases the rate of survival of fish or crustaceans (Sahu et al., 2008).

Few non-pathogenic isolates of *Vibrio alginolyticus* are prominently used for shrimp larvae cultivation. *Bacillus subtilis* can be immunized into shrimp culture basically to suppress the pathogenic vibrios, such as *Vibrio splendidus*, *Vibrio harveyi*, and *Vibrio parahaemolyticus* (Austin et al., 1995; Vaseeharan & Ramasamy, 2003). A bacterial strain *Lactobacillus* spp. isolated from chicken GI tract shows the effective growth and survival rates of young black tiger shrimp (*Penaeus monodon*) when fed continuously for 100 days (Phianphak et al., 1999). Inoculation of the saprophytic strain of *Bacillus* S11 increased the survival rate of post-larval black tiger shrimp that were dared by pathogenic luminescent bacterial culture (Rengpipat et al., 1998). The three bacterial strains isolated (*Bacillus* P64, *Vibrio* P62, and *Vibrio* P63) from the hepatopancreas of shrimp were found effective in white-leg shrimp (*Litopenaeus vannamei*). This bacterial strain showed an inhibitory effect against *V. harveyi* S2 under an in vivo environment with 58%, 83%, and 60% (Gullian et al., 2004). Another study showed that *Vibrio fluvialis* PM_{17} *Pseudomonas* spp. PM_{11} is isolated from the intestine of farm reader tiger shrimp, as these probiotics are effective in secreting extracellular macromolecule digestive enzymes (Alavandi et al., 2004). Based on their efficiency, few pharmaceutical companies launched commercial preparation probiotics aqua animal feed in the market, namely, Protexin, Spilac, and Aqualact (Sahu et al., 2008).

15.7.4 Probiotics in Salmonids

Salmonoids play an important role in fish production in many countries. *Aeromonas* sp. are the pervasive bacteria in both terrestrial and aquatic milieus. In salmonids, they are well known as the enteric pathogen responsible for fin rot, furunculosis, hemorrhagic septicemia, and soft tissue rot, resulting in major die-offs and fish kills. Few bacterial spp. such as lactic acid bacteria and bacillus increase the GI microflora that helps in the production of inhibitory components, increases immune response, aids digestive function, improves gastric morphology, inhibits virulence gene expression, and increases competition with potential pathogens. Therefore the advanced application of probiotics results in improved health status, body composition, and gut morphology; microbial harmony maintenance; improved disease resistance; and increased growth performance (Fečkaninová et al., 2017; Merrifield et al., 2010).

Another study showed that the *Carnobacterium* sp. isolated from the GI tract of Atlantic salmon had the potential effectiveness for salmonids. The in vitro studies demonstrated antipathy against *Flavobacterium psychrophilum*, *Streptococcus milleri*, *Photobacterium damselae* subsp. *piscicida*, *Aeromonas salmonicida*, *A. hydrophyla*, *Vibrio ordalii*, and *Vibrio anguillarum* but not for *V. harveyi*, *V. alginolyticus*, *Janthinobacterium lividum*, and *Debaryomyces hasenii* (Robertson et al., 2000).

15.7.5 Probiotics as an Animal Feed

The current outburst of food-borne disease emphasizes the need for the reduction of pathogenic bacteria in foods of animal origin because enteric pathogen from an animal is the only source for food contamination. The ban of antibiotics (as a growth promoter) is a challenge for animal nutrition, so there is a need for alternative techniques to minimize, control, and prevent the spread of such pathogenic bacteria and their colonization. New feed additives such as probiotic-incorporated feeds help to modulate the animal gut microbiota, which helps as a host protector (Gaggìa et al., 2010).

A study showed that *Bacillus velezensis* is a bacteria responsible for plant growth promotion, which inhibits the plant pathogen, and is an effective bacteria used in animal feed (Khalid et al., 2021). Another study showed that the administration of commercial strain *B. bifidum* was found to be operative in the treatment of cellulitis-infected broiler chicken, and *B. longum* PCB 133 suggestively reduced the number of *Campylobacters jejuni* in poultry feces (Estrada et al., 2001; Santini et al., 2010).

15.7.6 Prevention and Treatment of COVID-19

The WHO declared a viral infection, namely COVID-19 infection, a pandemic at the very beginning of 2020. COVID-19 is caused by SARS-CoV-2, which affects the epithelial cells of the human respiratory tract and leads to proinflammatory cytokines production and chronic lung inflammation (Singh & Rao, 2021).

A pilot study conducted over 15 patients with COVID-19 at the time of hospitalization showed a significantly altered fecal microbiome of deceased beneficial commensals and increased pathogens. A baseline profusion of *Coprobacillus* and a few species of *Clostridium* was found to correlate with COVID-19 severity. Similarly, the profusion of an anti-inflammatory bacterium *F. prausnitzii* was found inversely related to COVID-19 severity (Zuo et al., 2020). A similar study reported that there was a variation in gut microbiota and dysbiosis in COVID-19 patients, linked with disease severity and inflammatory markers (Liu et al., 2021; Yeoh et al., 2021).

GI symptoms were more prominent and associated with more severity; around 50–70% of COVID-19 patients were given antibiotics, and diarrhea was reported among 2–35% of them. The probiotic supplementation increased the colonic microflora. The probiotics such as *Lactobacillus* and *Bifidobacterium* uncertainly decreased the common cold, a symptom of COVID-19 infection (Xu et al., 2020). Another study reported that *Salmonella enterica* and its complement segmented filamentous bacteria could elevate the angiotensin-converting enzyme 2 (ACE2) and SARS-Cov-2 receptors (Liang et al., 2020). A similar study showed that both *Bacillus clausii* and *L. acidophilus* failed to reduce the coronavirus expression, after the treatment with *Salmonella* infection in the murine intestine (Kurian et al., 2021).

15.8 CONCLUSION

The effectiveness of probiotics on human health has caused a huge surge of interest in the current time. Generally, probiotics are considered safe when administered to humans in an adequate amount for an appropriate period of time, conferring several health benefits to the host. The mechanism involved behind the probiotic work is colonization and normalization of intestinal microbial content through competitive exclusion of pathogens, by producing bacteriocin and by modulating enzyme activity related to metabolization of toxic substances and carcinogens. The mechanism is also done by cell adhesion and mucin formation and moderation of the gut-related lymphoid tissues and immune system. Probiotics are generally used in a number of conditions such as neoplastic, allergy, inflammatory, and infectious conditions in both children and adults. But before introducing probiotics in daily routine dosage, proper evaluation is needed. Several standards and criteria should be followed regarding quality and reliability to meet benefits and effects. We have discussed the modern application of probiotics in many fields such as biomedicine preparation, aquaculture, salmonids, and animal feeds and in the most drastic conditions during the COVID-19 pandemic but not limited. Thus, placebo-controlled studies with validated results are needed in the future to adhere to the true health benefits of the product made, used by, or incorporated by probiotics.

BIBLIOGRAPHY

Alavandi, S. V., Vijayan, K. K., Santiago, T. C., Poornima, M., Jithendran, K. P., Ali, S. A., & Rajan, J. J. S. (2004). Evaluation of Pseudomonas sp. PM 11 and Vibrio fluvialis PM 17 on immune indices of tiger shrimp, Penaeus monodon. *Fish and Shellfish Immunology, 17*(2), 115–120. https://doi.org/10.1016/j.fsi.2003.11.007

Austin, B., Stuckey, L. F., Robertson, P. A. W., Effendi, I., & Griffith, D. R. W. (1995). A probiotic strain of Vibrio alginolyticus effective in reducing diseases caused by Aeromonas salmonicida, Vibrio anguillarum and Vibrio ordalii. *Journal of Fish Diseases, 18*(1), 93–96. https://doi.org/10.1111/J.1365-2761.1995.TB01271.X

Bazanella, M., Maier, T. V., Clavel, T., Lagkouvardos, I., Lucio, M., Maldonado-Gòmez, M. X., Autran, C., Walter, J., Bode, L., Schmitt-Kopplin, P., & Haller, D. (2017). Randomized controlled trial on the impact of early-life intervention with bifidobacteria on the healthy infant fecal microbiota and metabolome. *American Journal of Clinical Nutrition, 106*(5), 1274–1286. https://doi.org/10.3945/AJCN.117.157529

Bermudez-Brito, M., Plaza-Díaz, J., Muñoz-Quezada, S., Gómez-Llorente, C., & Gil, A. (2012). Probiotic mechanisms of action. *Annals of Nutrition and Metabolism, 61*(2), 160–174. https://doi.org/10.1159/000342079

Bordalo Tonucci, L., & Dos Santos, K. M. O. De luces Fortes Ferreira, C. L., Ribeiro, S. M. R., De Oliveira, L. L., & Martino, H. S. D. (2017). Gut microbiota and probiotics: Focus on diabetes mellitus. *Critical Review in Food Science and Nutrition. 57*(11), 2296–2309. https://doi.org/10.1080/10408398.2014.934438

Brodmann, T., Endo, A., Gueimonde, M., Vinderola, G., Kneifel, W., de Vos, W. M., Salminen, S., & Gómez-Gallego, C. (2017, September). Safety of novel microbes for human consumption: Practical examples of assessment in the European Union. *Frontiers in Microbiology, 8*, 289985. https://doi.org/10.3389/FMICB.2017.01725/BIBTEX

Castelli, V., D'Angelo, M., Quintiliani, M., Benedetti, E., Cifone, M. G., & Cimini, A. (2021). The emerging role of probiotics in neurodegenerative diseases: New hope for Parkinson's disease? *Neural Regeneration Research, 16*(4), 628–634. https://doi.org/10.4103/1673-5374.295270

Chae, C. S., Kwon, H. K., Hwang, J. S., Kim, J. E., & Im, S. H. (2012). Prophylactic effect of probiotics on the development of experimental autoimmune myasthenia gravis. *PLoS One, 7*(12), e52119. https://doi.org/10.1371/JOURNAL.PONE.0052119

Claes, A. K., Zhou, J. Y., & Philpott, D. J. (2015). NOD-like receptors: Guardians of intestinal mucosal barriers. *Physiology, 30*(3), 241–250. https://doi.org/10.1152/physiol.00025.2014

Cremonini, F., Di Caro, S., Nista, E. C., Bartolozzi, F., Capelli, G., Gasbarrini, G., & Gasbarrini, A. (2002). Meta-analysis: The effect of probiotic administration on antibiotic-associated diarrhoea. *Alimentary Pharmacology and Therapeutics, 16*(8), 1461–1467. https://doi.org/10.1046/J.1365-2036.2002.01318.X

Cunningham, M., Azcarate-Peril, M. A., Barnard, A., Benoit, V., Grimaldi, R., Guyonnet, D., Holscher, H. D., Hunter, K., Manurung, S., Obis, D., Petrova, M. I., Steinert, R. E., Swanson, K. S., van Sinderen, D., Vulevic, J., & Gibson, G. R. (2021). Shaping the future of probiotics and prebiotics. *Trends in Microbiology, 29*(8), 667–685. https://doi.org/10.1016/J.TIM.2021.01.003

D'Amelio, P., & Sassi, F. (2017). Gut microbiota, immune system, and bone. *Calcified Tissue International, 102:4, 102*(4), 415–425. https://doi.org/10.1007/S00223-017-0331-Y

Depommier, C., Everard, A., Druart, C., Plovier, H., Van Hul, M., Vieira-Silva, S., Falony, G., Raes, J., Maiter, D., Delzenne, N. M., de Barsy, M., Loumaye, A., Hermans, M. P., Thissen, J. P., de Vos, W. M., & Cani, P. D. (2019). Supplementation with Akkermansia muciniphila in overweight and obese human volunteers: A proof-of-concept exploratory study. *Nature Medicine*, *25*(7), 1096–1103. https://doi.org/10.1038/s41591-019-0495-2

Di Cerbo, A., & Palmieri, B. (2019). Review: The market of probiotics. *Pakistan Journal of Pharmaceutical Sciences, 28*(6), 2199–2206. https://pubblicazioni.unicam.it/handle/11581/431034

Doron, S., & Snydman, D. R. (2015). Risk and safety of probiotics. *Clinical Infectious Diseases, 60*(suppl_2), S129–S134. https://doi.org/10.1093/CID/CIV085

Estrada, A., Wilkie, D. C., & Drew, M. (2001). Administration of Bifidobacterium bifidum to chicken broilers reduces the number of carcass condemnations for cellulitis at the abattoir. *Journal of Applied Poultry Research, 10*(4), 329–334. https://doi.org/10.1093/JAPR/10.4.329

Fariq, A., & Saeed, A. (2016). Production and biomedical applications of probiotic biosurfactants. *Current Microbiology, 72*(4), 489–495. https://doi.org/10.1007/s00284-015-0978-4

Fečkaninová, A., Koščová, J., Mudroňová, D., Popelka, P., & Toropilová, J. (2017). The use of probiotic bacteria against Aeromonas infections in salmonid aquaculture. *Aquaculture, 469*, 1–8. https://doi.org/10.1016/J.AQUACULTURE.2016.11.042

Gaggìa, F., Mattarelli, P., & Biavati, B. (2010). Probiotics and prebiotics in animal feeding for safe food production. *International Journal of Food Microbiology, 141*(suppl_1), S15–S28. https://doi.org/10.1016/J.IJFOODMICRO.2010.02.031

Gasbarrini, G., Bonvicini, F., & Gramenzi, A. (2016). Probiotics history. *Journal of Clinical Gastroenterology, 50*(suppl_2), S116–S119. https://doi.org/10.1097/MCG.0000000000000697

Generally recognized as safe (GRAS) | FDA. (n.d.). Retrieved July 11, 2023, fromhttps://www.fda.gov/food/food-ingredients-packaging/generally-recognized-safe-gras

Genovese, K. J., Anderson, R. C., Harvey, R. B., & Nisbet, D. J. (2000). Competitive exclusion treatment reduces the mortality and fecal shedding associated with enterotoxigenic Escherichia coli infection in nursery-raised neonatal pigs. *Canadian Journal of Veterinary Research, 64*(4), 204–207. https://www.pmc/articles/PMC1189618/?report=abstract

Ghaisas, S., Maher, J., & Kanthasamy, A. (2016). Gut microbiome in health and disease: Linking the microbiome-gut-brain axis and environmental factors in the pathogenesis of systemic and neurodegenerative diseases. *Pharmacology and Therapeutics, 158,* 52–62. https://doi.org/10.1016/J.PHARMTHERA.2015.11.012

Gómez-Llorente, C., Muñoz, S., & Gil, A. (2010). Role of toll-like receptors in the development of immunotolerance mediated by probiotics. *Proceedings of the Nutrition Society, 69*(3), 381–389. https://doi.org/10.1017/S0029665110001527

Grölund, M., & Lehtonen, O. (n.d.). Fecal microflora in healthy infants born by different methods of delivery: Permanent changes in intestinal flora after cesarean delivery. *Journal of Pediatric Gastroenterology and Nutrition*. Retrieved July 7, 2023, from https://journals.lww.com/jpgn/Fulltext/1999/01000/Fecal_Microflora_in_Healthy_Infants_Born_by.7.aspx

Gullian, M., Thompson, F., & Rodriguez, J. (2004). Selection of probiotic bacteria and study of their immunostimulatory effect in Penaeus vannamei. *Aquaculture, 233*(1–4), 1–14. https://doi.org/10.1016/J.AQUACULTURE.2003.09.013

Gupta, V., & Garg, R. (2009). Probiotics. *Indian Journal of Medical Microbiology, 27*(3), 202–209. https://doi.org/10.4103/0255-0857.53201

Hashemi, A., Villa, C. R., & Comelli, E. M. (2016). Probiotics in early life: A preventative and treatment approach. *Food and Function, 7*(4), 1752–1768. https://doi.org/10.1039/C5FO01148E

Hempel, S., Newberry, S., Ruelaz, A., Wang, Z., Miles, J. N. V., Suttorp, M. J., Johnsen, B., Shanman, R., Slusser, W., Fu, N., Smith, A., Roth, B., Polak, J., Motala, A., Perry, T., & Shekelle, P. G. (2011). Safety of probiotics used to reduce risk and prevent or treat disease. *Evidence Report/Technology Assessment, 200,* 1–645. http://europepmc.org/books/NBK56091

Hesla, H. M., Stenius, F., Jäderlund, L., Nelson, R., Engstrand, L., Alm, J., & Dicksved, J. (2014). Impact of lifestyle on the gut microbiota of healthy infants and their mothers—The ALADDIN birth cohort. *FEMS Microbiology Ecology, 90*(3), 791–801. https://doi.org/10.1111/1574-6941.12434

Hevia, A., Delgado, S., Sánchez, B., & Margolles, A. (2015, November). Molecular players involved in the interaction between beneficial bacteria and the immune system. *Frontiers in Microbiology, 6,* 164790. https://doi.org/10.3389/FMICB.2015.01285/BIBTEX

Hill, C., Guarner, F., Reid, G., Gibson, G. R., Merenstein, D. J., Pot, B., Morelli, L., Canani, R. B., Flint, H. J., Salminen, S., Calder, P. C., & Sanders, M. E. (2014). The international scientific association for probiotics and prebiotics consensus statement on the scope and appropriate use of the term probiotic. *Nature Reviews. Gastroenterology and Hepatology, 11*(8), 506–514. https://doi.org/10.1038/nrgastro.2014.66

Hirano, J., Yoshida, T., Sugiyama, T., Koide, N., Mori, I., & Yokochi, T. (2003). The Effect of Lactobacillus rhamnosus on enterohemorrhagic Escherichia coli infection of Human intestinal cells in vitro. *Microbiology and Immunology, 47*(6), 405–409. https://doi.org/10.1111/J.1348-0421.2003.TB03377.X

Hirn, J., Nurmi, E., Johansson, T., & Nuotio, L. (1992). Long-term experience with competitive exclusion and salmonellas in Finland. *International Journal of Food Microbiology, 15*(3–4), 281–285. https://doi.org/10.1016/0168-1605(92)90059-C

Hojsak, I., Szajewska, H., Canani, R. B., Guarino, A., Indrio, F., Kolacek, S., Orel, R., Shamir, R., Vandenplas, Y., Van Goudoever, J. B., & Weizman, Z. (2018). Probiotics for the prevention of nosocomial diarrhea in children. *Journal of Pediatric Gastroenterology and Nutrition, 66*(1), 3–9. https://doi.org/10.1097/MPG.0000000000001637

Holzapfel, W. H., & Schillinger, U. (2002). Introduction to pre- and probiotics. *Food Research International, 35*(2–3), 109–116. https://doi.org/10.1016/S0963-9969(01)00171-5

Islam, S. U. (2016). Clinical uses of probiotics. *Medicine, 95*(5), e2658. https://doi.org/10.1097/MD.0000000000002658

Kailasapathy, K., & Chin, J. (2000). Survival and therapeutic potential of probiotic organisms with reference to Lactobacillus acidophilus and Bifidobacterium spp. *Immunology and Cell Biology, 78*(1), 80–88. https://doi.org/10.1046/J.1440-1711.2000.00886.X

Kałuzna-Czaplińska, J., & Błaszczyk, S. (2012). The level of arabinitol in autistic children after probiotic therapy. *Nutrition, 28*(2), 124–126. https://doi.org/10.1016/J.NUT.2011.08.002

Khalid, F., Khalid, A., Fu, Y., Hu, Q., Zheng, Y., Khan, S., & Wang, Z. (2021). Potential of Bacillus velezensis as a probiotic in animal feed: A review. *Journal of Microbiology, 59*(7), 627–633. https://doi.org/10.1007/s12275-021-1161-1

Kim, D. H., & Jin, Y. H. (2001). Intestinal bacterial β-glucuronidase activity of patients with colon cancer. *Archives of Pharmacal Research, 24*(6), 564–567. https://doi.org/10.1007/BF02975166

Kim, J., Choi, K. B., Park, J. H., & Kim, K. H. (2019). Metabolite profile changes and increased antioxidative and antiinflammatory activities of mixed vegetables after fermentation by Lactobacillus plantarum. *PLoS One, 14*(5), e0217180. https://doi.org/10.1371/JOURNAL.PONE.0217180

Kim, Y., Lee, D., Kim, D., Cho, J., Yang, J., Chung, M., Kim, K., & Ha, N. (2008). Inhibition of proliferation in colon cancer cell lines and harmful enzyme activity of colon bacteria by Bifidobacterium adolescentis SPM0212. *Archives of Pharmacal Research, 31*(4), 468–473. https://doi.org/10.1007/S12272-001-1180-Y

Konstandi, M., Voidarou, C., Papadaki, A., Tsiotsias, A., Kotsovolou, O., Evangelou, E., & Bezirtzoglou, E. (2009). Stress modifies the vaginal flora in cyclic female rats. *Microbial Ecology in Health and Disease. 18*(3–4), 161–169. https://doi.org/10.1080/08910600601072464

Kulkarni, N., & Reddy, B. S. (1994). Inhibitory effect of Bifidobacterium Iongum cultures on the azoxymethane-induced aberrant crypt foci formation and fecal bacterial β-glucuronidase. *Proceedings of the Society for Experimental Biology and Medicine. Society for Experimental Biology and Medicine, 207*(3), 278–283. https://doi.org/10.3181/00379727-207-43817

Kumar, M., Dhaka, P., Vijay, D., Vergis, J., Mohan, V., Kumar, A., Kurkure, N. V., Barbuddhe, S. B., Malik, S. V. S., & Rawool, D. B. (2016). Antimicrobial effects of Lactobacillus plantarum and Lactobacillus acidophilus against multidrug-resistant enteroaggregative Escherichia coli. *International Journal of Antimicrobial Agents, 48*(3), 265–270. https://doi.org/10.1016/J.IJANTIMICAG.2016.05.014

Kurian, S. J., Unnikrishnan, M. K., Miraj, S. S., Bagchi, D., Banerjee, M., Reddy, B. S., Rodrigues, G. S., Manu, M. K., Saravu, K., Mukhopadhyay, C., & Rao, M. (2021). Probiotics in prevention and treatment of COVID-19: Current perspective and future prospects. *Archives of Medical Research, 52*(6), 582–594. https://doi.org/10.1016/J.ARCMED.2021.03.002

Kwon, H. K., Kim, G. C., Kim, Y., Hwang, W., Jash, A., Sahoo, A., Kim, J. E., Nam, J. H., & Im, S. H. (2013). Amelioration of experimental autoimmune encephalomyelitis by probiotic mixture is mediated by a shift in T helper cell immune response. *Clinical Immunology, 146*(3), 217–227. https://doi.org/10.1016/J.CLIM.2013.01.001

Lee, J. W., Shin, J. G., Kim, E. H., Kang, H. E., Yim, I. B., Kim, J. Y., Joo, H. G., & Woo, H. J. (2019). Immunomodulatory and antitumor effects in vivo by the cytoplasmic fraction of Lactobacillus casei and Bifidobacterium longum. *Journal of Veterinary Science, 5*(1), 41–48. https://doi.org/10.4142/JVS.2004.5.1.41

Leuschner, R., & Robinson, T. (2010). *Qualified presumption of safety (QPS): A generic risk assessment approach for biological agents notified to the European food safety authority (EFSA)*. Elsevier. Retrieved July 7, 2023, from https://www.sciencedirect.com/science/article/pii/S0924224410001536

Li, S., Jiang, W., Zheng, C., Shao, D., Liu, Y., Huang, S., Han, J., Ding, J., Tao, Y., & Li, M. (2020). Oral delivery of bacteria: Basic principles and biomedical applications. *Journal of Controlled Release, 327*, 801–833. https://doi.org/10.1016/J.JCONREL.2020.09.011

Liang, W., Feng, Z., Rao, S., Xiao, C., Xue, X., Lin, Z., Zhang, Q., & Qi, W. (2020). Diarrhoea may be underestimated: A missing link in 2019 novel Coronavirus. *Gut, 69*(6), 1141–1143. https://doi.org/10.1136/GUTJNL-2020-320832

Lilly, D. M., & Stillwell, R. H. (1965). Probiotics: Growth-promoting factors produced by microorganisms. *Science, 147*(3659), 747–748. https://doi.org/10.1126/SCIENCE.147.3659.747

Liong, M. T. (2008). Roles of probiotics and prebiotics in colon cancer prevention: Postulated mechanisms and in-vivo evidence. *International Journal of Molecular Sciences*, *9*(5), 854–863. https://doi.org/10.3390/IJMS9050854

Liu, F., Ye, S., Zhu, X., He, X., Wang, S., Li, Y., Lin, J., Wang, J., Lin, Y., Ren, X., Li, Y., & Deng, Z. (2021). Gastrointestinal disturbance and effect of fecal microbiota transplantation in discharged COVID-19 patients. *Journal of Medical Case Reports, 15*(1), 1–9. https://doi.org/10.1186/S13256-020-02583-7/FIGURES/2

Ma, E. L., Choi, Y. J., Choi, J., Pothoulakis, C., Rhee, S. H., & Im, E. (2010). The anticancer effect of probiotic Bacillus polyfermenticus on human colon cancer cells is mediated through ErbB2 and ErbB3 inhibition. *International Journal of Cancer, 127*(4), 780–790. https://doi.org/10.1002/IJC.25011

Macfarlane, S., & Macfarlane, G. T. (2003). Regulation of short-chain fatty acid production. *Proceedings of the Nutrition Society, 62*(1), 67–72. https://doi.org/10.1079/PNS2002207

Mantegazza, C., Molinari, P., D'Auria, E., Sonnino, M., Morelli, L., & Zuccotti, G. V. (2018). Probiotics and antibiotic-associated diarrhea in children: A review and new evidence on Lactobacillus rhamnosus GG during and after antibiotic treatment. *Pharmacological Research, 128,* 63–72. https://doi.org/10.1016/J.PHRS.2017.08.001

Markowiak, P., & Ślizewska, K. (2017). Effects of probiotics, prebiotics, and Synbiotics on human health. *Nutrients, 9*(9). https://doi.org/10.3390/NU9091021

McFarland, L. V. (2015). From yaks to yogurt: The history, development, and current use of probiotics. *Clinical Infectious Diseases, 60*(suppl_2), S85–S90. https://doi.org/10.1093/CID/CIV054

McFarland, L. V., & Dublin, S. (2008). Meta-analysis of probiotics for the treatment of irritable bowel syndrome. *World Journal of Gastroenterology : WJG, 14*(17), 2650–2661. https://doi.org/10.3748/WJG.14.2650

Merrifield, D. L., Dimitroglou, A., Foey, A., Davies, S. J., Baker, R. T. M., Bøgwald, J., Castex, M., & Ringø, E. (2010). The current status and future focus of probiotic and prebiotic applications for salmonids. *Aquaculture, 302*(1–2), 1–18. https://doi.org/10.1016/J.AQUACULTURE.2010.02.007

Mokoena, M. P. (2017). Lactic acid bacteria and their bacteriocins: Classification, biosynthesis and applications against uropathogens: A mini-review. *Molecules, 22*(8), 1255. https://doi.org/10.3390/MOLECULES22081255

O'Toole, P. W., Marchesi, J. R., & Hill, C. (2017). Next-generation probiotics: The spectrum from probiotics to live biotherapeutics. *Nature Microbiology, 2*(5), 1–6. https://doi.org/10.1038/nmicrobiol.2017.57

Olivares, M., Díaz-Ropero, M. A., Gómez, N., Lara-Villoslada, F., Sierra, S., Maldonado, J. A., Martín, R., López-Huertas, E., Rodríguez, J. M., & Xaus, J. (2006). Oral administration of two probiotic strains, Lactobacillus gasseri CECT5714 and Lactobacillus coryniformis CECT5711, enhances the intestinal function of healthy adults. *International Journal of Food Microbiology, 107*(2), 104–111. https://doi.org/10.1016/J.IJFOODMICRO.2005.08.019

Orlando, A., Refolo, M. G., Messa, C., Amati, L., Lavermicocca, P., Guerra, V., & Russo, F. (2012). Antiproliferative and proapoptotic effects of viable or heat-killed Lactobacillus paracasei IMPC2.1 and Lactobacillus rhamnosus GG in HGC-27 gastric and DLD-1 colon cell lines. *Nutrition and Cancer, 64*(7), 1103–1111. https://doi.org/10.1080/01635581.2012.717676

Perraudeau, F., McMurdie, P., Bullard, J., Cheng, A., Cutcliffe, C., Deo, A., Eid, J., Gines, J., Iyer, M., Justice, N., Loo, W. T., Nemchek, M., Schicklberger, M., Souza, M., Stoneburner, B., Tyagi, S., & Kolterman, O. (2020). Improvements to postprandial glucose control in subjects with type 2 diabetes: A multicenter, double blind, randomized placebo-controlled trial of a novel probiotic formulation. *BMJ Open Diabetes Research and Care, 8*(1). https://doi.org/10.1136/BMJDRC-2020-001319

Phianphak, W., Rengpipat, S., Piyatiratitivorakul, S., & Menasveta, P. (1999). Probiotic use of Lactobacillus spp. For black tiger shrimp, Penaeus monodon. *Journal of Scientific Research, Chulalongkorn University, 24*(1). https://thaiscience.info/Journals/Article/CJSR/10324219.pdf

Plaza-Diaz, J., Ruiz-Ojeda, F. J., Gil-Campos, M., & Gil, A. (2019). Mechanisms of action of probiotics. *Advances in Nutrition, 10*(suppl_1), S49–S66. https://doi.org/10.1093/ADVANCES/NMY063

The prolongation of life: Optimistic studies/by Élie Metchnikoff; English translation edited by P. Chalmers Mitchell. | Wellcome Collection. (n.d.). Retrieved July 7, 2023, from https://wellcomecollection.org/works/a5439955

Rafter, J. (2004). The effects of probiotics on colon cancer development. *Nutrition Research Reviews, 17*(2), 277–284. https://doi.org/10.1079/NRR200484

Rastelli, M., Cani, P. D., & Knauf, C. (2019). The gut microbiome influences host endocrine functions. *Endocrine Reviews, 40*(5), 1271–1284. https://doi.org/10.1210/ER.2018-00280

Razmpoosh, E., Zare, S., Fallahzadeh, H., Safi, S., & Nadjarzadeh, A. (2020). Effect of a low energy diet, containing a high protein, probiotic condensed yogurt, on biochemical and anthropometric measurements among women with overweight/obesity: A randomised controlled trial. *Clinical Nutrition ESPEN, 35,* 194–200. https://doi.org/10.1016/J.CLNESP.2019.10.001

Reid, G., Jass, J., Sebulsky, M. T., & McCormick, J. K. (2003). Potential uses of probiotics in clinical practice. *Clinical Microbiology Reviews, 16*(4), 658–672. https://doi.org/10.1128/CMR.16.4.658-672.2003

Rembacken, B. J., Snelling, A. M., Hawkey, P. M., Chalmers, D. M., & Axon, A. T. R. (1999). Non-pathogenic Escherichia coli versus mesalazine for the treatment of ulcerative colitis: A randomised trial. *Lancet, 354*(9179), 635–639. https://doi.org/10.1016/S0140-6736(98)06343-0

Rengpipat, S., Phianphak, W., Piyatiratitivorakul, S., & Menasveta, P. (1998). Effects of a probiotic bacterium on black tiger shrimp Penaeus monodon survival and growth. *Aquaculture, 167*(3–4), 301–313. https://doi.org/10.1016/S0044-8486(98)00305-6

Ribet, D., & Cossart, P. (2015). How bacterial pathogens colonize their hosts and invade deeper tissues. *Microbes and Infection, 17*(3), 173–183. https://doi.org/10.1016/J.MICINF.2015.01.004

Robertson, P. A. W., O'Dowd, C., Burrells, C., Williams, P., & Austin, B. (2000). Use of Carnobacterium sp. as a probiotic for Atlantic salmon (Salmo salar L.) and rainbow trout (Oncorhynchus mykiss, Walbaum). *Aquaculture, 185*(3–4), 235–243. https://doi.org/10.1016/S0044-8486(99)00349-X

Sahu, M. K., Swarnakumar, N. S., Sivakumar, K., Thangaradjou, T., & Kannan, L. (2008). Probiotics in aquaculture: Importance and future perspectives. *Indian Journal of Microbiology, 48*(3), 299–308. https://doi.org/10.1007/S12088-008-0024-3

Sandhu, B. K., & Paul, S. P. (2014). Irritable bowel syndrome in children: Pathogenesis, diagnosis and evidence-based treatment. *World Journal of Gastroenterology, 20*(20), 6013–6023. https://doi.org/10.3748/WJG.V20.I20.6013

Santini, C., Baffoni, L., Gaggia, F., Granata, M., Gasbarri, R., Di Gioia, D., & Biavati, B. (2010). Characterization of probiotic strains: An application as feed additives in poultry against Campylobacter Jejuni. *International Journal of Food Microbiology, 141*(suppl_1), S98–S108. https://doi.org/10.1016/J.IJFOODMICRO.2010.03.039

Savignac, H. M., Tramullas, M., Kiely, B., Dinan, T. G., & Cryan, J. F. (2015). Bifidobacteria modulate cognitive processes in an anxious mouse strain. *Behavioural Brain Research, 287,* 59–72. https://doi.org/10.1016/J.BBR.2015.02.044

Schultz, M., Linde, H. J., Lehn, N., Zimmermann, K., Grossmann, J., Falk, W., & Schölmerich, J. (2003). Immunomodulatory consequences of oral administration of Lactobacillus Rhamnosus strain GG in healthy volunteers. *Journal of Dairy Research, 70*(2), 165–173. https://doi.org/10.1017/S0022029903006034

Shi, L. H., Balakrishnan, K., Thiagarajah, K., Mohd Ismail, N. I., & Yin, O. S. (2016). Beneficial properties of probiotics. *Tropical Life Sciences Research, 27*(2), 73–90. https://doi.org/10.21315/TLSR2016.27.2.6

Shori, A. B., Aljohani, G. S., Al-Zahrani, A. J., Al-sulbi, O. S., & Baba, A. S. (2022) Viability of probiotics and antioxidant activity of cashew milk-based yogurt fermented with selected strains of probiotic Lactobacillus spp. *LWT, 153,* 112482. https://doi.org/10.1016/j.lwt.2021.112482

Singh, K., & Rao, A. (2021). Probiotics: A potential immunomodulator in COVID-19 infection management. *Nutrition Research, 87,* 1–12. https://doi.org/10.1016/J.NUTRES.2020.12.014

Sireswar, S., Dey, G., Sreesoundarya, T. K., & Sarkar, D. (2017). Design of probiotic-fortified food matrices influence their antipathogenic potential. *Food Bioscience, 20,* 28–35. https://doi.org/10.1016/J.FBIO.2017.08.002

Snydman, D. R. (2008). The safety of probiotics. *Clinical Infectious Diseases: An Official Publication of the Infectious Diseases Society of America, 46*(suppl_2). https://doi.org/10.1086/523331

Soccol, C. R., Porto De Souza Vandenberghe, L., Spier, M. R., Bianchi, A., Medeiros, P., Yamaguishi, C. T., De, J., Lindner, D., Pandey, A., & Thomaz-Soccol, V. (n.d.). *The potential of probiotics: A review*. Retrieved July 12, 2023, from https://hrcak.srce.hr/en/file/92463.html

Soomro, T. M., Masud, T., & Kiran, A. (2001). Role of lactic acid bacteria (LAB) in food preservation and human health—a review. *Pakistan Journal of Nutrition, 1*(1), 20–24. https://doi.org/10.3923/PJN.2002.20.24

Stavropoulou, E., & Bezirtzoglou, E. (2020). Probiotics in medicine: A long debate. *Frontiers in Immunology, 11,* 554558. https://doi.org/10.3389/fimmu.2020.02192

Sun, J., Ling, Z., Wang, F., Chen, W., Li, H., Jin, J., Zhang, H., Pang, M., Yu, J., & Liu, J. (2016). Clostridium butyricum pretreatment attenuates cerebral ischemia/reperfusion injury in mice via anti-oxidation and anti-apoptosis. *Neuroscience Letters, 613,* 30–35. https://doi.org/10.1016/J.NEULET.2015.12.047

Szajewska, H. (2016). What are the indications for using probiotics in children? *Archives of Disease in Childhood, 101*(4), 398–403. https://doi.org/10.1136/ARCHDISCHILD-2015-308656

Toi, M., Hirota, S., Tomotaki, A., Sato, N., Hozumi, Y., Anan, K., Nagashima, T., Tokuda, Y., Masuda, N., Ohsumi, S., Ohno, S., Takahashi, M., Hayashi, H., Yamamoto, S., & Ohashi, Y. (2013). Probiotic beverage with soy isoflavone consumption for breast cancer prevention: A case-control study. *Current Nutrition and Food Science, 9*(3), 194–200. https://doi.org/10.2174/15734013113099990001

Tsiotsias, A., Voidarou, C., Skoufos, J., Simopoulos, C., Konstandi, M., Kostakis, D., & Bezirtzoglou, E. (2009). Stress-induced alterations in intestinal microflora. *Microbial Ecology in Health and Disease. 16*(1), 28–31. https://doi.org/10.1080/08910600410028632

Tuomola, E. M., Ouwehand, A. C., & Salminen, S. J. (1999). The effect of probiotic bacteria on the adhesion of pathogens to human intestinal mucus. *FEMS Immunology and Medical Microbiology, 26*(2), 137–142. https://doi.org/10.1111/j.1574-695X.1999.tb01381.x

Umbrello, G., & Esposito, S. (2016). Microbiota and neurologic diseases: Potential effects of probiotics. *Journal of Translational Medicine, 14*(1), 1–11. https://doi.org/10.1186/S12967-016-1058-7

Umu, Ö. C. O., Rudi, K., & Diep, D. B. (2017). Modulation of the gut microbiota by prebiotic fibres and bacteriocins. *Microbial Ecology in Health and Disease, 28*(1), 1348886. https://doi.org/10.1080/16512235.2017.1348886

Vanderhoof, J. A., & Young, R. J. (1998). Use of probiotics in childhood gastrointestinal disorders. *Journal of Pediatric Gastroenterology and Nutrition*, *27*(3), 323-332. https://doi.org/10.1097/00005176-199809000-00011

Vaseeharan, B., & Ramasamy, P. (2003). Control of pathogenic Vibrio spp. by Bacillus subtilis BT23, a possible probiotic treatment for black tiger shrimp Penaeus monodon. *Letters in Applied Microbiology, 36*(2), 83–87. https://doi.org/10.1046/J.1472-765X.2003.01255.X

Wang, Y., & Kasper, L. H. (2014). The role of microbiome in central nervous system disorders. *Brain, Behavior, and Immunity, 38,* 1–12. https://doi.org/10.1016/J.BBI.2013.12.015

Xu, K., Cai, H., Shen, Y., Ni, Q., Chen, Y., Hu, S., Li, J., Wang, H., Yu, L., Huang, H., Qiu, Y., Wei, G., Fang, Q., Zhou, J., Sheng, J., Liang, T., & Li, L. (2020). Management of corona virus disease-19 (COVID-19): The Zhejiang experience. *Zhejiang Da Xue Xue Bao. Yi Xue Ban/Journal of Zhejiang University, Medical Sciences, 49*(1). http://www.ncbi.nlm.nih.gov/pubmed/32096367; PubMed: 32096367

Yang, I., Corwin, E. J., Brennan, P. A., Jordan, S., Murphy, J. R., & Dunlop, A. (2016). The infant microbiome: Implications for infant health and neurocognitive development. *Nursing Research, 65*(1), 76–88. https://doi.org/10.1097/NNR.0000000000000133

Yeoh, Y. K., Zuo, T., Lui, G. C. Y., Zhang, F., Liu, Q., Li, A. Y. L., Chung, A. C. K., Cheung, C. P., Tso, E. Y. K., Fung, K. S. C., Chan, V., Ling, L., Joynt, G., Hui, D. S. C., Chow, K. M., Ng, S. S. S., Li, T. C. M., Ng, R. W. Y., Yip, T. C. F., . . . Ng, S. C. (2021). Gut microbiota composition reflects disease severity and dysfunctional immune responses in patients with COVID-19. *Gut, 70*(4), 698–706. https://doi.org/10.1136/GUTJNL-2020-323020

Yousefi, M., Movassaghpour, A. A., Shamsasenjan, K., Ghalamfarsa, G., Sadreddini, S., Jadidi-Niaragh, F., & Hojjat-Farsangi, M. (2015). The skewed balance between Tregs and Th17 in chronic lymphocytic leukemia. *Future Oncology, 11*(10), 1567–1582. https://doi.org/10.2217/FON.14.298

Zhu, Y., Wang, Z., Bai, L., Deng, J., & Zhou, Q. (2021). Biomaterial-based encapsulated probiotics for biomedical applications: Current status and future perspectives. *Materials and Design, 210,* 110018. https://doi.org/10.1016/J.MATDES.2021.110018

Zuo, T., Zhang, F., Lui, G. C. Y., Yeoh, Y. K., Li, A. Y. L., Zhan, H., Wan, Y., Chung, A. C. K., Cheung, C. P., Chen, N., Lai, C. K. C., Chen, Z., Tso, E. Y. K., Fung, K. S. C., Chan, V., Ling, L., Joynt, G., Hui, D. S. C., Chan, F. K. L., . . . Ng, S. C. (2020). Alterations in gut microbiota of patients with COVID-19 during time of hospitalization. *Gastroenterology, 159*(3), 944–955.e8. https://doi.org/10.1053/J.GASTRO.2020.05.048

Index

Note: Page numbers in *italics* indicate a figure and page numbers in **bold** indicate a table on the corresponding page.

A

B

C

D

E

H

M

N

R

S

T

U

V

W

X

Y

Z